Alternative and
Complementary Treatment in
NEUROLOGIC ILLNESS

MEDICAL GUIDES TO
Complementary & Alternative Medicine

Alternative and Complementary Treatment in NEUROLOGIC ILLNESS

MICHAEL I. WEINTRAUB, MD, FACP, FAAN
Clinical Professor
New York Medical College
Department of Neurology
Briarcliff, New York

Series Editor **MARC S. MICOZZI,** MD, PhD
Executive Director
The College of Physicians of Philadelphia
Adjunct Professor of Medicine and of Rehabilitation Medicine
University of Pennsylvania
Philadelphia, Pennsylvania

with 79 illustrations

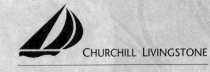

CHURCHILL LIVINGSTONE

A Harcourt Health Sciences Company
New York   Edinburgh   London   Philadelphia

CHURCHILL LIVINGSTONE

A Harcourt Health Sciences Company

The Curtis Center
Independence Square West
Philadelphia, Pennsylvania 19106

NOTICE

Pharmacology is an ever-changing field. Standard safety precautions must be followed, but as new research and clinical experience broaden our knowledge, changes in treatment and drug therapy may become necessary or appropriate. Readers are advised to check the most current product information provided by the manufacturer of each drug to be administered to verify the recommended dose, the method and duration of administration, and contraindications. It is the responsibility of the licensed prescriber, relying on experience and knowledge of the patient, to determine dosages and the best treatment for each individual patient. Neither the publisher nor the editor assumes any liability for any injury and/or damage to persons or property arising from this publication.

Library of Congress Cataloging-in-Publication Data

Alternative and complementary treatment in neurologic illness / [edited by] Michael Weintraub.

    p. cm.

    Includes index.

    ISBN 0-443-06558-6

    1. Nervous system—Diseases—Alternative treatment. I. Weintraub, Michael I.

RC346 .A42 2001
615.8'046—dc21
                                      00-065686

Editor-in-Chief: John A. Schrefer

Associate Editor: Kellie F. Conklin

Associate Development Editor: Jennifer L. Watrous

Editorial Assistant: Becky Swisher

Project Manager: Carol Sullivan Weis

Project Specialist: Christine Carroll Schwepker

Designer: Renée Duenow

Cover Image: © Dr. Dennis Kunkel/PHOTOTAKE

ALTERNATIVE AND COMPLEMENTARY TREATMENT IN NEUROLOGIC ILLNESS   ISBN 0-443-06558-6

Printed in the United States of America.

Last digit is the print number: 9 8 7 6 5 4 3 2 1

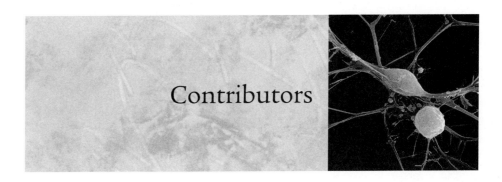

Contributors

R. LEA BORDEN, RN-C, BA
Critical Care Nurse, St. Helena Hospital
Napa Valley, California
Research Nurse, Kaiser Permanente
Santa Rosa, California

ELAINE CALENDA
Professional Member, American Massage Therapy Association
Nationally Certified in Therapeutic Massage and Bodywork
Clinical Education Director
Boulder College of Massage Therapy
Boulder, Colorado

EDWARD H. CHAPMAN, MD, DHt
Clinical Instructor, Harvard and Tufts Medical Schools
Newton, Massachusetts

REX L. CHENG, MD
Assistant Clinical Professor of Anesthesiology
UCLA School of Medicine, Department of Neurology
Harbor—UCLA Medical Center
Torrance, California

PEGGY CODDING, PhD
Professor, Music Therapy Department
Berklee College of Music
Boston, Massachusetts

JERRY COTT
Research Pharmacologist
Scientific Advisor to the Health Professions
College Park, Maryland

PAUL ESLINGER, PhD
Department of Neurology
Hershey Medical Center
Hershey, Pennsylvania

ADRIANNE FUGH-BERMAN, MD
Assistant Clinical Professor
Department of Health Care Sciences
George Washington University
School of Medicine and Health Sciences
Washington, District of Columbia

T.C. HAIN, MD
Associate Professor
Departments of Otolaryngology and Neurology
Northwestern University Medical School
Chicago, Illinois

SCOTT HALDEMAN, DC, PhD, MD
Clinical Professor, Department of Neurology
University of California, Irvine
Adjunct Professor, Los Angeles Chiropractic College
Private Practice
Santa Ana, California

D. CORYDON HAMMOND, PhD, ABPH
Professor, Physical Medicine and Rehabilitation
University of Utah School of Medicine
Salt Lake City, Utah

SUZANNE HANSER, EdD
Chair, Music Therapy Department
Berklee College of Music
Boston, Massachusetts

ANNE HARRINGTON, PhD
Co-Director, Harvard University Mind, Brain, Behavior
Inter-Faculty Initiative
Harvard University
History of Science Department
Cambridge, Massachusetts

A.R. HIRSCH, AR, MD
Neurologic Director
Smell and Taste Treatment Research Foundation
Chicago, Illinois

LINDA C. HOLE, MD
Faculty, American Academy of Pain Management
World Congress of Qi Gong
Private Practice
Spokane, Washington

PAUL HOOPER
Professor and Chair, Department of Principles and Practice
Southern California University of Health Sciences
Whittier, California

DORA T. HSU, MD
Associate Clinical Professor of Anesthesiology
UCLA School of Medicine, Department of Neurology
Harbor–UCLA Medical Center
Torrance, California

WAYNE B. JONAS, MD
Department of Family Medicine
Uniformed Services University of the Health Sciences
Bethesda, Maryland

SAM KABBANI, MD
East Tennessee Neurological Clinic
Knoxville, Tennessee

J. KOTSIAS, MS
Instructor of Tai Chi with American Tai Chi Tao
Caledonia, Minnesota

SIDNEY J. KURN, MD
Assistant Clinical Professor
University of California, San Francisco
Private Practice
Owner, Farmacopia
Santa Rosa, California

PAT LePORE, JD, MPA
ACP-ASIM
Compliance Officer
Main Line Health System
Devon, Pennsylvania

ERIC LESKOWITZ, MD
Pain Management Program
Spaulding Rehabilitation Hospital
Boston, Massachusetts

KLAUS LINDE, MD
Centre for Complementary Medicine Research
Department of Internal Medicine
Technische Universitaet
Munich, Germany

BALA V. MANYAM, MD
Director of Research, Department of Neurology
Scott & White Clinic
Texas A & M University
College Station, Texas

ANGELE McGRADY, PhD
Department of Psychiatry
Medical College of Ohio
Toledo, Ohio

TERRY OLESON, PhD
Chair, Department of Psychology
California Graduate Institute
Professor of Acupuncture
Emperor's College of Traditional Oriental Medicine
Samra University
Health Care Alternatives
Los Angeles, California

CLIVE PAI, PhD
Assistant Professor, Programs in Physical Therapy
Northwestern University
Chicago, Illinois

ROBYN ROSS, RYT
Advanced Certification, Integrative Yoga Therapy and Kripalu Yoga
Certified Holistic Health Educator
Founder and Co-Director, Living Yoga
New York, New York

KENNETH M. SANCIER, PhD
President, Qigong Institute
Menlo Park, California

GLENN N. WAGNER, DO, CHE
Deputy Director, Armed Forces Institute of Pathology
Washington, District of Columbia

SHARON WEINSTEIN, MD
Department of Neurology
University of Utah
Red Butte Pain Management Center
Salt Lake City, Utah

MICHAEL I. WEINTRAUB, MD, FACP, FAAN
Clinical Professor
New York Medical College
Department of Neurology
Briarcliff, New York

ALAN WITKOWER, EDD, CGP
Spaulding Rehabilitation Center
Boston, Massachusetts

To my family

For their love, understanding, and support

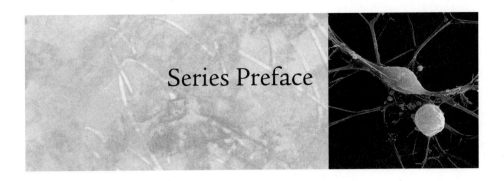

Series Preface

Complementary therapies in general have much application in addressing functional complaints and disorders. My basic text in this series, *Fundamentals of Complementary and Alternative Medicine,* second edition (Churchill Livingstone, 2001), describes the documented subjective improvements brought about by appropriate application of these therapeutic modalities over the ages.

Pain and headache (head pain) are perhaps the two most common functional disorders of the human condition, experienced by virtually everyone on an acute basis and by many on a chronic, episodic, or recurring basis. Much of the effort in human healing traditions throughout history has been directed at analgesia—the alleviation of pain—through discovery and development of materia medica (e.g., opiates, salicylates), manipulation (e.g., bone setting, chiropractic, traditional osteopathy, physical therapy), manual therapies (e.g., massage, yoga, acupuncture), and mind-body approaches, all of which are topics in this series. Energy healing represents a new frontier with ancient roots.

In the history of American medicine, alleviation of pain was one of the two central tenets of "rational medicine." Rational medicine in clinical practice was a conscious result of the Scottish Enlightenment of Adam Smith in economics. It was brought to the then-British Colonies by Drs. Morgan and Hutchinson from the University of Edinburgh to the College of Philadelphia (now the University of Pennsylvania), where they established the first school of medicine in what was to become the United States by charter from Colonial Governor Thomas Penn in 1765. The rest is history.

Today, pain is understood as a dynamic condition, not a static pathologic state or lesion. And although curing or removing a painful lesion eliminates the pain (with the curious exception of phantom pain, such as the "phantom limb" syndrome of amputees), pain exists in many other contexts where there is no "lesion" to cure or remove. Therefore the assessment and management of pain, whether alternative or mainstream, must lie in the interaction between mind and body, healer and patient, patient and therapy.

Pain is a subjective complaint, and therefore its improvement is also subjective yet associated with very high levels of patient satisfaction. That mind-body approaches are proving so successful in the management of pain is another sign that the Cartesian separation of mind and body has been an artificial accommodation to limited philosophical and naturalistic rationalizations. This outdated separation in Western civilization, which is not a problem in Asian civilization, for example, perhaps even influences how we are conditioned to experience and express pain itself. In traditional societies in Africa, for example, psychic pain is often "somatized" to a specific area of the body and presents as pain in a particular organ rather than a general mental state.

If the entire body is the organ of consciousness, as postulated by Candace Pert and others, mind-body distinctions begin to lose their meaning and a "gut feeling" is really being felt in the "gut." And some of the diffuse pain associated with chronic fatigue syndrome and fibromyalgia, for example, may ultimately be a conditioned response emanating from elsewhere. The successful alleviation of pain and treatment of other neurologic conditions cannot be considered "alternative" vs. mainstream; what works should simply be considered good medicine.

MARC S. MICOZZI, MD, PHD
Philadelphia, Pennsylvania
November 2000

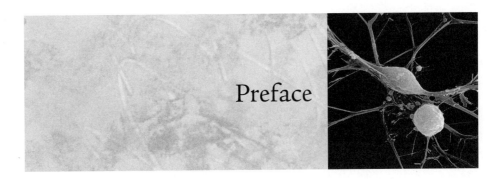

Preface

Complementary and alternative medicine is one of the fastest growing treatment areas in the United States. The public has embraced these approaches and subsequently fueled a revolution. The scientific community cannot ignore this exponential surge in public enthusiasm and confidence. Unfortunately, alternative medicine is a highly charged subject in the medical community, with both critics and proponents. Critics often may not understand or accept anecdotal statements without randomized placebo-controlled studies. Because alternative treatment is a challenge to their scientific training and beliefs, all positive responses are considered placebo. Thus the debate will continue until meaningful research clarifies the issues.

Alternative and Complementary Treatment in Neurologic Illness is a scholarly effort to educate neurologists and interested physicians regarding the major alternative and complementary therapies. It describes the cultural history and philosophy, discusses the strengths and weaknesses of clinical studies, and offers a practical approach to various neurologic symptoms and syndromes. This book also recognizes the shortcomings of conventional therapies and encourages the clinician to pursue and explore additional treatment options. Readers will be impressed and ed-

ucated by the data the distinguished authors have gathered. In addition, Dr. Wayne Jonas, former Director of the National Institutes of Health's Office of Alternative Medicine, puts this topic into proper perspective and advises how, in the absence of biological markers, clinicians can develop stronger protocols and methodologies. Further, Dr. Anne Harrington discusses the important role of placebo response and how patients can be influenced.

I am grateful to all of the experienced contributors, who have helped make this book a reality. I believe this publication is a major accomplishment, representing the first book dedicated to the treatment of neurologic symptoms and illness with complementary and alternative therapies.

At the beginning of this new millennium, the scientific community is presented an opportunity and a challenge to develop stronger protocols and test novel, nonpharmacologic approaches that may help individuals who suffer neurologic symptoms.

Michael I. Weintraub, MD, FACP, FAAN
Briarcliff, New York
November 2000

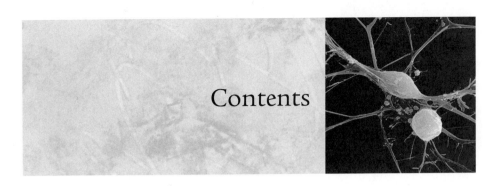

Contents

Alternative and
Complementary Treatment in
NEUROLOGIC ILLNESS

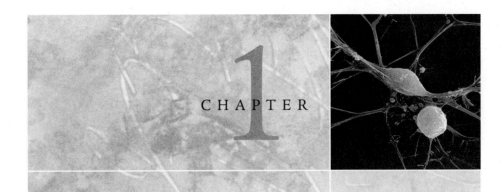

CHAPTER

1

Evaluating Research in Complementary and Alternative Medicine

WAYNE B. JONAS
KLAUS LINDE

Complementary and alternative medicine (CAM) is that subset of practices that is not an integral part of conventional health care but is still used by patients for the treatment and prevention of illness. Surveys done in 1990 and 1997 show an increase in CAM use of almost 45% in the United States during that time. Visits to CAM practitioners increased from 400 million per year to more than 600 million per year—surpassing the number of visits to primary care physicians. Out-of-pocket expenses for these practices rose from $14 billion to $27 billion in the last 7 years.[1] CAM is an important part of the public's health care. As its use rises, obtaining reliable information about the safety, effectiveness, and mechanism of these practices requires quality clinical investigation. This chapter addresses issues to be considered when conducting and evaluating research on these practices.

RESEARCH EVALUATION PRINCIPLES IN MEDICINE

Scientific Methods

Scientific methods have only recently been applied to medicine. Technologies for examining cellular functioning, the genetic regulation of life, and the mechanisms of infectious disease have been applied only in the last 100 years. The randomized controlled clinical trial (RCT) is just 50 years old and has

The views, opinions, and assertions expressed in this chapter are those of the authors and do not reflect official policy of the Department of the Army, Department of Defense, or the U.S. Government.

been an established standard for testing new drugs for only 25 years. Statistical principles have also only recently been applied to medicine. There are various types of research methods, including laboratory techniques, observational methods, RCTs, meta-analysis, qualitative research, and health services research. The use of these methods has provided better precision and more control over the body and the public's health than ever before. Which of these methods are essential for the clinical researcher to know, and how should they be integrated?

The Audience and the Evidence

When deciding whether or not to use a therapy, everyone wants to know if there is evidence that a therapy is safe and will work. Yet different groups often look for different types of evidence to make these decisions.

Patients

Patients or their family members may want to hear details about other individuals with similar illnesses who have used a treatment and recovered. If the treatment appears to be safe and there is little risk of harm resulting from it, these success stories may convince patients to use the treatment. This type of evidence is called *anecdotal* or, if more fully developed, a *case report*.

Practitioners

Physicians, who see many patients a day, often want a different type of evidence. They realize that what works in one case may not work in another, so they need more than a few patient recovery stories before they can recommend a therapy. They often want to know what the likelihood or probability is that a patient will recover or have an adverse effect based on a series of similar patients who have received the treatment. For example, out of 100 patients who received a specific treatment for a condition did 20% or 80% improve, and how many had side effects? They also want to know about the complexity of using the therapy, including its cost and inconvenience. This type of evidence comes from observational or clinical outcomes data.

Clinical Researchers

Scientists doing patient-oriented research may want a different type of evidence. They often want to know how much improvement occurred in a group who re-

ceived the treatment compared with another group who did not receive the treatment. For example, if 80% of the patients who received a treatment got better, but 75% of similar patients got better after only visiting a physician and getting any treatment, only 5% of the improved cases could be attributed to the treatment. This evidence is known as *comparative clinical trial evidence*. Some scientists will accept comparative evidence for a treatment only when it has come from an experiment in which blinding and randomization have been followed. This type of evidence is termed *clinical experimental* or *RCT evidence*.

Basic Scientists

Basic science investigators may want objective evidence supporting a mechanism of action. This evidence must be obtained in laboratory experiments that can explain the effects observed in clinical research or guide better clinical research. This is called *basic science evidence*.

Policymakers

Those in charge of determining public laws and health care policy often need definitive proof that a practice is safe and effective before applying it to large groups. They require evidence in which a high degree of confidence can be placed because policy errors can adversely affect millions of people and cost billions of dollars. This type of evidence comes from extensive evaluation and the synthesis of several research reports through systematic reviews, meta-analyses, and consensus evaluations performed by experts in the field.

Research Domains Relevant to Complementary and Alternative Medicine

The various types of information preferred by different audiences is obtained by different research methods. Figure 1-1 illustrates six types of research that are frequently used in the investigation of medicine and the general type of information that each of these approaches provides.

These types of research include the following:
1. **Qualitative research** includes such methods as detailed case studies and patient interviews that describe diagnostic and treatment approaches and that investigate patient preferences and relevance to those approaches. Qual-

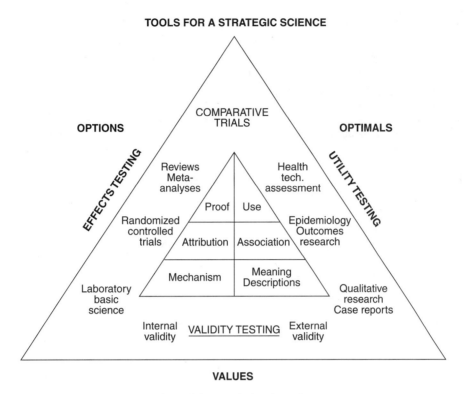

Figure 1-1 Knowledge domains.

itative approaches have been extensively developed in the nursing profession and are becoming increasingly common in primary care.

2. **Laboratory and basic science approaches** investigate the basic mechanisms and biological plausibility of practices. In vitro (cell culture and intracellular [e.g., with probe technology], in vivo (testing in normal, disease-prone, or genetically altered animals), and mixed approaches are now used extensively and are rapidly expanding into molecular realms.

3. **Observational studies,** such as practice audit and epidemiological research, outcomes research, and other types of observational research, describe associations between interventions and outcomes. Practice audits involve monitoring outcomes on all or a selected sample of patients receiving treatment. Patients are evaluated before and after an intervention to measure the effects. In these studies there may be no comparison group, or comparison groups may be developed by sampling patients

from other practices who have not been treated with the intervention or from the same practice before the intervention.

4. **RCTs** attempt to isolate or compare the specific contribution of different interventions on outcomes. In these studies researchers usually assign patients to one treatment group or another by using a method that ensures that the groups are comparable in all factors that might influence outcomes, except the treatments. Various methods, such as randomly selected numbers or computer-generated random assignment, are used. The treatment may be evaluated with or without knowledge of the assignments. The best approach is allocation concealment, where knowledge of which patients get which treatment at the time of assignment is concealed.

5. **Meta-analysis, systematic reviews, and expert review and evaluation** are methods for assessing the accuracy and precision of clinical research. Methods for expert review and summary

of research have evolved over the last several years through the use of systematic protocol-driven approaches, such as meta-analysis. These approaches are being used increasingly in place of subjective reviews to increase confidence in the idea that the effects found in clinical research are accurate and applicable across populations.

6. **Health technology assessment and health services research** examines the actual utility and impact of interventions in light of social factors, such as access, feasibility, costs, practitioner competence, patient compliance, and so forth. Often this type of research involves surveys or samplings from groups already undergoing interventions to determine the quality and costs of the treatment. Random sampling may or may not be used.

Goals of Research Types

Although certain groups may prefer one or more of these methods and the types of information they provide, information from all methods may be required for making clinical decisions. Laboratory research, RCTs, and systematic reviews or meta-analyses (left side of Figure 1-1) are usually used to determine the existence of a specific effect of an intervention or exposure or to support a theory about mechanisms. Qualitative research, observational trials, and health technology assessment (right side of Figure 1-1) are usually used to determine the probability, magnitude, and relevance of an effect in actual health care delivery. There is a tension between research performed to isolate specific effects (laboratory, RCTs, meta-analyses, etc.) and research that tries to investigate relevance and utility in the real world (qualitative, observational, health services, etc.). More than one question probably should not be investigated in a single research project, because designing research that attempts to address both specific and pragmatic questions simultaneously is difficult. To assess both specificity and utility, multiple research strategies are required. Consistent decision rules for the application of research methods are important for the development of science-based medicine.[2] In addition, the clinical researcher must understand what constitutes quality research within each of these evidence domains. Research quality criteria become the basis for evaluating any study or group of studies.[3]

Research Quality Criteria

Research quality can be assessed by using established criteria to determine the validity of information in research reports. For example, the validity of RCTs is evaluated with quality criteria that determine internal validity by assessing the likelihood that observed effects are due to bias. The general application of clinical research, including RCTs and observational trials, is evaluated with criteria that determine external validity or the likelihood that effects would occur in varied situations. There are numerous quality rating systems for evaluating clinical research. One of the best is the consort criterion, which is a widely adopted set of reporting guidelines for RCTs.[4,5] Most criteria emphasize the importance of allocation concealment, randomization, blinding, proper statistical methods, attention to dropouts, and other factors. Other guidelines exist for reporting meta-analysis, observational trials, and diagnostic tests.[6,7] Anyone evaluating clinical research should be familiar with those criteria.

In addition to internal and external validity, CAM research requires attention to model validity, or the likelihood that the research has addressed the unique taxonomy and context of the CAM system being investigated. Many CAM systems originate outside of Western medicine. Proper clinical research on these systems requires adequate expertise and experience in the CAM system.[8] Often the CAM system is examined in populations for which the practice is traditional and integral to the culture. However, there can be marked variations in response to treatments in different cultures. Results produced in one culture may not translate readily to another.[9] In addition, individual expectations and informed consent can have a significant effect on outcomes.[10,11] The evaluation of model validity in CAM requires that these items be considered when judging the quality of clinical research. Quality criteria for internal, external, and model validity of a CAM clinical trial are listed in Table 1-1.

The likelihood of validity evaluation (LOVE) system has been applied to the evaluation of several CAM clinical research sets. When examining clinical research, the practitioner can usually focus on the types of evidence dealing with clinical trials (middle two sections of Figure 1-1). These types of evidence address the questions "Is the treatment effective?" and "What is the magnitude of the treatment's effectiveness?"

TABLE 1-1

The Likelihood of Validity Evaluation Guidelines

Dimension	Main criteria
Internal Validity How likely is it that the effects reported are due to the independent variable (the treatment)?	**Randomization** (Was subject assignment to treatment groups done randomly and in a concealed manner?) **Baseline Comparability** (Were gender, age, and prognostic factors balanced?) **Change of Intervention** (Was there loss to follow-up, contamination, or poor compliance?) **Blinding** (Did the patients, practitioners, evaluators, or analysts know who got the treatment?) **Outcomes** (Was the objectivity, reliability, and sensitivity of the outcome assessed?) **Analysis** (Was the number treated large? Were p values significant? Were multiple outcomes measured and analyzed?)
External Validity How likely is it that the observed effects would occur outside the study and in different settings?	**Generalization** (Was there a range of patients as would be seen in practice, or were there multiple or narrow inclusions and exclusions? Was the study done at several sites with similar results?) **Reproducibility** (Was what was done clear? Were confidence intervals reported? Was the treatment transferable to other practitioners?) **Clinical Significance** (Was the effect size big enough to make a difference? Is the condition in need of this type of treatment? Were any preferences determined? Was adherence good?) **Therapeutic Interference** (Was there flexibility in varying the treatment? Was feedback on the outcomes available? Is the treatment feasible in most (or your) practice settings?) **Outcomes** (Were the outcomes clinically relevant? Were the outcomes checked for importance with the patients? Were any important outcomes missing?)

Continued

TABLE 1-1

The Likelihood of Validity Evaluation Guidelines—cont'd

Dimension	Main criteria
Model Validity How likely is it that the study accurately reflects the system under investigation?	*Representativeness/Accuracy* (Were the therapists well trained and experienced? Was the treatment strategy adequate? Was the treatment clearly described?) *Informed Consent* (Was the informed consent comprehensive? Was it effective? Did patients understand it? Did it generate expectations different from practice?) *Methodology Matching* (Were the goals of the study clear and limited? Did the investigators select the correct research method to achieve the goals?)* *Model Congruity* (Were the patients classified, was the treatment determined, and were the outcomes assessed according to the system of the practice being assessed?) *Context/Meaning* (Did the patients/practitioners believe in the therapy? How well was the intervention adapted to the culture, family, and meaning of the patient?)
Reporting Quality How likely is it that the report accurately reflects what was found in the study? How clear and accurate is the information presented?	*Comprehensive* (Can you address the above criteria?) *Clarity* (Could you reproduce this study?) *Conclusions* (Were the conclusions and reporting format [e.g., relative versus absolute improvement rates, strength of wording] appropriate to the data collected?)

*See the citation categories.

Is the Treatment Effective?

This question regarding efficacy is the main question to ask about all therapies. An intervention is effective if it changes the course of a disease in a beneficial way. Effectiveness includes a causal element (i.e., the treatment makes the difference) and a quantitative element (i.e., the degree of change). To determine whether a therapy is effective in a single patient, the researcher would have to compare the course of the disease in that patient both with and without the treatment. However, this type of comparison is not usually possible, and in most conditions the untreated course is variable. The next best way to evaluate effectiveness is by following two groups of comparable patients; one group receives the treatment, and the other receives no treatment. A placebo control group is included if the purpose of the study is to determine whether or not the treatment is effective. The study aims to find the proportion of specific effects attributable to a particular part of the intervention (e.g., needling a specific acupuncture point in a specific way) in comparison to the nonspecific effects resulting from treatment in general (e.g., the act of needling in general). This type of study provides information about the treatment's effectiveness over placebo, rather than its general effectiveness. This information may be important for the patient, depending on the risks, costs, feasibility, and other factors involved in the specific situation. However, placebo-controlled trials do not answer the question "Is the treatment effective?" because in actual practice patients are not given an option to get a placebo nor are they randomly selected to receive a treatment or not. Thus placebo-controlled trials can answer a theoretical question of whether a treatment is causally related to the outcome. However, such trials cannot address questions of comparative effectiveness when compared with no treatment or questions of relative effectiveness when compared with standard treatment. Answering these questions requires different controls and sometimes different study designs.

Is This the Most Effective Treatment?

Often the physician wants to know whether a therapy is the most effective treatment out of several options, which raises another question, namely, "Is this the most effective treatment?" Answering this question requires directly comparing two active treatments to examine their relative merits, or comparative effectiveness. In such studies, randomization is preferred to ensure that the groups are comparable before treatment. Outcomes measured should be relevant for the patient. Study methods should minimize the influence of chance and error, but they also should balance this goal with the goal of delivering the treatment in the same way it is delivered in practice.

Summarizing Research

Keeping up with the literature even in a small subspecialty is a daunting task. There are at least 80 major databases and more than 400 journals on CAM worldwide. Systematic, consistent, and rational reviews of the literature are therefore needed. Research summaries can come to markedly different conclusions because of publication bias, incomplete access to the literature or selection of different studies, poor quality of clinical research, variable evaluation standards, and differing beliefs in the practice.[7,12] The Cochrane Collaboration, an international network that does reviews in health care, provides the best current approach to clinical research summary.[13] Other summary methods, such as those used for practice guidelines and the NIH Consensus Conference method, although adequate for their purposes, are usually inadequate for deciding on individual treatment in the clinic.

DEVELOPING RESEARCH STRATEGIES FOR CAM

Matching Goals and Methods of Research

Research must be rigorous but also relevant. The tools chosen to investigate an area must be appropriate for the information sought and the purposes for which it will be used. Clearly defining the questions being asked and the goals those questions seek to fulfill and applying the appropriate methods necessary to answer those questions is crucial for understanding the role of research in medicine.[14] Each method has its own purpose, value, and limitations. The quality of a study should be judged in relation to these goals and to the questions being asked.[15] For example, for assessing the relevance of outcome measures across a population, qualitative methods with in-depth interviews and content analysis are most appropriate. When seeking to determine the incidence, prevalence, and rates of practices, surveys or cross-sectional and longitudinal studies are the most useful. For identifying the impact of complex interventions, clinical context, pragmatic trials, and outcomes approaches should be used. When attempting to isolate the specific causal effect of treatment on specific outcomes, randomized controlled trials are best. The relationship among study goals, the type of information needed, and the type of methodology used are shown in Figure 1-2. When evaluating CAM research, ensure that the question asked and the method selected are appropriate. Once selected, each method should be evaluated for quality using the criteria previously outlined, such as in the LOVE approach shown in Table 1-1.

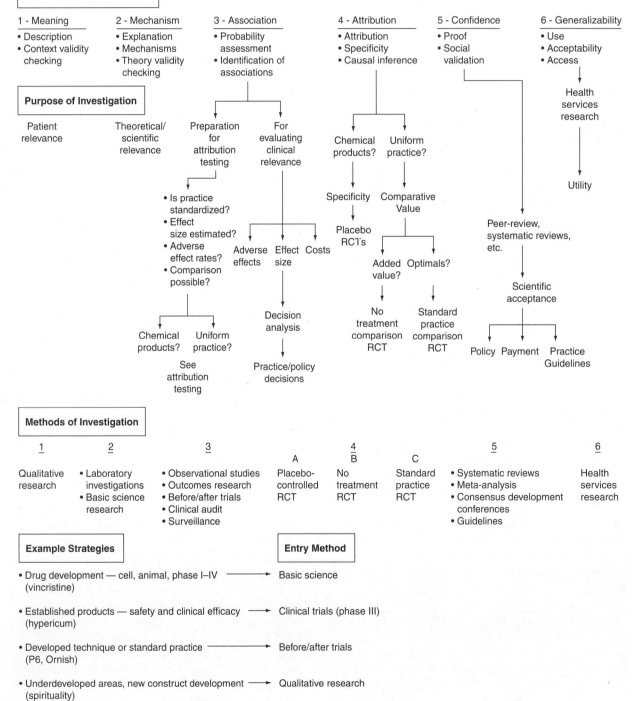

Unit of Investigation

- Components
- Products
- Techniques (simple)
- Modalities (complex)
- Systems (organized rule-driven combinations)
- Professional practice
- Practice combination interest

Type of Information Sought

1 - Meaning
- Description
- Context validity checking

2 - Mechanism
- Explanation
- Mechanisms
- Theory validity checking

3 - Association
- Probability assessment
- Identification of associations

4 - Attribution
- Attribution
- Specificity
- Causal inference

5 - Confidence
- Proof
- Social validation

6 - Generalizability
- Use
- Acceptability
- Access

Health services research

Utility

Purpose of Investigation

Patient relevance

Theoretical/ scientific relevance

Preparation for attribution testing

For evaluating clinical relevance

Chemical products?

Uniform practice?

Specificity

Comparative Value

Placebo RCTs

- Is practice standardized?
- Effect size estimated?
- Adverse effect rates?
- Comparison possible?

Adverse effects

Effect size

Costs

Added value?

Optimals?

Peer-review, systematic reviews, etc.

Chemical products?

Uniform practice?

Decision analysis

No treatment comparison RCT

Standard practice comparison RCT

Scientific acceptance

See attribution testing

Practice/policy decisions

Policy

Payment

Practice Guidelines

Methods of Investigation

1	2	3	A	4 / B	C	5	6
Qualitative research	• Laboratory investigations • Basic science research	• Observational studies • Outcomes research • Before/after trials • Clinical audit • Surveillance	Placebo-controlled RCT	No treatment RCT	Standard practice RCT	• Systematic reviews • Meta-analysis • Consensus development conferences • Guidelines	Health services research

Example Strategies

Entry Method

- Drug development — cell, animal, phase I–IV ⟶ Basic science
  (vincristine)

- Established products — safety and clinical efficacy ⟶ Clinical trials (phase III)
  (hypericum)

- Developed technique or standard practice ⟶ Before/after trials
  (P6, Ornish)

- Underdeveloped areas, new construct development ⟶ Qualitative research
  (spirituality)

Figure 1-2 CAM research strategy chart.

Ensuring Research Quality

Several quality criteria are described in this chapter. These methods do not function in isolation nor are they always in a particular fixed hierarchy. To predefine a hierarchy from more to less important methods without specifying the goal of the research is both illogical and dogmatic. Both experimental and observational data are required to assess the validity and value of CAM concepts and assumptions. Experts in both conventional and CAM fields are needed to conduct this research, which can lead to new fields and discoveries. For example, psychoneuroimmunology (PNI) developed when psychologists and immunologists began to explore parallel effects, bringing together their respective laboratory and clinical research methods. Other cross-disciplinary fields are likely to develop if scientists conduct multidisciplinary projects that cut across research domains. This research could produce a scientific basis for therapeutic diversity in management decisions for patients with chronic disease and could improve the value of science in making those decisions.

Balancing Rigor, Relevance, and Realism

Evaluation of the effectiveness of CAM practices can be complex. A few rigorous large-scale randomized trials will not provide all the necessary answers to questions about CAM or even the most important ones. Despite growing resources, systematic research will not be available in the foreseeable future even for the most commonly used interventions. Still, CAM use continues to increase. There are several different audiences, and the results of research must serve each audience, with different but overlapping information needs and priorities. We cannot afford to have a single research method or goal in CAM; we must use a variety of methods that balance between relevance, scientific rigor, and feasibility. Knowing how various groups use research information can guide the evaluation of research on CAM (Figure 1-2).

Modifying the Evidence Pyramid

The evidence pyramid described in Figure 1-1 can help explain the main types of research needed. This evidence pyramid is a modification of the one usually used in which attributional research (RCTs) is the primary goal of all investigation. In attributional research the RCT is the gold standard. In this pyramid the value of a particular approach depends on a number of factors, including attribution. These factors are as follows:

- The simplicity or complexity of the condition and therapy being investigated
- The type of information sought, whether causal, descriptive, associative, attributional, etc.
- The purpose for which a particular audience will use the information
- The methods of investigation that are available, ethical, and affordable

The purpose of the research and the main audience it addresses can be used to determine whether the appropriate research method has been used (Figure 1-2). In complex or skill-based practices, observational data and outcomes research are the best initial approach. In well-described CAM practices, observational data used with decision analysis often may be adequate. In natural product research in which the active constituents are unknown, basic laboratory characterization is necessary before clinical research is done. Well-characterized natural products need to undergo RCTs, provided their potential public health impact justifies such an investment. Placebo studies of natural products are more useful for making regulatory decisions (e.g., product marketing, public claims) than individual decisions. The U.S. National Institutes of Health's study on the efficacy of the herb St. John's Wort for the treatment of depression is an example of this approach. The study is a large, three-armed, multicentered, placebo-controlled, and standard therapy–controlled trial.

When physicians consider referring a patient for acupuncture, they want to know what kind of patients the local acupuncturists see, how patients are treated, whether patients are satisfied with treatment, and what the outcomes are. This kind of information comes from practice audit, which is observational research. Such information is more valuable when making referral decisions than are the results of small-scale, randomized placebo-controlled trials that may have been done in another country with patients who are quite different from those the physician sees. Methods for simple practice-based observational studies have been neglected in the effort to conduct randomized trials for a few popular CAM products. Certain aspects of observational studies must be performed as carefully as experimental studies, so efficient systems for conducting such studies must be developed. When theories and observations (e.g., psychic healing, homeopathy) do not fit into the current assumptions of Western medicine a rational strategy for approaching them is needed. Given the high public interest in many of these areas and the implications for science if some of them turn out to have merit, it is irresponsible for the scientific community to ignore them.[8]

Complementary and Alternative Medicine and the Evolution of the Scientific Method

The investigation of unconventional medicine has often resulted in improvements in the scientific method. For example, the current methods of blinding and randomization in orthodox medicine developed more than 50 years ago after having first been applied to unorthodox practices, such as mesmerism, psychic healing, and homeopathy.[16] Traditional and cross-cultural medicine challenges us to better define the concept of quality in biomedical science (such as model validity) and to explore the evidence on which current quality criteria are based. Research in CAM will undoubtedly lead to improved research and the development of a better strategic scientific approach to the global medicine of the future.

Most conventional or complementary therapies will never be fully evidence based; that is, all six evidence domains from Figure 1-1 will never be filled in. What is needed is not complete evidence, however, but sufficient evidence for particular purposes, such as individual choices, practice decisions, regulatory rules, public health implications, and so forth. To do this a more careful examination of science's role in the management of chronic disease and in the investigation of unconventional paradigms is required. Research answers incremental and isolated questions, and thus science can never answer all questions that are of interest. Because skepticism about unorthodox practices is higher than for conventional practices, there is often a demand for rigorous evidence before CAM practices are accepted. The continuing interface between orthodox and unorthodox medicine provides the opportunity for new research strategies and

methodologies to arise. If a creative tension between the established and the frontier can be maintained, scientific methods can be advanced and the role and boundaries of science in medicine elucidated.

References

1. Eisenberg DM: Trends in alternative medicine use in the United States 1990-1997: results of a follow-up national survey, *JAMA* 280:1569-1575, 1998.
2. Eddy DM: *Clinical decision making: from theory to practice: a collection of essays from JAMA,* Boston, 1996, Jones & Bartlett.
3. Jonas WB: Evaluating unconventional medical practices, *Journal of NIH Research* 5:64-67, 1993.
4. Begg C: Improving the quality of reporting of randomized controlled trials, *JAMA* 276:637-639, 1996.
5. Moher D: CONSORT: an evolving tool to help improve the quality of reports of randomized controlled trials, *JAMA* 279:1489-1491, 1998.
6. Stroup DF: Meta-analysis of observational studies in epidemiology *JAMA* 283:2008-2012, 2000.
7. Egger M, Davey SG, Altman DG: *Systematic reviews in health care: meta-analysis in context,* London, 2000, BMJ.
8. Jonas WB: Researching alternative medicine, *Nature Medicine* 3:824-827, 1997.
9. Moerman DE: Cultural variations in the placebo effect: ulcers, anxiety, and blood pressure, *Med Anthropol Q* 14:51-72, 2000.
10. Bergmann J et al: A randomized clinical trial of the effect of informed consent on the analgesic activity of placebo and naproxen in cancer pain, *Clinical Trials and Meta-Analysis* 29:41-47, 1994.
11. Kirsch I: *How expectancies shape experience,* Washington, DC, 1999, American Psychological Association.
12. Oxman AD, Guyatt GH: Guidelines for reading literature reviews, *CMAJ* 138:697-703, 1988.
13. Bero L, Rennie D: The Cochrane collaboration, *JAMA* 274:1935-1938, 1995.
14. Feinstein AR: Models, methods and goals, *J Clin Epidemiol* 42:301-308, 1989.
15. Linde K, Jonas WB: Evaluating complementary and alternative medicine: the balance of rigor and relevance. In Jonas WB, Levin JS, editors: *Essentials of complementary and alternative medicine,* Philadelphia, 1999, Lippincott Williams & Wilkins.
16. Kaptchuk TJ: Intentional ignorance: the history of blind assessment and placebo controls in medicine, *Bull Hist Med* 72:389-433, 1998.

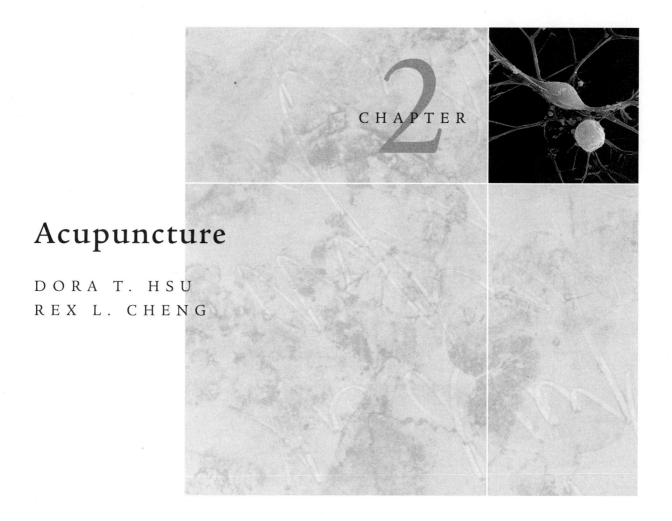

CHAPTER 2

Acupuncture

DORA T. HSU
REX L. CHENG

Acupuncture has been used to treat a variety of medical and surgical conditions. Over the years it has been increasingly and successfully incorporated as one of the treatment modalities in today's multidisciplinary approach to the management of pain and other medical disorders. Even though acupuncture's origin was not based on scientific data, it has survived thousands of years because it effectively ameliorates pain and the symptoms of many medical conditions. This treatment modality is widely accepted in East Asia, and in 1971 gained much publicity in the United States after the late *New York Times* columnist James Reston's remarkable article was published.[1] Reston described his personal experience with severe postappendectomy pain and how this pain was successfully controlled with acupuncture needles, which were applied in Beijing by a practitioner.

The past decade has seen the discipline evolve into a defined subspecialty of alternative medicine that is increasingly being accepted as complementary to mainstream medicine. Guidelines and regulations for training, education, and practice in the field have been formulated, established, and implemented. Several professional acupuncture societies[2] on the state, national, and international levels currently represent physicians' interests. In the United States a specialty board examination has evolved and is conducted annually.

Acupuncture is based primarily on traditional Chinese medicine (TCM) conceptualized from the Taoist philosophy that the human body is in a state of dynamic interaction with nature—the environment or the universe—which in turn is in a state of continuous change. The changes, arising from an inherent dynamism of cyclical patterns, are constant. For example, there are four seasons in the year, the sun rises in the East and sets in the West, and a biological being passes through the four stages of birth, maturation, senescence, and death. Dating from the Han dynasty (second century B.C.) the well-known ancient medical text, the *Huang Di Nei Jing* (meaning "yellow Emperor's inner classic"), is the bible of all Chinese medical philosophy. It describes the human body, explaining that it is a part of the universe, and emphasizes the importance of preserving and maintaining a harmonious energy balance within the body and in relation to the environment. Any imbalance in the energy state will bring about ailments. The observations of the natural phenomena gave rise to two theories: the Yin-Yang and the Five Phases. The *Nei Jing* is said to provide the first written documentation of the theory of acupuncture therapy.

A subsequent ancient medical text, the *Nan Jing* (meaning "classic of difficult issues"), was written in the second century A.D. It addresses the cause and diagnosis of ailments, the theories for point needling, and energy channels and their use in the treatment of disease states.

PRINCIPLES OF TRADITIONAL CHINESE MEDICINE

Laotse, a philosopher of the fifth century B.C. and the founder of Taoism, describes Tao as the natural law that is the absolute source of all creation in this universe. From this primal state emanate two complementary energy fields called *yin* and *yang* (Figure 2-1). These energy fields represent two opposing but balancing forces that exist in any natural phenomenon (e.g., heat is yang and cold is yin, day is yang and night is yin) and account for the relationship of an entity with its surroundings and the universe. The two opposing forces are not always absolute and may be construed as relative opposites in the framework of the phenomenon. Thus time can be divided into day (yang) and night (yin), and morning is yang within yang and afternoon is yin within yang. With respect to the human body, the organs are similarly categorized under their respective opposing forces. All associated organ activities are interdependent and in balance with one other.

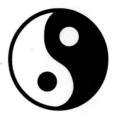

Figure 2-1 Yin and yang symbol.

The Five Phases is another organizational system for the patterns of phenomena. The five natural resources—wood, fire, earth, metal, and water—represent the phases. Each entity is interdependent and in balance with the others. Each phase is also associated with certain qualities and functions. Each of the major organs in the body is categorized in one of the five phases and interacts dynamically with the others. Disturbance in an organ may arise from the hyperactivity or hypoactivity of the modulating organ to which it is related (Figure 2-2).

When the body is in balance, there is unobstructed flow of normal "Qi," the vital energy that penetrates the entire body and protects, maintains, and nourishes the organs and tissues. There are three kinds of normal Qi: Original Qi (Yuan-Qi), which is inherited at birth and stored in the kidneys; acquired Qi (Gu-Qi), which is derived from the metabolism of food; and natural air Qi (Kong-Qi), which is derived from the air via the lung. A healthy person has sufficient Qi, whereas a sick person has weak or deficient Qi. The Qi energy flows through a system of imaginary lines (meridians) that run longitudinally in and around the body. Each set of lines is functionally connected to corresponding yin and yang organs. The longitudinal lines are interconnected via collaterals, which run transversely. There are 12 major meridians, each associated with an organ. The heart, pericardium, lung, spleen, liver, and kidney are yin organs; and the gall bladder, stomach, small intestine, large intestine, bladder, and "triple energizer" are yang organs (Table 2-1). Each of the major meridians is symmetrically represented in the body and follows a distinct pathway. Acupuncture points are located along the major meridians. There are a total of 361 classic acupuncture points. This network of channels serves as a pathway for the Qi energy to move through the muscles, organs, and other parts of the body.

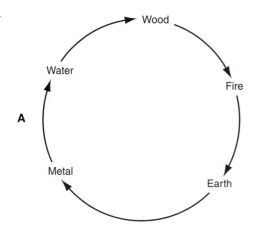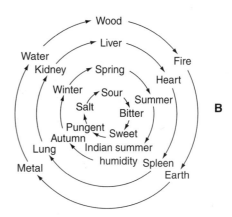

Figure 2-2 **A,** The Five Phases. **B,** The Five Phases and their corresponding entities. (Courtesy Robert Amaral.)

TABLE 2-1

Standard International Nomenclature for the 12 Major and 2 Collateral Meridians

Name of meridian	Alphabet code	
	Agreed	Former
Lung	LU	Lu,P
Large intestine	LI	CO,Co,IC
Stomach	ST	S,St,E,M
Spleen	SP	Sp,LP
Heart	HT	H,C,Ht,He
Small intestine	SI	Si,IT
Bladder	BL	B,Bi,UB
Kidney	KI	Ki,R,Rn
Pericardium	PC	P,Pe,HC
Triple energizer	TE	T,TW,SJ,3H,TB
Gallbladder	GB	G,VB,VF
Liver	LR	Liv,LV,H
Governor vessel	GV	Du,Du Go,Gv,Tm
Conception vessel	CV	Co,Cv,J,REN,Ren

Adapted from Filshie J, White A: Medical acupuncture: a western scientific approach, London, 1998, Churchill Livingstone p. 439.

Insufficient, overabundant, and/or obstructed flow of Qi causes disharmony, which leads to illness. In TCM the diagnosis parameters involve assessment of symptoms, physical examination of the patient's countenance and tongue, and palpation of the pulse quality in both hands. From this assessment an energy disharmony of a specific organ or meridian line is identified. Treatment is formulated to restore the body to its balanced state. Therapy modalities include acupuncture, herbal medicine, diet regulation, Qi Gong, and massage (Tui Na).

ACUPUNCTURE POINTS

The classic points are usually but not always situated in the skin areas of low electrical resistance.[3,4] They are found near major nerve bundles[5,6] and are located on the major meridians. Because of their strategic position, the classic points serve as access areas where the Qi energy may be externally modulated. For example, the classic upper respiratory tract infection is caused by wind invading the body. Treatment involves needling GB 20 (Fengchi), also known as the *wind pond,* to dispel the wind pathogen.

Point location is often described in relation to the surrounding surface anatomical landmarks. The common reference structures used include the hairline, brow ridge, inner and outer canthi, tragus of the ear, spinous process of the vertebrae, major skin crease, umbilicus, and pubic symphysis. The large intestine 4 point (Hegu) and lung 7 point (Lieque) are identified by the thumb and index finger, respectively, on specified anatomical areas as illustrated in Figure 2-3. The Chinese unit of measurement is the cun, and the patient's finger measurements are used as the reference source. One cun is equivalent to the width across the first interphalangeal joint of the

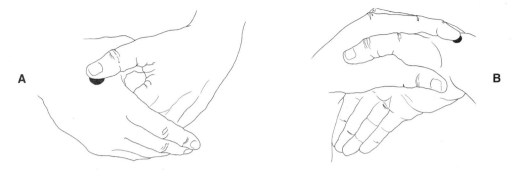

Figure 2-3 **A**, Large intestine 4 (Hegu) is located where the thumb touches the dorsum of the hand between the first and second metacarpal bones when the transverse crease of the interphalangeal joint of the thumb is approximated to the web margin of the other hand. **B**, Lung 7 (Lieque) is located distal to the styloid process of the radius. (Courtesy Robert Amaral.)

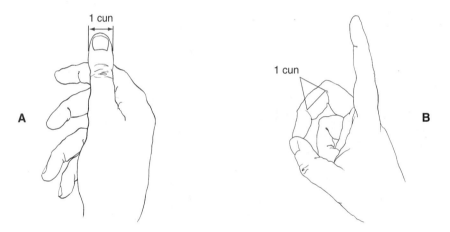

Figure 2-4 Cun measurement. **A**, One cun is equivalent to the width across the first interphalangeal joint of the thumb. **B**, One cun is equivalent to the distance between the two interphalangeal joints measured at the proximal crease lines with the middle finger flexed. (Courtesy Robert Amaral.)

thumb (Figure 2-4, *A*) or the distance between the two interphalangeal joints measured at the proximal creases of the middle finger when flexed (Figure 2-4, *B*). The width across the dorsal surface of the index and middle fingers held together and measured at the level of the proximal interphalangeal crease of the middle finger (Figure 2-5) equals 1½ cun. Likewise, 3 cun is equivalent to the width across the dorsal surface of the four fingers measured at the level of the proximal interphalangeal crease of the middle finger (Figure 2-6).

Nomenclature of the acupuncture points is based on the meridian on which the points are lo-cated. Points on the same meridian are given serial numbers with the same prefix. In addition, each retains its intrinsic Chinese name. For example, P6 (Neiguan) is the sixth point on the pericardial meridian and is located 2 cun proximal to the transverse crease of the wrist between the palmaris longus and flexor radialis tendons (Figure 2-7). Similarly, P7 (Daling) is the seventh point on the pericardial meridian, and is located on the transverse crease of the wrist between the same tendons but distal to P6 (Figure 2-7). As reference guides, a variety of acupuncture atlases of the meridians and points are available from several publishers.[7]

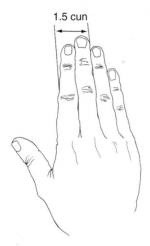

Figure 2-5 Cun measurement. One and one half cun is equivalent to the width across the dorsal surface of the index and middle fingers held together, measured at the level of the proximal interphalangeal crease of the middle finger. (Courtesy Robert Amaral.)

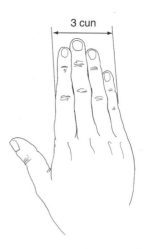

Figure 2-6 Cun measurement. Three cun is equivalent to the width across the dorsal surface of the four fingers at the level of the proximal interphalangeal crease of the middle finger. (Courtesy Robert Amaral.)

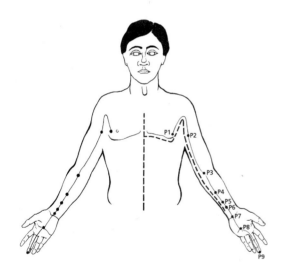

Figure 2-7 Location of P6 (Neiguan) and P7 (Daling) on the pericardial meridian. The solid line indicates external pathway; the dotted line indicates internal pathway. (Courtesy Robert Amaral.)

NEEDLES

As a tool, the needle has come a long way. In ancient times, needles were carved out of stone, animal bones, bamboo splinters, or any raw material that would yield a cutting point for easy skin penetration. Later, needles were made of elemental gold, silver, copper, and alloys, such as tin and bronze. For economic reasons these needles were reused. Modern technology has allowed the mass production of stainless steel needles at a fraction of the cost of the elemental ones. These needles are now the accepted standard. However, because some specialists still believe that the elemental needles are more effective, they continue to be an important part of the acupuncturist's armamentarium.

The standard needle consists of three parts—the handle, shaft (body), and tip (Figure 2-8). The needle width ranges from 0.22 to 0.45 mm, corresponding to gauge 34 to 26, respectively. The length may vary from 15 to 125 mm. Short, fine needles are reserved for use on children or the delicate sites on the adult face and ears. Long, wide-gauge needles are used for the deeper, thick skin areas. In general for adults the common needle size is 32 gauge, with a width of 0.25 mm and a length of 40 mm. The depths of needle penetration vary from a few millimeters to 5 cm.

Single-use and reusable needles are available. Because of the risk of infection transmission, reusing needles is strongly discouraged. The stainless steel needles presently available in the United States are imported from China, Japan, Korea, and Italy. They come prepackaged in boxes, containing 100 needles; each needle is sterilized and individually blister packaged. The needles are intended for single use only.

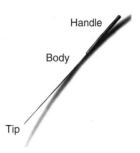

Figure 2-8 A disposable acupuncture needle. (Courtesy Robert Amaral.)

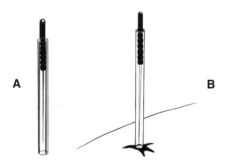

Figure 2-9 **A,** Acupuncture needle with insertion tube. **B,** Acupuncture needle with insertion tube on the skin. The insertion tube puts tension on the skin resulting in easy and nearly painless penetration. (Courtesy Robert Amaral.)

Some manufacturers place the individual needle in a plastic insertion tube, thus limiting the acupuncturist's point of contact to the handle tip (Figure 2-9).

PATIENT POSITIONING AND NEEDLING TECHNIQUES

It is essential that the patient be comfortable and relaxed during acupuncture because the treatment may last from 15 minutes to an hour. Frequent changes in posture while needles are in place are strongly discouraged because of the possibility of needle dislodgement or displacement. The ideal posture is such that the target points are easily accessible. Because of the remote possibility of a vasovagal event, the recumbent position in supine, prone, and lateral form is preferred.

Several methods for point identification are practiced. The most common method is palpating for the appropriate anatomic landmarks and using the traditional cun measurement. In another method the point locator is used to measure the lowered skin resistance. At the identified points, the locator emits a signal in the

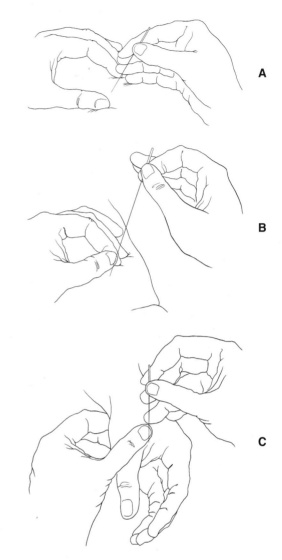

Figure 2-10 Right-handed needling showing various position placements of the left hand. (Courtesy Robert Amaral.)

form of light or sound. This method is limited in that not all acupuncture points have lowered skin resistance. Palpating for point tenderness is yet another way to localize insertion sites. Although these tender areas are not the classic points, this technique is often used in the treatment of musculoskeletal problems.

The ultimate goal is accurate needle placement with minimal discomfort. To avoid infection, the skin site is cleaned with alcohol. The different hand positions are illustrated in Figure 2-10. The common angle for needle insertion is perpendicular or oblique to the skin (Figure 2-11). Near-horizontal insertion is re-

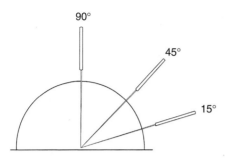

Figure 2-11 Different angles for needle insertion. (Courtesy Robert Amaral.)

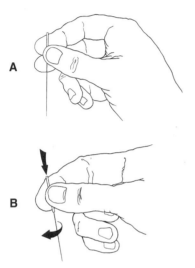

Figure 2-12 **A,** Right-handed needle positioning for a near 90-degree angle insertion. **B,** Needle position for a near 90-degree angle penetration showing quick insertion with a simultaneous twirling motion. (Courtesy Robert Amaral.)

served for areas where the skin is thin, such as the face and anterior chest. To minimize pain, a quick insertion with a simultaneous twirling motion is recommended (Figure 2-12). A slow insertion increases pain. The needle depth can vary from a few millimeters to 5 cm. An accurate site with proper depth placement will elicit De Qi sensation, often described as achiness, heaviness, fullness, and numbness, but not pain. Needles may be left in place to drain off excess energy or may be stimulated manually or electrically to boost energy in the respective meridians. Manual stimulation is labor intensive, involving combinations of lifting, twirling, thrusting, or plucking the needle periodically, and thus has been replaced by electrical

stimulation. A precise stimulation frequency between 1 and 500 Hz, with differing intensities, can be accurately delivered for a specified time. There is an added option of modifying the pulse width and duration. Currently, several types of battery-operated units are available. For a person who has never had an acupuncture treatment, the initial therapy should last no longer than 20 minutes. Excessive treatment leads to generalized body fatigue.

PRECAUTIONARY MEASURES

On the day of therapy patients are advised to avoid consumption of heavy meals or alcohol because of the possibility of nausea and vomiting. Previous steroid therapy may attenuate the body's response to effective acupuncture. To maximize efficacy, treatment ideally is delayed for 1 to 2 months after steroid therapy has been discontinued, thus giving the adrenals time to recover. Relative contraindications include anticoagulant therapy and pregnancy. Blood thinning medications may prolong bleeding from the needling points. One patient ended up in the hospital emergency department when multiple hematomas developed several hours after treatment. The acupuncturist had not elicited the patient's medication history, which included prolonged warfarin (Coumadin) therapy. Acupuncture treatment during pregnancy can induce preterm labor[8] and hence is best avoided. If acupuncture is used at all during pregnancy, a milder treatment involving selected ear points is the only alternative. Direct needling into blood vessels, major body organs (e.g., the heart or lung), the eyeball, open wounds, and abscesses is strictly prohibited. To date, there have been no reports of harmful side effects when treatment has been given in the presence of coexisting medical problems, such as ischemic heart disease, diabetes mellitus, or renal failure.

Patients should be forewarned that their original symptoms will be exacerbated 24 to 48 hours after a treatment. This rebound phenomenon may be bothersome but transient before symptomatic improvement is seen. General fatigue and sleepiness are common side effects that may be immediate or delayed for several hours. Therefore patients are advised to refrain from making major legal decisions, driving automobiles, and operating complex machinery after treatment. So far, there have been no reports to indicate that the general fatigue and sleepiness resulting from acupuncture are problematic for patients taking concomitant medications or undergoing other pain management procedures. For example, patients taking sedatives, anticonvulsants, or opioid analgesics or undergoing nerve blocks after receiving acupuncture therapy have not experienced respiratory depression.

COMPLICATIONS

Several technical and reported medical problems deserve mention, including a bent or broken needle shaft or the inability to remove a needle (Table 2-2). The improvements in the alloy and the manufacturing process and the advent of single-use needles have diminished the incidence of needle damage. Occasionally, when a patient is extremely anxious, a needle may become difficult to remove. Anxiety causes intense muscle spasms at the insertion site. If reassurance and relaxation are encouraged, often the needle can be extracted uneventfully. In cases in which relaxation is insufficient to allow needle removal, gentle massage around the site or counterirritation with another needle insertion in the vicinity relieves the surrounding spasm.

Syncope occurring during treatment is uncommon. This phenomenon usually occurs in young, healthy, muscular male patients receiving treatment while in the upright posture.[9] Accompanying symptoms include pallor, nausea, dizziness, cold sweats, and bradycardia. Symptoms resolve when the patient moves to a supine posture. After a syncopal episode, removal of all needles is advised and constant verbal contact is essential. If symptoms do not resolve, aggressive supportive measures, including parenteral hydration and anticholinergics, may have to be pursued.

Other reported major medical problems are related to transmission of hepatitis B[10] and human immunodeficiency virus (HIV)[11] during needling therapy. In 1980 there was a hepatitis B outbreak among a Florida chiropractor's patients because the sterilization process used at the office was inadequate. The isolated incident of HIV infection occurred in a young man who was already at high risk for the disease. Dermatitis resulting from needle contact is uncommon. Two case reports of dermatitis (one occurring after insertion of a permanent needle[12] and the other after insertion of a nickel needle[13]) resolved uneventfully.

Poor technique and inadequate fundamental knowledge of anatomy may result in hematoma or organ and tissue damage. Proficient training minimizes complications.

ACUPUNCTURE SYSTEMS

Several schools of acupuncture exist. Despite the universal acceptance of the classic points and meridians, each school has its preferred combination of choice points and practice styles. Some examples of the different systems are the TCM, the 5-Element Theory,[14] French Energetics,[15] Japanese Meridian Theory,[16] auriculotherapy,[17] Korean hand acupuncture, and scalp acupuncture. In general, acupuncture systems can be categorized into four groups.

Traditional Acupuncture and Its Derivatives

Traditional acupuncture is based on the TCM principle of maintaining a harmonious, balanced energy state that allows the smooth flow of *Qi*. Harmony may be restored through acupuncture of classic points in conjunction with herbal medicine, diet regulation, *Qi Gong*, and massage (Tui Na). Similar illnesses in different individuals require tailored classic acupuncture points depending on each person's unique constitution. The balanced energy principle of TCM brought about other systems, such as the 5-Element Theory,[14]

TABLE 2-2

Common Complications Associated with Acupuncture Needling

Technical problems	Reported medical problems
Bent needle	Muscle spasm
Broken needle	Vasovagal symptoms
Inability to remove needle	Hematoma
	Dermatitis
	Infection (hepatitis B, HIV)
	Organ, tissue damage
	Premature labor

From Hsu Dora T: Acupuncture: a review, *Reg Anes* 21(4): 364, 1996.

French Energetics,[15] and Japanese Meridian Theory.[16] The universal emphasis is on the restoration of wholeness to the individual.

Formula Acupuncture

In formula acupuncture, fixed sets of classic points are used for the management of a defined pathological problem irrespective of the individual's constitutional makeup. This type of acupuncture is commonly practiced in research settings in the Western hemisphere where well-designed clinical studies require objectivity and uniformity for evaluating therapeutic outcome.

Symptomatic Acupuncture

In symptomatic therapy, needles are placed along or around the problem area. Classic points are not used. This type of acupuncture may be the close equivalent of present-day myofascial trigger point injections. This treatment modality is commonly used for pain management.

Auriculotherapy and Hand and Scalp Acupuncture

The commonality among auriculotherapy and hand and scalp acupuncture is that the entire body may be somatotopically represented in a defined external body part, namely, the ear, hand, or scalp. Needling of the points in these external structures has a similar, though milder effect when compared with that of traditional body acupuncture. Auriculotherapy is often used in conjunction with the traditional system for enhancement.

BASIC RESEARCH

In an attempt to identify acupuncture's mechanism of action, the majority of initial work was done in acupuncture analgesia. Near the end of the 1970s, physiologists from the People's Republic of China demonstrated the importance of an intact somatosensory pathway for acupuncture to be effective.[18] A decade later, after reviewing the scientific literature and findings from his own laboratory work, Pomeranz pub-

lished his hypothesis that acupuncture analgesia is mediated through the release of endorphins produced by the indirect activation of the spinal cord, the midbrain, and the hypothalamopituitary centers via acupuncture stimulation.[19] Han and co-workers further showed that different frequencies of stimulation (e.g., 100 Hz versus 4 Hz)[20,21] released different types of endorphins. Other researchers have provided evidence that monoamines, such as norepinephrine and serotonin, also may play a role in acupuncture analgesia.[22] Neuropeptides with antiopioid activity have been discovered in the brain.[23] Their existence may explain why some individuals respond more efficaciously to acupuncture than do others. More research is required to identify the role of these neuropeptides in the brain.

CLINICAL RESEARCH

In a clinical trial to prove the efficacy of a medication or treatment modality, comparable controls are required to allow evaluation of the outcome measures. Over the years there have been many clinical studies on acupuncture treatment. Most had study designs with major flaws, sample sizes with inadequate controls, and outcome measures with inadequate follow-up. The trials either yielded equivocal results or were unable to substantiate the efficacy of the treatment modality. Following are some of the common problems encountered in clinical acupuncture research for which there are still no good answers.

Choice of Points

Traditional acupuncture requires assessment of the patient's symptoms, countenance, complexion, and pulse quality and the condition of the tongue. The energy imbalance along a specific meridian, organ, or both is identified, and a treatment course is instituted with the ultimate goal of restoring wholeness and balance, thus achieving health. At each visit the energy balance of the individual is reassessed, and classic points are chosen accordingly. Treatment is individualized, and different points are stimulated at subsequent visits. Formula acupuncture, commonly practiced by Western-trained physicians, is used in present-day clinical research. Based on the diagnosis a consistent group of points is used throughout the treatment course; that is, individuals with the same ailment receive treatment at the same points. This method is not consistent with the concept of TCM.

Control Groups

Appropriate controls allow the evaluation of outcome measures. Though not ideal, controls in the form of transcutaneous electrical nerve stimulation (TENS) or "sham acupuncture" (superficial or deep) have been used with varying success. TENS is known to have a therapeutic effect.[24,25] Sham acupuncture involves insertion at points that are theoretically ineffective. Lewith showed that sham point treatment provided analgesia in 40% to 50% of patients,[26] and therefore its use as a control in pain studies is of limited value.

Blinded Trials

A double-blind trial eliminates researcher bias. However, difficulties arise when a trained acupuncturist can identify a real point versus a sham point. In addition, patients who have had acupuncture treatment before are aware that stimulation of the sham points does not result in De Qi. To circumvent this problem, a single-blind trial may be the solution. However, to avoid affecting patient response, the researchers must have no bias toward the true or the sham form of treatment.

Number and Duration of Treatments

Until now, the number of treatments and the duration of each course have been empirical. There has been no evidence in the scientific literature defining the frequency and number of treatments required for a therapeutic trial. Recent clinical trials have used one to two treatments per week for a course duration of 2 to 4 months.[27-29]

Outcome Measurement

Both objective and subjective assessments of the outcome are essential. Additional multidimensional measurements must be considered to address the physiological and behavioral effects that can occur while the patient is undergoing treatment.

RECOGNITION OF ACUPUNCTURE

In a consensus workshop on acupuncture in April 1994, U.S. Food and Drug Administration (FDA) authorities valued the amount of basic and clinical research data available to support acupuncture as a form of therapeutic intervention. However, they voiced their concern regarding the inadequacy of sham points as good controls. The shortfall and limitations of control groups prompted some of the regulatory officials to recommend future randomized clinical studies comparing the efficacy of acupuncture with that of conventional therapies rather than with placebo controls.[30] Outcome studies would then be more clinically informative and conclusive.

The U.S. National Institutes of Health (NIH) held a Consensus Development Conference in November 1997 during which a panel reviewed and evaluated existing data on clinical research.[31] The panel concluded that acupuncture treatment is effective for postoperative and chemotherapy-associated nausea and vomiting, nausea in pregnancy, and postoperative dental pain. Although there is inadequate scientific support data, acupuncture also may serve as adjunct or possibly alternative therapy for headaches, stroke rehabilitation, low back pain, fibromyalgia, addiction, carpal tunnel syndrome, tennis elbow, menstrual cramps, and asthma.

ACUPUNCTURE FOR THE MANAGEMENT OF CERTAIN CONDITIONS

Neurologic Ailments

There is a tremendous amount of research work and established information in China that requires translation for review in the Western hemisphere. Until then the available information from the MEDLINE database, though extensive, is still limited.

There are about 360 classic points distributed along the 12 principal, minor, and collateral meridians. Different points may be used to treat the same health problem in a patient population. In general, experienced TCM acupuncturists limit the use of points to no more than five per session. Western-trained acupuncturists may require 10 or more. The goal is to use as few points as possible.

Headache

To date there has been a considerable amount of anecdotal information and to a lesser extent scientific literature supporting the therapeutic effect of acupuncture in the management of headaches. The majority of studies involve migraine and tension headaches. Although earlier migraine studies[32,33] showed that acupuncture resulted in some improvement, there were no controls and the subjects were not followed long enough to allow for conclusive evidence. Clinical studies with acceptable controls failed to show a significant therapeutic advantage of acupuncture over a placebo. Both Dowson's group[34] in 1985 and Hesse's group[35] in 1994 showed a decreased frequency in headaches for both the control and the study arms. There was no significant, favorable outcome in the acupuncture group. Hesse's group showed that metoprolol was significantly better than acupuncture in reducing headache frequency.

Similarly, other outcome findings related to acupuncture and tension headaches did not show a definite advantage to treatment with this modality. Vincent's[36] 1990 study revealed decreased frequency and pain scores in both the control and study arms, and Carlsson's[28] 1994 findings also showed a decrease in pain intensity in both the acupuncture treatment group and the physical therapy control group.

Syncope and Fainting

According to TCM, syncope may arise from either yang or yin deficiency[37] or from disturbance in the flow of Qi and blood. Therapeutic measures include reinforcing the deficiency state, decreasing the excess condition (heat or cold), and using herbs. Manual needling or acupressure, if no needle is available, of GV 26 (Ren Zhong) often arouses the patient to consciousness. GV 26 is a very strong stimulation point. Follow-up therapy is based on the presence of symp-

toms and signs that were prevalent around the time of syncope. There are no controlled studies to prove acupunctures efficacy in treating syncopal episodes.

Epilepsy and Convulsion

Prolonged stagnation of Qi in the heart and liver creates fire that rises to affect the mind. Seizure activity is a sudden, transient imbalance of yin and yang. Treatment may be categorized as abortive or as maintenance therapy to control the frequency of attacks. During a seizure, manual stimulation of GV 26 often successfully aborts the episode and, according to Stux and Pomeranz, is effective in 80% to 90% of patients.[38] Maintenance therapy involves the following points: GV 20 (Bahui), HT 7 (Shenmen), KI 1 (Yongquan), GB 34 (Yanglingquan), LI 4 (Hegu), and Yintang. Acupuncture alone is inadequate to maintain complete control of seizures. During the start of maintenance acupuncture therapy, antiepileptic medications are continued and adjusted downward if there is a good response to treatment. The ultimate goal is to prevent or minimize seizure episodes.

Stroke

Disequilibrium in the yin and yang, and a Qi-blood deficiency of the heart, liver, and kidney results in obstruction and wind invasion of certain meridians and collaterals. The end result is paresis, paralysis, or both. The TCM treatment objective is to remove the blood and Qi stagnation, thus activating free flow. Point selections include GB 20 (Fengchi), GB 21 (Jianjing), LI 15 (Jianyu), LI 4 (Hegu), LI 10 (Shousanli), ST 36 (Zusanli), BL 23 (Shenshu), and BL 40 (Weizhong).

In 1990 Chen and Fang[39] retrospectively reviewed 108 cases of hemiplegia and concluded that treatment initiated within the first 3 weeks after the cerebral insult was statistically more successful than treatment started more than 3 weeks after the episode. Magnusson's 1994[40] study of stroke patients showed that sensory stimulation improved recovery in the form of regaining normal or near-normal dynamics of human postural control. Other earlier studies implied that acupuncture performed soon after stroke improved patients' performance in daily life activities. However, Gosman-Hedstrom's 1998[41] randomized study does not support these studies findings. His results showed no significant difference between the control and the acupuncture groups.

Painful Peripheral Neuropathy

A MEDLINE search revealed few studies on the use of acupuncture to treat HIV and painful diabetic neuropathy. The diabetic study by Abuaisha[42] revealed an improvement in 67% of the individuals receiving acupuncture for long-term (1 year) pain relief. Studies of HIV were not too convincing. One study conducted by the Terry Beirn Community Programs for Clinical Research[43] showed neither acupuncture nor amitriptyline was effective.

Tinnitus

Several double-blind, placebo-controlled studies were conducted in the Scandinavian countries.[44,45] Traditional points TE 21 (Ermen), TE 17 (Yifeng), ST 36 (Zusanli), LI 4 (Hegu) were used. Even though the combination of points differed in each of the studies, the outcome was the same. No significant differences were found between the acupuncture group and the placebo group.

Parkinson's Disease

There is scant translated clinical data regarding the treatment of Parkinson's disease in TCM. In laboratory research, however, the rat model has shown that a combination of acupuncture and herbal medicine increases dopamine levels in the midbrain and caudate nucleus.[46]

Hiccups

The reverse flow of Qi in the stomach, liver, or both causes hiccups. Other causes include prolonged debilitation of the stomach, with a resultant yang deficiency, and the excessive consumption of spicy or greasy food causing blockage of Qi in the middle burner or heater. Several uncontrolled trials have shown a favorable outcome using auriculotherapy and body acupuncture. Further studies are required

to validate this claim of efficacy. TCM therapy involves the regulation and restoration of stomach Qi with the following body points: ST 25 (Tianshu), ST 36 (Zusanli), ST 40 (Fenglong), PC 6 (Neiguan), BL 17 (Geshu), BL 21 (Weishu), and BL 25 (Dachangshu). Auriculopoints, such as the Shenmen, stomach, liver, and spleen, are commonly used.[47,48]

Sleep Disorders and Insomnia

Excessive mind activity depletes nourishment for the heart and leads to unrest in the mind. An improper diet causes stagnation of stomach and spleen Qi, whereas a kidney yin deficiency results in hyperactive fire. Many disturbances cause fire to rise and affect the mind with ensuing insomnia. A 1999 German study,[49] using polysomnography in a sleep laboratory, demonstrated that insomniacs receiving acupuncture experienced a statistically significant improvement in the quality of their sleep as compared with a control group. Diagnosis was based on TCM principles, and each patient received individualized acupuncture treatment. For excessive types of imbalance the following acupuncture points are often used: GV 20 (Bahui), HT 7 (Shenmen), EX 8 (Anmian I), and EX 9 (Anmian II). For kidney deficiency, moxibustion along the BL 22 (Sanjiaoshu) and BL 23 (Shenshu) and stimulation of kidney points along the medial ankle are helpful.

Foot Drop and Wrist Drop

Treatment for nerve palsy usually consists of stimulation of localized and distal points on the meridians in the affected area. Although there are no well-defined acupuncture outcome studies reported in Western literature, this treatment pattern has been used extensively in China.

Foot drop is the result of common peroneal nerve pathology. Manifestations include inversion of the foot; foot drop; and the inability to dorsiflex the ankle, extend the toes, and evert the foot. There also may be an accompanying area of hypoaesthesia, anesthesia over the lateral aspect of the leg, or both. Prolonged pathology of the nerve leads to wasting of the anterior tibial muscle. Treatment involves stimulation of points in the problem area along the stomach, gall bladder, bladder, and kidney meridians, namely, ST 36

(Zusanli), ST 38 (Tiaokou), ST 341 (Jiexi), GB 34 (Yanglinquan), GB 39 (Xuanzhong), BL 62 (Shenmai), and KI 6 (Zhaohai).

Radial nerve palsy is manifested by wrist drop, thumb abduction with hypoesthesia, or anesthesia over the posterior radial aspect of the hand, metacarpals of the thumb, and index and middle fingers. Points used in acupuncture of patients with wrist drop include LI 11 (Quchi), LI 5 (Yangxi), LI 4 (Hegu), TE 5 (Waiguan), TE 4 (Yangchi), and ST 36 (Zusanli).

Multiple Sclerosis

When conventional therapies are unable to offer a cure for a disease, such as multiple sclerosis, patients seek alternate resources. Not surprisingly, because of the increasing popularity of alternative therapies in the form of aquatic therapy, therapeutic touch, yoga, and acupuncture they have become adjuncts to mainstream treatment. In a 1994 study[50] 30% of multiple sclerosis patients responded that their quality of life had improved as a result of alternative therapy.

The inherent nature of multiple sclerosis makes acupuncture outcome studies particularly difficult to evaluate. The remission and relapsing characteristics of the disease together with the possibility of spontaneous recovery render less than convincing evidence of the efficacy of acupuncture as a treatment modality. To date, only one outcome study[51] has addressed the effect of acupuncture on patients with multiple sclerosis; this study noted specific irritability of the acupuncture points on needle insertion, leading to spasm, clonus, and even tonic-clonic contractions of the limb muscles. This response is specific to this illness and may serve as a herald sign for the disease. Further studies are required to prove this hypothesis and substantiate this observation.

Neck Pain with and without Radiculitis

There are innumerable causes of neck pain. Common causes include occipital neuralgia, cervical spondylopathy, torticollis, and myofascial trigger points. The predominant prescription is stimulation of points located in the meridians of the involved area, with occasional stimulation of distal points of the affected meridian.

Occipital Neuralgia

Pain along the distribution of the greater and lesser occipital nerve may be mitigated by stimulation of the following prescription points in the problem area: GB 12 (Wangu), GB 19 (Naokong), GB 20 (Fengchi), SI 3 (Houxi), BL 10 (Tianzhu), and BL 60 (Kunlun).

Cervical Spondylopathy

Pain may be localized near the midline or on the side of the neck, with radiation down the upper extremity. Midline pain involves the small intestine and bladder meridians, whereas pain off of the midline involves the Sanjiao and gall bladder meridians. Recommended acupuncture points include SI 3 (Houxi), SI 5 (Waiguan), SI 12 (Bingfeng), BL 11 (Dashu), BL 60 (Kunlun); GB 20 (Fengchi), GB 21(Jianjing), GB 34 (Yanglingquan), and SJ 5 (Waiguan).

Torticollis and Myofascial Problems

Symptoms of torticollis are related to wind invasion of the local meridians with stagnation of the flow of Qi and blood. The treatment objective is to remove the obstructive element (wind) and reestablish the free flow of Qi and blood. Prescription points include SI 3 (Houxi), SI 11 (Tianzong), TE 5 (Waiguan), and Ashi points.

Low Back Pain with and without Radiculitis

According to TCM, back pain arises when there is an invasion of wind and dampness or when there is a lack of kidney energy and liver blood nourishing the respective channels. The objective is to promote the circulation of Qi and blood. When the cause is a deficiency syndrome, needling together with moxibustion is indicated.

Low back pain may be localized on or off of the midline of the lumbar spine. The main meridians involved are the bladder (for midline pain) and the gallbladder (for lateral pain). Prescription points include BL 25 (Dachangshu), BL 26 (Guanyushu), BL 40 (Weizhong), BL 60 (Kunlun), GB 30 (Huantiao), GB 31 (Fengshi), GB 34 (Yanglingquan), and GB 39 (Xuanzhong).

Richardson and Vincent[52] evaluated published results of controlled and uncontrolled clinical therapeutic acupuncture studies on pain control that had been conducted between 1973 and 1985. The most common disorders were headache and back pain. Other less studied conditions included acute postoperative pain, phantom limb pain, rheumatoid arthritis, osteoarthritis, and neck pain. In general, 50% to 80% of the patients in the controlled studies showed therapeutic response supporting the short-term effectiveness of the treatment. The follow-up period ranged from 2 weeks to 4 months. There was not enough data available for analysis of the long-term effectiveness (6 months or longer). The few studies lasting longer than 6 months were uncontrolled studies that showed nearly a 50% relapse rate in patients who had a favorable response initially. Carlsson and Sjolund[53] in 1994 looked at the long-term effectiveness of acupuncture on various subtypes of chronic pain. They showed that individuals with nociceptively mediated low back pain benefited most; 49% experienced pain relief compared with 32% in the neurogenic and 15% in the psychogenic groups. Of the nociceptive pain responders, only half continued to have pain relief 6 months after one course of treatment, which consisted of one to two treatments per week for a mean of 7.8 treatments.

Carpal Tunnel Syndrome

The entrapment of the median nerve in the carpal canal causes numbness and pain in the index, middle, and ring fingers. Timely release of the flexor retinaculum minimizes atrophy of the thenar muscles and the loss of sensation on the radial aspect of the thumb and index, middle, and ring fingers.

There has been only one recently reported outcome study[54] in which laser and needle acupuncture were used together with herbal medication. The results were extraordinary in that 91.6% of patients had no pain or had reduced pain. Long-term follow-up for 1 to 2 years was promising in that only 8.3% of the patients 60 years of age and younger had recurrence of pain. These patients were successfully treated, with resolution of symptoms.

Dysphagia

In TCM, dysphagia is a disorder amenable to acupuncture treatment. Vasointestinal peptide is one of the main neurotransmitters that relaxes the lower esophageal sphincter.[55] In 1994, Tusheng[56] conducted a controlled, nonrandomized trial to treat achalasia using GB 21 (Jianjing) and supplemental points PC 6 (Neiguan), CV 12 (Zhongwan), CV 17 (Shanzhong), and ST 36 (Zusanli). Based on a barium swallow study, Tusheng showed that acupuncture of these points improved swallowing, though this improvement was inversely related to the duration and severity of the symptoms.

Stuttering

There have been several anecdotal reports regarding stuttering and several claims of cure resulting from acupuncture. A pilot study was undertaken in 1995 by the Department of Health Services[57] in New South Wales, Australia, to look into acupuncture's effectiveness in the treatment of stuttering. Two subjects were studied, both of whom had stuttered since childhood. There was no difference in the baseline and posttreatment measurements of stuttering frequency, speech rate, naturalness of speech, or anxiety level. Claims that acupuncture reduces stuttering must be carefully evaluated. The authors caution that a definitive conclusion cannot be drawn regarding the ineffectiveness of this modality because only two subjects were studied. A larger sample size is needed for future research.

Pain Syndromes Secondary to Trauma, Cancer, and Illness

Pain as defined in 1994 by the International Association for the Study of Pain is "an unpleasant sensory and emotional experience, associated with actual or potential tissue damage or expressed in terms of such damage." Categorically there are four major types of pain:
1. Nociceptive pain
2. Neuropathic (central and peripheral) pain
3. Sympathetically mediated pain (complex regional pain syndrome)
4. Psychogenic pain

In pain conditions a combination of the aforementioned types of pain may coexist. How effective is acupuncture in the management of pain? For acute pain, stimulation of the following points has provided temporary relief: LI 4 (Hegu) and ST 44 (Neiting). However, effective, long-term pain control is unproven.

SUMMARY

Acupuncture has been used for a variety of neurologic ailments. Some scientific outcome studies support the efficacy of this treatment modality for some of these ailments. Further well-designed studies are required to validate its short- and long-term effects on migraine headaches, rehabilitation after stroke, and seizure control. Acupuncture therapies for peripheral neuropathies, tinnitus, vertigo, and sleep disorders are based on anecdotal communications with insufficient support of scientific evidence. Until additional outcome studies providing positive evidence are presented, practitioners and patients should be cognizant of the therapy's present limitations. For practitioners, counseling patients appropriately concerning the realistic expectations of a cure resulting from acupuncture is a must.

ACKNOWLEDGMENTS

The authors thank Robert Amaral, a medical illustrator from the University of Southern California, for his patience, hard work, and excellent production of the figures.

Due acknowledgment is also extended to the publishers who have kindly given us permission to use their work (quoted or reproduced) in this chapter.

Suggested Further Reading

Filshie J, White A: *Medical acupuncture: a western scientific approach*, New York, 1998, Churchill Livingstone.
Helms JM: *Acupuncture energetics: a clinical approach for physicians*, Berkeley, California, 1995, Medical Acupuncture.
Kaptchuk T: *The web that has no weaver*, Berlin/Heidelberg, 1983, Congdon and Weed.
Stux G, Pomeranz B: *Basics of acupuncture*, ed 4, New York, 1997, Springer.

References

1. Reston J: *Now about my operation in Peking*, The New York Times, p. 1, 6, July 26, 1971.
2. Hsu DT, Diehl DL: The west gets the point, *Lancet* 352:1, 1998.
3. Pomeranz B: Scientific basis of acupuncture. In Stux G, Pomeranz B, editors: *Basics of acupuncture*, rev ed 4, New York, 1997, Springer.
4. Baldry PE: The deactivation of trigger points. In Baldry PE, editor: *Acupuncture, triggerpoints and musculoskeletal pain*, London, 1993, Churchill Livingstone.
5. Heine H: Zur Morphologie der Akupunkturpunkte, *Dtsch Z Akupunkutur* 30:75, 1987.
6. Heine H: Anatomie Strukutur der Akupunkturpunkte. *Dtsch Z Akupunkutur* 31:26, 1988.
7. Mann F: Points and meridians in relation to surface anatomy. In Mann F, editor: *Atlas of acupuncture*, Hertford, UK, 1990, Heinemann.
8. Dunn PA, Rogers D, Halford K: Transcutaneous electrical nerve stimulation at acupuncture points in the induction of uterine contractions, Obstetrics Gynecology 73:286-290, 1989.
9. Chen FP, Hwang SJ, Lee HP, Yang HY, Chung C: Clinical study of syncope during acupuncture treatment, *Acupuncture Electrother Res* 15(2): 107-119, 1990.
10. Hepatitis B associated with acupuncture, *MMWR* 30:1-31, 1981.
11. Vittecoq D, Mattetal JF, Rouzioux, Bach JF, Acute HIV infection after acupuncture treatments, N Engl J Med 32:250-251, 1989.
12. Romaguera C, Grimalt F: Contact dermatitis from a permanent acupuncture needle, *Contact Dermatitis* 7:156-157, 1981.
13. Romaguera C, Grimalt F: Nickel dermatitis from acupuncture needles, *Contact Dermatitis* 5:195, 1979.
14. Moss CA: Five elements and medical acupuncture, *AAMA Rev* 3:21-26, 1991.
15. Helms J: Acupuncture energetics. In Helms J, editor: *Clinical approach for physicians*, ed 1, Berkeley, 1995, Medical Acupuncture.
16. Denmai S: *Introduction to meridian therapy*, Seattle, 1990, Eastland.
17. Nogier PFM: Foundations of auriculotherapy. In Nogier PFM, editor: *From auriculotherapy to auriculomedicine*, Maisonneuve, S.A., France, 1983.
18. Han JS, Terenius L: Neurochemical basis of acupuncture analgesia, *Annu Rev Pharmacol Toxicol* 22:193-220, 1982.
19. Pomeranz B: Scientific basis of acupuncture. In Stux G, Pomeranz B, editors: *Basics of acupuncture*, rev ed 4, New York, 1998, Springer.
20. Han JS: Differential release of enkephalin and dynorphin by low and high frequency electroacupuncture in the central nervous system, *Acupuncture Sci Int J* 1:19-27, 1990.
21. Han JS, Wang Q: Mobilization of specific neuropeptide by peripheral stimulation of identified frequencies, *News Physiol Sci* 7:176-180, 1992.
22. Cheng R, Pomeranz B: Monoaminergic mechanism of electroacupuncture analgesia, *Brain Res* 215:77-92, 1981.
23. Ungar G et al: Brain peptides with opiate antagonistic action: their possible role in tolerance and dependence, *Psychoneuroendocrinology* 2:1-10, 1977.
24. Langley GB, Shepperd H, Johnson M, Wigley RD: The analgesic effects of transcutaneous electrical stimulation and placebo in chronic pain patients, *Rheumatol Int* 2:1-5, 1984.

25. Thornsteinsson G et al: The placebo effect of transcutaneous electrical stimulation, *Pain* 5:31-41, 1978.

26. Lewith GT, Machun D: On evaluation of clinical effects of acupuncture, *Pain* 16:111-127, 1983.

27. Gosman-Hedstrom G et al: Effects of acupuncture treatment on daily life activities and quality of life, *Stroke* 29:2100-2108, 1998.

28. Carlsson CP, Sjolund BH: Acupuncture and subtypes of chronic pain: assessment of longterm results, *Clin J Pain* 10:290-295, 1994.

29. Christensen BV et al: Acupuncture treatment of severe knee arthrosis: a long term study, *Acta Anaesthesiol Scand* 36:518-525, 1992.

30. Vickers A: Acupuncture and the US food and drug administration: how should complementary therapies be regulated? *Complement Ther Med* 5:27-28, 1997.

31. Hsu DT, Diehl DL: The west gets the point, *Lancet* 352 (Suppl IV):1, 1998.

32. Poitinen PJ, Salmela ND: Acupuncture treatment of migraine. In Sicuteri F, editor: *Headache new vistas,* Florence, 1977, Biomedical.

33. Boivie J, Bratteberg G: Are there long lasting effects on migraine headaches after one series of acupuncture treatment? *Am J Chin Med* 15:69-70, 1987.

34. Dowson D, Lewith G, Machin D: The effects of acupuncture versus placebo in the treatment of headache, *Pain* 21:35-42, 1985.

35. Hesse J, Mogelvang B, Simonsen H: Acupuncture versus metoprolol in migraine prophylaxis: a randomized trial of trigger point inactivation, *J Int Med* 235:451-456, 1994.

36. Vincent CA: The treatment of tension headache by acupuncture: a controlled single case design with time series analysis, *J Psychosom Res* 34:553-561, 1990.

37. Deng S: Acupuncture treatment of syncope based on differentiation of signs and symptoms, *J Tradit Chin Med* 10(3):182-188, 1990.

38. Stux G, Pomeranz B: Neurological disorders. In Stux G, Pomeranz G, editors: *Basics of acupuncture,* rev ed 4, New York, 1997, Springer.

39. Chen Y, Fang Y: 108 cases of hemiplegia caused by stroke: the relationship between CT scan results, clinical findings and the effect of acupuncture treatment. *Acupunct Electrother Res* 15:9-17, 1990.

40. Magnusson M, Johansson K, Johansson B: Sensory stimulation promotes normalization of postural control after stroke, *Stroke* 25:1176-1180, 1994.

41. Gosman-Hedstrom G et al: Effects of acupuncture treatment on daily life activities and quality of life, *Stroke* 29:2100-2108, 1998.

42. Abuaisha B, Costanzi J, Boulton A: Acupuncture for the treatment of chronic painful peripheral diabetic neuropathy: a long term study, *Diabetes Res Clin Pract* 39:115-121, 1998.

43. Shlay J et al: Acupuncture and amitriptyline for pain due to HIV-related peripheral neuropathy: a randomized controlled trial, *Denver Community Programs for Clinical Research on AIDS,* jshlay@dhha.org.

44. Nielsen O, Moller K, Jorgensen K: The effect of traditional Chinese acupuncture on severe tinnitus: a double-blind, placebo-controlled clinical study with an open therapeutic surveillance, *Ugeskr Laeger* 161:424-429, 1999.

45. Axelsson A, Andersson S, Gu LD: Acupuncture in the management of tinnitus: a placebo-controlled study, *Audiology* 33:351-360, 1994.

46. Zhu W, Xi G, Ju J: Effect of acupuncture and Chinese medicine treatment on dopamine level of MPTP-lesioned C57BL mice, *Chen Tzu Yen Chiy* 21:46-49, 1996.

47. Li F, Wang D, Ma X: Treatment of hiccoughs with auriculoacupuncture, *J Tradit Chin Med* 11:14-16, 1991.

48. Li X, Yi J, Qi B: Treatment of hiccoughs with auriculoacupuncture and auriculopressure: a report of 85 cases, *J Tradit Chin Med* 10:257-259, 1990.

49. Montakab H: Acupuncture and insomnia, *Forsch Komplementarmed* 1(Suppl 6):29-31, 1999.

50. Fawcett J et al: Use of alternative health therapies by people with multiple sclerosis: an exploratory study, *Holis Nurs Pract* 8:36-42, 1994.

51. Steinberger A: Specific irritability of acupuncture points as an early symptom of multiple sclerosis, *Am J Chin Med* 14:175-178, 1986.

52. Richardson P, Vincent C: Acupuncture for the treatment of pain: a review of evaluative research, *Pain* 24:15-40, 1986.

53. Carlsson C, Sjolund B: Acupuncture and subtypes of chronic pain: assessment of longterm results, *Clin J Pain* 10:290-295, 1994.

54. Branco K, Naeser M: Carpal tunnel syndrome: clinical outcome after low-level laser acupuncture, microamps transcutaneous electrical nerve stimulation, and other alternative therapies—an open protocol study, *J Altern Complement Med* 5:5-26, 1999.

55. Dichl D: Acupuncture for gastrointestinal and hepatobiliatary disorders, *J of Alternative and Complementary Medicine* 5(1):27-45, 1999.

56. Tusheng S: Acupuncture and Jianjing for treatment of achalasia of the cardia, *J Tradit Chin Med* 14:174-179, 1994.

57. Craig A, Kearns M: Results of a traditional acupuncture intervention for stuttering, *J Speech Lang Hear Res* 38:572-578, 1995.

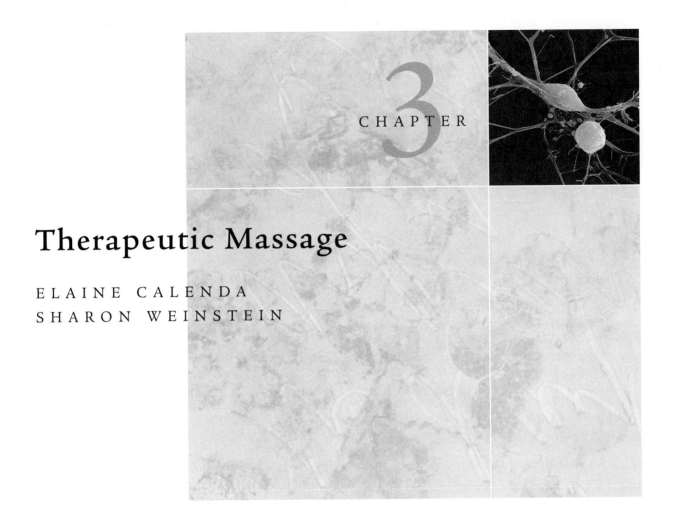

CHAPTER 3

Therapeutic Massage

ELAINE CALENDA
SHARON WEINSTEIN

HISTORY

Massage is an ancient teaching art, with written records dating back to 3000 B.C. As archeologists continue to unearth remains of ancient civilizations, more evidence of the practice of manual medicine is revealed. Mummies recently uncovered in the Gobi desert are the most perfectly preserved to date. Scientists theorize that the corpses were anointed with oils and wrapped in cloth before burial. These oils probably were used by the living to protect their skin from the elements, as well as to prevent the skin of the dead from disintegrating in the arid climate. This kind of anointing dates back thousands of years and must have relieved the daily stresses that challenged the existence of these ancient nomads.

The discovery of these mummies was significant also because they were Caucasian. What were Caucasians doing in Asia thousands of years ago? They probably traveled by horseback from Europe, forging a union with the Asian people they encountered and sharing their knowledge and culture. Natural disaster eventually buried them in the sand, like the dinosaurs, and nature's attempt to join the European and Asian cultures came to an end—until now.

In the last century, thousands of practitioners traveled from East to West and back again to study manual medicine in hopes of reestablishing these important ties. Historical accounts of the uses of manual therapies have been unearthed in all civilizations. The Egyptians, Greeks, and Romans developed forms of massage similar to techniques used today, including

27

traction, rubbing the muscles, and passively moving joints. Massage also was well documented in China, dating back to 2000 B.C. The words *Tui-na* and *Anma,* meaning "to rub" and "to press," are found in Chinese literature. *Romi-romi* is the term used by the Polynesians to describe their method of manual healing, and Hawaiians use the term *Lomi-lomi.* Although many names have been used to denote massage, the translation generally produces similar meanings, such as rubbing, pressing, lifting, beating, and stretching. Roman Olympians were prepared for events by being rubbed with oil and sand mixtures and then being beaten with the hands to relieve fatigue, much like modern boxers during a fight.

Modern methods of massage and bodywork also are known by many names. The European styles are credited to the work of Per Henrik Ling of Sweden and Dr. Johann Mezger of Holland. The Swedish system developed by Ling is still the most recognized by the Western world. Ling attempted to scientifically systematize massage as a medical therapy. He organized exercises and the basic elements of traditional massage technique according to the principles of anatomy and physiology as they were understood at the time. Thus the system became known as *Swedish massage and remedial gymnastics.*[1]

Massage combined with heat and exercise was a fundamental technique used by physical therapists during the polio epidemic. From 1920 to 1950 numerous works on the effects of massage were published, including Harvey Kellogg's *Art of Massage,*[2] which is still in publication.

As the field of physiotherapy, or physical therapy, made advances in the treatment of neurologic diseases, higher education became necessary. However, when physical therapists were required to learn neuroanatomy, neurophysiology, and kinesiology, the practice of massage decreased. During the 1950s, modern modalities, such as galvanic stimulation, automated traction, and other treatments performed by machinery emerged in physical medicine, leading to a further decline in the use of massage. Though the machines proved effective and saved time, a vital personal element of health care was lost.

In the years that followed the practice of massage was confined to health clubs and spas, and its practitioners were referred to as *masseuses* and *masseurs.* Training, offered by only a handful of schools, fell under the auspices of vocational education. One of these schools was the Swedish Institute in New York City,

founded in 1916. Its original program of 1000 hours of training, 888 of which were conducted in a hospital setting, was nearly abandoned in the 1960s. Fortunately, the Eckardt family inherited the school during the physical fitness craze of the early 1970s, and the program was resurrected. Today the school is thriving, offering a 1260-hour Associate of Occupational Studies (A.O.S.) degree program. Other schools throughout America are developing similar programs in higher education. The Boulder College of Massage Therapy in Colorado offers an A.O.S. degree along with 200-hour certification programs in specializations, such as sports and orthopedic massage, shiatsu, and energy medicine. These progressive schools are laying the groundwork for the resurgence of a profession that was once nearly extinct.

At present, state education and licensing requirements for massage therapists vary. Some states do not regulate the legitimate practice. In other states, massage therapy is considered an allied health profession, and strict guidelines exist for training, licensure, and professional practice. In Texas the Department of Public Safety certifies massage therapists. It is difficult to determine the national scope of practice, given that not all massage therapists are officially registered. The American Massage Therapy Association, the nation's largest professional organization of massage therapists, has more than 16,000 members.[3]

Providers with other credentials also may offer massage. Soft tissue manipulation may be included in chiropractic care. Osteopathic physicians, once uniformly trained in soft tissue manipulation, may or may not incorporate this therapy into their medical practices. Swedish massage technique is used in the standard "back rub" taught in nursing schools. Physical therapists employ Swedish massage, trigger point stimulation, and myofascial manipulation. Podiatrists may practice foot massage. Cosmetologists give facial, scalp, and neck massages. Many other bodywork techniques that may properly fall under the category of soft tissue manipulation, such as reflexology, Feldenkrais, Rolfing, and shiatsu (acupressure), are practiced without regulation. Mechanical massage devices are used routinely for specific medical indications, such as to prevent thrombosis of the veins of the lower extremities during convalescent care and to reduce postmastectomy lymphedema.

Despite widespread use of massage and some scientific progress in demonstrating its physiologic effects, there are few studies of its clinical application. In the 1950 American Medical Association's *Handbook of Physical Medicine and Rehabilitation,* Pemberton stated, with regard to massage, "there is probably no other measure of equal known value in the entire armamentarium of medicine which is so inadequately understood and utilized by the profession as a whole."[4] Currently, massage therapy remains largely outside the realm of standard medical practice; it is considered "unconventional" or "alternative" care. The extent to which the American public seeks such care may be quite remarkable, as evidenced by out-of-pocket dollars spent.[5]

STATUS OF THE PROFESSION

Education

The number of massage and shiatsu training programs has tripled in the last decade in part because of an increasing public demand for more natural approaches to health care. A number of regulating bodies govern the practice of massage and bodywork. Education requirements vary, tremendously in some cases, from state to state and thus from school to school. The national mean educational requirement is 500 hours of training. In the last 5 years programs providing 1000 hours of training and associate degree programs (equivalent to 2-year college programs) have become more common.

Massage therapy and bodywork schools teach communication skills, Eastern and Western bodywork modalities and philosophies, anatomy, physiology, pathophysiology, kinesiology, business practices, ethics, and first aid/cardiopulmonary resuscitation. In addition to the classroom studies, students gain experiential knowledge by participating in supervised clinical internships. Some schools and colleges require externships as well, which generally take place in hospitals, hospices, assisted care organizations, athletic departments, and corporations.

Massage therapists and bodyworkers must possess healthy interpersonal skills along with sensitivity and empathy. Furthermore, massage therapists with minimal training should not treat patients until they have received specialized training. All practitioners of massage therapy must adhere to a code of ethics and the standards of practice and must respect the scope of practice.

Credentialing

There are a number of professional massage and bodywork organizations and associations in the United States and Canada. The American Massage Therapy Association (AMTA), founded in 1943, now has more than 44,000 members. The AMTA supports its members by providing continuing education through regional and national conferences and conventions and by offering liability insurance. The National Certification Board for Therapeutic Massage and Bodywork (NCBTMG) developed the first national examination in therapeutic massage and bodywork, which is used by several states as a credentialing requirement. Furthermore, massage and bodywork schools throughout the country undergo regular site visits from organizations like the Accrediting Commission of Career Schools and Colleges of Technology (ACCSCT), the Accrediting Council for Continuing Education and Training (ACCET), the Council on Occupational Education (COE), and the Commission on Massage Therapy Accreditation (COMTA).

DEFINITIONS

Massage

From the Latin word *massa,* meaning "to knead," massage describes a means of touch that manipulates the skin and muscle against the bones with a kneading action. Massage therapy, or therapeutic massage, is described as the practice of skilled touch for the purposes of reducing pain brought about by injury, disease, or prolonged stress. It includes muscular rehabilitation and preventive care.

Myofascial Release

Myofascial release is a technique that works on the principle of thixotropy (from the Greek words *thingein* [stem: thix-], meaning "to touch," and *tropy,* meaning "a turn or change") and the sol to gel principles. *Sol* is a term used to describe the warm fluid environment of the body during activity, and *gel* denotes the negative solidifying effects of disuse. The heat generated by the hands of the practitioner during manipulation of the muscles and fascia promotes the gel to sol reaction. The technique is divided into three components:

broad-base approach, general approach, and specific approach. The system is designed to release the skin from the fascia and the fascia from the muscle to establish the optimal cellular environment and increase joint range of motion.

Muscle Energy Techniques

Muscle energy techniques fall into the category of neuromuscular therapy. These techniques are similar to Ling's Swedish gymnastics in that they require the patient's active participation through a series of controlled muscle contractions. The techniques include proprioceptive neuromuscular facilitation, pandiculation, and active isolated stretching. Other techniques are based on Sherrington's law of reciprocal inhibition and use postisometric relaxation and reciprocal inhibition.

Hydrotherapy and Cryotherapy

Hydrotherapy is a term used to describe the therapeutic use of water in the form of hot or cold applications or emersions. *Cryotherapy* refers to the use of ice or ice massage.

Zen Shiatsu

Developed by Shizuto Masunaga, zen shiatsu is one of several forms of Asian and Oriental bodywork. Shiatsu (Japanese for "finger pressure") is a Japanese bodywork modality that approaches the human form in both health and disease according to ancient Asian and Oriental beliefs and methodologies. Shiatsu directly affects the meridian systems that govern the organs of the body. The manipulation of Qi (life force) by skillful and intuitive contact of the tsubos (points) along meridians is the basis of treatment. The needs of the patient are assessed by an evaluation of the Hara* before, during, and after the session. Shiatsu is mentioned throughout this chap-

ter when a more energetic approach may be indicated, particularly if the patient cannot tolerate much movement against the body.

STATE OF KNOWLEDGE

Physiologic and Psychological Effects

Massage may be studied in terms of the physiologic basis of its effects (the psychological effects; the effects of different techniques; and the effects on tissue, organ, or system) or its application as a treatment for a specific condition. Mennell categorized the mechanisms of the effects of massage as mechanical, chemical, reflex, and psychological.[7] Pemberton and Scull summarized the physiologic effects of massage in 1944.[8] Beard reviewed the scientific literature over the 10 years before 1972.[9] What follows is a summary of the relevant findings as documented in the medical literature over the last few decades:

- Massage improves the circulation of blood and lymph.[10-17]
- Massage effectively reduces lymphedema in cancer patients.[18]
- Massage speeds recovery of fatigued muscles,[19-21] may improve joint range of motion,[22,23] induces muscle relaxation,[24-27] may be used to break down joint adhesions,[28] and improves neuromuscular function after spinal cord injury.[29]
- Serum myoglobin levels rise after massage in patients diagnosed with fibrositis.[30]
- Massage improves ventilation.[31,32]
- Massage may result in a transient increase in sympathetic nervous tone in healthy and critically ill patients.[33-35]
- Changes in skin temperature and function are observed after massage.[36,37]
- Changes in serum enzymes, urinary hormones, and cerebrospinal fluid enzymes have been noted as a result of massage.[38-40]
- Serum endorphins may transiently rise in humans after massage.[41,42]
- The neuroendocrine effects of touching the skin have been investigated in nonhuman primates and human infants; it has been demonstrated that touch is vital to growth and development.[43,44]

---

*Hara is the "vital center" that expresses the state of the entire being. The trained practitioner can "read" and assess the Hara by palpating the abdomen. The Japanese and Chinese also examine the tongue and several different pulses in the differential diagnosis. Whereas Westerners struggle to connect the body and the mind, Easterners have never taken them apart. Therefore a simple explanation of the Hara is equal to a quick description of the universe.[6]

- Rats handled early in infancy show better responses to stress and fewer aging changes in the brain.[45]
- Lowered glucocorticoid levels have been demonstrated in preterm infants after massage.[46,47]

Skin is the primary organ through which psychological nurturing occurs.[48] A person receiving massage may enter a "hypnagogic" state of deep relaxation resembling sleep. The psychological accompaniment of this effect may be the release of psychological defenses, allowing the individual to feel cared for and nurtured. Massage reduces anxiety.[49,50] Physiological changes accompanying relief of anxiety also have been shown.[51-58] Massage has been used as an adjunctive treatment for chemical dependency.[59]

NEUROLOGIC SYMPTOMS AND THEIR TREATMENT

Pain

Pain is a function of the nervous system. Nociceptive (pain) signals are transduced in specialized neural receptors, transmitted along neurons, modulated at all levels of the nervous system, and finally processed in the higher cortical centers. Pain is defined as a complex perceptual phenomenon, a dynamic product of multiple neural circuits. There is no known "pain center" in the brain.

Acute pain is the result of active tissue damage and the release of inflammatory and algesic mediators. Nociception may arise in any pain-sensitive tissue (somatic, visceral, or connective). Chronic pain states may result from a number of different processes occurring in the peripheral and central nervous tissues. Chronic pain may result from an abnormal peripheral or central pain "generator." This type of pain is generally termed *neuropathic.*

Somatic back pain syndromes may derive from musculoskeletal tissues of the spine, such as ligaments, facets, and intrinsic muscles. All of these structures, including the intervertebral disks, are considered pain sensitive. Pain arising from these areas does not appear to be caused by neurologic compromise or nerve root compression but rather by inflammatory or degenerative processes resulting from injury, disease, or normal wear and tear. Orthopedic assessment tests assist the practitioner in the formulation of a treatment plan for the individual and as a means of noting progress.

Preliminary data on the use of massage therapy in the treatment of cancer-related pain are limited.[60] Small studies of patients with nonmalignant pain have demonstrated that massage results in lowered pain intensity scores and reduced analgesic consumption.[61-65]

The term *myofascial pain syndrome* refers to that type of pain induced when muscle and soft tissue are inflamed and pressure is applied. Pressure applied directly on an active trigger point in the levator scapulae muscle often elicits pain in the midback and along the spine of the scapula. Postural and mechanical problems contribute to the formation of trigger points which are nodules of fibrous tissue that have become ischemic. Trigger points also are related to holding patterns and the pain/spasm/pain cycle. Treatment of trigger points is most successful when a combination of direct digital pressure followed by thorough passive stretching is used.

Posttraumatic pain may have several sources. Examples include pain that follows physical injury resulting from an accident, assault, poisoning, near-drowning, and recovery from surgery. Psychological trauma also must be addressed in these patients because some degree of mental anguish coincides with the cause of their pain. For treatment to be fully successful, therefore, the individual must pursue help on all levels by participating in physical therapy that includes massage and psychological, emotional, or spiritual counseling.

Headache and Migraine

A comfortable, quiet, and dimly lit environment is helpful during massage treatments, particularly when trying to combat a headache. If a migraine is already in progress, even the most gentle massage may be too disturbing. Most headaches, including migraines, are relieved or greatly reduced by massage of the cranium, cervical region, and facial structures. Shiatsu point pressure on the cranium can quell even the worst pounding headache in minutes. The relief from pain may last for hours or days, depending on the causative factors. One study of patients with chronic headache showed that massage produces analgesia accompanied by improvement in mood.[66] Massage may abort migraine headache,[67] and patients may readily accept massage therapy.[68]

There are nine studies of the efficacy of massage for pain relief, representing more than 500 patients.

These studies are best described as well-designed quasiexperimental studies, well-designed nonexperimental studies, and case series. The limitations of these studies include lack of specificity of the condition treated, limited details of the treatment applied, and lack of standardized pain assessments. As judged by the general outcome criteria of self-reported reduced pain, reduced analgesic requirement, and improved physical functioning, these studies provide weak evidence to suggest massage may be beneficial for some chronic pain conditions, including tension headache, migraine with aura, postconcussive headache, nonspecific low back pain, nonspecific neck pain, inflammatory joint pain, and regional muscle pain.

A parasympathetic response is achieved by gently stroking in rhythmic patterns. The patient can participate by breathing slowly and deeply during the session. Guided imagery is helpful for patients who find it difficult to release muscle tension. Lymphatic drainage, traction of the cervical vertebrae, and friction at the temporal and occipital regions are extremely beneficial for the reduction of muscle tension and fluid retention. Gentle vibratory percussions promote drainage of the sinuses and thus reduce pain. Massage of the abdomen, the lower extremities, and reflex points on the feet also has been effective as part of a more complete approach to the treatment of headache.

MOTOR SYMPTOMS

Weakness/Spastic Paralysis

The primary goals when treating paralysis are to enhance the patient's comfort, to assist venous return, and to inhibit spasticity through the application of rhythmic kneading, compression, and percussion.

Increased Tone
One of the symptoms of subacute paralysis is increased muscle tone. The violent muscle contraction and severe pain are controlled by muscle relaxants. Massage can be beneficial as a means of promoting circulation, but care must be taken not to disrupt brittle fibers. Medium pressure should be used to prevent a hyperreflexive reaction.

Decreased Tone
One of the symptoms of long-term paralysis is decreased muscle tone. The limbs lay flaccid, and tissue wasting is evident. Gentle massage that includes skin rolling and lifting can promote hydration of the tissues.

Weakness
Massage combined with muscle energy techniques can retard the progression of atrophy and improve function at the neuromuscular junction.

Loss of Coordination

Lack of coordination is a common symptom of nervous system disorders, especially those that affect the cerebellum or the inner ear. A systematic massage of the entire body that includes passive movements like those used in patients recovering from stroke is similarly beneficial for patients with muscular disorders.

MUSCULAR DISORDERS

Cramps

A muscle cramp is a type of sustained muscle contraction caused in part by a disturbance in blood and lymph flow. Cramps tend to occur during periods of rest. Dehydration, faulty alignment, microscopic tears, and poor walking or running habits contribute to the incidence of cramps. Fibrous formations resulting from previous injuries can interfere with normal activity and circulation.

During a severe cramp, reciprocal inhibition and intermittent percussions are generally successful as first aid pain relief. When the cramp subsides, muscular kneading promotes better circulation. As soon as it can be tolerated, friction should be applied to disrupt excessive collagen formation. Passive stretching is used to stretch the muscles, nerves, and fascia in the affected area. The stretching facilitates the optimal flow of lymph and blood through the tissues.

Multiple Sclerosis

The etiology of multiple sclerosis is unknown, but viral infection is suspected. Symptoms vary from mild loss of motor function to severe dysfunction of the lung or bladder. Complications in these organs can cause death. Symptoms arise in individuals between the ages of 20 and 40 years, and episodes may last only a few years and then spontaneously subside. For others the disease is more progressive and completely debilitating. Insults to the nervous system caused by multiple spinal traumas (i.e., whiplash) may exacerbate symptoms.

Muscular symptoms include a feeling of weakness in the extremities, especially in the lower limbs; cramping at the proximal hamstring; and ataxia.

Common symptoms of the nervous system include numbness and neuralgia, which may be severe or mild. In mild cases massage treatment can be administered for up to 1 hour and should include passive range of motion, as tolerated, to relieve stiffness. The fingertips can be used to rake the muscles from the proximal to the distal attachments and stimulate motor excitement. In addition, general massage that lifts the muscle from the bone or rolls muscle onto bone effectively improves circulation, sensation, and strength. Very light massage may frustrate patients and leave them feeling restless. The massage therapist must explore different pressures and track how much time is spent on each area to determine the best therapy for each patient. The beneficial effects of massage may last for several hours or days, depending on the stage of disease.

MOVEMENT DISORDERS

Rigidity

Lymphatic drainage therapy is beneficial for decreasing edema. Myofascial release and cross-fiber friction of the ligaments facilitate increased movement and diminish stiffness of the tissues.

Tremor

Massage and muscle energy techniques have been successful in decreasing the fatigue factor associated with tremors.

Bradykinesia

Massage and reciprocal inhibition techniques can be helpful as long as some voluntary movement is present.

Parkinson's Disease (The Shaking Palsy)

Parkinson's disease begins as a slow degeneration of the central nervous system, initially destroying the substania nigra neurons that produce the neurotransmitter dopamine. In primary parkinsonism the pigmented cells of the substania nigra that are dispersed along the putamen and caudate nucleus die off. These cells are important structures in the basal ganglia that control muscle coordination. Once these cells die, balance and muscular control diminish. The disease generally presents between the ages of 40 and 60 years, but juvenile parkinsonism can occur in younger persons. Although the exact cause is unknown, drugs that block dopamine receptors or cause metallic toxicity are contributing factors.

Treatment is directed toward decreasing rigidity. Rigidity is present whenever tremor is not. As the disease progresses, fine tremors of the head, hand, or foot develop. General massage and muscle energy techniques are beneficial.

Amyotrophic Lateral Sclerosis

Massage is indicated for relief of muscle spasms and fatigue. Gentle kneading, jostling, and stretching temporarily relieve symptoms and promote a feeling of increased strength. Shorter treatments several times per week are most productive.

CEREBROVASCULAR DISEASE

Cerebrovascular accidents (or strokes) affect hundreds of thousands of people each year. Stroke is related to cardiovascular disease, as in cerebral insufficiency, or results from hypertension or atherosclerosis. Massage therapists must have medical clearance before working with individuals who have had strokes.

Massage therapy can be extremely helpful in assisting patients with deficient circulation and can restore a sense of calm after such an episode. However, the practitioner must be aware of any blood clot or emboli before undertaking the case. Knowledge of the side effects of the patient's medications is also an important consideration, especially if analgesics are being administered. The massage therapist must take care not to massage too vigorously or apply deep pressure. The primary goals are to provide comfort, assist venous return, and reduce stress.

PERIPHERAL NEUROPATHY

Neuralgia

The nerves most commonly affected by neuralgia are the trigeminal (third cranial), sciatic, and brachial nerves. Myofascial release and nerve release techniques effectively alleviate pain but only temporarily in some cases. Neuralgia is often a symptom of muscular atrophy or hypertrophy, which may be further aggravated by unhealthy blood chemistry. Viral infection also can produce neuralgic pain, and in these cases many nerves may be affected. Myofascial release and percussion along the course of the nerve are extremely helpful. The underlying cause, however, should determine the treatment. Patients in the acute phase react differently to direct pressure. Some patients respond positively to direct pressure, but for others the effect is quite adverse and may exacerbate symptoms. This extreme difference in reaction may be a result of the individual's pain tolerance and how the nerve is situated in the soft tissues.

NERVE ENTRAPMENT

Carpal Tunnel Syndrome

Carpal tunnel syndrome is described as a compression of the median nerve where it passes through the carpal tunnel at the wrist and through the volar surface of the hand. Causative factors include narrowing of the space between the carpal bones and the transverse carpal ligament (flexor retinaculum) and laxity of the carpal ligaments resulting from repetitive motion, strain, the intrusion of certain hormones, and maintaining static wrist positions. Differential diagnostic testing is essential to rule out other causes and syndromes. To date, Tinel's and Phalen's tests continue to be reliable and widely used.

Signs and Symptoms

Impingement of the median nerve causes a sharp shooting pain that starts at the proximal wrist flexors and extends into the wrist. Pain often begins after activity and can disturb sleep. Chronic impingement causes atrophy of the thenar muscle. Practitioners must conduct physical assessment tests to determine whether other impingements exist. Some of the commonly associated areas of neurovascular compression, such as the cervical, interscalene, subclavicular, pectoral, cubital, and Luyon's canal (ulnar nerve), should be explored. These areas must be investigated in treatment because they are factors in most cases. To be successful, treatment also must address the holding patterns that can develop. The shrug mechanism is the most common type of muscular contracture and can

limit recovery if not treated. The other holding pattern is the tendency to splint the arm, which impedes axillary circulation and interferes with the healing process.

Treatment

Treatment should include general massage and lymphatic drainage techniques to prepare the patient for deeper pressure. Myofascial release and specific nerve release techniques are used in areas where nerves are compromised or compressed. Squeezing the ulna and radius at the wrist during passive movement improves ligamental tone and helps restore the carpal arch. Passive mobilization of the neck, shoulder, elbow, and wrist ensures complete coverage of related areas.

Cubital Tunnel Syndrome (Ulnar Neuropathy)

Cubital tunnel syndrome responds to the treatment outlined for carpal tunnel syndrome, but the ulnar nerve release technique must be added to the regimen. This technique involves thrusting with a "plucking" motion the flexor carpi ulnaris muscle from the medial surface of the ulna, from just below the elbow, through Luyon's Canal and the hypothenar muscle.

Radial Tunnel Syndrome (Posterior Interosseous Nerve Syndrome)

Techniques that thrust the extensor carpi radialis longus and extensor carpi radialis brevis muscles medially from the posterior surface of the radius should be performed from the proximal to the distal portions of the bone. Vigorus friction along the interosseus membrane is also helpful.

Thoracic Outlet Compression Syndrome

Thoracic outlet compression syndrome involves an interference of proper pulsation and blood flow through the subclavian artery as it passes through the interscalene triangle. This condition can result from a variety of mechanical impingements and osseous compressions. Myofascial release of neurovascular compression at the interscalene triangle, subclavicular area, and pectoralis minor muscle has been quite successful in conservative and postsurgical care.

CONVULSION/SEIZURE DISORDER

When working with seizure patients, massage therapists should be prepared to move the patient to a safe place if he or she has a seizure during a session. The patient should be helped from the massage table onto the floor, all objects should be removed from the area, and an ambulance should be called if the seizure does not subside quickly. General massage is indicated to relax muscles and decrease anxiety.

PANIC ATTACK

Panic attacks are common, but most people recover without medication or physical treatment. If panic attacks occur frequently and appear to worsen over time, additional medical attention should be sought. The panic reaction to stress usually begins at an early age and may disappear in adulthood, only to return during periods of great stress. During a panic attack the individual experiences both psychological terror and physical discomfort.

A variety of symptoms are associated with a panic attack, but a true panic attack must include several of the following symptoms: increased perspiration, feeling of terror, difficulty breathing or shortness of breath, uncontrollable yelling or screaming, tightness in the chest, dizziness, uncontrollable muscle trembling or contraction, fear of dying, fear of losing control, thoughts of going insane, "out of body" experience, and other similar sensations related to the "flight or fight" response of the autonomic nervous system.

Persons pursuing massage therapy for panic attacks can benefit from the soothing effect massage has on the nervous system. The treatment should consist of gentle strokes performed in rhythmic, predictable patterns. Deep and continuous breathing should be encouraged and monitored throughout the session.

SLEEP DISORDERS (INSOMNIA)

Sleep disorders, including difficulty sleeping and insufficient sleep, are often associated with chronic pain, anxiety, and dietary factors. Ideally the treatment should be given late in the day or even just before the patient's usual bedtime. Gentle, predictable,

and repetitive strokes can induce sleep. Massage of the face, spine, and feet has a particularly hypnotic effect on the CNS.

HICCOUGH (SINGULTUS)

Hiccoughs are involuntary repetitive spasmodic contractions of the diaphragm, followed by a sudden closure of the glottis. Low levels of carbon dioxide (CO_2) increase the incidence of hiccoughs, whereas high blood levels of CO_2 inhibit it. Deep tissue massage temporarily increases the release of CO_2 from the body tissues, often causing patients to hold their breath. Although breath holding is strongly discouraged during massage, it is the body's instinctive attempt to balance the blood gases.[2] Thus the therapist may try using flushing strokes during consistent breathing patterns and sustained pressures and squeezing techniques during breath holding.

Several other massage techniques can be used to treat hiccoughs; however, specialized training is mandatory before performing any of the following techniques:

Squeezing the cervical musculature to increase vagal stimulation

Applying judicious pressure to the phrenic nerves behind the sternoclavicular joints

Applying intermittent and sustained carotid sinus pressure

Slowly, steadily compressing the sternum as many as 12 times

Massaging the diaphragm just below the xiphoid process and continuing to just above the umbilicus in four to six passes, with each pass gradually becoming deeper

Using intermittent flipping frictions up from under the costal arch to achieve myofascial release

DYSPHAGIA (DIFFICULTY SWALLOWING)

Before undertaking any of the suggested treatments for dysphasia, the practitioner should complete specialized training beyond the standard 500 hours. General massage for relaxation should precede the medical portion of the treatment for dysphagia and should be used throughout the session to reduce anxiety. Placing the hand on the forehead as a method of distraction and tapping lightly on the sternum after a challenging technique calms patients. Facial and cranial massage is useful to reduce rigidity of the muscles. A tongue depressor is used to urge the tongue to elongate; the patient is instructed to push the tongue up against the depressor for 8 to 10 seconds and then slowly relax. This technique is beneficial for those who habitually press the tongue to the roof of the mouth, sometimes throughout the night, which eventually weakens the tongue muscle and may cause the gums to recede. The patient is then asked to protrude the tongue from the mouth as far as possible and is taught techniques for self-massage of the interoral structures. Massage may continue, using myofascial techniques that elongate the platysma. Direct digital pressure is placed against the myohyoid beneath the mandible until relaxation is perceived. The same procedure may be used to achieve a similar effect on the geniohyoid and digastric muscles. The subhyoidal structures also must be treated, but direct pressure should be applied with great caution. Using the tips of the thumb and first and second digits, the practitioner pulls and collects small portions of the skin covering the trachea as a way of gently massaging the trachea. This technique is followed with transverse mobilization of the trachea from the thyroid cartilage to just above the sternum. Slow, firm pressures on the sternum are followed through to the epigastric region, elongating the stomach and duodenum. The practitioner frequently returns to the submandibular, sublingual, and parotid glands, applying upward and circular massage to stimulate salivary secretions. This procedure facilitates swallowing as well.

URINARY INCONTINENCE (INVOLUNTARY LEAKAGE OF URINE)

Massage of the lower extremities and systemic circulatory massage indirectly stimulates urine production and urgency. When massaging a patient with bladder dysfunction (incontinence), the practitioner must place a special mattress pad under the treatment sheet on the bed or massage table. Use of this pad protects the treatment surfaces, puts the patient at ease, and helps avoid unnecessary embarrassment. If the patient has increased urinary urgency and frequency, the practitioner must ensure that a restroom or other ac-

commodation is nearby. Because massage stimulates urine output, the therapist may choose to limit the session to 30 minutes.

SPECIFIC TREATMENT FOR THE BLADDER

The bladder is situated just behind the pubic bone in the pelvis. Undue direct digital pressure on the bladder should be avoided.

The patient is in the supine position with the bolster under the knees so the abdominal muscles relax. General myofascial lifting, with the whole surfaces of the hands placed at the lower *abdomen,* should be performed during the patient's full inspiration and exhalation.

ANOSMIA (LOSS OF THE SENSE OF SMELL)

Gentle massage of the head and neck initially stimulates the flow of saliva. If there has been physical damage to the olfactory bulbs, the senses of smell and taste are not likely to return. The mood-enhancing effect of massage may relieve some of the anger and frustration related to this sensory loss. It also facilitates the body's attempt to heal the damaged tissue by containing edema. Before any work is done inside the mouth or the nostrils, the procedure and its beneficial outcomes must be fully explained to and understood by the patient. Use of a skull to demonstrate the techniques is helpful. After the procedure has been explained, the patient must be allowed to choose whether or not to submit to the treatment. Vinyl or powder-free latex gloves must always be worn by the practitioner performing oral and nasal massage.

Massage of the platysma, sternocleidomastoid, and scalene muscles and the submandibular area should precede interoral work. Gentle facial massage is relaxing and can be repeated throughout the session to reduce the patient's anxiety.

Patients who have had extensive plastic surgery may require special consideration because of scarring, altered sensitivity and tolerance, and surgical implants (plastic or dental). Open communication with the patient is essential. Describing the procedure and the expected beneficial effect is strongly advised.

Interoral procedures can be accomplished by using a tongue depressor and the digits. The tongue depressor can be inserted horizontally and turned to a vertical position as it is pressed against the inner wall of the cheek. The tissue is gently stretched laterally, with upward and downward movements. Techniques are executed on both sides, and vibration is used to "finish" the area before the tongue depressor or the practitioner's fingers are removed from the oral cavity. Digital palpation and pressure should be used to explore areas of muscle tension and to reduce the rigidity of the temporomandibular joints. Other structures involved in the restriction of movement include the pterygoid, digastric, and superior and inferior hyoid muscles. Extreme caution should be exercised at all times, and stimulation of the gag reflex should be avoided as much as possible.

THE NASAL REGION: THE NARES

The treatment generally consists of inserting a fingertip into the nare and sustaining digital pressure against the maxilla for several seconds, then repeating in the other nostril. Not all patients consent to nasal massage even though massage therapists do not penetrate past the nasal bone. In these instances an attempt is made to teach patients to perform self-massage using a cotton-tipped swab to apply gentle pressure in a circular movement just inside the nostrils. The same is true of interoral massage. It should be encouraged as part of an oral hygiene program.

PSYCHIATRIC SYMPTOMS

Massage therapists lack the education to treat patients with severe neurosis; however, practitioners who have pursued degrees in psychology may be better equipped to handle such cases. Massage therapists are trained to recognize common neuroses, such as dissociation, the physical symptoms of eating disorder, hypochondriasis, and the like. Such patients are then referred for psychological counseling. Some massage therapists work in psychiatric facilities where they serve as apprentices acting under direct supervision.

SAFETY OF MASSAGE

When performed by a trained professional, massage therapy is safe. Isolated case reports of complications of massage include sigmoid perforation, aggravation of thyrotoxicosis, communication of herpes-zoster virus, and arterial dissection. The general contraindications to massage are an open skin lesion, bleeding diathesis, fever, and hemodynamic instability; the sites of tumors and fractures should not be massaged.

References

1. Travell J: *Myofascial pain and dysfunction: the trigger point manual, upper half of the body,* vol 1, 1983, Williams & Wilkins.
2. Kellogg J: *The art of massage,* Brushton, NY, 1999, TEACH Services.
3. American Massage Therapy Association (AMTA) Houston Unit Newsletter, p 4, May 1993, The Association.
4. Pemberton R: The physiology of massage. In *American Medical Association handbook of physical medicine and rehabilitation,* Philadelphia, 1950.
5. Eisenberg DM et al: Unconventional medicine in the United States: prevalence, costs, and patterns of use, *N Engl J Med* :246-252, Jan 28, 1993.
6. MatSumoto K, Birch S: *Hara diagnosis: reflections on the sea,* Brookline, Mass, 1988, Paradigm.
7. Mennell JB: *Physical treatment,* ed 5, Philadelphia, 1945.
8. Pemberton R, Scull CW: Massage. In Glasser O, editor: *Medical physics,* Chicago, 1944, Yearbook.
9. Wood C: *Beard's massage principles and techniques,* ed 2, Philadelphia, 1974, WB Saunders.
10. Hovind N, Nielsen SL: Effect of massage on blood flow in skeletal muscle, *Scand J Rehabil Med* 6(2):74-77, 1974.
11. Hansen TI, Kristensen JH: Effect of massage, shortwave diathermy and ultrasound upon 133Xe disappearance rate from muscle and subcutaneous tissue in the human calf, *Scand J Rehabil Med* 5(4):179-182, 1973.
12. Ek AC, Gustavsson G, Lewis DH: The local skin blood flow in areas at risk for pressure sores treated with massage, *Scand J Rehabil Med* 17(2):81-86, 1985.
13. Wyper DJ, McNiven DR: Effects of some physiotherapeutic agents on skeletal muscle blood flow, *Phys Ther* 62(3):83-85, 1976.
14. Severini V, Venerando A: The physiological effects of massage on the cardiovascular system, *Europa Medicophys* 3:165-183, 1967.
15. Severini V, Venerando A: Effect on the peripheral circulation of substances producing hyperemia in combination with massage, *Europa Medicophys* 3:184-198, 1967.
16. Mortimer PS et al: The measurement of skin lymph flow by isotope clearance—reliability, reproducibility, injection dynamics, and the effect of massage, *J Invest Dermatol* 95(6):677-682, 1990.
17. Xujain S: Effect of massage and temperature on the permeability of initial lymphatics, *Lymphology* 23(1):48-50, 1990.

18. Gray B: Management of limb oedema, *Nurs Times* 83(49):39-41, 1987.
19. Cafarelli E et al: Vibratory massage and short-term recovery from muscular fatigue, *Int J Sports Med* 11(6):474-478, 1990.
20. Rodenburg JB et al: Warm-up, stretching and massage diminish harmful effects of eccentric exercise, *Int J Sports Med* 15:414-419, 1994.
21. Smith LL et al: The effects of athletic massage on delayed onset muscle soreness, creatine kinase, and neutrophil count: a preliminary report, *J Orthop Sports Phys Ther* 19(2):93-99, 1994.
22. Crosman LJ, Chateauvert SR, Weisberg J: The effects of massage to the hamstring muscle group on range of motion, *J Orthop Sports Phys Ther* 6(3):168-172, 1984.
23. Wiktorsson-Meller et al: Effects of warming up, massage and stretching on range of motion and muscle strength in the lower extremity, *Am J Sports Med* 11(4):249-252, 1983.
24. Goldberg J, Sullivan SJ, Seaborne DE: The effect of two intensities of massage on H-reflex amplitude, *Phys Ther* 72(6):449-457, 1992.
25. Morelli M, Seaborne DE, Sullivan SJ: H-reflex modulation during manual muscle massage of human triceps surae, *Arch Phys Med Rehabil* 72(11):915-919, 1991.
26. Sullivan SJ et al: Effects of massage on alpha motoneuron excitability, *Phys Ther* 71(8):555-560, 1991.
27. Matheson DW et al: Relaxation measured by EMG as a function of vibrotactile stimulation, *Biofeedback Self Regul* 3:285, 1976.
28. Hammer WI: The use of transverse friction massage in the management of chronic bursitis of the hip or shoulder, *J Manipulative Physiol Ther* 16:107-111, 1993.
29. Goldberg J et al: The effect of therapeutic massage on H-reflex amplitude in persons with a spinal cord injury, *Phys Ther* 74(8):728-737, 1994.
30. Danneskold-Samse B et al: Regional muscle tension and pain ("fibrositis"): effect on massage on myoglobin in plasma, *Scand J Rehabil Med* 15(1):17-20, 1983.
31. Chopra SK et al: Effects of hydration and physical therapy on tracheal transport velocity, *Ann Rev Resp Dis* 115(6):1009-1014, 1977.
32. Petersen LN et al: Foot zone therapy and bronchial asthma—a controlled clinical trial, *Clin Trial* 154(30):2065-2068, 1992.
33. Naliboff BD, Tachiki KH: Autonomic and skeletal muscle responses to nonelectrical cutaneous stimulation, *Percept Mot Skills* 72(2):575-584, 1991.
34. Tyler DO et al: Effects of a 1-minute back rub on mixed venous oxygen saturation and heart rate in critically ill patients, *Heart Lung* 19(5Pt2):562-565, 1990.
35. Barr JS, Taslitz N: The influence of back massage on autonomic functions, *Phys Ther* 50(12):1679-1691, 1970.
36. Olson B: Effects of massage for prevention of pressure ulcers, *Decubious* (4):32-37, 1989.
37. Bogdan FL et al: Epithelial mesenchymal interrelations at the skin level, *Morphol Embryol* 28(1):3-9, 1982.
38. Jian H, Yang Z: Influence of finger pressing massage on cAMP and cGMP in the cerebrospinal fluid in prolapsed intervertebral disc, *Chin J Mod Dev Tradit Med* 10(1):27-29, 1990.
39. Arkko P, Pakarinen AJ, Kari-Koskinen O: Effects of whole body massage on serum protein, electrolyte and hormone concentrations, enzyme activities and hematologic parameters, *Int J Sports Med* 4(4):265-267, 1983.
40. Bork K, Karling GW, Faust G: Serum enzyme levels after "whole body massage," *Arch Dermatol Forsch* 240:342-348, 1971.
41. Kaada B, Tosteinbo O: Increase of plasma beta-endorphins in connective tissue massage, *Gen Pharmacol* 20(4):487-489, 1989.
42. Day JA, Mason RR, Chesrown SE: Effect of massage on serum level of b-endorphin and B-lipotropin in healthy adults, *Phys Ther* 67(67):926-930, 1987.
43. Wheeden A et al: Massage effects on cocaine-exposed preterm neonates, *Dev Behav Pediatr* 14(5):318-322, 1993.
44. Scafidi F et al: Factors that predict which preterm infants benefit most from massage therapy, *Dev Behav Pediatr* 14(3):176-180, 1993.
45. Meaney MJ et al: Effect of neonatal handling on age-related impairments associated with the hippocampus, *Science* 239:766-768, 1987.
46. Acolet D et al: Changes in plasma cortisol and catecholamine concentrations in response to massage in preterm infants, *Arch Dis Child* 68(Suppl 1):29-31, 1993.
47. Rice RD: Premature infants respond to sensory stimulation, APA Monitor, 6(11):8-9, 1975.
48. Montagu A: *Touching: the human significance of the skin,* New York, 1978, Harper & Row.
49. Fraser J, Kerr JR: Psychophysiological effects of back massage on elderly institutionalized patients, *J Adv Nurs* 18(2):238-245, 1993.
50. McKechnie AA et al: Anxiety states: a preliminary report on the value of connective tissue massage, *J Psychosom Res* 27(2):125, 1983.
51. Longworth JC: Psychophysiological effects of slow stroke back massage in normotensive females, *ANS* 4(4):44-61, 1982.
52. Ho KH et al: Reduction of post-operative swelling by a placebo effect, *J Psychosom Res* 32(2):197-205, 1988.
53. Zanolla R et al: Evaluation of the results of three different methods of postmastectomy lymphedema treatment, *J Surg Oncol* 26:210-213, 1984.
54. Meek SS: Effects of slow stroke back massage on relaxation, *Image J Nurs Sch* 25(1):17-21, 1993.

55. Platania SA et al: Relaxation therapy reduces anxiety in child and adolescent psychiatric patients, *Acta Paedopsychiatr* 55(2):115-120, 1992.
56. Field T et al: Massage reduces anxiety in child and adolescent psychiatric patients, *J Am Acad Child Adolesc Psychiatry* 31(1):125-131, 1992.
57. Bumpus S et al: The effect of caring touch on the psychological well-being of selected residents of a long-term care facility, *SC Nurs* 8(1):26-27, 1993.
58. Groer M et al: Measures of salivary secretory immunoglobulin A and state anxiety after a nursing back rub, *Appl Nurs Res* 7(1):2-6, 1994.
59. Milkman H, Metcalf D, Reed P: An innovative approach to methadone detoxification, *Int J Addict* 15(8): 1199-1211.
60. Weinrich SP, Weinrich MC: The effect of massage on pain in cancer patients, *Appl Nurs Res* 3(4):140-145, 1990.
61. Konrad K et al: Controlled trial of balneotherapy in treatment of low back pain, *Ann Rheum Dis* 51(6):820-822, 1992.
62. Koes BW et al: Randomised clinical trial of manipulative therapy and physiotherapy for persistent back and neck complaints: results of one year follow up, *Br Med J* 304(6827):601-605, 1992.
63. Koes BW et al: The effectiveness of manual therapy, physiotherapy, and treatment by the general practitioner for nonspecific back and neck complaints, *Spine* 17(1):28-35, 1992.
64. Marin I et al: Postoperative pain after thoracotomy: a study of 116 patients, *Rev Mal Respir* 8(2):213-218, 1991.
65. Jensen OK, Nielsen FF, Vosmar L: An open study comparing manual therapy with the use of cold packs in the treatment of post-traumatic headache, *Cephalalgia* 10(5):2241-2250, 1990.
66. Puustjarvi K, Airaksinen O, Pontmen PJ: The effects of massage in patients with chronic tension headache, *Acupunct Electrother Res* 15(2):159-162, 1990.
67. Lipton SA: Prevention of classic migraine headache by digra massage of the superficial temporal arteries during visual aura, *Ann Neurol* 19(5):515-516, 1986.
68. Engel JM et al: Value of physical therapy from the viewpoint of the patient: results of a questionnaire, *Z Rheumatol* 46(5):250-255, 1987.
69. Travell J: *Myofascial pain and dysfunction: The trigger point manual, the lower extremities,* vol 2, 1983, Williams & Wilkins.

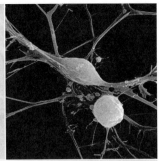

CHAPTER 4
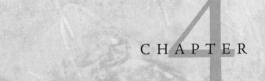

Herbs and Dietary Supplements for Neurologic Problems

ADRIANE FUGH-BERMAN
JERRY COTT

A telephone survey of 2055 English-speaking adults found that 42.1% had used at least one alternative therapy in 1997.[1] Herbal and dietary supplement use is extremely common. In the same survey, of adults who regularly take prescription medication, 18.4% reported the concurrent use of at least one herbal product or high-dose vitamin. Only 39.8% of those surveyed who saw an unconventional practitioner discussed their experience with their physician. Herbal use is particularly popular; however, interaction problems may arise when herbs are combined with other drugs.[2] The pharmacologic effect of herbs is not surprising; many of the drugs in clinical practice are derived from plants. Lidocaine and novocaine are derived from the coca plant (*Erythroxylum coca*), opioids from the poppy (*Papaver somniferum*), and aspirin from meadowsweet (*Spirea ulmaria*) whence the "spir" part of

its name derives. Digoxin comes from foxglove (*Digitalis lanata*), and warfarin is a derivative of dicoumarin found in sweet clover (*Melilotus officinalis*).

According to an industry survey, sales of single herbal preparations in natural products stores grew by 4.7% from December 1997 to December 1998 to a total of $412.9 million. Sales of these preparations in grocery, drug, and mass merchandise stores increased an average of 50% to reach a total of $286.5 million.[3] The majority of these sales represent botanical products that are purported to have therapeutic actions on the brain and central nervous system; however, vitamins, amino acids, and other dietary supplements are also popular.[4] Some data indicate that dietary supplements may hold promise for the treatment of several neurologic problems. Following are summaries of selected trials in this area.

MIGRAINES

Magnesium

Magnesium, which is essential for all reactions using adenosine triphosphate (ATP), is the fourth most common cation in the body. Magnesium deficiency is quite common. According to estimates of magnesium intake based on the Third National Health and Nutrition Examination Survey (1988 to 1994), magnesium intake was lower than the recommended daily allowance (RDA) in males and females between 12 and 60 years of age in all racial and ethnic groups, except non-Hispanic white males.[5] The incidence of deficiency is even higher among hospitalized patients; 65% of those in intensive care, up to 12% in general wards, and 30% of hospitalized alcoholics have hypomagnesemia.[6]

Several trials have indicated that magnesium supplementation may be a helpful treatment for migraine. Although the exact mechanism of magnesium's effects is unclear, it may interrupt the process at the vasoconstriction stage by interacting with serotonin and N-methyl-D-aspartate receptors, nitrous oxide synthesis and release, other migraine-related receptors, and neurotransmitters.[7]

Some studies suggest that patients with low ionized serum magnesium levels are more likely to respond to initial magnesium treatment than those with normal serum magnesium levels. In one study of 40 patients with acute migraine attacks,[8] 35 had at least 50% pain relief within 15 minutes after iv infusion of 1g magnesium sulfate. In 18 of 21 patients whose pain relief lasted at least 24 hours, serum magnesium levels initially were below normal (0.54 to 0.65 mmol/l).

Excess magnesium causes diarrhea, an effect that was seen in every trial in which these data were collected. Inorganic forms of magnesium (magnesium oxide, magnesium chloride) may be more likely to cause diarrhea than organic forms (magnesium citrate, magnesium aspartate), but diarrhea can result from administration of any preparation.

Prevention

In another multicenter, randomized, double-blind study, 81 adult migraine patients, with a mean migraine frequency rate of 3.6 per month, received either oral magnesium (24 mmol trimagnesium dicitrate,

equivalent to 600 mg/day) or placebo for 12 weeks.[9] In the last 4 weeks, frequency of migraine attacks was reduced by 41.6% in the magnesium group compared with 15.8% in the placebo group. The number of days with migraine was also significantly decreased in the magnesium group. No significant changes were noted in the duration or intensity of migraine attacks nor in drug consumption during an attack. Diarrhea was reported in 18.6% and gastric irritation in 4.7% of patients receiving magnesium.

A third placebo-controlled, double-blind trial of 69 subjects with migraine showed no benefit of magnesium supplementation over placebo.[10] Patients were treated for 12 weeks with either magnesium (10 mmol twice daily, equivalent to 500 mg/day) or placebo. Endpoints were reduction of intensity or duration of migraines by at least 50%. This trial, originally designed to enroll 150 patients, was stopped after the interim analysis of 69 patients showed no benefit for the patients receiving magnesium. An equivalent number of patients in each group (28.6% of those receiving magnesium and 29.4% of those receiving placebo) experienced a reduction in the intensity or duration of migraines. Mild adverse effects were experienced by 45.7% of those receiving magnesium and 23.5% of those on placebo. Diarrhea or soft stool was the most common complaint in the magnesium group. It is extremely unusual to stop a trial at interim analysis in such a case; usually trials are brought to an end only when there is such a large difference in either benefit or risk between the groups that it is deemed unethical to continue in the face of what is known at that point.

Prevention of Menstrual Migraine

In a randomized trial of 24 women with menstrual migraine,[11] the women received 360 mg/day of magnesium pyrrolidine carboxylic acid or placebo from the fifteenth day of their cycles until menses. During this phase of the trial, both groups reported a reduction in pain total index (a measure of both frequency and intensity of attacks). Women receiving magnesium had significantly less pain than the placebo group, and the number of days with headache decreased only in the magnesium group. After 2 months, the trial became an open-label trial in which magnesium was given to all patients for an additional 2 months. Significant decreases in pain total index were seen in both groups between the second and fourth months. Although subjects in this trial apparently were not routinely asked about side effects, two (one from each group) of four dropouts were attributed to side effects.

Riboflavin

Riboflavin is a B vitamin that is a necessary enzyme cofactor in the production of ATP. Although gross riboflavin deficiency is rare in Western countries, marginal deficiency is relatively common, especially among older adults and adolescents.

A randomized, placebo-controlled, 3-month trial of 55 patients with migraine found that 400 mg of riboflavin taken daily was superior to placebo in reducing attack frequency and headache days.[12] The proportions of patients who improved by at least 50% were 59% in the riboflavin group and 15% in the placebo group. Two of three patients who reported mild adverse effects of polyuria and diarrhea were in the treatment group. The dose of riboflavin used in this trial was quite high—about 300 times higher than the RDA. However, riboflavin is extraordinarily benign.

Feverfew (Tanacetum parthenium)

Several trials indicate that feverfew (Figure 4-1) may be effective in migraine prophylaxis. A small double-blind study tested feverfew withdrawal in regular users. Seventeen patients who regularly used feverfew to prevent migraine were randomized and given either freeze-dried feverfew powder or placebo.[13] Those who received placebo had a significant increase in the frequency and severity of headache, nausea, and vomiting, whereas those in the feverfew group showed no change in the incidence of migraines. In a larger crossover study, 72 migraine patients were given either one capsule of dried feverfew or placebo daily for 4 months, and then received the other therapy for 4 more months.[14] Patients receiving feverfew had fewer migraines, less severe attacks, and less emesis, although the duration of migraines that did occur remained the same. A review of five randomized, controlled trials of feverfew in migraine prevention found that although the majority of studies favored feverfew over placebo, the clinical effectiveness had not yet been proven beyond a reasonable doubt.[15]

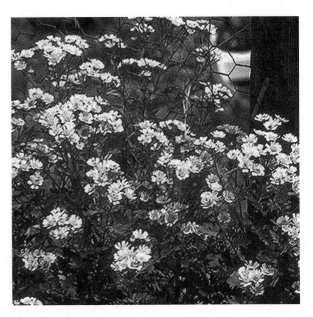

Figure 4-1 Feverfew. (From Blake: Alternative Remedies CD-ROM, St. Louis, Mosby, 1998.)

CARPAL TUNNEL SYNDROME AND VITAMIN B₆

A review of the literature on vitamin B_6 and carpal tunnel syndrome[16] concluded that there is no convincing evidence that vitamin B_6 is adequate as the sole treatment of carpal tunnel syndrome but that it may be useful as adjunctive treatment to conservative therapy.

NEUROPATHY AND CHILI PEPPERS (CAPSICUM SPECIES)

Topical capsaicin may be useful in the treatment of diabetic neuropathy. One placebo-controlled study of 252 patients with diabetic neuropathy[17] found that 69.5% of patients treated with 0.075% capsaicin cream reported less pain compared with 53.4% of those on placebo. A controlled trial of 32 elderly patients with postherpetic neuralgia[18] found that almost 80% of the capsaicin-treated patients experienced some relief from their pain after 6 weeks.

A 4-week, placebo-controlled study found that, of 45 patients treated with 0.025% topical capsaicin or placebo for fibromyalgia,[19] those receiving capsaicin reported less tenderness at their trigger points. There was no significant difference in visual analog pain scores. A significant increase in grip strength in the capsaicin group was also noted.

A recent review found that topical capsaicin is effective for treatment of psoriasis, pruritus, and cluster headache and can help relieve itching and pain in patients with postmastectomy pain syndrome, symptoms of oral mucositis and cutaneous allergy, loin pain in those with hematuria syndrome, neck pain, amputation stump pain, and cutaneous pain associated with skin tumor. It may also be helpful for patients with neural dysfunction, including detrusor hyperreflexia and reflex sympathetic dystrophy.[20] The authors note that the placebo-controlled studies did not use a "burning" placebo and that this may have compromised blinding.

ANXIETY AND KAVA (PIPER METHYSTICUM)

A psychoactive member of the pepper family, the root of the Kava plant is used widely in Polynesia, Micronesia, and Melanesia as a ceremonial, tranquilizing beverage. It is used medicinally for anxiety and insomnia in Europe and the United States and is approved and registered in Germany for the treatment of "states of nervous anxiety, tension, and agitation" in doses of 60 to 120 mg of kavalactones for up to 3 months' duration.[21,22] Kava appears to be a safe herbal remedy for short-term relief of stress and anxiety. Several placebo-controlled trials have shown significant anxiolytic activity.

In a randomized, double-blind, placebo-controlled trial, 58 patients with various anxiety and neurotic disorders as diagnosed per the International Classification of Diseases received 70 mg of kavalactones or placebo three times daily for 4 weeks. Compared with those receiving placebo, the kava group demonstrated a significant reduction in anxiety as assessed by the Hamilton anxiety scale.[23] In a second randomized, double-blind, placebo-controlled multicenter study, 101 outpatients with anxiety disorders (agoraphobia, specific phobia, generalized anxiety disorder, or adjustment disorder with anxiety) as diagnosed per the third, revised *Diagnostic and Statistical Manual of Mental Disorders* (DSM-IIIR) were treated with a kava extract for 24 weeks.[24] The results showed significant reductions in anxiety as assessed by the Hamilton anxiety scale in the kava group. Several other controlled, double-blind trials on kava extracts or the isolated compound DL-kawain have been published in the

German literature.[21] In one placebo-controlled trial, 58 patients with anxiety received 210 mg kava or placebo daily for 1 month.[25] Compared with those receiving placebo, those receiving kava had significantly greater reductions in Hamilton Anxiety Scale (HAMA) scores, with improvements beginning within 1 week.

INSOMNIA AND VALERIAN (VALERIANA OFFICINALIS)

Valerian is a popular European medicine used for its mild sedative and tranquilizing properties. The drug's central nervous system activity is largely ascribed to the valepotriates and sesquiterpene constituents of the volatile oils. The German Commission E recommends 2 to 3 g of the dried root one or more times a day for "restlessness and nervous disturbance of sleep."[22] Valerian is a popular sleep remedy, despite the fact that few clinical trials on sleep or other parameters can be found in the literature.[26]

One study of 128 subjects compared the effects of an herbal preparation containing *Valeriana officinalis* as one of a mixture of herbs, a valerian-only extract (400 mg), and placebo in subjects with varying sleep difficulties.[27] Both valerian preparations produced a significant decrease in subjectively evaluated sleep latency scores and improved sleep quality. In another study, 27 patients with sleep difficulties received two pills that they took on consecutive nights.[28] Both pills contained hops and lemon balm, but one pill contained only 4 mg of valerian and the other contained a full 400-mg dose. Seventy-eight percent of the subjects preferred full-dose valerian, 15% preferred the low-dose valerian, and 7% had no preference.

DIABETIC NEUROPATHY

Vitamin E

In a randomized double-blind trial, 21 subjects with type II diabetes were assigned to receive either 900 mg vitamin E or placebo for 6 months.[29] Nerve conduction, measured by electrophysiologic tests, was the main outcome measure. Nerve conduction velocity in the median motor nerve fibers and tibial motor nerve distal latency improved significantly in the treatment group. The other 10 electrophysiologic parameters did not change.

Thiamine

In Tanzania, diabetic peripheral neuropathy is associated with thiamine deficiency. In a controlled study comparing thiamine (25 mg/day) and pyridoxine (50 mg/day) therapy with placebo (containing 1 mg each thiamine and pyridoxine), significant improvement in pain, numbness, parasthesia, and impairment of sensation in the legs was noted in the treatment group. The severity of signs of peripheral neuropathy decreased in 48.9% of the treatment group compared with 11.4% in the placebo group.[30]

Alpha-Lipoic Acid

In the study on alpha-lipoic acid use in patients with diabetic neuropathy, 328 patients with type II diabetes and symptomatic peripheral neuropathy were randomly selected to receive placebo or three different doses of intravenous alpha-lipoic acid (1200, 600, or 100 mg) over 3 weeks.[31] Total symptom scores were significantly reduced in groups receiving 600 or 1200 mg alpha-lipoic acid.

RESTLESS LEGS SYNDROME AND IRON

Iron deficiency, whether or not it results in anemia, appears to be an important factor in the development of restless legs syndrome (RLS) in older adults. In one study, 26 of 27 patients with severe RLS had ferritin levels less than or equal to 50 mcg/ml.[32] Lower ferritin levels correlated with greater severity of RLS symptoms and decreased sleep efficiency. In another study, serum ferritin levels were lower in 18 RLS patients (33 mcg/l) compared with 18 controls (59 mcg/l).[33] Lower serum ferritin levels correlated significantly with greater RLS severity, and improvement was noted after iron repletion.[33]

DISORDERS OF TASTE AND SMELL AND ZINC

Acute, severe zinc deficiency can cause hypogeusia (decreased sensitivity of taste). Two uncontrolled studies of patients with renal disease and hypogeusia found that taking 50 mg of elemental zinc a day significantly improved the patients' sense of taste. A single-blind study of 103 patients with idiopathic hypogeusia found that 100 mg zinc taken daily resulted in improvements.[34] However, an earlier double-blind crossover trial evaluated zinc (100 mg/day) in the treatment of hypogeusia in 106 patients with taste and smell dysfunction (of various etiologies) and found no effect.[35] It has been pointed out that these patients were on a variety of medications that may have affected the results.[34]

Zinc may be effective only in those individuals with low serum zinc levels. The 98 patients in one placebo-controlled trial were divided into four groups, depending on the etiology of their hypogeusia (zinc deficient, idiopathic, drug induced, and other). All received zinc gluconate (22.6 mg tid) for 4 months. Zinc benefited the zinc deficient and idiopathic groups but not the groups of patients whose conditions were drug induced or fell into other categories.[36]

In another study, patients with sensorineural olfactory disorder were treated with usual therapy, zinc sulfate, or both. Of patients with posttraumatic olfactory disorder, those in the zinc sulfate groups had significantly higher improvement rates than did those in the group that received the usual therapy.[37] For patients with disorders of postviral or unknown etiology, there were no significant differences in improvement among the three groups. In this study, pretreatment serum zinc concentrations were not significantly related to improvement rates.

Treatment for head and neck cancer often causes taste alterations. In a randomized, placebo-controlled study, 18 patients receiving external radiation to the head and neck were randomly chosen to receive zinc sulfate (45 mg tid) or placebo at the onset of taste alterations. The treatment was continued for 1 month after the radiation therapy had ended.[38] Patients treated with placebo experienced a greater loss in taste acuity during radiation treatment compared with those treated with zinc. In addition, those treated with zinc had a faster recovery of taste acuity than those receiving placebo.

DEMENTIA

Ginkgo (Ginkgo biloba)

The ginkgo tree is one of the oldest living species (Figure 4-2). The use of ginkgo has greatly increased since 1994 when Germany approved a standardized form of leaf extract (EGb 761) for the treatment of

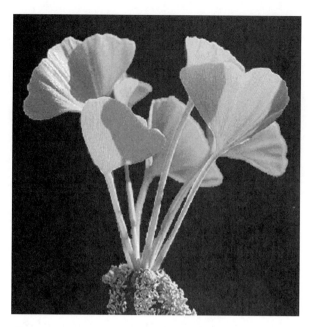

Figure 4-2 Leaves of the ginko biloba tree. (From Blake: Alternative Remedies CD-ROM, St. Louis, Mosby, 1998.)

dementia. The standardized extract contains 22% to 27% flavonoid glycosides (including quercitin and kaempferol and their glycosides) and 5% to 7% terpene lactones (consisting of 2.8% to 3.4% ginkgolides A, B, and C and 2.6% to 3.3% bilobalide).[21]

A randomized, double-blind, placebo-controlled trial of 309 patients with Alzheimer's disease or multi-infarct dementia found that patients who received EGb 761 (120 mg/day) scored higher on the Alzheimer's Disease Assessment Scale-Cognition sub-scale (ADAS-Cog).[39] After 1 year of treatment, 29% of patients receiving ginkgo showed at least a 4-point improvement on the test compared with 14% of those receiving placebo. Although improvement was not apparent according to the Clinician's Global Impression of Change, beneficial treatment effects were apparent to caregivers as measured by the Geriatric Evaluation by Relative's Rating Instrument.

A randomized, double-blind, placebo-controlled 6-month trial of 216 patients with Alzheimer's disease or multi-infarct dementia found that patients who were given 240 mg/day of a standardized ginkgo extract had significant improvements in memory, attention, psychopathology, and behavior compared with patients who were given placebo.[40]

In another randomized, double-blind, controlled trial of 40 Alzheimer's patients, those given 240 mg/day

of standardized ginkgo extract for 3 months showed significant improvements in memory, attention, and psychopathology compared with those given placebo after 1 month.[41]

Ginkgo may also have beneficial effects on memory impairment that is not related to Alzheimer's disease. In one double-blind study, 31 outpatients who were older than 50 years and had mild to moderate memory impairment were given 120 mg of ginkgo a day. As evidenced by tests of digit copying and speed of response in a classification task, researchers noted a beneficial effect of the therapy; however, no improvement was noted on other tests of cognitive function at 12 and 14 weeks.[42]

A recent meta-analysis by Oken et al.[43] attempted a summary of all published studies in which ginkgo was given for dementia. Only randomized, double-blind, and placebo-controlled trials were included in the analysis. The patients were sufficiently characterized with a diagnosis of Alzheimer's disease by either DSM-III or National Institute of Neurological Disorders and Stroke-Alzheimer's Disease and Related Disorders Association criteria, or the article contained enough clinical detail for the reviewer to assign diagnosis. The trials excluded patients with depression or other neurologic disease and excluded use of other central nervous system–active medications. They included studies that used standardized ginkgo extract at any dose, had at least one outcome measure that was an objective assessment of cognitive function, and contained sufficient statistical information for meta-analysis. Although more than 50 articles were identified, the majority did not meet inclusion criteria because of a lack of clear diagnoses of dementia and Alzheimer's. Of the four studies that met all inclusion criteria, there were 212 subjects in each of the placebo and ginkgo treatment groups. Overall, there was a significant effect ($P<0.0001$) that translated into a 3% difference in ADAS-Cog scores. The authors concluded that 3 to 6 months of treatment with 120 to 240 mg ginkgo has a small but significant effect on objective measures of cognition in patients with Alzheimer's disease.

Choline and Lecithin

Neurochemical studies of Alzheimer's disease suggest a cholinergic deficit. Therefore there is a theoretical basis for treatments that enhance cholinergic activity. However, choline and lecithin supplementation has generally been ineffective.[44] Providing precursors of acetylcholine in this way is probably insufficient to boost cholinergic activity to a meaningful level; inhibiting the catabolism of acetylcholine with cholinesterase inhibitors is the current therapeutic alternative.

Phosphatidylserine

Although numerous studies, such as that by Cenacchi et al.[45] support a therapeutic effect of bovine-derived phosphatidylserine given to patients with dementia, these products are no longer available because of concerns about mad cow disease. Currently-available preparations are derived from soy, but no studies involving these new products have been published in the scientific literature.

COGNITION AND VITAMIN STATUS

Subclinical malnutrition may play a small role in the reduced cognitive function in some older individuals. Folic acid deficiency, one of the most common nutritional deficiencies worldwide, has often been associated with cognitive disorders.[46] In elderly patients the incidence of deficiency is particularly marked and may be as high as 90%.[47]

Folate and vitamin B_{12} are required for the methylation of homocysteine to methionine and for the synthesis of S-adenosylmethionine. S-adenosylmethionine plays a role in numerous methylation reactions involving proteins, phospholipids, deoxyribo-nucleic acid, and neurotransmitter metabolism. Folate and vitamin B_{12} deficiency may cause similar neurologic and psychiatric disturbances, including depression, dementia, and a demyelinating myelopathy.[46,48] Supplementation may be beneficial in deficient individuals, but more definitive studies are ongoing.[49]

In an observational study, Goodwin et al.[50] evaluated the association between nutritional status and cognitive function in 260 noninstitutionalized men and women older than 60 years who had no known physical illnesses and were taking no medications. Nutritional status was evaluated based on 3-day food records and the participants' blood levels of specific nutrients. Cognitive status was evaluated by the Halstead-Reitan categories test (a nonverbal test of abstract thinking ability) and by the Wechsler memory test. Subjects with low blood levels of vitamins C or B_{12} had lower scores on both tests. Subjects with low levels of riboflavin or folic acid had lower scores on the categories test. These differences remained significant after controlling for age, gender, level of income, and amount of education.

TINNITUS AND GINKGO

Ten ear, nose, and throat specialists conducted a multicenter, double-blind, placebo-controlled study involving 103 outpatients with tinnitus over a 3-month treatment period.[51] Patients, all of whom had had tinnitus for 1 year or less, were either given ginkgo or placebo. The groups were comparable in regard to duration and intensity of symptoms and degree of impairment. Comparison of the groups revealed that a significantly greater percentage of the ginkgo-treated group experienced either resolution of symptoms or distinct improvement, regardless of the duration of symptoms, whether the tinnitus was bilateral or unilateral, and whether symptoms were constant or intermittent.

Holgers et al.[52] designed a study in two parts. The first part was an open-label trial ($n = 80$) of ginkgo (Seredrin, approximately 30 mg/day) in subjects with persistent, severe tinnitus; the second part was a double-blind, placebo-controlled study ($n = 20$). Of 21 patients who reported that the ginkgo supplementation had a positive effect on their tinnitus in the open study, 20 were included in a double-blind, placebo-controlled crossover study ($n = 20$). Seven patients preferred ginkgo, seven preferred placebo, and six had no preference. This study failed to confirm that consumption of ginkgo affects tinnitus; however, the dose was much smaller than that used in other studies.

Coles[53] published a brief correspondence describing an open trial of 23 tinnitus patients given 120 mg EGb 761 for 12 weeks. Eighteen of these patients had experienced tinnitus for more than 3 years; the median duration was 8 1/2 years. Two patients did not complete the trial. Of the 21 who remained, 11 reported no change, 2 reported that severity of symptoms was lessened, and 2 reported that severity was slightly lessened. A total of 5 patients reported that their tinnitus was worse. There were no changes in audiometric measurements. The author concluded that ginkgo was ineffective in this trial.

Von Wedel et al.[54] reported a placebo-controlled trial in 155 patients with chronic tinnitus of at least 6 months' duration and one or more failed treatments. The design included four groups treated with one of the following: an investigational technique involving soft-laser irradiation of the cochlea, a ginkgo extract given intravenously, both treatments combined, or a double-placebo control. Nineteen patients in the combined therapy group dropped out; six of them did so because the tinnitus worsened. The dropouts were not included in the analyses. Treatment consisted of 12 sessions 2 to 3 days apart. Patients in the combined-therapy group received 5 ml ginkgo intravenously (concentration or formulation was not provided) before the laser treatment. There were no differences among the groups, including the group receiving placebo. The conclusion of the authors was that neither treatment was effective.

In conclusion, there are mixed data on the efficacy of ginkgo in patients with tinnitus. There is a possibility that ginkgo may have significant potential only in patients with recent-onset tinnitus, such as those in the Meyer study.[51]

ACUTE HEARING LOSS AND GINKGO

In a therapeutic trial of acute cochlear deafness, Dubreuil[55] reported a randomized, double-blind, controlled study of EGb 761 (320 mg/day) and a standard alpha-blocker (nicergoline) given for 30 days. The rationale for the study was that ischemia may underlie acute cochlear deafness, regardless of the triggering event. Nine patients in each group, which were comparable in pathology at the beginning of the study, completed the treatment. From the tenth day until the end of the trial, improvement appeared to be greater in the ginkgo group, although both groups improved. The audiometric gain in the ginkgo group ranged between 6 and 15 decibels greater than in the nicergoline group; however, no formal statistical analysis was performed.

Hoffmann et al.[56] reported the results of a randomized comparison study on 80 patients with idiopathic sudden hearing loss (of no more than 10 days' duration). EGb 761 (175 mg intravenous infusion plus 160 mg oral/day) was compared with the vasodi-

lating, antiserotonergic drug, naftidrofuryl (400 mg intravenous infusion plus 400 mg oral/day). The primary outcome was audiometric data, measured as relative hearing gain. After 1 week of observation, 40% of the patients in each group showed a complete remission of hearing loss. This percentage is consistent with expected rates of spontaneous recovery. After 2 and 3 weeks of observation, there was no difference between groups in relative hearing gain, yet there was a borderline benefit of ginkgo ($p = 0.06$) over naftidrofuryl. Although no side effects were attributed to ginkgo, some patients in the naftidrofuryl group developed orthostatic blood pressure changes, headache, or sleep disturbances.

VERTIGO AND GINKGO

Haguenauer and others [57] enrolled 70 patients with vertigo of recent onset and undetermined origin in a multicenter study. In a randomized, double-blind trial conducted over a 3-month period, subjects received either 160 mg/day EGb 761 or a placebo. The effectiveness of ginkgo on the intensity, frequency, and duration of the disorder was statistically and clinically significant by the end of the first month. After 3 months, 47% of the ginkgo-treated patients were asymptomatic, compared with 18% of those who received placebo.

NEUROLOGIC AND PSYCHIATRIC DISORDERS AND OMEGA-3 FATTY ACIDS

Omega-3 polyunsaturated fatty acids are long-chain, polyunsaturated fatty acids (PUFAs) found in plant and marine sources. These essential fatty acids, particularly docosahexaenoic acid (DHA), are necessary for proper membrane function and may be etiologic factors in depression, bipolar disorder, schizophrenia, and other psychiatric and neurologic disorders.[58-62] The Western diet contains considerably high amounts of omega-6 fatty acids and lesser amounts of omega-3 fatty acids. Fish oil is high in PUFAs, DHA, and eicosapentaenoic acid. Neuronal membranes contain high concentrations of DHA, as well as arachidonic acid (AA). Both of these acids are crucial components of the phospholipid bilayer; each comprises approximately 25% of the phospholipid content.[63] Neurotransmitter receptors lie embedded in the matrix of this membrane, and their three-dimensional conformation is dependent on the fatty acids that give structure to the membrane.[64]

Biochemical studies have shown that high doses of omega-3 fatty acids lead to the incorporation of these compounds into the neuronal membrane phospholipids, which are crucial for cell signaling.[65,66] Phosphatidylinositol-associated second messenger activity is also suppressed.[67] Dietary supplementation with large amounts of omega-3 fatty acids is related to a general dampening of signal transduction pathways associated with phosphatidylinositol, AA, and other systems.[66,68]

Some have suggested an association between depression and multiple sclerosis.[69] This relationship is based on a meta-analysis of published studies and is consistent with essential fatty acid depletion, especially DHA and to a lesser extent AA, in both white matter[70-72] and plasma.[73] DHA is apparently completely absent in the adipose tissue of patients with multiple sclerosis.[74]

The relationship between abnormal concentrations of omega-3 and omega-6 fatty acids and the occurrence of other neurologic disorders, such as Huntington's disease and tardive dyskinesia, also has been noted.[75,76]

SUMMARY

Limited but intriguing evidence is available regarding the possible benefits of certain alternative therapies as sole or adjunctive therapy in patients with some neurologic disorders. Magnesium (for migraine), ginkgo (for various vascular disorders), and essential fatty acids (for psychiatric and neurologic disorders) seem particularly promising. Naturally, more research must be done in these areas. Although these treatments may be considered alternative or complementary, testing them would be quite straightforward. These treatments would all lend themselves to standard clinical trial design, and perhaps testing them should be considered a higher priority.

References

1. Eisenberg DM et al: Trends in alternative medicine use in the United States, 1990-1997: results of a follow-up national survey, *JAMA* 280:1569-1575, 1998.

2. Fugh-Berman A: Herb-drug interactions, *Lancet* 355:134-138, 2000.

3. Johnson BA: Herbal formulas show market growth, *HerbalGram* 46:57, 1999.

4. Fugh-Berman A, Cott J: Dietary supplements and natural products as psychotherapeutic agents, *Psychosom Med* 61:712-728, 1999.

5. Shils ME: Magnesium. In Shils ME et al: *Modern nutrition in health and disease*, ed 9, Baltimore, 1999, Williams & Wilkins.

6. Weisinger JR, Bellorin-Font E: Magnesium and phosphorus, *Lancet* 352:391-396, 1998.

7. Mauskop A, Altura BM: Role of magnesium in the pathogenesis and treatment of migraines, *Clin Neurosci* 5:24-27, 1998.

8. Mauskop A et al: Intravenous magnesium sulfate relieves migraine attacks in patients with low serum ionized magnesium levels: a pilot study, *Clin Sci* 89:633-636, 1995.

9. Peikert A, Wilimzig C, Kohne-Volland R: Prophylaxis of migraine with oral magnesium: results from a prospective, multi-center, placebo-controlled and double-blind randomized study, *Cephalalgia* 16:257-263, 1996.

10. Pfaffenrath V et al: Magnesium in the prophylaxis of migraine—a double-blind, placebo-controlled study, *Cephalalgia* 16:436-440, 1996.

11. Facchinetti F et al: Magnesium prophylaxis of menstrual migraine: effects of intracellular magnesium, *Headache* 31:298-301, 1991.

12. Schoenen J, Jacquy J, Lenaerts M: Effectiveness of high-dose riboflavin in migraine prophylaxis, *Neurology* 50:466-470, 1998.

13. Johnson ES et al: Efficacy of feverfew as prophylactic treatment of migraine, *BMJ* 291:569-573, 1985.

14. Murphy JJ, Heptinsall S, Mitchell JRA: Randomized double-blind placebo-controlled trial of feverfew in migraine prevention, *Lancet* Vol. ii 189-192, 1988.

15. Vogler BK, Pittler MH, Ernst E: Feverfew as a preventive treatment for migraine: a systematic review, *Cephalalgia* 18:704-708, 1998.

16. Jacobson MD, Plancher KD, Kleinman WB: Vitamin B_6 (Pyridoxine) therapy for carpal tunnel syndrome, *Hand Clin* 12:253-257, 1996.

17. Capsaicin Study Group: Treatment of painful diabetic neuropathy with topical capsaicin, *Arch Intern Med* 151:2225-2229, 1991.

18. Watson CPN, Evans RJ, Watt VR: Post-herpetic neuralgia and topical capsaicin, *Pain* 33:333-340, 1988.

19. McCarty DJ et al: Treatment of pain due to fibromyalgia with topical capsaicin: a pilot study, *Semin Arthritis Rheum* 23 (suppl 3):41-47, 1994.

20. Hautkappe M et al: Review of the effectiveness of capsaicin for painful cutaneous disorders and neural dysfunction, *Clin J Pain* 14:97-106, 1998.

21. Schultz V, Hansel R, Tyler VE: *Rational phytotherapy: a physician's guide to herbal medicine,* ed 3, Berlin, 1998, Springer-Verlag.

22. Blumenthal M, Goldberg A, Brinckmann J: *Herbal medicine: expanded commission E monographs,* Newton, MA, 2000, Integrative Medicine Communications.

23. Lehmann E, Kinzler E, Friedemann J: Efficacy of a special Kava extract (Piper methysticum) in patients with states of anxiety, tension, and excitedness of non-mental origin—a double-blind placebo-controlled study of four weeks treatment, *Phytomedicine* III:113-119, 1996.

24. Volz HP, Kieser M: Kava-kava extract WS 1490 versus placebo in anxiety disorders—a randomized placebo-controlled 25-week outpatient trial, *Pharmacopsychiatry* 30:1-5, 1997.

25. Kinzler E, Kromer J, Lehmann E: Wirksamkeit eines Kava-Spezial-Extraktes bei Patienten mit Angst-, Spannungs- und Erregungszustanden nicht-psychotischer Genese, *Arzneimittelforschung* 41:584-588, 1991.

26. Wagner J, Wagner ML, Hening WA: Beyond benzodiazepines: alternative pharmacologic agents for the treatment of insomnia, *Ann Pharmacother* 32:680-691, 1998.

27. Leathwood PD et al: Aqueous extract of valerian root improves sleep quality in man, *Pharmacol Biochem Behav* 17:65-71, 1982.

28. Lindahl O, Lindwall L: Double blind study of a valerian preparation, *Pharmacol Biochem Behav* 32:1065-1066, 1989.

29. Tutuncu NB, Bayraktar M, Varli K: Reversal of defective nerve conduction with vitamin E supplementation in type 2 diabetes: a preliminary study, *Diabetes Care* 21:1915-1918, 1998.

30. Abbas ZG, Swai AB: Evaluation of the efficacy of thiamine and pyridoxine in the treatment of symptomatic diabetic peripheral neuropathy, *East Afr Med J* 74:803-808, 1997.

31. Ziegler D, Gries FA: Alpha-lipoic acid in the treatment of diabetic peripheral and cardiac autonomic neuropathy, *Diabetes* 46 (Suppl 2):S62-66, 1997.

32. Sun ER et al: Iron and the restless legs syndrome, *Sleep* 21:371-377, 1998.

33. O'Keefe ST, Gavin K, Lavan JN: Iron status and restless legs syndrome in the elderly, *Age Ageing* 23:200-203, 1994.

34. Heyneman CA: Zinc deficiency and taste disorders, *Ann Pharmacother* 30:186-187, 1996.

35. Henkin RI et al: A double-blind study of the effects of zinc sulfate on taste and smell function, *Am J Med Sci* 272:285-299, 1976.

36. Yoshida S, Endo S, Tomita H: A double-blind study of the therapeutic effect of zinc gluconate on taste disorder, *Auris Nasus Larynx* 18:153-161, 1991.

37. Aiba T et al: Effect of zinc sulfate on sensorineural olfactory disorder, *Acta Otolaryngol Suppl (Stockh)* 538:202-204, 1998.

38. Ripamonti C et al: A randomized, controlled clinical trial to evaluate the effects of zinc sulfate on cancer patients with taste alterations caused by head and neck irradiation, *Cancer* 82:1938-1945, 1998.

39. Le Bars P et al: A placebo-controlled, double-blind, randomized trial of an extract of Ginkgo biloba for dementia, *JAMA* 278:1327-1332, 1997.

40. Kanowski S et al: Proof of efficacy of the Ginkgo biloba special extract EGb 761 in outpatients suffering from mild to moderate primary degenerative dementia of the Alzheimer type or multi-infarct dementia, *Pharmacopsychiatry* 29:47-56, 1996.

41. Hofferberth B: The efficacy of Egb 761 in patients with senile dementia of the Alzheimer type, a double-blind, placebo-controlled study on different levels of investigation, *Human Psychopharmacology* 9:215-222, 1994.

42. Rai GS, Shovlin C, Wesnes KA: A double-blind, placebo-controlled study of Ginkgo biloba extract ("Tanakan') in elderly outpatients with mild to moderate memory impairment, *Curr Med Res Opin* 12:350-355, 1991.

43. Oken BS, Storzbach DM, Kaye JA: The efficacy of Ginkgo biloba on cognitive function in Alzheimer disease, *Arch Neurol* 55:1409-1415, 1998.

44. Rathmann KL, Conner CS: Alzheimer's disease: clinical features, pathogenesis, and treatment, *Drug Intelligence and Clinical Pharmacy* 18:684-691, 1984.

45. Cenacchi T et al: Cognitive decline in the elderly: a double-blind, placebo-controlled multicenter study on efficacy of phosphatidylserine administration, *Aging (Milano)* 5:123-133, 1993.

46. Reynolds EH: Interrelationships between the neurology of folate and vitamin B_{12} deficiency. In *Folic acid in neurology, psychiatry, and internal medicine,* New York, 1979, Raven.

47. Thornton WE, Thornton BP: Geriatric mental function and serum folate: a review and survey, *South Med J* 70:919-922, 1977.

48. Hutto BR: Folate and cobalamin in psychiatric illness, *Compr Psychiatry* 38:305-314, 1997.

49. Nilsson-Ehle H: Age-related changes in cobalamin (vitamin B_{12}) handling: implications for therapy, *Drugs Aging* 12:277-292, 1998.

50. Goodwin JS, Goodwin JM, Garry PJ: Association between nutritional status and cognitive functioning in a healthy elderly population, *JAMA* 249:2917-2922, 1983.

51. Meyer B: Multicenter randomized double-blind drug vs. placebo study of the treatment of tinnitus with Ginkgo biloba extract, *Presse Med* 15:1562-1564, 1986.

52. Holgers KM, Axelsson A, Pringle I: Ginkgo biloba extract for the treatment of tinnitus, *Audiology* 33:85-92, 1994.

53. Coles R: Trial of an extract of Ginkgo biloba (EGB) for tinnitus and hearing loss, *Clin Otolaryngol* 13:501-502, 1988.

54. Von Wedel et al: Soft-laser/Ginkgo therapy in chronic tinnitus: a placebo-controlled study, *Adv Otorhinolaryngol* 49:105-108, 1995.

55. Dubreuil C: Therapeutic trial in acute cochlear deafness: a comparative study of Ginkgo biloba extract and nicergoline, *Presse Med* 15:1559-1561, 1986.

56. Hoffmann F et al: Ginkgo extract EGb 761 (Tebonin)/HAES versus naftidrofuryl (Dusodril)/HAES: a randomized study of therapy of sudden deafness, *Laryngorhinootologie* 73:149-52, 1994.

57. Haguenauer JP: Treatment of equilibrium disorders with Ginkgo biloba extract: a multicenter double-blind drug vs. placebo study, *Presse Med* 15:1569-1572, 1986.

58. Hibbeln JR, Palmer JW, Davis JM: Are disturbances in lipid-protein interactions by phospholipase-A2 a predisposing factor in affective illness? *Biol Psychiatry* 25:945-961, 1989.

59. Hibbeln JR, Salem N Jr: Dietary polyunsaturated fatty acids and depression: when cholesterol does not satisfy, *Am J Clin Nutr* 62:1-9, 1995.

60. Hillbrand M, Spitz RT, VandenBos GR: Investigating the role of lipids in mood, aggression, and schizophrenia, *Psychiatr Serv* 48: 875-876, 1997.

61. Hibbeln JR et al: Do plasma polyunsaturates predict hostility and depression? *World Rev Nutr Diet* 82:175-186, 1997.

62. Stoll AL et al: Omega-3 fatty acids in bipolar disorder: a preliminary double-blind, placebo-controlled trial, *Arch Gen Psychiatry* 56:407-412, 1999.

63. Mahadik SP, Evans DR: Essential fatty acids in the treatment of schizophrenia, *Drugs of Today* 33:5-17, 1997.

64. Mitchell DC et al: Why is docosahexaenoic acid essential for nervous system function? *Biochem Soc Trans* 26:365-370, 1998.

65. Medini L et al: Diets rich in n-9, n-6 and n-3 fatty acids differentially affect the generation of inositol phosphates and of thromboxane by stimulated platelets, in the rabbit, *Biochem Pharmacol* 39:129-133, 1990.

66. Sperling RI et al: Dietary omega-3 polyunsaturated fatty acids inhibit phosphoinositide formation and chemotaxis in neutrophils, *J Clin Invest* 91:651-660, 1993.

67. Kinsella JE: Lipids, membrane receptors, and enzymes: effects of dietary fatty acids, *Journal of Parenteral and Enteral Nutrition* 14:200s-217s, 1990.

68. Tappia PS et al: The influence of membrane fluidity, TNF receptor binding, cAMP production and GTPase activity on macrophage cytokine production in rats fed a variety of fat diets, *Mol Cell Biochem* 166:135-143, 1997.

69. Schubert DS, Foliart RH: Increased depression in multiple sclerosis patients. A meta-analysis. *Psychosomatics* 34(2):124-30, 1993.

70. Gerstl B et al: Alterations in myelin fatty acids and plasmalogans in multiple sclerosis, *Ann NY Acad Sci* 122:405-407, 1965.

71. Kishimoto Y et al: Gangliosides and glycerophospholipids in multiple sclerosis white matter, *Arch Neurol* 16:41-54, 1967.

72. Wilson R, Tocher DR: Lipid and fatty acid composition is altered in plaque tissue from multiple sclerosis brain compared with normal brain white matter, *Lipids* 26:9-15, 1991.

73. Cunnane SC, Ho SY, Dore-Duffy P, Ells KR, Horrobin DF: Essential fatty acid and lipid profiles in plasma and erythrocytes in patients with multiple sclerosis. *Am J Clin Nutr* 50(4):801-6, 1989.

74. Nightingale S, Woo E, Smith AD, French JM, Gale MM, Sinclair HM, Bates D, Shaw DA: Red blood cell and adipose tissue fatty acids in mild inactive multiple sclerosis. *Acta Neurol Scand* 82(1):43-50, 1990.

75. Nilsson A et al: Essential fatty acids and abnormal involuntary movements in the general male population: a study of men born in 1933, *Prostaglandins Leukot Essent Fatty Acids* 55:83-87, 1996.

76. Vaddadi KS: Essential fatty acids and movement disorders. In Peet M, Glen I, Horrobin DF, editors: *Phospholipid spectrum disorder in psychiatry,* Carnforth, UK, 1999, Marius.

Additional Readings

Kleijnen J, Knipschild P: Ginkgo biloba for cerebral insufficiency, *Br J Clin Pharmacol* 34:352-358, 1992.

Kleijnen J, Knipschild P: Ginkgo biloba, *Lancet* 340:1136-1139, 1992.

Linde K et al: St. John's wort for depression—an overview and meta-analysis of randomized clinical trials, *BMJ* 313:253-258, 1996.

Reynolds EH, Carney MW, Toone BK: Methylation and mood, *Lancet* 2:196-198, 1984.

Schoenen J, Lenaerts M, Bastings E: High-dose riboflavin as a prophylactic treatment of migraine: results of an open pilot study, *Cephalalgia* 14:328-329, 1994.

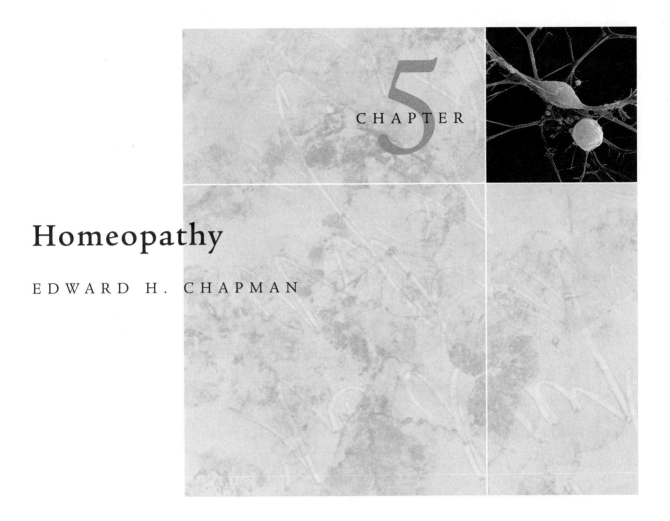

CHAPTER 5

Homeopathy

EDWARD H. CHAPMAN

The current interest in complementary and alternative medicine (CAM) by the general public and the medical professions has arisen largely from the public's frustration with the limits of conventional (allopathic) medical care.[1] Preliminary data from randomized clinical controlled trials support the efficacy of a homeopathic approach in a number of conditions for which people seek the services of a neurologist. The conditions include mild traumatic brain injury,[2] stroke,[3] Parkinson's disease,[4] vertigo,[5,6] fibromyalgia,[7] and migraine headache.[8] This chapter presents the principles of homeopathic medicine, the controversy surrounding homeopathy, a summary of the evidence supporting the activity of homeopathic medicines, a review of the clinical research relevant to neurology,

and a detailed clinical example to illustrate the homeopathic experience.

The 3.8 million Americans[9] who use homeopathy do so when conventional therapy has had no benefit or limited benefit; the risk of conventional therapies is high, such as during pregnancy; side effects limit the usefulness of conventional medications; or reduction of the dose of allopathic medications in the management of chronic conditions would be beneficial.[10] Homeopathy treats the whole person, mobilizing the individual's innate healing capacity. The following discussion covers the fundamental principles of homeopathy and the research supporting the efficacy of homeopathy. The nature of homeopathic assessment, as well as the individualized nature of the homeopathic prescription, is discussed in detail.

WHAT IS HOMEOPATHY AND WHAT IS A HOMEOPATHIC MEDICINE?

Homeopathy is a system of therapy based on the observation that a medicine can cure the same symptoms in an ill person that it produces in healthy subjects. Known as the *principle or law of similars,* this correlation was articulated 200 years ago in Germany by Samuel Hahnemann.[11] A homeopathic medicine is one that acts according to this principle. Homeopaths understand symptoms to be clues to the workings of the body's homeostatic mechanisms. These symptoms arise spontaneously within a person during illness, or they can be induced by administering medicines during experiments called *homeopathic drug provings* (HDPs).[12-14] Homeopathic therapy depends on finding a homeopathic preparation with "proving symptoms" that are similar to the symptoms of the ill person. The homeopathic medicine's capacity to stimulate this innate healing capacity of an organism is person specific rather than diagnosis specific.

The homeopathic approach differs from other therapeutic systems that are in use. Other mechanisms include suppressing bodily responses or external disease agents (allopathy); replacing substances the body is failing to produce (replacement therapy [e.g. hormones, insulin]); or using attenuated doses of disease-producing agents to sensitize or desensitize the immune system (isopathy or treatment by the same substance [e.g. immunization or allergy desensitization]). Homeopathy relies on the inherent capacity of an organism to heal itself. The homeopathic prescription provides the information the organism needs to bring about a healthier functional state using the minimum dose necessary.

Homeopathic medicines are prepared by a process of serially agitated dilution (SAD).[15] The extreme dilution of these preparations (10^{-6} to $10^{-200,000}$ molar) makes skeptics attribute any action of homeopathic medicines to the placebo effect. Based on the concept of Avogadro's number (10^{23} molecules/gram molecular weight), dilutions below 10^{-23} molar have an infinitesimal probability of containing any molecules of the original substance. However, high-quality research has clearly established that the action of homeopathic medicines cannot be explained by the placebo effect.[54]

The preparation of homeopathic medicines follows a rigorous process. For soluble substances, one part of the original plant, mineral, or animal substance is diluted in water or lactose on a decimal [(X) 1 part: 10 parts], centesimal [(C) 1:100] scale, or 50 millesimal scale [(LM) 1:50,000]. Each dilution is then vigorously agitated. Insoluble substances are serially diluted in lactose and ground in a mortar and pestle at each dilution. This process is referred to as *trituration*. Eventually the lactose triturate is dissolved in water, and the process of potentization is continued using the liquid medium. Homeopaths call these dilutions *potencies*, referring to the extent of dilution, or *remedies*. Low-potency remedies range from 2X (0.01 molar) to 30C; high potencies range from 200X ($10^{-200 \text{ molar}}$) to 100,000C ($10^{-200,000}$ molar). Therefore a 30C potency is diluted 1:99 30 times, which is equivalent to a 10^{-60} molar dilution of the original substance. A 12X is diluted 1:10 12 times and has a dilution of 10^{-12} molar.

The major controversy surrounding homeopathy is how medicines containing no molecules of the substance from which they are derived can affect biologic systems. Very few data are available about the mechanism of action of homeopathic preparations, but the most favored hypothesis involves memory of water, which is discussed later in the chapter. Homeopaths' experience suggests that homeopathic medicines act as catalysts. Catalysts are small quantities of a substance that initiate a reaction. Although a specific mechanism of action has yet to be determined, the biologic effects of a homeopathic medicine are inferred from the subjective and objective changes that occur after the administration of a dose.

The effect of pheromones is a good example of the catalytic action of low dilutions in biologic systems. Pheromones are molecules secreted by animals. A single molecule of a pheromone can stimulate specific receptors in animals of the same species, resulting in dramatic changes in the physiology and behavior of the animal. In much the same way, the homeopathic dose initiates an effect on the homeostatic forces inherent to the organism. Once the desired response is initiated, the body itself completes the healing process. The dose needs to be repeated only when there is evidence that further stimulation is required. Consequently the medicine may not need to be repeated for months after a curative response to a single dose. The dose of homeopathic medicines is so minute that the risk of serious side effects or allergic reactions is minimal. Relative to conventional drugs, the cost of homeopathic medicines—pennies a dose—is also miminal.

Homeopathic pharmacopoeias standardize the preparation of homeopathic drugs, so the clinician knows what is safe to prescribe. The *Homeopathic Pharmacopoeia of the United States*[16] *(HPUS)* was one of two pharmacopoeias grandfathered into the 1938 Food and Drug Act that created the U.S. Food and Drug Administration (FDA). With few exceptions, these homeopathic medicines are classified and sold as over-the-counter (OTC) medicines.[17] They are regulated by the FDA in consultation with the Homeopathic Pharmacopoeia Convention of the United States (HPCUS), the body responsible for setting standards for the manufacture of homeopathic medicines. Because of their safety, these medicines are available to the general public for self-prescribing. Exceptions to the OTC categorization include medicines in low potency (1X to 3X) containing molecules that could have toxic effects; medicines formulated for injectable use; and medicines made from pathogenic organisms or labeled for indications not considered OTC. These types of medicines require a prescription.

Two general categories of homeopathic medicines exist: single remedies and combination, or complex, remedies. The FDA's labeling requirements poorly reflect the therapeutic reality of the medicines. Currently, single remedies, those constituted from only one medicine, are inaccurately labeled with common indications, such as headache and runny nose. Labeling a single homeopathic medicine with a single indication is misleading. Prescribing single remedies accurately depends on assessing the totality of the patient's mental, emotional, and physical symptoms and then prescribing the one medicine or simillimum (the most similar remedy) that best matches that totality. Prescribing single homeopathic medicines is a skill that requires specific training and a basic understanding of homeopathic principles.

Classic homeopathy is based on a specific homeopathic principle—the law of similars. Prescribing single homeopathic medicines using this principle employs data that are patient specific rather than disease specific. The minimum dose principle of homeopathy refers to the use of medicines produced by SAD. SADs can also be prescribed using a pathologic approach. The process of prescribing single or complex (combination) medicines using diagnosis-specific, allopathic indications is referred to as *homeopathic pathologic prescribing.* A number of schools of homeopathic prescribing use the following pathologic approaches: homotoxicology, anthroposophy, biochemistry according to Schussler, spagyric therapy according to Krauss/Zimpel, gemmotherapy, lithotherapy, and resonance homeopathy. Some clinicians use data from the readout of skin-resistance biofeedback instruments, pendulums, or muscle testing to choose the appropriate medicine.

Drug products supplied by homeopathic manufacturers are referred to as *homeopathic,* reflecting the specific manufacturing process of SAD. Because the FDA regulates homeopathic medicines, most of which are sold OTC, the word *homeopathic* is sometimes loosely applied to herbal or nutritional OTC products also. Though the majority of homeopathic medicines are derived from plants, they are not the same as herbal medicines. The two types of medicines are often confused by the public because the common names on the label are sometimes the same (e.g., chamomilla or hypericum). However, herbal preparations are loose, compressed, or encapsulated plant materials or alcohol tinctures of the fresh plant. In addition, herbs cannot use the *HPUS* designation on their labels. Most herbal preparations, like vitamins and minerals, are regulated as dietary supplements.

Complex homeopathic remedies combine several low potency (usually 1X to 12C, but occasionally 200C) remedies commonly prescribed as single remedies for specific pathologic conditions. One assumption behind homeopathic pathologic prescribing is that one of the ingredients in a complex formulation will act as a simillimum for the patient. Such medicines act like a shotgun shell as opposed to a carefully aimed single bullet. It is also possible that the ingredients will act synergistically as do many conventional OTC pharmacologic products. Their design allows prescription for allopathic, diagnosis-based indications, such as premenstrual syndrome (PMS), sinusitis, allergy, cramps, and vertigo. Although labeling suggests efficacy for specific conditions, unfortunately, few manufacturers have tested the products for the specific indications for which they are sold. Prescribing homeopathic preparations based on diagnostic or syndrome-based indications facilitates their use for the public and for allopathic-trained health care providers who approach health and healing from this perspective. Consequently, complex homeopathic products represent 80% to 90% of the sales of homeopathic medicines in the United States.[18]

SOCIAL AND HISTORIC CONTEXT

Samuel Hahnemann (Figure 5-1) first articulated the law of similars (*similia similibus curantur*, or like curelike) in Germany in 1796. His observations and a discussion of this system of healing were described in the *Organon of the Medical Art,* first published in 1810.[11] Six editions were printed during his career, the last in 1842, the year before his death. He also discovered that by serially diluting and succussing (vigorously shaking) medicines, the therapeutic efficacy could be increased and the adverse effects of larger doses could be limited. He also developed protocols, which he called *homeopathic drug provings,* for testing new medicines on healthy volunteers. Minute doses of medicines were given in repeated doses to healthy subjects. The symptoms that provers developed were recorded and published between 1825 and 1833 in the six volumes of *Materia Medica Pura.*[19] Through these experiments he increased the number of homeopathic medicinal agents used in the treatment of chronic and acute illness.

Hahnemann gathered around him a committed group of disciples who assisted him and continued his work. Some of these students emigrated to the Americas where homeopathy flourished during the rest of the nineteenth century.[20] In 1825, Hans Graham was the first homeopathic physician to come from Europe to the United States. He was soon followed by Constantine Hering, who in 1844 helped found the American Institute of Homeopathy (AIH) to promote the practice of homeopathy by the medical profession. The AIH, which was founded 2 years before the American Medical Association (AMA), is the oldest national medical organization in the United States. It continues to represent the interests of homeopathic medical professionals to the government and the public.

During this century, many of the original provings of Hahnemann and his disciples have been repeated and new substances have been tested. These provings, together with toxicologic and clinical observations of the medicines' effects, have been compiled in materia medicas. The most famous of these are The *Encyclopedia of Pure Materia Medica*[21] and *Guiding Symptoms,*[22] both of which are used daily by modern homeopaths. James Tyler Kent authored *Lectures on Homeopathic Philosophy,*[23] *Lectures on Homeopathic Materia Medica,*[24] and *Kent's General Repertory.*[25] Kent's *Repertory,* an index of the symptoms contained in various materia medica, has changed the way homeopathy is practiced. Kent's format for indexing the vast amount of information contained in the published materia medica forms the basis for computerized repertorization systems that have been developed in the past 20 years.

A contentious relationship existed between homeopathic and allopathic physicians during the nineteenth century. The code of ethics of the AMA was designed to prevent medical practitioners from associating with homeopaths, as is shown in the following excerpt:

No one can be a regular practitioner, or fit associate in consultation, whose practice is based on an exclusive dogma, to the rejection of the accumulated experience of the profession, and of the aids actually furnished by anatomy, physiology, pathology, and organic chemistry.[26]

By 1900, 8% of American physicians had incorporated homeopathy into their practices and 20 homeopathic medical schools had been established,[27] including Boston University, Hahnemann Medical School, New York Medical, and University of Michigan. With the changes toward more scientifically-based medical education catalyzed by the Flexner Report in 1910 and the discovery of antimicrobials,

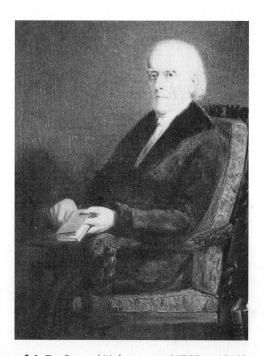

Figure 5-1 Dr. Samuel Hahnemann (1755 to 1843).

however, the popularity of homeopathy suffered a steep decline. Homeopathic schools either closed or, to maintain government funding and attract students, converted to the modern scientific paradigm espoused by the authors of the Flexner Report. The last Hahnemann Medical School issued its final homeopathic diploma in 1950.

Although the demise of homeopathic medical schools left a vacuum in homeopathic education and research in the United States, homeopathy continued to flourish in Europe, India, Mexico, Argentina, and Brazil. In the United States only a handful of medical doctors were practicing homeopathy by the 1960s. However, the presence of an enthusiastic lay population, which continued self-prescribing OTC homeopathic products, kept the homeopathic manufacturing pharmacies alive.

The 1970s saw a resurgence of interest in homeopathy by medical professionals and the public. It was prompted by a widespread feeling that the current medical model had limitations, including high costs, adverse side effects, lack of a personal relationship with the provider, and ineffectiveness in treating many chronic and acute conditions. Since the 1980s, sales of homeopathic medicines, 85% of which were sold OTC,[17] increased an average of 20% a year.

Currently an estimated 500 homeopathic physicians practice in the United States, and many more physicians use homeopathy on a limited basis.[28] Extrapolation of data reported in December 1998 in the *Journal of the American Medical Association*[9] suggested that 8.5 million Americans used homeopathic medicines. Of these, about 16.5% actually visited homeopaths in 1997.

Even during the 1950s and 1960s when interest in homeopathy waned, combination prescribing kept homeopathy alive in the United States. At the same time, homeopathy was being investigated and used worldwide. In the late 1940s, German physician Reinhold Voll developed a method for choosing homeopathic medicines based on changes elicited in the galvanic skin resistance measured at various acupuncture and skin points. Voll's homeotherapeutic method, which is practiced worldwide, is known as *electro-acupuncture according to Voll*[29] (EAV). In the United States, proponents of this method have been instrumental in passing homeopathic licensing laws in Arizona and Nevada.

Interest among health care professionals has spurred an increase in homeopathic educational opportunities. To date the only federally accredited, undergraduate professional educational program teaching homeopathy is the naturopathic college at Bastyr University in Seattle. In addition to four naturopathic colleges, homeopathic education is available through postgraduate programs that educate existing medical professionals in the use of homeopathic medicines. Basic courses consist of 30 to 100 classroom hours. To achieve specialty status requires a minimum of 500 hours supplemented with preceptorships to develop homeopathic competence. Educational programs in homeopathy are accredited by the Council for Homeopathic Education.

Board certification is available for medical (MD) and osteopathic physicians (DO) through the American Board of Homeotherapeutics (ABHT) founded in 1959, for naturopaths by the Homeopathic Association of Naturopathic Physicians, and for other licensed and unlicensed homeopathic professionals by the Council for Homeopathic Certification. An entry-level Primary Homeopathic Certification for physicians, nurse practitioners (RN-C), and physician assistants (PA-C) was inaugurated in 1997 by the ABHT. Nevada, Arizona, and Connecticut have separate homeopathic licensure for physicians; other health care professionals, including medical physicians, osteopathic physicians, nurse practitioners, physician assistants, acupuncturists (LicAc), and chiropractors (DC), practice within their conventional licenses.

As part of a growing movement founded in the British tradition of "professional homeopathy," homeopathy is being practiced as a separate profession with certification but without licensure. Represented by the North American Society of Homeopaths (NASH) and arguing that homeopathy is safe in the hands of non–medically trained professionals, this group is petitioning for legislative change that would allow homeopathic practice outside of medical licensing statutes.

HOMEOPATHIC PHILOSOPHY

Three principles are at the heart of homeopathic philosophy: the law of similars, the minimum dose, and the totality of symptoms. In addition, the entire phenomenon of homeopathy is rooted in vitalism. Vitalism assumes an inherent, active, responsive intelligence that guides the workings of the living organism. Unlike the molecules and organs of the body, this vital force[30] cannot be directly measured. It is known only by its influence on the functions and expressions of the organism through the language of physical signs, symptoms, emotion, and thought. When homeopaths refer to treating the totality of a person, they are referring indirectly to a unique constellation that is greater than the sum of the individual symptoms and signs of illness. These expressions are specific to each individual; no two individuals with the same illness present with the same manifestations. These vitalistic roots give homeopathy its capacity to transcend the mind-body dualism of the biomolecular model and allow homeopathy to connect with the ambiguous and complex world of systemic thinking and chaos theory.[31]

Homeopaths determine the capacity of each substance to heal through four sources: toxicologic data, information gained in HDPs, clinical research, and accumulated clinical experience. Pharmacologic and toxicologic data and information gathered from using substances in indigenous healing systems often provide an initial idea of the scope of a medicine. To further elucidate the scope of the drug, provings are done to test a single substance. The substance is administered in a homeopathic potency, usually 30C, to a group of healthy volunteers called *provers* in a controlled clinical trial. The medicine expresses itself in the symptoms these subjects develop. The provers' symptoms are recorded to form the basic symptom picture of the medicine. Symptoms that are repeatedly cured by the homeopathic medicine in clinical cases are added to the symptom picture to complete the full expression of each remedy. These data sets are combined into remedy pictures that are unique for each medicine in the same way that each person is unique. Traditionally the symptoms have been recorded in homeopathic materia medica and organized using an anatomic structure, such as mind, vertigo, head, or eye. Symptom records are also available in other formats in computer databases.

Knowledge of the totality of symptoms for both a medicinal substance and a patient can be approached but never understood completely. The homeopath seeks to understand what is to be healed in a patient, that is, the dysfunction that is represented by the noxious sensation and disturbances of feeling and thinking that cause suffering to the patient. Recognizing how patients' symptom clusters correspond to known pathogenetic patterns of medicines allows the law of similars to be applied. For instance, in the medicine belladonna the active ingredient is atropine. Atropine

produces signs of cholinergic stimulation, including lack of perspiration, flushing and hot skin, dilation of the pupils, and visual hallucinations. Provers also develop throbbing pains, usually right sided, that come on suddenly and are associated with agitation. These symptoms and signs are similar to those that a young healthy child with an acute febrile illness or an adult with a cluster headache might experience. Therefore belladonna is frequently prescribed in these cases. A detailed clinical example of the prescribing process is presented later in this chapter.

How homeopathic medicines act in the body is unknown. Hahnemann believed that the medicine creates an artificial disease[11] in the patient, which is similar in character to the natural disease. As the body mobilizes its defenses to eliminate the artificial disease, the natural disease is also extinguished because of its resemblance to the medicinal disease. This metaphor can be partially understood by considering the biologic response to immunization or allergy desensitization. In homeopathy a medicinal substance and a disease are related by the similarity of the symptoms they produce. This phenomenon of the therapeutic action of similar medicines is observable in conventional medicines, such as methylphenidate (Ritalin). The seemingly paradoxic action of methylphenadate produces a hyperkinetic state in healthy people but helps modify the same symptoms in a person with attention-deficit hyperactivity disorder. Colchicine treats gout in material doses and SADs, but it produces symptoms of gout in homeopathic drug provings. Digitalis can produce any arrhythmia it can cure; the differing effects depend on the dose.

At the center of the debate concerning the efficacy of homeopathy is the lack of a defined mechanism of action for homeopathic medicines. "When a homeopathic medicine contains no molecules of the medicine, what plausible mechanism of action can there be?" ask the critics. There is no answer to that question at this time, only hypotheses. The memory of water theory proposes that through the process of serial dilution and succussion, information contained in the original solute is transferred to the solvent. There it is maintained beyond dilutions in which molecules of the original substance can be measured. This information is transferred to the organism by the homeopathic medicine.

SADs carry information transferred from the solute to the aqueous solvent. Agitating the solution adds potential energy stored in altered bonding of the diluent molecules and determined in part by characteristics of the solute. Information necessary for the catalytic property of homeopathic medicines is encoded in the altered molecular bonding of the medicine. This process of encoding information in seemingly inert substances is analogous to the record and playback function of an audiotape or videotape. When the tape is passed under the magnetic recording head, digital or analog information is encoded in the altered bonding angles of the ferrous emulsion on the tape. Although chemically unaltered, an enormous amount of information is carried on the tape, which, when passed through a tape deck, is transformed into visual and auditory images. Likewise the information encoded in the water that is used to prepare homeopathic medicines can be read by biologic systems and can result in transformation of the physiologic processes of an organism. The specific mechanism by which the transfer of information occurs has yet to be clearly defined.

HOMEOPATHIC RESEARCH

Research in homeopathy is in its infancy in many respects. A community of sophisticated homeopathic researchers that has evolved in the last decade is fostering a new respect for homeopathy within the scientific community. A recent publication edited by Ernst and Hahn[32] provided an up-to-date description of the status of homeopathic researchers and the issues they are facing. The most important question to the scientific community is whether homeopathic medicines, which are so highly diluted, can have biologic activity or efficacy in the treatment of disease. In other words, are they anything more than elaborate placebos? The general thrust of homeopathic research is currently focused on answering that question. Most high-quality homeopathic research has been done in Europe, but active research efforts are ongoing in India and the Americas. Evidence for the possible effectiveness of homeopathic medicines comes from a number of sources, including epidemiologic, clinical, and basic science studies.

In the realm of epidemiology, Eisenberg[9] reported in 1998 that 3.4% of Americans used homeopathy, an increase of more than 300% since 1991. Only 16.5% of these Americans saw homeopathic providers, suggesting that approximately 85% of users self-prescribe OTC remedies. This estimate corresponds closely with the

homeopathic manufacturers' figures for their percentage of OTC sales.[17] According to the homeopathic pharmaceutical industry, sales of homeopathic medicines are increasing by 20% each year.[17] Berman[33] surveyed American primary care physicians and found that 13.8% refer to homeopaths, 15.9% use homeopathy, and 49% want training in homeopathy. A survey[1] of homeopathic use in the Los Angeles area from 1994 to 1995 described the population seeking homeopathic services as predominantly white, well educated, female, and in fair to good health. Subjects indicated that they were seeking care for more than one medical problem, most of which were chronic, and for which they had already attempted conventional treatment. After 4 months of homeopathic treatment, 70% reported improvement and 18% complete resolution of their complaints; 60% had improvement in general health status markers. These statistics indicate that the public and medical professionals have a growing perception that homeopathy is effective and should be tried.

BASIC SCIENCE RESEARCH

Laboratory research has demonstrated the activity of SAD beyond Avogadro's number in a variety of biologic systems. Many of the significant experiments from this research are reviewed in three recent publications.[34,35,37] A meta-analysis[36] of 135 experiments in toxicology found that 80% of the experiments showed positive outcomes. There was an average 20% greater protective effect in SAD-treated animals than in those given placebo. For example, mice were pretreated with a SAD derived from the hearts and livers of mice that had died from tularemia. Thirty-seven of the mice were then exposed to tularemia organisms, a universally fatal disease in mice, and 20% of the mice survived.

In 1988 *Nature* published a report[38] from a team headed by Jacques Benveniste in which human basophils were shown to degranulate when exposed to antiserum against immune globulin E (IgE) at dilution of 10^{-120}. The accompanying editorial[39] summarized the incredulity of the scientific community to the suggestion that solutions containing no molecules of the substance from which they were derived could affect biologic systems:

The principle of restraint which applies is simple: that when an unexpected observation requires that a substantial portion of our intellectual heritage should be thrown out it is prudent to ask whether the observation is correct.

The disbelief of Benveniste's results led to a questionable investigation and subsequent rebuttal of this preliminary research by *Nature*. In 1999 the findings of the Benveniste team were confirmed in a series of studies[40-42] that demonstrated the in vitro activity of dilutions below 10^{-23} molar.

Despite the cumulative evidence for the action of SADs, the lack of a defined mechanism of action for homeopathic medicines generates skepticism among modern scientists. Among the potential mechanisms proposed, the most probable is that the original source material leaves a memory in the water in which it is serially agitated and diluted by altering the bonding of water molecules. Experimental data supporting this theory come from documentation of clathrates[43] and discoveries arising from research in catalyst chemistry.[44,45] SAD solutions contain aggregated water molecules. These 3-nm "IE crystals" form in response to the electrostatic forces around individual ions in solution. As the solution is serially diluted and then agitated, these molecules sheer off the parent compound and reaggregate into increasingly independent stable structures. These structures are stable over a wide range of pH and temperature and can be measured using ultraviolet spectroscopy, electron microscopy, and atomic phase microscopy. At dilutions of 10^{-7} these IE crystals become self-replicating and increasingly stable; at dilutions of 10^{-16} they may compose almost 4% of the solution. The physical characteristics of the aggregates appear to be dependent on the characteristics of the initial solute.

From this data it could be surmised that the SAD antiserum in Benveniste's experiments contained IE crystals that were capable of triggering the cell surface receptors on the basophils, resulting in degranulation. IE crystals act as catalysts in a variety of systems, from enhancing the combustion of gasoline to inducing the production of cytokines by white blood cells.[46,47] These IE crystals are a proprietary product. The physicists who developed them have not yet tested any manufactured homeopathic products. However, they have inferred by the similarity of their production process that homeopathic products may contain structure similar to IE crystals.

CLINICAL EVIDENCE

Randomized controlled clinical trials (RCCTs) in homeopathy number approximately 200. The bulk of this research has been done in Europe where homeopathic researchers have the support of governments, the Euro-

pean Economic Community, a well-established pharmaceutical industry, and private foundations. Recognizing the deficiency in funding for research in homeopathy and other alternative and complementary therapies, the Office of Alternative Medicine (OAM) at the National Institutes of Health (NIH) was created by Congress in 1992. This was the first time U.S. federal funding became available for research into any alternative therapies. Consequently, two homeopathic clinical trials[65] received funding from the federal government. Only three[2,45,49] have been published in peer-reviewed medical journals. In 1998 the OAM was upgraded by congress to the status of a center (the National Center for Complementary and Alternative Medicine, or NCCAM) with independent granting authority. OAM's 1998 budget of $12 million was increased to NCCAM's $50 million budget in 1998. The NCCAM has provided an invaluable service by legitimizing the links between academic institutions and alternative medicine providers.

As a consequence of increased funding and interest, clinical research in homeopathy has increased in the last decade and a number of promising research efforts are underway in the United States. High-quality, peer-reviewed RCCTs[54] have suggested efficacy in a wide variety of conditions, including diarrhea,[48] asthma,[50] seasonal rhinitis,[57] mild head trauma,[2] otitis media,[52,53] fibrositis,[7] and migraine.[8] Three meta-analyses[54-56] of homeopathic RCCTs have reached similar conclusions: The activity of homeopathic potencies cannot be explained by placebo and the lack of large-scale, independently replicated trials limits the conclusions that can be drawn from single studies.[51]

Since the inception of homeopathy, clinical research has been conducted in the form of HDP. In Hahnemann's time these HDPs were informal experiments to test the potential therapeutic value of medicines based on information from toxicologic reports or folk use. Contemporary HDPs employ modern methodology and statistics[32] to define a set of symptoms that characterize each medicine and can be used to make homeopathic prescriptions.

CLASSIC HOMEOPATHIC RESEARCH IN TOPICS OF RELEVANCE TO NEUROLOGY

Several areas of homeopathic clinical research are of interest to neurologists, including headache, Parkinson's disease, vertigo, mild traumatic brain injury (MTBI), chronic pain, acute soft tissue injury, and stroke. The size, quality, and lack of independent replication of the following pilot studies make definitive interpretation of this research premature.

Migraine Headache

Brigo and Serpelloni[8] demonstrated that patients (n = 30) treated with classic homeopathy compared with those given placebo (n = 30) showed significant reductions in the intensity ($p < 0.000001$), duration ($p < 0.001$), and frequency ($p < 0.000001$) of migraine headaches. This study used an individualized classic approach. Remedies in a 30C potency were administered four times, at 2-week intervals for 6 weeks. Patients were followed for a total of 4 months. Two attempts[57,58] to replicate this trial in patients with chronic headaches, not specifically migraine, failed to find benefit for homeopathic treatment. Differences in methodology such as the use on prescription by a consensus of experts and inclusion of chronic headache patients rather than migraine subjects may account for the differences in outcome.

Broca's Aphasia

There is evidence of the efficacy of homeopathic medicines for Broca's aphasia,[3] an aphasic syndrome characterized by deficits in motor, verbal, and executive language functions associated with a dominant hemisphere stroke. A controlled clinical trial was performed in Bombay, India, and the outcomes were presented at an international symposium in 1980. A randomized group of patients with a diagnosis of aphasia were treated with the appropriate homeopathic medication or placebo. After 120 days, 22 of 24 patients in the verum group improved, compared with 3 of 12 in the placebo group, based on a bedside neurologic examination and speech evaluation. Although the data suggest benefit from homeopathic treatment, no formal statistical analysis or characterization of the nature of improvements was performed on this data.

Bothrops lanceolatus, a remedy derived from the venom of a snake, was used in more than 50% of the cases. The symptoms produced by exposure to this venom are described in the *Homeopathic Recorder*[59] as "Inability to articulate without any affection of the tongue. Hemorrhages, the blood being fluid and black. . . . Paralysis of one arm or one leg only." The

similarity of these symptoms to those of a patient with Broca's aphasia is the key to the successful homeopathic prescription. The dilution of the venom by the homeopathic pharmaceutical process to potencies in the range of 10^{-60} to 10^{-400} make it safe while maintaining the desired effect. Unfortunately, this trial has never been replicated. The promising pilot data, the lack of other treatment for this condition, and homeopathy's safety would make it an excellent candidate for an RCCT.

Parkinson's Disease

Potencies (6X, 12X, and 30X) of a nerve growth factor, neurotrophin, derived from cobra venom, were tested in 20 Parkinson's disease patients using a double-blind crossover methodology.[4] All subjects had previously responded to intranasal doses of neurotrophin (750 μg), with responses appearing after 28 days. Using homeopathic potencies, the response occurred after 4 to 5 days and was characterized by significant reduction in tremor ($p = 0.005$), bradykinesia, ($p = 0.005$), rigidity ($p = 0.004$), confusion ($p = 0.003$), on/off phenomena ($p = 0.005$), and medication dosage ($p < 0.05$). The authors postulate that the action of this homeopathic preparation could be explained by receptor activation.

The same research team demonstrated improvements in mentation, language, behavior, and intellectual function in five patients with Down syndrome treated for 60 days with neurotrophin (6C, 12C, 30C).[60]

Chronic Pain (Fibromyalgia)

A study of fibrositis[7] showed statistically significant outcomes in patients with chronic musculoskeletal pain (fibromyalgia) treated with a single medicine, *Rhus toxicodendron* (poison ivy). This study was an attempt to emulate a single-agent pharmaceutical trial. Only patients whose pains were similar to the symptoms of individuals exposed to *Rhus toxicodendron* were selected for inclusion in the trial. Those symptoms included becoming worse from cold, wet weather and better from heat and continued motion. Of potential subjects, 42% met these criteria and were treated with *Rhus toxicodendron* (6C twice a day) in a double-blinded, placebo-controlled crossover design. Subjective scoring of pain and sleep and clinician-rated mean number of tender points were significantly reduced ($p < 0.005$). A multicenter replication of this study is planned.

Head Injury

MTBI is a devastating function disturbance that persists in 5% to 15% of patients with mild closed head injury, resulting in considerable social and economic disruption. Apparent efficacy of homeopathic treatment of MTBI[2] was observed in a pilot study of 50 patients conducted between 1994 and 1996 at Spaulding Rehabilitation Hospital in Boston. Statistically significant reductions in patients' symptom intensity ($p = 0.01$) and difficulty functioning ($p = 0.0008$) were found. Because there is no conventional pharmacologic therapy that stimulates the global recovery observed in patients in this study, the possibility that homeopathy could be helpful in MTBI patients needs further confirmation. The interpretation of the findings of this pilot study was limited because of the small sample size, duration of treatment, and questions about the validity and reliability of the measures used. A multicenter collaborative study is planned to validate the findings of the pilot study.

Vertigo

In a study[6] conducted in Athens, Greece, 74 subjects were randomized to treatment with dimenydrinate (50 mg four times a day) or classically prescribed homeopathic medication. Beginning at 1 week and continuing for the duration of the 6 months of treatment, the homeopathic group had a significant reduction in the frequency of episodes of vertigo ($p < 0.001$) and in concomitant medical and psychological complaints ($p < 0.01$).

Weiser and Strosser[5] treated patients (n = 59) with vertigoheel, an oral combination formula for vertigo of various etiologies. The patients faired equally well when compared with others receiving active treatment (n = 60) with the antihistamine drug betahistine hydrochloride, a conventional drug used widely in Europe. This RCT was done in 15 general practice centers in Germany and measured the frequency, duration, and intensity of vertigo attacks during the 6-week treatment period. Both treatments were tolerated well.

Acute Soft Tissue Injury

The primary, single remedy used in clinical practice to treat acute trauma is Arnica montanna. A recent meta-analysis[61] of clinical trials using Arnica showed that the outcomes of half of the trials were positive and half were negative. The authors of this meta-analysis point out that most of the trials had severe methodologic flaws and conclude that "the claim that Arnica is efficacious is not supported by rigorous clinical trials." Given the widespread clinical use of Arnica and the perception of benefit by patients and clinicians using it, the issue defined by this meta-analysis was the need for rigorous trials to settle the issue of efficacy of Arnica. This has been the conclusion of all the meta-analyses of homeopathic clinical trials done to date.

Homeopathic researchers have begun to explore several areas of interest to neurologists. These pilot studies are intriguing but need confirmation through larger, high-quality, independently replicated clinical trials. The findings represent a subset among the many areas in which integration of homeopathy into the treatment of neurologic disease is actually used in practice.

CLINICAL EXAMPLE: A PATIENT WITH MTBI

The theoretical and research backgrounds of homeopathy have been outlined; a clinical example will further illustrate the nature of homeopathic treatment. The following case concerning a subject who was in the active treatment group of a study of homeopathic treatment for MTBI exemplifies the homeopathic prescribing process.

Case Description

A 32-year-old woman entered the study 2½ years after a head-on automobile accident. At the time of the accident, she lost consciousness for several minutes and sustained fractures to her knees, cervical spine, clavicle, shoulder, and ribs, resulting in a 4-week hospitalization. She was heavily medicated for pain, and although she recovered, her intelligence was affected and she lost many skills. These losses prevented her from resuming gainful employment.

Before the accident the woman did desktop publishing, but after her MTBI she could not remember how to turn on a computer. Her math skills were severely affected; for instance, she was unable to conceptualize 3 inches and no longer knew multiplication tables. Her hand trembled when she wrote, and she was unable to concentrate. She could not think and speak at the same time, and her short-term memory was poor.

The subject slept 19 hours a day for a year after the accident. The sleepiness, imbalance, and tremor were due at least partly to effects of prescribed medications. Amitriptyline, alprazolam (Xanax), clonazepam (Klonopin), fluoxetine (Prozac), and butorphanol nasal spray (Stadol NS) were cumulatively prescribed to manage problems with mood and pain. She was weaned from these medications at an inpatient pain treatment unit. At enrollment in the study, she was taking no medications for MTBI but was using oral contraceptive pills (OCPs), co-trimoxazole (Bactrim) and nitrofurantoin for urinary tract infection prophylaxis, and vitamins.

She complained of left-sided headaches secondary to neck injury. Movement of her eyes caused pain, and her head felt as if it would explode. Symptoms were aggravated by excitement, stress, stooping, noise, light, and the odor of perfumes, smoke, and paint. The symptoms were alleviated by relaxation and quiet.

She experienced back pain and paresthesias in the legs when she sat. The sounds of voices irritated her, and she felt driven. She believed that everything had to be on time and "things must be done now." She felt impatient when anything was out of order. Before the accident she had been happy-go-lucky and friendly. She did not like to spoil others' fun so she did not say much about her symptoms, and then she told only her close friends. "Life was very limited."

Nine months after her accident, the subject was admitted to a psychiatric hospital. While attending an auction she suddenly became catatonic. She was not frightened—just blank, like a zombie. For 3 months afterward she could not be left alone. After a second accident she experienced a flashback of the original accident with subsequent panic attacks. She was again hospitalized, which prompted her husband to call a meeting of her nine doctors and arrange for her transfer to a regional, inpatient pain treatment center. She feared driving in a car; her worst fears

came true when she was involved in a second accident. She had frightening dreams, she feared taking drugs, and she started from sudden noise. Since the injury she felt chillier and had night sweats, and her sex drive had disappeared.

Assessment

The patient was a 32-year-old woman who had sustained an MTBI. She was in an oversensitive state that had appeared after treatment with polypharmacy allopathic medications. Her headaches and mental state were aggravated by stimulation of all kinds. She was impatient and intolerant, and felt chillier than usual.

The process of a homeopathic prescription involves translating the patient's expressions of symptoms into the language of the homeopathic repertories and materia medica. The repertory[62] contains symptoms, or rubrics, indexed by the body part of function. Each rubric is associated with a list of homeopathic medicines that have produced a specific symptom in provings or have cured clinical cases. The following rubrics were chosen to represent her symptoms. The numbers in parentheses indicate the number of remedies in that rubric.

MIND; IMPATIENCE (138)
MIND; HURRY, haste; tendency (138)
MIND; STARING, thoughtless (17)
MIND; MEMORY; weakness, loss of; mental exertion; from (14)
MIND; MEMORY; weakness, loss of; words, for (64)
MIND; MISTAKES, makes; calculating, in (21)
MIND; MEMORY; weakness, loss of; say, for what he is about to (41)
HEAD PAIN; GENERAL; injuries, after mechanical (24)
HEAD PAIN; GENERAL; noise, from (98)
HEAD PAIN; GENERAL; excitement of the emotions, after (58)
HEAD PAIN; GENERAL; odors; strong, from (22)
HEAD PAIN; GENERAL; stooping; from (140)
HEAD PAIN; LOCALIZATION; sides; left (197)
BLADDER; INFLAMMATION; chronic (53)
GENERALITIES; MEDICAMENTS, allopathic medicine; oversensitive to (18)
EXTREMITIES; NUMBNESS, insensibility; lower limbs; sitting; while (22)
GENERALITIES; INJURIES, blows, falls and bruises; concussion; actual or tendency (61)

	Sulph.	Nux-v.	Puls.	Nat-m.	Sil.	Calc.	Bell.	Lyc.	Lach.	Ph-ac.	Arn.
Total	29	28	23	22	21	20	20	19	19	17	16
Rubrics	14	13	12	11	12	12	9	14	11	11	9
Family											
MIND; IMPATIENCE (138)	3	3	2	2	3	2	1	2	2	1	
MIND; HURRY, haste; tendency (138)	3	2	2	3	3	1	2	1	2	2	
MIND; STARING, thoughtless (17)			2								
MIND; MEMORY; weakness, loss of; mental exertion, from (14)	3	3	1	2	2	2			2	1	
MIND; MEMORY; weakness, loss of; words, for (64)	2	2	1	2	1	1		2	2	2	2
MIND; MISTAKES, makes; calculating, in (21)		2				1		2	1		
MEMORY; weakness, loss of; say, for what he is about to (41)	2			2				1		2	2
HEAD PAIN; GENERAL; injuries, after mechanical (24)	1		1	2		1	2				2
HEAD PAIN; GENERAL; noise, from (98)		2		1	2	3	4	1	2	2	1
HEAD PAIN; GENERAL; excitement of the emotions, after (58)	1	3	3	3	1	2	2	2	2	3	2
HEAD PAIN; GENERAL; odors; strong, from (22)	2	1			2		2	2			
HEAD PAIN; GENERAL; stooping; from (140)	3	2	3	2	2	2	3	1	1	1	1
HEAD PAIN; LOCALIZATION; Sides; left (107)	2	2	1	1	1	2		1	2	1	2
BLADDER; INFLAMMATION; chronic (53)	2		2					1			
NUMBNESS, insensibility; Lower Limbs; sitting; while (22)	1	1			1		1			1	
INJURIES, blows, falls and bruises; concussion; actual or ... (61)	1	2	2	2	2	2	2	1		1	3
MEDICAMENTS, allopathic medicine; oversensitive to (18)	3	3	3		1					2	1

Figure 5-2 Chart illustrating the symptoms of the patient with MTBI graphed against the remedies included under each rubric.

The graph in Figure 5-2 is generated when these symptoms are graphed against the remedies included under each rubric.

Repertorization

The patient's symptoms are listed to the left on the graph; abbreviations of remedies run across the top. The intensity of the correlation between the remedy and the symptom is graded from 1 to 4: white is lowest (0), yellow is second (1), green is third (2), and pink is highest (3). The row labeled *Rubrics* indicates the number of rubrics that matched for each remedy. The row labeled *Total* indicates the total score for each remedy. The remedy prescribed was Nux vomica despite its not having the numerically highest score. Repertorization gives the homeopathic prescriber a sense of the remedies that might fit the case. However, the actual selection is based on the study of materia medica, which leads to the prescription of the most similar remedy for the case. Prescribing is not simply matching specific symptoms; it is matching the characteristic *state* that is represented by the totality of these symptoms, sometimes referred to as a *remedy* or *constitutional picture*. The following materia medica description of Nux vomica[63] shows a marked similarity to the essence of the case presented.

It is frequently the first remedy, indicated after much dosing, establishing a sort of equilibrium of forces and counteracting chronic effects. Nux vomica is pre-eminently the remedy for many of the conditions incident to modern life. The typical Nux patient is rather thin, spare, quick, active, nervous, and irritable. He does a good deal of mental work; has mental strains . . . which lead to use of stimulants, coffee, wine, possibly in excess, and . . . rich and stimulating food. A thick head, dyspepsia, and irritable temper are the next day's inheritance. These conditions produce an irritable nervous system, hypersensitive and overimpressionably, which Nux vomica will do much to soothe and calm. Convulsions and consciousness; aggravated touch, moving; . . . patients are easily chilled, avoid open air, etc. Nux vomica always seems to be out of tune. Inharmonious spasmodic action. . . . Tense contracted feeling. . . . Bruised soreness . . . of abdomen, brain, etc. . . . Contractive pains throughout the body. General bruised feeling in the morning in bed. . . . Great debility, & oversensitiveness of all the senses. Everything makes too strong an impression. Stitches in jerks throughout the whole body. . . . Trembling all over; mostly of hands, esp. in morning; in drunkards.

Plan

The similarity of this portrait to the patient's case, together with the matching of most of the specific symptoms displayed in the repertorization graph, led to the prescription of Nux vomica 200C, 1 dose daily for 7 days.

One-Month Follow-Up

The improvement was fairly sudden. The patient felt better, her mind was working again, and she stated that she could remember more things. She felt ready to try the computer and had bought one within 2 weeks. She could read manuals and follow directions. Her husband said, "She is sharper across the board." She had not tried math but still had difficulty conceptualizing 3 inches.

Her general energy level was changed; she was able to work from 8:00 AM to 3:30 PM on a computer. She was tired by evening and went to bed early. Her headaches had improved, coming on after maintaining steady concentration for 2 days or after significant excitement. After the remedy her back pain had worsened initially, peaked that same week, and then gradually improved. The initial worsening was an example of a homeopathic aggravation.

She was in a better mood and felt more useful, although the driven feeling was still there. Her insomnia and diminished sexual desire persisted. Performing multiple simultaneous tasks was still difficult, and she continued to complain of chilliness.

Assessment

The subject rated her symptoms in three areas (on a scale of intensity in which 10 was worst and 0 was none) as follows: cognitive dysfunction from 10 to 4 and continuing to improve; physical dysfunction from 10 to 8, continuing to have back pain; and emotional distress from 10 to 0. She stated her sense of usefulness had returned. There was a clear and dramatic improvement in her overall state.

Plan

Do nothing. Homeopathic medicines act as catalysts and do not need repetition unless the remedy reaction ceases. She was asked to call if she relapsed or stopped improving.

Two-Month Follow-Up

The patient had a mild relapse of her symptoms 2 weeks after the visit and repeated the Nux vomica 200C, taken diluted in water daily for 3 days. After this dose she continued to improve.

Three-Month Follow-Up

The subject had to repeat the remedy, diluted in water, several times with minimal improvement. She repeated the remedy when her energy level was lower, and she had fewer useful hours in the day. She was self-employed 5 to 6 hours a day, 3 days a week. Memory remained an issue; she was unable to remember to take her OCP or antibiotic. She had an unpleasant dream about a friend having a heart attack and not knowing what to do while someone else was drowning. In describing the dream she said, "I'm there and can't help." She had drenching night sweats at 1 or 2 AM. She felt hot all over but especially on her chest and thighs and radiated heat when she was asleep. She left the window open. Her moods were more stable and less cranky, agitated, and frustrated. She craved fat, pizza, hot spices, and creamy foods.

Assessment

She was better but had reached the maximal benefit from the 200C potency of Nux vomica. The driven feeling and dreams of fatal accidents are characteristic of patients taking Nux vomica. Under routine circumstances the potency would be increased to 1000C (1M), but the study protocol allowed only the 200C potency. Some fundamental shifts in her state had begun to appear, including body warmth, desire for spices, and an increase of night sweats. The warmer body temperature was a return to a state that had been normal for her before the accident.

Plan

In the absence of a higher potency of Nux vomica she was given a complementary remedy that covered the new symptoms: sulfur 200C, daily for 7 days.

Four-Month Follow-Up

The patient said, "I'm excellent and have returned to work on my own schedule, building up slowly, now averaging

20 hours per week." After taking the second remedy, the sulfur 200C, she developed intensive headaches, so she repeated Nux vomica 200C in water and gradually improved. In general she felt great. She went to bed by 9:30 PM and awoke at 6:30 AM with an alarm. On weekends she slept until 8 AM. She was still waking at 1 to 2 AM with night sweats, and she still had nightmares. Her bladder was stable; she planned to speak to her primary care physician the next week about going off antibiotics. The "discs in her back felt swollen" in wet weather. A bad cold and possible pneumonia resolved using echinacea. Her short-term memory was still limited.

Assessment

The patient was improved overall. She had an initial aggravation by the sulfur during which she took Nux vomica. It was unclear whether the subsequent improvement was due to the sulfur or to repeating the Nux vomica.

Plan

This patient was terminated from the study after the prescribed 4-month treatment period and referred to a local homeopathic physician for follow-up. Ideally a higher potency of Nux vomica will be given, possibly followed by sulfur if indicated but starting with a lower potency than previously given. Herbal support for her urinary tract infections might allow her to discontinue the antibiotics, which could be interfering with the homeopathic medicine.

SUMMARY

From the discussion of homeopathic principles and research and from the clinical example presented in this chapter it is apparent that homeopathy has an important therapeutic role in conditions commonly treated by neurologists. Two potential approaches exist for using homeopathy: classic and complex, or combination. Each approach has its merits and limitations. The combination approach allows the physician to practice in an allopathic mindset. Although the results are likely to be palliative, the few published trials of these products compare favorably with allopathic alternatives.

The application of the classic approach may lead to long-term, curative effects but requires in-depth training in homeopathic prescribing. Achieving competence in the classic methods has traditionally taken years of study. Recent initiatives in homeopathic training have emphasized the recognition of key patterns for remedies prescribed in conditions commonly seen in primary care. Physicians trained in this way have achieved clinically significant outcomes in 60% to 70% of their cases.[64]

An evidence-based approach is appropriate for using the findings from clinical research in areas of interest to neurologists, such as head trauma, stroke, fibromyalgia, and Parkinson's disease. Homeopathic research must focus on identifying prescribing indications of homeopathic medicines in specific clinical syndromes. This research could lead to a simplification of homeopathic prescribing by non–homeopathically trained clinicians using algorithms. Alternatively these data could be used to rationally design combination products that could then be tested for effectiveness.

These approaches to simplifying the classic homeopathic prescribing process would facilitate the use of homeopathic medicines in appropriate cases seen by neurologists.[65] The efficacy of prescribing algorithms or combination products could be tested against both conventional alternatives and the classic homeopathic method. The curative potential of homeopathic medicines, together with their low cost and the minimal incidence of adverse reactions resulting from their use, make collaboration between the neurology and homeopathic communities an intriguing possibility.

References

1. Goldstein MS, Glick D: Use of and satisfaction with homeopathy in a patient population, *Altern Ther Health Med* 4(2):60-65, March 1998.
2. Chapman E et al: The homeopathic treatment of mild traumatic brain injury, *J Head Trauma Rehabilitation*, 14(6): 521-542, December 1999.
3. Ericsson AD: *Homeopathic neutrophin: treatment of Parkinson's disease,* Houston, Institute of Biological Research. Houston, TX. Unpublished research.
4. Master FJ: Scope of homeopathic drugs in the treatment of Broca's aphasia. Proceedings of the forty-second Congress of LMHI, Arlington, Va. 1987. Published proceedings of the LMHI, 330-334.
5. Tsiakopoulis I et al: Comparative study of homeopathic and allopathic treatment of benign paroxysmal positional vertigo. Proceedings of the forty-third Congress of the International Homeopathic Medical League, Athens, Greece, 1988. Published proceedings of the LMHI, 94-97.
6. Weiser M, Strosser W, Klein P: Homeopathic versus conventional treatment of vertigo, *Arch Otolaryngol Head Neck Surg* 124:879-885, August 1998.

7. Fisher P et al : Effect of homeopathic treatment on fibrositis, *Br Med J* 299:365-366, 1989.

8. Brigo B, Serpelloni G: Homeopathic treatment of migraines: a randomized double blind controlled study of sixty cases, *Berl J Res Homeopathy* 1:98-105, 1991.

9. Eisenberg DM, Davis RB: Trends in alternative medicine use in the United States, 1990-1997: results of a follow-up national survey, *JAMA* 280(18):1569-1575, 1998.

10. Jonas W, Jacobs J: *Healing with homeopathy,* New York, Warner Books, 1996.

11. Hahnemann S. In W.B. O'Reilly, ed: *Organon of the medical art,* Redmond, Wash., Bird Cage Books.

12. Riley D: Contemporary homeopathic drug provings, *J Am Inst Homeopathy* 84:144-148, 1994.

13. Weiland F: The role of drug provings in the homeopathic concept. In Ernst E, Hahn J, editors: *Homeopathy: a critical appraisal,* Oxford, 1998, Butterworth, Heinemann.

14. Dantas F, Fisher P: A systematic review of homeopathic pathogenetic trials ('provings') published in the United Kingdom from 1945 to 1995. In Ernst E, Hahn J, editors: *Homeopathy: a critical appraisal,* Oxford, 1998, Butterworth, Heinemann.

15. Kayne SB: *Homeopathic pharmacy: an introduction and handbook,* Edinburgh, 1997, Churchill Livingstone.

16. Homeopathic Pharmacopoeia Convention of the United States: Homeopathic Pharmacopoeia Convention of the United States abstracts, 1995, Washington DC, HPCUS.

17. United States Food and Drug Administration: Compliance Policy Guide 7132.15, *Conditions under which homeopathic medicines may be marketed,* 1988, U.S. Government.

18. Borneman JP: Homeopathy in the United States and Canada: an analysis of the self-medication market for homeopathic drugs. In *Improving the success of homeopathy,* January 23, 1997, Royal London Homeopathic Hospital, NHS, pp. 82-89. Proceedings of meeting.

19. Hahnemann S: *Materia medica pura, vol 1 and 2,* New Delhi, 1980, Jain (Translated by RE Dudgeon).

20. Coulter HL: *Divided legacy: a history of the schism in medical thought,* vol 3, Science and ethics in American medicine: 1800-1914, Washington DC, 1973, McGrath.

21. Allen TF: *The encyclopedia of pure materia medica: a record of the positive effects of drugs upon healthy human organism,* 12 vols, Indian Edition, New Delhi, 1982, Jain.

22. Hering C: *The guiding symptoms of our materia medica,* 10 vols, Indian Edition, New Delhi, 1972, Jain.

23. Kent JT: *Lectures on homeopathic philosophy, memorial edition,* Chicago, 1929, Ehrhart & Karl.

24. Kent JT: *Lectures on homeopathic materia medica,* ed 4, Philadelphia, 1956, Boericke & Tafel.

25. Kent JT: *Kent's repertorium generale,* Berg, Germany, 1987, Barthel & Barthel. (Edited by Kunzli von Fimmelsberg, J.)

26. Rothstein WG: *American physicians in the 19th century,* Baltimore, 1984, Johns Hopkins University Press.

27. Ernst E, Kaptchuk T: Homeopathy revisited, *Arch Intern Med* 159:2162-2164, September 28, 1996.

28. Ullman, D: *Discovering homeopathy: medicine for the 21st century,* Berkley, CA, 1991, North Atlantic Books.

29. Voll R: The phenomenon of medicine testing in electro-acupuncture according to Voll, *Am J Acupuncture* 8:97-104.

30. Vithoulkas G: *The science of homeopathy,* New York, 1980, Grove Press.

31. Bellavite P, Signorini A: *Homeopathy - a frontier in medical science,* Berkley, 1995, North Atlantic Books (translated by A Steele).

32. Ernst E, Hahn EG, editors: *Homeopathy: a critical appraisal,* Oxford, 1998, Butterworth, Heinman.

33. Berman B et al: Homeopathy and the US primary care physician, *Br Homeopathic J* 86:131-138, July 1997.

34. Endler PC, Schulte J: *Ultra high dilution physiology and physics,* Boston, 1994, Kluwer Academic Publishers.

35. Bastide M: *Signals and Images,* Boston, 1997, Kluwer Academic Publishers.

36. Linde K et al: Critical review and meta-analysis of serially agitated dilutions in experimental toxicology, *Hum Exp Toxicol,* 13:481-492, 1994.

37. Jonas WB, *Do homeopathic nosodes protect against infection? An experimental alternative therapy,* 1999; 5(5): 36-40.

38. Davenas E, Beauvais F, Amara J: Human basophil degranulation triggered by very dilute antiserum against IgE, *Nature* 333:816-18, 1988.

39. Editorial, When to believe the unbelievable, *Nature* 333:787, June 30, 1988.

40. Belon P et al: Inhibition of basophil degranulation by successive histamine dilutions: results of a European multi-center trial, *Inflamm Res* 48(suppl)1:S17-S18, 1999.

41. Sainte-Landy J, Belon P: Application of flow cytometry to the analysis of the immunosuppressive effect of histamine dilutions on human basophil activation, *Inflammation Research,* 46(suppl)1:S27-S28, 1997.

42. Sainte-Landy J, Belon P: Analysis of immunosuppressive activity of serial dilution of histamine on human basophil activation by flow cytometry, *Inflammation Research,* 45(suppl)1:S33-S34, 1996.

43. Anagnostatos GS et al: Theory and experiments on high dilutions. In Ernst E, Hahn EG, editors: *Homeopathy: a critical appraisal,* Oxford, 1998, Butterworth, Heinman.

44. Lo, SY: Anomalous state of ice, *Modern Physics Letters B* 10(19):909-919, 1996.

45. Lo, SY: Physical properties of water with IE structures, *Modern Physics Letters B* 10(19):921-930, 1996.

46. Bonavida B: Induction and regulation of human peripheral blood TH1-TH2 derived cytokines by IE water preparations and synergy with mitogens. Proceeding of the first international symposium of the physical, chemical and biological properties of IE clusters, 1997, pp 4-6. [Online: http://www.atcg.com/randd/workshop.html, April 29, 1998].

47. Sinitsyn AP: Effect of IE solutions on enzymes and microbial cells. Proceeding of the first international symposium of the physical, chemical and biological properties of IE clusters, 1997, pp 6-7. [Online: http://www.atcg.com/randd/workshop.html, April 29, 1998].

48. Jacobs J et al: Treatment of acute diarrhea with homeopathic medicine: a randomized clinical trial in Nicaragua, *Pediatrics* 93(5):719-725, May 5, 1994.

49. Davidson J: Homeopathic treatment of depression and anxiety, *Altern Ther Health Med* 3(1):46-49, 1997.

50. Reilly DT et al: Is evidence for homeopathy reproducible? A controlled trial of allergic asthma, *Lancet* 344(8937):161-6, Dec 10, 1995.

51. Reilly DT et al: Is homeopathy a placebo response? Controlled trial of homeopathic potency, with pollen in hayfever as model, *Lancet* ii:881-885, 1986.

52. Jacobs J: Homeopathic treatment of acute otitis media in children—a randomized placebo-controlled trial (submitted for publication, 1998).

53. Friese KH et al: The homeopathic treatment of otitis media in children—comparisons with conventional therapy, *Int J Clin Pharmacol Ther* 35(7):296-301, 1997.

54. Linde K et al: Are the clinical effects of homeopathy placebo effects? A meta-analysis of placebo controlled trials, *Lancet* 350:834-843, 1997.

55. Boissel JP et al: Overview of data from homeopathic medicine trials: report on the efficacy of homeopathic interventions over no treatment of placebo. Report of the Homeopathic Medicine Research Group, Brussels, 1996, European Commission.

56. Kleijnen, J et al: Clinical trials in homeopathy, *Br Med J* 302:316-23, 1991.

57. Walach H et al: Classical homeopathic treatment of chronic headaches, *Cephalalgia* 17:119-26, 1997.

58. Whitmarsh THE: Double-blind randomized placebo-controlled study of the homeopathic prophylaxis of migraine, *Cephalalgia* 17:600-604, 1997.

59. Roberts, HA: *Homeopathic Recorder*, 1938;53(5):3.

60. Ericsson AD: *Down syndrome: Treated with homeopathy*, Houston, Institute of Biological Research (submitted for publication 1999).

61. Ernst E, Pittler MH: Efficacy of homeopathic Arnica: a systematic review of placebo-controlled clinical trials, *Arch Surg* 133:1187-1190, 1998.

62. Warkentin DK, van Zandvoort R: *The complete repertory*, San Anselmo, Calif, 1992, MacRepertory 3.4.

63. Morrison R: *Desktop guide to keynotes and confirmatory symptoms*, Albany, Calif, 1993, Hahnemann Clinic Press.

64. Reilly DT: Is homeopathy a placebo response? What if it is? What if it is not? In Ernst E, Hahn EG, editors, *Homeopathy: a critical appraisal*, Oxford, 1998, Butterworth, Heinamann.

65. Chapman E, Woo E, Weintraub R, Milburn M, Neal-Pirozzi T. The homeopathic treatment of mild traumatic brain injury, *J Head Trauma Rehabil*, 1999: 14(6): 521-542. Jacobs #65. Jacobs J. Is Homeopathy Effective for Hot Flashes and Other Estrogen-Withdrawal Symptoms in Breast Cancer Survivors? United States Army Medical Research and Materiel Command, Breast Cancer Research Program, Grant # BC981184.

Resources

The National Center for Homeopathy
801 Fairfax Street, Suite 306
Alexandria, VA 22314
(703) 548-7790 www.homeopathic.org
Information on homeopathy and homeopathic practitioners for the general public.

American Institute of Homeopathy
801 Fairfax Street, Suite 306
Alexandria, VA 22314
(703) 246-9501 www.healthy.net/aih
The oldest national medical professional organization in the United States.

American Board of Homeotherapeutics
801 N Fairfax Dr, Suite 306
Alexandria, VA 22314
(703) 548-7790
Provides specialty and primary care certification for MDs, DOs, RN-Cs, PA-Cs.

Council for Homeopathic Education
3 Main St
Chatham, NY 12037
(518) 392-7975
Accredits and maintains listing of homeopathic education programs.

American Homeopathic Pharmaceutical Association
Box 174
Newtown, PA 19073
(610) 325-7464
Information on manufacturing and distribution of homeopathic medicines.

Homeopathic Pharmacopoeia Convention of the United States
PO Box 2221, Southeastern, PA 19399-2221
www.hpus.com
The complete HPUS or Abstracts.

Books/Tapes/Software
Homeopathic Educational Services
2124 Kittredge St
Berkeley, CA 94794
(800) 359-9051

Kent Homeopathic Associates, Inc.
710 Mission Ave, San Rafael, CA 94901
(415) 457-0678
Homeopathic software for the professional. The ReferenceWorks Library includes every notable homeopathic book published in the past 175 years.

Minimum Price Homeopathic Books
PO Box 2187
Blaine, WA 98231
(800) 663-8272
World Wide Web Resources
http://altmed.od.nih.gov/nccam
Searches the National Institutes of Health, Center for Complementary and Alternative Medicine.

Further Reading

Castro M: *The complete book of homeopathy*, New York, NY, 1990, St. Martins Press.

Hahnemann, S: *Organon of the medical art*, Redmond, Wash, 1996, Birdcage Books (Edited by WB O'Reilly).

Jonas W, Jacobs J: Healing with homeopathy: the complete guide, 1996, Warner Books.

Kayne SB: *Homeopathic pharmacy—an introduction and handbook*, Edinburgh, 1997, Churchill Livingston.

Bellavite P, Signorini A: *Homeopathy—a frontier in medical science*, Berkley, 1995, North Atlantic Books (Translated by A Steele).

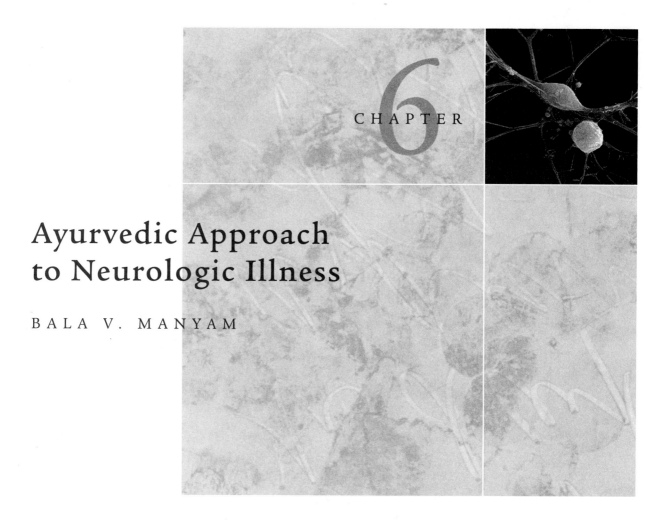

6

Ayurvedic Approach to Neurologic Illness

BALA V. MANYAM

The ancient Indian medical system, Ayurveda (*Ayu* = life, combined state of body, senses, mind, and soul; *Veda* = science; Ayurveda = science of life, Sanskrit) is the oldest system of medicine in the world based on scientific principles.[1] It is the only system of medicine that can be compared to cosmopolitan medicine, that is, allopathy or Western medicine. Like cosmopolitan medicine, Ayurveda is a complete system composed of all branches of medicine, such as surgery, diagnosis, drug treatment, physical therapy, and psychiatry and basic sciences, such as anatomy, pharmacology, and toxicology. Neurologic diseases were recognized in Ayurveda. Before discussing specific neurologic diseases, however, it is important to understand the basis of Ayurveda.

Ayurveda is derived from *Atharvaveda*, one of four *Vedas*. The other three *Vedas* are *Rigveda*, *Yajurveda*, and *Samaveda*. The *Vedas* are the oldest books in the library of humans.[2] The basic concepts of Ayurveda were refined and advanced as they evolved during the Vedic Period (1500 BC). Ayurveda considered disease or disorder to be emanating from derangement from body; mind; external factors (such as toxins, pathogens); and intricate causes, such as metabolic derangement, altered immune response, or host resistance. Ayurveda was divided into eight specialties, namely, *kayachikitsa* (internal medicine or therapeutics), *shalyatantra* (surgery), *shalakyatantra* (diseases of eyes, ears, nose, tongue, oral cavity, and throat), *balatantra* or *kaumaraabhritya* (pediatrics, including antinatal and postnatal baby care, and care of mother before conception and after pregnancy), *agadatantra* (toxicology, dealing with poisons of various types and their antidotes, including environmental and water pollution), *bhutavidaya* (psychiatry or demonic disease), *rasayana* (geriatrics, including knowledge of procedures for arresting the process of mental and physical decay, and rejuvenation), and *vajikarnatantra* (science dealing with toning the weakened organs of reproduction to increase virility).[3] As time progressed, a number of treatises in Ayurveda were composed, resulting in the creation of full-fledged specialties. From them, two large specialties developed that resulted in two distinct schools—the school of medicine and the school of surgery.

The major treatise of the school of medicine is *Caraka Samhita,* originally written by Atreya in approximately 1000 BC. Subsequently, Caraka and later Drdhrabala improved on it. The text continues to be called *Caraka Samhita.* The major treatise of the schools of surgery is *Susruta Samhita,* which was originally written by Susruta between 1000 BC and 500 BC. Susruta devoted the greatest portion of his work to anatomy, surgical instruments and procedures, inflammation, surgical diseases, military medicine (care of the king and his troops in the battlefield), obstetric procedures, and poisoning.[4]

In Ayurveda, diseases are described under *nidana* (etiology), *samprapti* (pathogenesis), *purvarupa* (prodrome), *rupa* (signs and symptoms), *upasaya* (therapeutic suitability), and *ausadha* (therapeutics). Caraka says that one should examine the patient, consider the drug, and thereafter proceed with the treatment.[5] Pharmaceutic processes and preparations that involved fermenting, extracting, preparing inhalant substances, filtrating, heating in a closed cavity, purifying, and making pills are described.[6]

Ayurveda has drawn its basic concepts from the different philosophic systems of ancient India. The *Samkya-Patanjala* (*Samkya* = discriminative) systems and the *Nyaya-Vaisesika* (*Nyaya* = logical) system have considerably influenced the physical, physiochemical, physiologic, and pharmacologic theories of Ayurveda. The *Samkya-Patanjala* system accounts for the creation of the universe and composition of matter on the principles of cosmic evolution. The *Nyaya-Vaiseska* system lays down the methodology of scientific studies and elaborates on the concepts of mechanics, physics, chemistry, and medical sciences.[6] The manifested world, according to the *Samkya-Patanjala* system, is an evolution of the unmanifested *prakreti* or primordial matter, which is conceived as formless and undifferentiated, limitless and ubiquitous, indestructible and nondecaying, ungrounded and uncontrolled, and

without beginning or end. It is an undifferentiated manifold of three attributes called the *sattva,* the *rajas,* and the *tamas.* The *sattva* attribute is the medium of reflection of intelligence. The *rajas* represent the energy through which work overcomes resistance. The *tamas* is the mass or inertia in which the effects of rajas and sattva, in the form of energy and conscience, respectively, are manifested. The *rajas,* in combination with the *sattva,* help the creation of the sensory and motor faculties, including the mental faculty.

There are nine *dravyas* or categories of matter. Of these nine, five are together referred to as *mahabhutas,* namely, *prthvi* (earth), *ap* (water), *tejas* (heat), *vayu* (air), and *akasa* (universe). The remaining four *dravyas* are *dik* (direction or space), *kala* (time), *atman* (soul), and *manas* (mind). *Panchamahabhutas* (*pancha* = five) are five great elements that originated from subtle vibrations. The primordial sound (Om) created the first element, space. As space became mobile, its movement created the second element, air. The friction produced from these movements created heat and light engendering the third element, fire. The heat of the fire element dissolved and liquefied portions of the space and air elements, as well as a portion of itself, and manifested the water element. Some portion of the water element condensed to form the fifth element, earth. From these five basic elements—space, air, fire, water, and earth—all organic life was not only created, but continues to play a major role in the maintenance of health. In humans, fire is expressed as a metabolic process of the body's trillions of cells, each generating heat and energy, and maintaining body heat and various chemical processes. Water forms a major component of the human body, comprising as much as 78% of total body weight in an average individual. Water is a vital part of cytoplasm, digestive secretions, and various biologic fluids, including cerebrospinal fluid, blood, and lymph. Oxygen from the air forms the vital component for survival of tissue. The component of earth can be compared to various bones, tendons, skin, hair, nails, and other solid structures, which often contain various minerals and other elements.

Mahabhutas are present in the biologic world, including the human body, in a particular proportion. The human body grows during young age, attains a plateau during adulthood, and reaches a decayed or reduced state during old age. During all these stages of human life, the *mahabhutas* remain in a particular proportion in a state of equilibrium in the human body. Because the activities of life force are represented in the action of *agni,* or enzymes, the natural consequence is that the *mahabhutas* are consumed to generate energy and heat during the different stages of life. This natural loss is replenished and normal growth and stability are achieved by the supplementing *mahabhutas* through intrinsic and extrinsic sources. These sources include food, drink, air, light, and mental activities. If there is any change in this equilibrium of *mahabhutas* in the human body, disease and decay result. To correct this state of imbalance, patients are given various types of drug, food, and drink regimens that help maintain a state of equilibrium. This, in brief, is the concept underlying the basis for selecting a drug for the treatment of a disease in Ayurveda.

However, it is very difficult to ascertain the nature of the *mahabhutas* that have undergone changes in the body. It is also difficult to determine the quantum of *mahabhutas* present in a particular drug, diet, or regimen. For this reason the theoretical concept in Ayurveda is simplified with a view to enable the physician to determine with ease and convenience the nature of the disturbance in the body and the type of drug and diet regimen required for the person in health or disease.

The five *mahabhutas,* which participate as composition of the human body, are classified into three categories—*doshas, dhatus,* and *malas. Doshas* govern the physiologic and physio-chemical activities of the body and are three in number, namely, *vatha, pitta,* and *kapha* (these are not to be translated as wind, bile, and phlegm, respectively). *Vatha* is responsible for all the movements and sensations, including motor actions and propagation of nerve impulses. *Pitta* is responsible for all physio-chemical activities of the body in the form of metabolism (production of heat and energy). *Kapha* is the substance that maintains compactness or cohesiveness in the body by providing it with the fluid matrix. *Vatha* is considered the most important of the three *doshas* because it provides the movement for the other two relatively immobile *doshas.* The *dhatus* are the seven tissue elements of the body. They are *rasa* (chyle or plasma), *rakta* (red blood corpuscles), *mamsa* (muscle), *medas* (fat tissue), *asthi* (bone), *majja* (bone marrow), and *sukra* and *rajas* (sperm and ovum, respectively). Nervous tissue is considered *medas.* The *malas,* or the waste products, consist of feces, urine, and sweat. The catabolic products of the body in the form of unwanted *mahabhutas* are eliminated through the waste products.

According to Ayurvedic concepts, these *doshas* are in a state of homeostasis during health. Any disturbance of the homeostasis of *doshas* can lead to disease.

The type of disease or signs and symptoms depends on the type of disturbance. For example, nervous and mental disorders are said to originate from a disturbance of *vatha* humor. An individual is born with a predominant *dosha,* which contributes to his or her constitution *(prakarti).* In addition to the genetic influence, a person's constitution is affected by environment, diet, and age. The three *doshas* are subdivided into numerous sub-*doshas* with different locations and functions throughout the body. During health there is a balance of the three *doshas.* Any disturbance or imbalance of one *dosha* with respect to the others results in disease or disorder. *Vatha* imbalance predisposes an individual to disorders such as diseases of the nervous system, chronic pain, cardiac arrhythmia, rheumatic disorders, anxiety, and insomnia. *Pitta* governs digestion, assimilation, metabolism, temperature regulation, hunger, and thirst. Individuals with *pitta prakarti* (*pitta* constitution) are predisposed to peptic ulcers, hypertension, inflammatory bowel disease, skin diseases, and allergic reactions. *Kapha* in its healthy state removes cohesiveness in the body and gives stability, lubrication, strength, resistance to immunologic diseases, tranquility of mind, and emotional stability. *Kapha* imbalance predisposes a person toward diseases of the upper respiratory system, sinusitis, diabetes melitis, obesity, and cancer.[7]

NEUROSCIENCES

The brain was differentiated from the head even in the *Atharvaveda.* Susruta studied anatomy by dissecting cadavers and considered the brain *(mastiska* or *hrt)* to be the only organ that made the function of all other organs possible. The *Atharvaveda* referred to nervous tissue as *nadidhatu* and included such terms as intelligence-carrying channels *(buddhivaha sira)* and psycho-cortical routes *(marovaha srotas).* The spinal cord is referred to as *susumna* and the vertebral column as *prsthavamsa.* Bhela, a contemporary of Caraka, considered the brain to be the center of mind.[8] Mind *(manus)* is considered to be connected with cognitions and is associated with the brain being located between palate and vertex (frontal lobe). *Manus* is given considerable importance in Ayurveda and is the basis of mind-body medicine. Autonomic nervous system and various plexus were recognized in Ayurveda. In its highest level, yoga is learning to voluntarily control autonomic functions such as cardiac and respiratory rate, body temperature, and blood pressure.

Sensory symptoms were recognized in Ayurveda. Numbness of feet was referred to as *padasuptala;* numbness of both hands and feet was called *karapada-suptala*. The loss of sensation was referred to as *supti;* the loss of sensation to touch was called *sparsajnatva;* and the loss of sensation to cold was *sitasparsavedana*. Peripheral neuropathy was referred to as *packa daha* and radiculopathy as *giddhasi*.

Coma was *synnyasa,* and stupor *tandra*. Excessive drowsiness was called *tandratiyoga,* and lethargy was *dirghasutrata*. Syncope was referred to as *murccha,* and vertigo and dizziness as *bhrama*. Signs of death were known and were called *arista*.

Ayurveda is based on concepts that are explainable using contemporary scientific principles. Although a disease might have been present in only one organ or the entire individual with the realization that the whole individual was affected physically, mentally, and spiritually. Nevertheless, specific diseases, such as depression, epilepsy, migraine, Parkinson's disease, and others, and their treatments were recognized and treated. Discussion of a few neurologic conditions follows.

HEADACHE

The headache is well recognized in Ayurveda and is referred to as *shirah shoola*. Migraine and tension headaches are two separate disorders. The cause is considered to be an imbalance of the three humors (*vatha, pitta,* and *kapha*). Migraine is referred to as *ardha-vabhedaka; Sankhak* is severe bitemporal headache. The frontal headache is called *lalatabheda,* and the fronto-temporal headache is *shankhabheda*. Headaches secondary to central nervous system (CNS) infections, head injury, tumors, and blood-related disorders are also described. Treatments include use of various herbal decoctions, massages to the head, and avoidance of stress and excessive alcohol intake. A middle path is recommended with less stressful occupation, meditation, and stress reduction by yoga practice.

AGING AND DEMENTIA

In Ayurveda, geriatrics falls under *Rasayana* and encompasses a comprehensive discipline aimed at promoting longevity, imparting immunity against disease, and furthering mental competence. This includes improving memory, skin luster, voice, and sexual vigor, and promoting a healthy state of all organs. *Rasayana* is not only a drug therapy but also a regimen covering the general mode of life, social conduct, behavior, diet, and use of specific restorative remedies. *Rasayana* is a process by which all of the body tissues regenerate and various organs are toned to delay the aging process and promote a healthful long life. The word *Rasa* means normalcy of health. The practice of *Rasayana* therapy is advocated to improve a number of specific conditions, such as individual constitution (*Prakrati*), aging, tissue restoration (*Satmya*), microcirculation (*Spotasa*), digestion and metabolism (*Agni*), and vitality (*Ojas*). It is said that this process should begin in late adulthood or midlife. It will not be effective if it is started too late because many of the approaches are preventive rather than curative. *Vajikarana* includes restoring sexual potency and improving resistance to disease (immunity). Therapeutics in *Rasayana* are derived from a wide variety of plants, minerals, and dairy products.

Cognitive function is well recognized in Ayurveda. The mind (*manus*) is thought to be the inner instrument for perception. Mind, ego, and intellect together form an internal organ whose chief function is to receive impulses from the external environment and respond suitably. The system includes sensory and motor organs as accessories. The whole apparatus, consisting of the internal organ and its several accessories, corresponds to the brain and the nervous mechanisms associated with its function, which is similar to concepts in modern psychology.[9] Intelligence is referred to as *Buddhi;* dementia is termed *Cittinasa* (loss of mind). The *Caraka Samhita* outlines seven factors that promote the emergence of memory: perception of cause, perception of form, similarity, contrast, predominance of practice, constant thinking, and repeated hearing. Thus memory is defined as the recollection of what is seen, heard, and experienced.[10]

Rasayana is a method of systemic rejuvenation. It is a broad-based approach to analyzing the aging process and the drugs that may help treat dementia disorders, as described in *Medhya. The Materia Medica of Ayurveda* contains several herbal drugs (botanicals) that have been used to treat dementia for several centuries. They are considered to be both safe and effective.[11]

The Ayurvedic approach to mental function is considered to result in improved memory, intelligence, concentration, and clarity of speech.[5] The emphasis was on delaying the onset of age-related disorders, including dementia. Preventive treatment is to be started in late youth or middle age and should focus on a combination of herbal preparations, diet, exercise, and social behavior. If treatment is started after the onset of symptoms, it is believed to be less effective or ineffective. Details of this treatment are reviewed in the *Journal of Complementary and Alternative Medicine*.[11]

MOVEMENT DISORDERS

Descriptions of various movement disorders are scattered throughout Ayurveda (Table 6-1). Parkinson's disease, under the term *kampavata*, is described in more detail.[12] Various signs and symptoms describing *kampavata* are found among Ayurvedic treatises.[13] These symptoms include dyskinesia, rigidity, tremor, drooling, depression, somnolence, reptilian stare, and stammering. A more precise description is found in Chapter 6 of *The Basavarajiyam*, written in 1400 AD. It stated that a "tremor of hand and feet, difficulty in body movements, disturbed sleep and dementia are symptoms of kampavata."

Ayurveda has described 35 different formulations for the treatment of *kampavata*.[14] At least 18 of these contained *Mucuna pruriens (Atmagupta)*. Not until 1937 was the presence of levodopa in *Mucuna pruriens* known.[15] In 1978 the first clinical trial of *Mucuna pruriens* seed powder was attempted for treatment of paralysis agitans.[16] Using a 6-Hydroxydopamine rat model and rotameter, *Mucuna pruriens* seed powder was compared to synthetic levodopa. Dose for dose, *Mucuna pruriens* was found to be twice as effective as synthetic levodopa.[17] A dose-response evaluation was made of acute and chronic toxicity studies in rabbits and rats, including hematologic, hepatic, and renal

function (complete blood cell count, blood chemistry, and urine analysis) and tissue examination at necropsy (gross and histologic). *Mucuna pruriens* failed to reveal any adverse effects.[18] In a multicenter clinical trial of HP200 (a commercial product containing *Mucuna pruriens* manufactured by Zamdu Pharmaceutical Works, Mumbai, India), 60 patients with Parkinson's disease (46 men and 14 women) with a mean (± SD) age of 59 (± 9) years were treated in an open study for 12 weeks. Of these, 26 patients were taking synthetic levodopa/carbidopa formulations before treatment with HP200. The remaining 34 were levodopa naive. HP200, a powder supplied as a 7.5-g sachet, was mixed with water and given orally. The Unified Parkinson's Disease Rating Scale (UPDRS) was used at baseline and periodically during the 12-week evaluation. Statistically significant reductions in Hoehn & Yahr stage and UPDRS scores were seen from baseline to the end of the 12-week treatment ($p < 0.0001$, t-test). The group mean (± SD) dose for optimal control of symptoms was 6 (± 3) sachets. Adverse effects were mild and were mainly gastrointestinal in nature.[19] An Ayurvedic formulation named *Masabaladi Pacana* contains beans of *Mucuna pruriens* and is used in disorders of *vata*, including *kampavata*.[20] Other Ayurvedic preparations, such as *Chyavanprash* and *Abhayamalaki aveleha*, also contain *Mucuna pruriens* and they, too, are used in the treatment of *kampavata*. Preparations such as *Jatiphatadi churna* and *Parasikyavani churna* are advocated for parkinsonian tremor, but no data are available as to the specific alkaloids present in them.[13] Toxic effects of Atmagupta were also recognized in Ayurveda. These included headache (*Sirah suta*), dystonia (*manyastambha*), fatigue (*srama*), tremor (*kampa*), syncope (*murcha*), and thirst (*trsa*).[4]

TABLE 6-1

Ayurvedic Equivalent Terms for Movement Disorders

Disorder	Ayurvedic Term
Paralysis agitans	Kampavata
Torticollis	Manyagroha
Blepharospasm	Vartmatambha
Tic	Vyariddha spandana
Tremor	Kampa
Head tremor	Sirahkampa

EPILEPSY

Epilepsy is referred to as *apasmara* in Ayurveda. The prefix *apa-* means negation or loss of, and *-smara* means consciousness or memory. The cause of epilepsy was considered to be due to both endogenous and exogenous factors. Among the exogenous factors were internal hemorrhage; high fever; excessive sexual intercourse; disturbances of the body caused by fast running, swimming, and jumping; eating foods that are contaminated; nonhygienic practices; and extreme mental agitation caused by anger, fear, lust, or anxiety. An endogenous disturbance refers to a metabolic derangement in the form of a disturbance of *doshas,* which are aggravated and lodged in the channels of *hrt* (brain). It was also recognized that epilepsy could be secondary to other diseases. Epilepsy *(apasmara)* was distinguished from seizures *(graha),* and both were distinguished from pseudoseizures *(apatantraka).*[21] Aura was recognized and was called *apasmara poorva roopa.* An actual attack of seizures was said to occur when the patient saw nonexistent objects (visual hallucinations), fell down, and had twitching in the tongue, eyes, and eyebrows with jerky movements in the hands and feet associated with excessive salivation. After the paroxysm was over, the patient awakened as if from sleep.[5]

Epilepsy was classified into four types. The *vatika* type is characterized by frequent seizures with uncontrollable crying, unconsciousness, trembling, gnashing of teeth, and rapid breathing. Upon regaining consciousness, the patient has a headache. In *pattika* epilepsy the patient becomes agitated, has sensations of heat and extreme thirst, and has an aura of the environment being on fire. These symptoms are followed by frequent seizures accompanied by groaning and frothing at the mouth and, finally, falling. In *kaphaja* epilepsy the onset of convulsions is delayed and is preceded by an aura during which the patient feels cold and heavy and sees objects as blank. The seizure is accompanied by falling and frothing at the mouth. The fourth type, *sannipatika,* is due to a combination of all of the above. This type occurs in older people, is considered incurable, and results in emaciation.

The first step in the treatment was awakening the patient from unconsciousness by using drastic measures to clear the *doshas* that blocked channels of the mind. After the patient was awake, drug formulations to alleviate epilepsy were administered. Several formulations, including the amount of each ingredient and method of preparation were mentioned in various texts of Ayurveda, such as *Caraka Samhata, Susrata Samhita,* and others. The ingredients of these preparations included sulfur *(gandhaka),*[6] aged ghee (butter fat), and many herbs, such as *Achyranthes aspena, Holanthena antidysenterica, Alstonia scholaris,* and *Ficus carica.* Blends of herbal formulations, such as *Pancamula* and *Triphala,* were also named. General measures to correct exogenous factors, such as proper hygiene and balanced diet, were recommended. Persons with epilepsy, like the insane, were to be protected from deep water, fire, treetops, and hills as a safety measure.

CEREBROVASCULAR DISEASES

Susruta described hemiplegia *(pakshaghata)* as "when extremely agitated vata produces pathologic conditions in the *dhamanis* (nerve chains), which spread either in the left or right side of the body whether in the upward, downward, or lateral direction, making them lax and with no vigor and in which the joints of the other side of the body become useless and inoperable." Table 6-2 lists terms in Sanskrit used for various forms of motor defects. Prognosis was considered poor for paralysis during pregnancy, puerperium, childhood, or old age or in an emaciated person. Paralysis of hemorrhagic origin or paralysis associated with unconsciousness, limb or generalized edema, sensory loss, and severe pain, was expected to have a fatal outcome. Treatment included physical exercise or therapy *(vyayama)* and massage *(abhyangana).* A form of medicated warm oil massage referred to as *panchakarma* was administered for 21 to 30 days depending on the degree of paralysis or spasticity. Massage was the most common form of therapy administered. Those with prior good health and no complications were considered good candidates for rehabilitation *(prakrtisthapana).*

SUMMARY

In conclusion, Ayurveda recognized various neurologic disorders, as well as neuroanatomy and neurophysiology. Yoga, a system that is an outcome of

TABLE 6-2

Ayurvedic Equivalent Terms for Motor Disorders

Disorder	Ayurvedic Term
Paralysis	Jihwastambha
Monoplegia	Ekangaghata
Hemiplegia	Pakshaghata (Syn: Pakshavadha, Pakshata)
Paraplegia	Pangh (Syn: Pangulva)
Quadriplegia	Sarvangaroga
Facial paralysis	Ardita
Foot drop	Padabhrunsa
Stiffness of body part	Angagraha
Contracture	Khalli

Ayurveda, is based on the autonomic nervous system. Meditation is a form of autonomic self-control of the reaction to stress. At its highest form, yoga allows one to control the heart rate or vary the body temperature. It often takes years of practice to attain that level of control. Treatment in Ayurveda is often directed at correcting the balance of metabolic derangement through the use of herbal preparations, dietary regimen, physical therapy, and surgery. Preventive measures are emphasized. In the Western world, Ayurveda is perceived as an alternative medicine; however, in some cultures it has been the mainstream medicine for centuries. Even today in rural India and in several Asian countries, cosmopolitan or Western medicine is considered the alternative medicine, making the terms relative. Medicine knows no geographical boundaries, nationality, race, or religion.

ACKNOWLEDGMENTS

The editorial assistance of Glen Cryer and Lisa Blaschke, the Scientific Publication Office, Scott & White Clinic, and Memorial Hospital, is greatly appreciated.

References

1. Kurup PNV: *Birds-eye-view on indigenous systems of medicine in India,* Delhi, 1977, Depak.
2. Siddhantalankar S: *Heritage of Vedic culture,* Bombay, 1969, Taraporevala & Sons.
3. Jee BS: *A short history of Aryan medical science,* ed 2, Gondal, 1927, Shree Bhabyat Singh Jee Electric Printing Press.
4. Dutt VC: *Materna medica of the Hindus,* Varanasi, 1980, Chowkhmba Saraswalibhawan.
5. Sharma PV, editor-translator: *Caraka-Samhita,* vol. 1, Varanasi, 1981, Chaukhambha Orientalia.
6. Dash VB, Kashyap VL: *Materia medica of Ayurveda,* New Delhi, 1980, Concept Publishing.
7. Sharma HM, Triguna BD, Chopra D: Maharashi Ayur-Veda: modern insights into ancient medicine, *JAMA* 265:2633-2634, 1991.
8. Das Gupta SN: *A history of Indian philosophy,* ed 2, Cambridge, Mass., 1952, Cambridge University Press.
9. Hiriyanna M: *The essentials of Indian philosophy,* London, 1960, Allen & Unwin.
10. Sharma PV: *Charaka-samhita text with English translation,* vol II, Varanasi, 1981, Chaukhambha Orientalia.
11. Manyam BV: Dementia in Ayurveda-Indian medical system, *J Comp. Alt Med* 5:81-88, 1999.
12. Manyam BV, Sanchez-Ramos JR: Traditional and complementary therapies. In Stern G, editor: *Parkinson's disease,* Philadelphia, 1999, Lippincot-Raven.
13. Manyam BV: Paralysis agitans and levodopa in "Ayurveda," ancient Indian medical treatise, *Mov Dis* 5:47-44, 1990.
14. Bhatt NS: Personal communication, 1993.
15. Damodaran M, Ramaswamy R: Isolation of L-dopa from the seeds of Mucuna pruriens, *Biochem* 31:2149-2151, 1937.
16. Vaidya AB, Rajogopalan TG, Mankodi NA et al: Treatment of Parkinson's disease with the Cowhage plant—Mucuna pruriens bak, *Neurol India* 26:171-176, 1978.
17. Hussain G, Manyam BV: Mucuna pruriens proves more effective than L-DOPA in Parkinson's disease animal model, *Phytotherapy Res* 11:419-423, 1997.
18. Manyam BV: HP-200: An affordable and effective treatment for Parkinson's disease, *Neurol India* 42(Suppl):37, 1994.
19. Manyam BV et al: HP-200: An "alternative medicine" treatment for Parkinson's disease, *J Altern Complement Med* 1:249-255, 1995.
20. Sharma PV: Personal communication, 1991.
21. Singhal GD, Tripathi SN, Sharma KR: *Ayurvedic clinical diagnosis based on Madhava-Nidana, part 1,* Varanasi, 1985, Singhal.

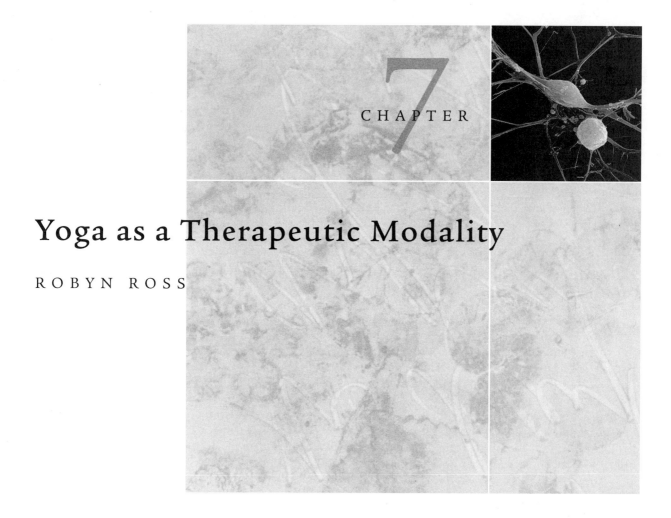

CHAPTER 7

Yoga as a Therapeutic Modality

ROBYN ROSS

Yoga is emerging as a valuable holistic health program for the next millennium. People from all walks of life and many celebrities have publicly touted the benefits of yoga in their lives. As a result of yoga's increasing popularity, influences from yoga can be seen in today's fashions and in advertising, television, and movies. In view of this exposure, many patients may be interested in learning how yoga can be incorporated into their current treatment plan.

Yoga is a philosophy of life, a powerful system of self-improvement. It is not a religion. Therefore such diverse groups as local YMCAs, universities, corporations, community centers, churches and synagogues, and major medical institutions sponsor yoga classes.

Physically, yoga is a low-impact activity so people of all ages, shapes, sizes, and conditions can practice it with relative ease and comfort.

As an eminently pragmatic culture, it makes sense that a major attraction of yoga in this country is its documented capacity to support good health and well being. There is mounting scientific and clinical evidence to support the medical benefits of yoga.[1,2] This chapter illustrates how yoga can be applied as an effective form of therapy for certain neurologic disorders.

In the future, mind-body programs such as yoga will play a complementary role in disease management models that focus on self-care.[3] With the growing interest in alternative medicine, this is the time to approach healthcare with an integrative perspective.

The author would like to thank the photographer, Joan Tedeschi, and models Jason Frome, Ellen Wallach, and Margaretta (Maji) Richards for joining her in demonstrating the postures depicted in this chapter.

WHAT IS YOGA?

In Sanskrit, yoga translates literally as *yuj,* meaning to yoke together, to make whole. Most commonly, however, yoga is translated as union—union of the mind, body, and soul and union of the self to the divine. In the West, yoga has taken many different forms. The most recognizable form today is called *Hatha Yoga,* the physical postures. The Sanskrit root, *Ha,* means sun or positive aspect, and *tha* means moon or negative aspect. It represents the relationship of opposites, such as dark to light, male to female, and yin and yang. *Hatha Yoga* seeks to unite polarities and resolve conflicts into a state of balance, harmony, and union. According to ancient yogis, disease occurs when the body is out of balance. Yoga then comes to mean a way to bring the body into a state of balance, homeostasis, and optimal health.

There are many other paths of yoga, including *Raja Yoga,* which is the way to balance and union through meditation and control of the mind. *Jnana Yoga* is knowledge or study; *Bhakti Yoga* is about devotion and selfless love. *Karma Yoga* is union through service, work, and action, and *Mantra Yoga* is union through sound, vibration, and speech.

This chapter focuses on classic *Hatha Yoga.* This path provides a unique form of physical therapy to help students on their journey toward a broadening knowledge of self and the needs of the mind and body. This therapy will help the student achieve and maintain good physical and mental health and spiritual harmony.

Yoga uses a combination of techniques, including physical postures, breathing exercises, relaxation methodologies, and meditation to reach optimal physical and mental health. Following is a brief overview of the components and benefits that make up a classic yoga session:

- **Centering and meditation** begins the session to bring the student into the present. The student begins to connect inward, to develop concentration, and to focus the mind for the session ahead.
- **Breath control (*Pranayama*)** is a voluntary regulation of breathing to oxygenate the blood and release carbon dioxide buildup. A series of techniques is used to stimulate, balance, or relax the entire system.
- **Warm-ups and stretching** lubricate the joints and start to release muscle tension and increase circulation throughout the body. Warming up increases the range of motion and begins to cultivate body awareness.
- **Postures (*Asanas*)** strengthen the musculoskeletal system and increase flexibility. The postures reeducate the alignment of the bones, ligaments, and tendons. Each posture series is designed to move the body in all planes of motion. It causes an increase of blood to the specific target organ or gland. Increasing the mobility of the spine can ensure a clear pathway of nerves out to the body.
- **Relaxation (*Yoga Nidra* or *Shavasana*)** integrates the system into a state of balance, or homeostasis, giving the student time to let go of physical and emotional tension and to rest deeply.
- **Affirmation and visualization** are sometimes included to recondition the subconscious mind away from negative habitual thoughts. Visualizing health in a certain area brings *prana* (life energy) to that area.
- **Meditation** ends each session to create stillness, a sense of nondoing, and a reconnection to the essential self. Meditation helps create clarity and peace of mind and is a major component of a full yoga practice.

When all these approaches are synthesized, a consistent practice of yoga can create a powerful state of vitality and rejuvenation, a formula for health and healing. Yoga refers to the disease process as *dis-ease,* which means a disturbance in the natural ease or balance of the body. Also contributing to this dis-ease is any form of constriction in the flow of vital life energy, known as *Prana.* Therefore one of the key purposes of yoga is to increase and/or regulate the flow of *Prana* and maintain an environment of organic stability.

Hatha Yoga and meditation, as adjunctive therapies for promoting and maintaining wellness, offer an excellent example of the mind-body connection at work. *Hatha Yoga* creates balance, both physically and emotionally, as it opens the door to self-actualization to create the perfect union of mind, body, and spirit.[4]

HISTORY AND PHILOSOPHY

Yoga, which began about 5000 years ago in India, may be the oldest mind-body health system known today. According to an article in *YogaWorld,* "It is that the great sages spontaneously practiced yoga, evolving out of their relationship and harmony with nature. Using their deepest intuition, intelligence, and experience, they became familiar and instinctual about the energy flowing throughout all life forms. They developed natural ways to access, build, nurture and direct the energy for greater health and awareness."[5]

There is no one historical reference to the beginning of yoga, so there is no one manuscript to explicate yoga. Several ancient texts contribute to the body of knowledge about yoga and its history. Among these are the *Vedas,* the *Upanishads,* the *Bhagavad Gita,* and the *Yoga Sutras.*

The Hindu scriptures, *Vedas* (knowledge), which are the oldest written tradition in India (second century AD), explore the possibilities of the human spirit and discuss the purpose and meaning of life. The *Ayru Vedas* contain early writings about health and medical treatments; *Ayurveda* is the *Vedic* science of healing that uses yoga as one of its modalities.

The *Upanishads,* possibly dating as far back as the middle of the second millennium BC, are philosophical poems that explore the nature of the universal soul; that is, they are a collection of metaphysical speculations. The *Upanishads* (meaning to sit down close to one's teacher) is a reference to the mode in which esoteric knowledge is transmitted by word of mouth from teacher (guru) to student (disciple).[6] The *Maitri Upanishad* in particular outlines the essential practices of yoga.

The *Bhagavad Gita* (Lords Song) from the third or fourth century BC is one of yoga's core sacred texts. Written as a dialog between Lord Krishna and his devotee, Arjuna, it is a story of the battle between good and evil within us. It also discusses the various yogic paths toward liberation, such as *Jnana Yoga, Karma Yoga, Bhakti Yoga,* and *Hatha Yoga.*

The *Yoga Sutras of Pantanjali* (aphorisms on yoga) from the second century BC presents yoga in a coherent and systematized format. Most modern yogis regard it as an authoritative text on yoga, and all the different schools of yoga recognize it. The *Yoga Sutras* are a philosophical compilation with direct techniques for spiritual advancement. Included is the eight-fold path of yoga or eight limbs:

1. *Yama:* social ethics, restraints
2. *Niyama:* personal ethics, observances
3. *Asana:* discipline of the body
4. *Pranayama:* discipline of the breath
5. *Pratyahara:* withdrawal of the senses
6. *Dharana:* mental concentration
7. *Dhyana:* contemplation, meditation
8. *Samadhi:* bliss, union with the supreme.

Various schools of yoga emphasize different techniques, but the goal of *union* is always the same. *Hatha Yoga* uses practices mentioned in the sutras, such as breath control, meditation, and physical postures as the path to awaken spiritual awareness. This awakening ultimately leads to self-realization and vital health.

Georg Feuerstein wrote, "Yoga is comprised of so many different approaches and schools that one is justified in calling it the most versatile spiritual tradition in the world."[7] Classic yoga as we know it emerged as a tradition about 500 BC. A strong influence of yoga can also be seen in Buddhism, but even though yoga was originated within the Hindu culture, today Christians, Jews, Muslims, and Hindus all practice yoga while maintaining devotion to their traditional religious beliefs. It cannot be emphasized enough that yoga is not a religion but instead a practical science of self-improvement.

Guided by these texts, the various paths, and accomplished teachers, the aim of the yogi is to eventually experience liberation, that is, self-realization and self-knowledge. Liberation or freedom comes when the yogi breaks the bond of old mental habits, destructive patterns, and physical disease, thereby achieving the ability to live in harmony, vitality, and peace of mind. Yoga is a valuable philosophy to apply to everyday life. One of the primary reasons that yoga is so effective as a healing tool is that it is not just a dynamic system of physical exercise and health promotion. Rather, yoga is about a deeper understanding of the self.

Yoga can then be described as a true holistic concept, one involving the whole person and affecting the mind, body, and spirit. The yoga teacher simply helps students take control of their body, breath, and mind and thereby begin to take control of their lives.

THERAPEUTIC YOGA

The power of yoga to affect healing should not be underestimated, however, because its efficacy is well documented in the scientific literature. Yoga techniques are being used increasingly as an adjunct to medical management. Many major medical institutions and physicians in private practice now refer their patients to qualified yoga teachers who can use yoga as a restorative modality. Yoga has become extremely adaptable and effective in aiding the process of healing and can be easily executed in a chair, in bed, or even in a wheelchair. The ancient postures can be modified in many creative ways, and the results have been very encouraging.

The various components that make up a yoga session can be useful for patients with particular neurologic aliments. Using yoga for rehabilitation has diverse applications. Studies show that many physically handicapped subjects had restorations of some degree of functional ability after practicing yoga.[8]

As discussed, breathing techniques, postures, meditation, and relaxation are specifically designed to bring the student into a profound understanding of the self. This understanding leads to *a deeper awareness and understanding of the body,* which will eventually be the ultimate teacher for the student. They will be better suited to communicate their symptoms in specific and clear terms, which means that patients can be better partner physicians for a more integrative approach to their recovery. Studies reveal that patients are motivated to pursue complementary approaches to become active participants in their own healing process, which can also help patients cope with their disease.[9]

The objective is to use yoga as a therapeutic technique. Yoga therapists (YTs) evaluate the best way to help clients with their particular difficulties and disabilities and adapt the yoga postures accordingly. The YT takes a personal and medical history and then draws upon available resources, as well as personal experience, knowledge, and intuition, to help the client. Various yogic techniques are incorporated along with props and/or hands-on assistance when necessary. Sessions in restorative yoga can be very nurturing and can heal the effects of chronic stress.[49] Each session is specifically designed to include breathing techniques, gentle movements, and relaxation and meditation routines that accurately address the patient's problems and provide support on the path toward health and wholeness.

Special emphasis must be expressed to the patient to approach the exercises with compassion and to listen deeply to the body's messages. What makes yoga different from traditional physical therapy is the intense one-pointed concentration on the task at hand and the deep yogic breathing that is incorporated into every movement. The client learns never to strive or to push the body past its limitations. The postures are all executed with steadiness and ease (*sthria* and *sukha*),

and without strain or struggle. Yoga is eventually performed with "effortless effort." A nonjudgmental attitude is also key and should be encouraged throughout the session. Individuals should begin to practice accepting the body as it is in the present, from one moment to the next. Movements must be slow and gentle, completely conscious, and always coordinated with the breath. An inner awareness develops, so patients learn where the joints and muscles feel restricted and where they feel more flexible. From there patients begin their healing journey.

YOGA FOR STRESS REDUCTION

In a society addicted to stress, and with its tendency to overactivate the sympathetic high-arousal system, many serious stress-related illnesses have developed. According to medical statistics, 70% of all diseases are stress related. Because its purpose is to relax, rejuvenate, and restore the body, mind, and spirit, yoga is one of the most powerful tools to counteract the stress response. Yoga postures, combined with meditation and *pranayama* (breath control), can neutralize this overarousal by using clinically proven techniques to help elicit the parasympathetic functions and decrease sympathetic discharges. Postures and breath work can begin to equalize and alter autonomic responses; thus yoga can create a time for the body to recover from the imbalance stress can place on the body and mind.

Numerous studies have shown a statistically significant fall in both systolic and diastolic blood pressure[11] and a reduction of the heart rate with the practice of yoga.[12] Moreover, significant clinical differences can be observed concerning coping with stress and mood elevation at the end of experiments using yoga.[13] *Pranayama* (breath control), for instance, appears to alter autonomic responses by increasing vagal tone[10] (see Breathing Techniques). A regular practice of yoga can therefore be used as an essential recuperative tool for dealing with the effects of stress. According to I.S. Chohan, "Yoga is known to induce beneficial effects on physiological, biochemical and mental functions in man."[14] It is also important to note that yoga may be used to stimulate sympathetic activity when it is therapeutically indicated.

To maintain health and well being, life's challenges must be balanced with periods of rest and relaxation. Sleep disturbances, headaches, and muscle spasms, to name only a few, are often symptomatic of a person's inability to fully relax. Brownstein and Dembert wrote, "Relaxation training, of which yoga is one type, has been reported in the medical literature to have wide clinical application. It should be considered as a nonpharmacological therapy adjunct or alternative for medical disorders."[15]

Jamiel described yoga this way:

In day to day life, the mindful awareness that yoga cultivates can allow a patient to become more readily aware of any quickened respiration, muscular tension and other physical symptoms of stress. This awareness gives one the ability to consciously interrupt the habitual stress response by doing something as simple as taking a breath or moving the body. Hence, the integration of the yogic breathwork, focused awareness and relaxation during day to day life may afford the greatest opportunity for stress reduction. Like traditional Chinese and Tibetan medicine, the Indian system views health as a state of balance sustained by diet, lifestyle and mental attitudes. The traditional view maintains that when this delicate balance is disturbed, various disorders may arise. Yoga is not a medicine, per se, but a system of practices that can restore and maintain this balance.[16]

POTENTIAL BENEFITS OF YOGA

Following are some of the beneficial clinical outcomes of the practice of yoga:
- Decreased blood pressure
- Reduced heart rate
- Decreased sympathetic stimulation
- Increased parasympathetic tone
- Increased joint range of motion
- Increased body strength, stamina, and flexibility
- Improved balance
- Decreased symptoms of carpal tunnel syndrome
- Enhanced mental alertness, memory, concentration, and focus
- Better circulation and oxygenation of the blood
- More efficient breathing
- Decreased muscle stiffness

Beneficial anecdotal outcomes of the practice of yoga include the following:
- Relief of constipation and stimulation of digestion
- Improved body awareness of physical posture
- Decreased muscular fatigue

- Relief of back pain and joint pain
- Reduced pain
- Stress reduction and relaxation
- Improved posture and muscle tone
- Decreased emotional tension
- Decreased premenstrual and menopausal symptoms
- A more positive outlook on life

POTENTIAL RISKS

Because of the demand for yoga and the many yoga classes that are appearing, it is more important than ever to find a qualified YT. Since yoga uses the body in ways that are perhaps new to most people, there is always a chance for injury. Depending on the patient's condition, it may be advantageous for him or her to have private yoga sessions with a certified YT or qualified teacher. For those who are new to yoga, it is advisable to start with a class designed specifically for beginners, regardless of athletic background. The postures must be taught clearly and safely. The teacher must be attentive and involved in each students' participation. The student should not simply be expected to follow along. Just as in the selection of a physician, care must be taken to determine the training and experience of the teacher (see Finding a Yoga Teacher). Presently YTs are not licensed in this country, and the length of training necessary to be certified varies from years to as little as one weekend.

Inadequately supervised yoga practice has resulted in injuries ranging from simple strains to a case of sciatic neuropathy in the thigh, resulting from prolonged sitting in the lotus posture.[47]

There are general precautions and contraindications that can be followed to prevent undue injury. Certain inverted postures, those that bring the head below the heart, are contraindicated for people with untreated or malignant hypertension, heart conditions, some nervous disorders, and pregnancy. Recent surgeries and certain chronic conditions or severe inflammation may prohibit specific movements. During acute sciatica or a herniated disk, certain movements should be prohibited. When balance is impaired from multiple sclerosis (MS) or Parkinson's, special modifications are used for balancing postures. When necessary, yoga can even be performed in a wheelchair or in bed.

As mentioned, the advantage of yoga is that it can be modified to meet the needs of even high-risk individuals. Because of its gentle nature, yoga can be applied even when a patient is recovering from a serious injury. The author was on staff as a yoga therapist at Columbia-Presbyterian Medical Center in New York City for 3 years developing a yoga program for cardiac patients, 3 days postoperative. She worked with these patients bedside or they came to a group chair yoga class. Even with the inherent risks involved, she was able to devise a protocol to guide them through a complete experience of simple yoga postures, breathing techniques, meditation, and relaxation. Patients were able to move their bodies in a safe and gentle way after this invasive major surgery. Many patients reported that following the yoga session they felt a decrease in postoperative pain, a mood elevation, increased energy, and a reconnection to the body. It also had a relaxing and calming effect. D. MacArthur, a heart transplant patient, gratefully reported that "the yogic breathing and stretching was an adaptable tool that I was able to draw upon whenever I needed it during my recuperation. I was also able to incorporate the breathing tools into my life, especially within stressful situations." MacArthur race walked the last two New York City marathons and used his yogic breathing as an important addition to his training, as well as during the race. Looking back at the experience at the hospital, the author is once again amazed at the adaptability and efficacy of yoga for high-risk individuals.

CLINICAL APPLICATIONS

Yogis have always used themselves as empirical research laboratories. In fact, the brilliance of yoga is that it integrates the spiritual with the empirical. Spiritual practices that lead to desired outcomes are integrated into the discipline, and those that do not are eliminated. The result is a system designed over thousands of years to promote the outcome of good health. In clinical applications, we take much the same empirical approach that is used by yogis. Postures are suggested based on past successes, the yogic literature, and the growing body of evidence-based research; however, client outcome always determines the efficacy of the treatment plan. Since the essence of yoga is developing awareness, beginning to incorporate it can be as straightforward as paying attention to one's breath for a few minutes each day.[16]

Nadis and the Nervous System

It is fascinating to note that a system in yoga called the *Nadis* bears a remarkable resemblance to modern anatomic descriptions of nerves and plexus. The ancient manuals of yoga anatomy describe a network of several thousand *Nadis* that are considered to be energy channels, tubes, or pathways throughout the gross and subtle body.[17] They have been compared to the nerve plexi, which controls the autonomic nervous system.

One of the many ways that *prana* (life energy) passes through the physical body is via the *nadis* (nerve plexus). To accomplish this the *prana* is absorbed and then flows via this plexus throughout the nervous system to the rest of the body. According to Hindu scriptures, there are 350,000 energy channels in the system (Figure 7-1).[18] Of these channels the *Sushumna, Ida,* and *Pingala* are the most important. The main channel is the *Sushumna,* or line of energy, which stems from the root of the tailbone and goes up the spine. The *Ida* and the *Pingala* are two major energy channels that intertwine up the spine. They are usually pictured as two snakes coiling up a centerline. The coils meet and cross at seven spinning energy centers called the *Chakras.* Illustrations of the *Sushumna* with the *Ida* and *Pingala* are an identical representation of the caduceus, which is used as a symbol of the medical model today (Figure 7-2).

It is easy to see how these ancient texts parallel the modern. For instance, the *Pingala* represents the sympathetic nervous system (SNS), which is responsible for the left brain functions, the right nostril breathing,[19,20] the solar energy, or the fight or flight. The *Ida,* representing the parasympathetic nervous system (PNS), is responsible for the right brain functions, the left nostril breathing,[19] the lunar energy, or the relaxation response. Various yoga postures, sounds, and *pranayama* techniques are used to open and balance the vital flow of energy through these *Nadis.* This is a complicated and subtle practice.

Treatments

There can be no standard treatment plan for yoga. Any program that is prescribed is a synthesis of what a client is able and willing to do and what is appropriate for the client at that moment. The ability to modify traditional postures whenever it is necessary to fit the client's need is vital. It is also important that each program be de-signed to move all joints within a pain-free range of motion. The YT assesses the patient and prescribes the appropriate treatments specific to the problem.

Whenever feasible, it would be helpful for the YT to maintain a working relationship with the student's physician during the yoga treatment. This integrative form of health care can lead to strong support for the patient. The following treatments provide basic ideas that can be used to treat certain disorders. Please note that for clarity, the classic Sanskrit terminology is not used when referring to the yoga postures in this section. Examples of certain yoga postures are provided in this chapter.

Breathing Techniques

Proper breathing is the foundation of yoga and may be used by itself as treatment for many disorders. Life force is called *Prana,* to master or control is *Ayama.* Therefore to master the life force through breath control is translated as *Pranayama.* The system of *Hatha Yoga asanas* (postures) and breathing is based on balancing and increasing the flow of *Prana* in the body. The key to understanding *Prana* and energy is breath. Yoga postures without the awareness of breath are just movement, not yoga.

There are many *pranayama* techniques that can be incorporated into a yoga practice. The following are recommended:

The way one breathes has a profound effect on health. Many people breathe short, shallow, rapid breaths that actually elicit the SNS. The **three-part yogic breath** *(Dirgha)* is full deep breathing that allows the abdominal area to expand, then opens the rib cage area, and brings the breath all the way up to the clavicular region. The breath then releases from the chest, or rib cage area, and finally the abdominals are contracted to promote full exhalation.

This type of breathing encourages the diaphragm, the lower ribs, and the muscles in the back to expand, thereby opening up more space and massaging the abdominal organs. Barbara Phillips, MD, a professor of pulmonary and critical care medicine at the University of Kentucky College of Medicine in Lexington notes, "As you breathe more slowly and fully with awareness, that brings more oxygen to the body, slowing the heart rate and triggering the PNS creating a

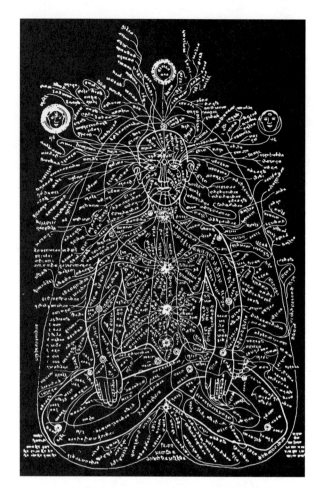

Figure 7-1 Ancient Hindu drawing of the Nadis and Chakras. (From Hills C, editor: *Energy, Matter & Form,* Boulder Creek, Calif., 1977, University of the Trees Press, p. 238.)

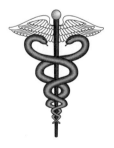

Figure 7-2 "The caduceus, modern symbol for healing, traces the path of Chakras and Nadis, with the Ida & Pingala emanating from the base to the two winged petals at the top." (From Anodea J: *Wheels of Life,* St Paul, Minn., 1987, Llewellyn.)

feeling of relaxation and calm." Breathing is clinically shown to influence the PNS and the SNS.

The control of *Prana* is the regulation of inhalation and exhalation. By adjusting the ratio of inhalation to exhalation we can adjust and influence the relative emphasis given to each activity. John Clark, MD, Harvard Medical School and board certified in cardiology, family practice, and internal medicine writes, "The technique of 2-to-1 breathing for instance, where the exhalation is twice as long as the inhalation will indicate a drop in the arousal level of the SNS and increase the influence of the PNS."[21] One can also count the number of breaths to provide a focus for the mind, simply doubling the number of exhalations to inhalations.

Another technique involves **alternate nostril breathing** (ANB), or *Nadi Shodhanam* and *Anuloma Viloma.* There are many variations of ANB, each with a particular purpose; yet they all have the common theme of alternating the flow of breath between two nostrils.[22] This is done by simply closing off one nostril with the thumb or ring finger of the right hand, inhaling through one nostril and exhaling through the alternate nostril, back and forth. This is a continuous, long, silent relaxed flow of air. Studies suggest that ANB has a balancing effect on the functional activity of the left and right hemisphere of the brain.[23] Left nostril breathing showed a reduction of the SNS; right nostril breathing showed an increase in metabolism due to increased sympathetic discharge to the adrenal medulla. These results indicate that breathing selectively through either nostril could have a marked activating effect or relaxing effect on the SNS.[19] Therapeutic implications to alter metabolism by changing the breathing pattern may also be hypothesized.[24]

Kapalabhati pranayama, referred to as **the breath of fire,** is a technique of rapid respiration. The technique demonstrates a unique unilateral effect on sympathetic stimulation of the heart that may have therapeutic value.[25] This form of *pranayama* employs quick abdominal contractions and expulsion of air through both nostrils upon exhalation. Using this technique will increase physical and mental energy. According to Dharma Singh Khalsa, MD, in his book *Brain Longevity,* "It is believed to be effective because it stimulates the splanchnic nerves in the abdominal cavity. Stimulation of these nerves causes the release of epinephrine and norepinephrine."[26]

The *Ujjayi* breath, also known as the **ocean-sounding breath,** is another *pranayama* technique used to relax the nervous system. This is done by constricting the epiglottis slightly and creating a hissing sound at the back of the throat. Ujjayi pranayama is deeply soothing and centering. The mind becomes absorbed and focused by the sound which induces meditation. This technique can be applied to all of the treatments listed.

Thoughts and feelings influence breath; therefore in yoga breath is thought to influence emotions and attitudes. These basic-breathing techniques are the simplest and most effective of the stress-management techniques. They can be done anytime, anywhere.

Learning how to breathe effectively has a profound balancing effect on the nervous system. Scientific evidence indicates that a yoga therapy program can result in a significant increase in pulmonary function and greater exercise tolerance as well.[27] The adequate flow of breath constantly supports good physical health.[28,29,30]

Additional Readings

Benson H: *The relaxation response,* New York, 1975, Avon Books.

Migdow J, Loehr JE: *Breath in, breath out,* New York, 1999, Time Life.

Ornish D: *Dr. Dean Ornish's program for reversing heart disease,* New York, 1996, Ballantine.

MULTIPLE SCLEROSIS

Stress and tension play a part in an attack of MS. When muscle tension increases spasticity, spasms and clumsiness also increase. Problems with balance and movement tend to make the body compensate by using other muscles, which can also add to chronic muscle tension. Yoga can aid in relaxing the entire body to help reduce this stress and mental stress as well. This awareness is the hallmark of yoga, representing centuries of wisdom. The patient should begin with very slow movements and deep awareness to help locate the muscles that are weak or inflexible and therefore inhibiting movement. The patient can then begin to increase the number of movements, expending the least effort. Through that awareness the patient can work to bring strong and weak muscle groups into balance. The body then becomes less awkward and strain is alleviated.

Yoga *asanas* (postures) tone the neuromuscular system and may help to correct postural abnormalities, a crucial aspect of proper walking. Postures can also help return joints to their proper alignment. Yogic stretching and strengthening postures can return a degree of usefulness to a limb that has lost its ability to function. Howard Kent, director of The Yoga for Health Foundation in Bedfordshire, England, states, "We have evidence that where people are effectively maintaining a yoga practice both mentally and physically, it is rare for us to find deterioration in patients with MS. By the correct use of breathing, mental relaxation and postures, I have seen people move legs with control, which have not moved in years."[31] In addition, studies have shown improvement in the degree of plasticity in motor control systems with the practice of yoga.[32] Certain stretching exercises may also be useful for temporarily relieving pain.

Because this disease brings on inefficient breathing patterns, it is important to incorporate deep rhythmic breathing into this routine for oxygenation of the cells, relaxation, and energy. These postures can be practiced on the floor, seated in a chair, or standing with support.

Postures
Cat/dog (see illustrated box on p. 85)
Supine butterfly
Half locust
Leg lifts
Cobra (modified), sphinx (see illustrated box on p. 85)
Bridge (modified)
Boat (modified)
Seated mountain, seated half moon (see illustrated box on p. 84)
Hug both knees in chest
Mountain with wall support
Wind reliever and circle knees
Legs on wall
Seated spinal twist (see illustrated box on p. 84)
Warrior with chair
Forward bend on floor/chair
Triangle with wall
Breathing
Three-part yogic breath
Alternate nostril breathing
Meditation on breath

To what extent these postures can be practiced depends on the individual and the degree of disability. At first patients may find certain movements difficult, but with steady practice they may accomplish actions they would not have thought possible. The routine is very simple and adaptable. Props can be used to aid in safety and stability and to prevent added stress or fatigue. Because people dealing with MS are often advised not to get overheated, yoga can also be done in a pool, where props, such as blocks and ropes, can help the patient hold poses longer. A student with MS, Eric Small, later became a YT. He claimed to feel stronger and less fatigued, his digestion improved, he could walk farther, and he felt more centered after beginning yoga. His depression, which is often associated with MS, lifted. It has been 25 years since he has had a serious attack.[33]

CARPAL TUNNEL

With the growing use of computer keyboards, there has been a high incidence of carpal tunnel syndrome (CTS) during the past 10 years. Repetitive stress injuries (RSI) can also occur in many other occupations, from musicians and athletes to construction workers. To prevent RSI and CTS the individual must take awareness breaks throughout the day. One of the most beneficial aspects of yoga is the cultivation of body and breath awareness. Patients should be encouraged to apply the awareness they have developed during the yoga session to their body alignment, breath, and repetitive movements.

The easiest way to prevent CTS and RSI is with simple yoga postures concentrating on hand, arm, and body movements coordinated with breath. It is important to establish a routine and to execute it on a regular basis throughout the workday. Exercising the wrists and fingers eases stiffness and tenderness. It is important to focus on upper body yoga postures to improve flexibility and decrease muscle tension. Frequent yoga breaks are crucial since prolonged repetitive physical actions cause this syndrome. It is also important to get up from the desk intermittently, move around, and do some yoga stretches for the entire body. Proper working posture and correct positioning of everything on the desk also aids in the prevention of CTS because poor posture creates added stress on arms and wrists. Yoga emphasizes correct posture and teaches students techniques for sitting, standing, and moving in proper alignment. Correcting alignment of hands, wrists, arms, and shoulders; stretching; and increasing awareness of optimal joint position during use are all preventative measures for CTS.[34]

Yoga Postures

The following photos illustrate various Yoga postures discussed in this chapter.

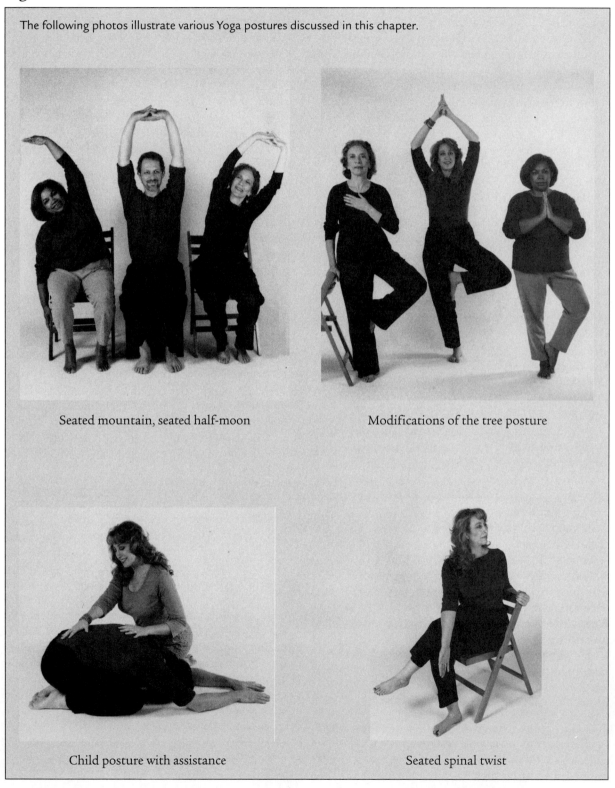

Seated mountain, seated half-moon

Modifications of the tree posture

Child posture with assistance

Seated spinal twist

Yoga Postures—cont'd

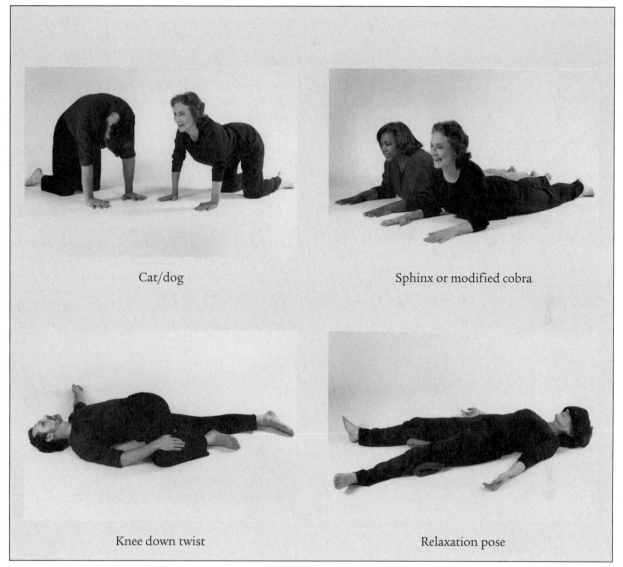

Cat/dog

Sphinx or modified cobra

Knee down twist

Relaxation pose

A recent study published in *JAMA* shows how yoga and relaxation techniques can alleviate pain and tenderness and increase the range of motion for patients with CTS. In this randomized trial, subjects were assigned 11 yoga postures designed for strengthening, stretching, and balancing each joint on the upper body. They were also given relaxation techniques. Patients in the control group were offered a wrist splint to supplement their current treatment. The subjects in the yoga group had significant improvement in grip strength and pain reduction. Changes in grip strength and pain were not significant in the control group.[34]

A study conducted at Cedars-Sinai Medical Center in Los Angeles also found yoga to be helpful for people with CTS and RSI.[35] Yoga stretches and strengthens muscles, nerves, and tendons, which may help untangle spasms and prevent other spasms from developing. Stretching the muscles and tendons seems to stave off more spasms, thus relieving pain.

Proper posture, correct positioning, body awareness, office yoga stretch breaks, and breathing techniques can help prevent and perhaps alleviate CTS symptoms. The following postures should be practiced frequently:[36,37,38,39]

Postures
Rotate wrists in both directions
Press hand forward and back, stretching wrists and forearms
Spider pushups with fingers spread
Make prayer hands, turning front and back
Shake out hands and arms to increase circulation
Massage palm side of each hand
Move joints in fingers and wrists
Clench hands in a fist, then open; repeat opening and closing
Eye movements (additional)
Reach arms overhead, interlace fingers, and stretch upward and side to side (seated mountain and half moon)
Interlace hands behind body to stretch shoulders and open chest
Chair twists
Dog pose with chair
Standing mountain
Half moon
Shoulder stretch on wall
Ragdoll
Child
Relaxation pose
Breathing
Three-part yogic breath
Kapalabhati breath
2-to-1 breath
Alternate nostril breath

Additional Readings

Anderson, B: *Stretching at your computer or desk,* Bolinas, Calif., 1997, Shelter.
Brody JE: Carpal tunnel syndrome: some new treatment, *New York Times,* Feb 28, 1996.
Freedman, M, Hankes J: *Yoga at work,* Rockport, Mass., 1996, Element.
Lusk JT: *Desk top yoga,* New York, 1998, Berkley.

BACK PAIN

There are many causes of low back pain, ranging from spinal disk injury, nerve damage, and impingement to muscle sprain and tension. Many yoga postures relieve back pain by relaxing muscle tension while releasing pressure on affected nerve centers.[40] For treatment, certain yoga postures can be used to strengthen the muscles that support the back and increase abdominal strength and the surrounding hip flexibility. Yoga has a series of gentle and safe stretches that also stretch the paraspinal muscles. These stretches may increase the intervertebral space, improving the range of motion of the spinal column. Yoga contributes to reeducating and restructuring the postural alignment. As mentioned, yoga can increase the patient's body awareness and the structural understanding of how to stand, sit, and lift correctly to avoid possible strain.

In the case of sciatic pain from intervertebral disk syndrome, the YT must be very careful not to exacerbate the injury. Anterior or posterior stretches may be contraindicated. However, if the sciatica is due to pirformis syndrome, certain yoga postures can offer great relief by relaxing and gently stretching the overcontracted muscle that may be impinging upon the sciatic nerve root.[47]

The use of gentle yoga postures for back pain may offer the patient a safe and natural alternative to back surgery.

Postures
Cat/dog (see illustrated box on p. 85)
Child posture (see illustrated box on p. 84)
Easy forward bend
Sphinx or modified cobra (see illustrated box on p. 85)
Half locust
Bridge
Knees to chest and wind reliever
Knee down twist or seated twist (see illustrated box on p. 85)
Pigeon and hero; piriformis stretches
Mountain
Half moon
Relaxation pose (see illustrated box on p. 85)
Breathing
Three-part yogic breath
Alternate nostril breathing
2-to-1 breath
Ocean-sounding breath
Meditation/visualization

Additional Readings

Schatz MP: *Back care basics,* Berkely, Calif., 1992, Rodmell.
Weller S: *The yoga back book,* Hammersmith, London, 1993, HarperCollins.

NECK PAIN

Stretching and relaxing the neck muscles allows for better circulation and improved posture. Again, gentle movements coordinated with breath performed slowly and with awareness can begin to reduce stiffness and promote mobility of the cervical spine. Special emphasis should be placed on lengthening the neck to temporarily increase the space between the vertebrae, thereby causing less stress on the cervical disks and facet joints and freeing nerve compression. Movements that exacerbate or create pain, numbness, or radicular pain are contraindicated. Special care must be taken to perform movements in a pain-free range of motion. These movements can be practiced anywhere to help prevent and relieve neck pain. Following are gentle neck and shoulder movements to relieve neck pain. Isolated cervical movements without rolling the neck are recommended.

Postures
Chin to chest
Ear to shoulders (lateral movements)
Head forward and slightly back (posterior, anterior movements)
Trace outline of circle with nose and/or figure 8s
Shoulder squeeze
Rotate shoulders
Facial movements (especially to release tension in jaw)
Cow's head
Eagle arms
Lying down in relaxation pose turn head from side to side; unclench teeth and relax jaw
Relaxation pose (see illustrated box on p. 85)
Breathing
Three-part yogic breath
Alternate nostril breathing
2-to-1 breath
Ocean-sounding breath
Meditation/visualization

ANXIETY AND PANIC ATTACK

Anxiety disorders can vary greatly in their severity; they may be mild or completely immobilizing. The yogic three-part breath is an extremely effective tool in reducing panic reactions and a useful and valuable tactic for anyone who finds him or herself in a frightening or anxious situation. During most panic reactions the patient has the sensation of hyperventilation or loss of breath. Therefore, incorporating slow, long, deep yogic breath at the time of an attack can be very beneficial in easing the fear. Visualization, affirmation, and meditation can counteract intruding negative thoughts that add to the attack and can help the patient return his or her focus to healthy thoughts.

Inducing deep relaxation of nerves and muscles can help to eliminate the buildup of tension in both mind and body. Studies have shown that yoga postures followed by a period of deep relaxation can help normalize the blood pressure, calm the mind, and relax the symptoms of the fight or flight reactions. Clinical evidence indicates that yoga practice has proven most effective with a wide range of psychosomatic and psychiatric disorders.[41] Decreases in both self-reported anxiety and anxious behavior, as well as a decrease in cortisol levels in psychiatric patients were noted after the practice of yoga.[42] Yoga groups showed markedly higher scores in life satisfaction and high spirits and lower scores in excitability, aggressiveness, and somatic complaints.[13]

Postures
Mountain posture (stand, seated)
Tree (see illustrated box on p. 84)
Spinal twist (see illustrated box on p. 84)
Sphinx (see illustrated box on p. 85)
Easy forward bend
Child
Legs up on wall or chair
Relaxation pose (see illustrated box on p. 85)
Progressive relaxation technique (relaxing body parts head to toe, using body scanning)
Breathing
Three-part yogic breath
Alternate nostril breathing
Counting breath
Ocean-sounding breath
Meditation on breath/visualization

Additional Readings

Munro R, Nagarathna, HR Nagendra, R Nagarathna: *Yoga for common ailments,* New York, 1990, Fireside.
Weller S: *Yoga therapy,* Hammersmith, London, 1995, HarperCollins.

Anecdotal Case History

A YT is currently working with a 70-year-old woman who has been housebound for 2 years. Through the teacher's work with this woman, she was able to shift her attention away from falling down the stairs to a primary focus on her breath. This allowed her to take her first steps. Within 6 months she was down the flight of stairs and outside for the first time in 2 years. This is a good example of the relationship between anxiety and breath. In this work, the goal is not to deny the fear or to change the fear in any way. The focus is simply shifted to the breath and to the observation of the experience.

TENSION HEADACHES

Yoga can offer a holistic form of treatment for pain associated with tension headaches caused by an over-contraction of the head, neck, and shoulder muscles. Gentle stretching (see Neck Pain Treatment), relaxation pose and alternate nostril breathing (see Breathing Techniques), and meditation can calm emotional and physical tension, providing an alternative to painkillers.

MIGRAINE HEADACHES

Migraines are more deeply rooted than tension headaches, involving the flow of blood to the brain. Treatments that have been mentioned for neck pain and tension headaches may be helpful for the sufferer, but sometimes even the slightest movement can be too painful or cause nausea and visual disturbances. Instead, a period of relaxation using *yoga nidra* and the corpse pose *(shavasana)* may be beneficial. The corpse pose is the relaxation pose (see illustrated box on p. 85) that is done by lying on the floor or bed, giving the full weight of the body to the earth. The arms are spread, palms open, so they are 18 inches out from the body. The feet are 8 to 12 inches apart with the ankles relaxed. Placing a pillow under the knees will reduce the gap in the lower back. Also recommended is a dark room or a soft dark cloth placed over the eyes, and rest. The goal of the *shavasana* is for the body and mind to be still and fully relaxed. With the eyes closed, a technique of autogenic relaxation can be used (see In-

somnia Treatment). "Deep breathing and progressive relaxation, can help stave off stress," according to Joseph Kandel, MD, and David B. Sudder, MD, in their book, *Migraine: What Works!*[43,44,45,46] Watching the gentle flow of breath such as the 2-to-1 breath (see Breathing Techniques) may also help soothe and relax tension.

Additional Readings

Kandel J, Suddert DB: *Migraine: what works!* 1996, Rocklin, Calif., Prima.
Reilly R.: Acute and prophylactic treatment of migraine, *Nurs Times* 90(29): 20-26; 35-36, 1994.

INSOMNIA

Yoga can provide a natural solution to the problem of insomnia caused by excessive tension and anxiety. Here again, using simple yogic techniques can calm the body, slow the mind, and reduce anxiety.

A gentle routine of stretching and breathing before retiring to bed will increase the PNS tone and relax muscle tension. While in bed the patient may also try deep yogic-related relaxation techniques, such as autogenic self-suggestive phrases to help induce sleep naturally. The patient concentrates on the different parts of the body from the toes to the head. Using phrases such as "relax the toes, allow them to get warm and heavy, …" relaxes every region of the body systematically. Each time the mind wanders, it should be brought back to the task at hand. A regular practice of yoga will help eliminate the muscle tension buildup that prevents relaxing at bedtime. It is also important to take breathing breaks periodically throughout the day to release stress buildup. Yoga helps the student train the wandering mind to reduce internal mental stimulation that often creates anxiety and tension and keeps the student from "switching off" the brain at night.

Postures
Neck stretches
Knees to chest, circle knees
Knee down twist, seated twist (see illustrated box on p. 85)
Wind reliever
Cat and dog (see illustrated box on p. 85)
Child (See illustrated box on p. 84)
Relaxation pose (see illustrated box on p. 85)

Breathing
Three-part yogic breath
Counting breath
Ocean-sounding breath
Meditation on breath/ visualization

Additional Reading

Munro R, Nagarathna, Nagendra HK, R. Nagarathna: *Yoga for common ailments*, New York, 1990, Fireside.

VERTIGO AND DISEQUILIBRIUM SYNDROME: ANECDOTAL CASE HISTORY

A YT recently worked with an 83-year-old woman who had fallen repeatedly during the previous year and wanted to increase her strength. During the initial screening, marked ataxia was discovered, and the client was immediately referred to a neurologist for assessment. The physician suspected that the woman had myelin sheath degeneration, but the client's daughter did not want her mother to be subjected to the medical testing required to confirm the diagnosis. The neurologist suggested that the woman continue gentle yoga without restrictions, but he did not express much hope for improvement. In working with the client, it became evident that in addition to the unbalanced gait she became easily distracted while walking. While she worked on basic yoga postures and strength-building practices, the major focus was on the breath and concentration. The primary yoga practice consisted of walking meditation in which the client focused on her breath and the sensation on the sole of each foot as it touched down. This created a dramatic change in her ability to even out her erratic gait. She then purchased a treadmill, which she used daily for 5 to 10 minutes to practice her meditative walking. These treadmill meditations increased her focus and strength, and helped reduce her number of falls. After 6 months the client asked her daughter to watch as she walked briskly in a straight line across the length of her lobby. Her daughter wanted to know what new drug she was taking that had finally cured her terrible gait. However, it was a combination of increased strength along with improved mental focus that supported her change.

MUSCLE WEAKNESS, MYOPATHY, AND MUSCULAR DYSTROPHY

As discussed previously, yoga *asanas* (postures) may be used therapeutically for most neuromuscular disorders. Using clinically proven techniques to relax the mind and body while strengthening the muscular system can be very effective. The YT should first assess the patient's weaknesses and strengths, then check the range of motion and, finally, design a routine that can address the affected areas. Again, yoga is a profound way for the patient to become aware and therefore understand his or her own body's strengths and weaknesses and begin the process of integration and healing.

ATTENTION DEFICIT DISORDER, LEARNING DISABILITY, AND HYPERACTIVITY SYNDROME

Yoga can help enhance mental alertness, concentration, and focus, and its relaxation techniques can calm the body and the nervous system. These qualities make yoga therapy an important tool in dealing with attention deficit disorder, learning disability, and hyperactivity. Some children respond remarkably well to a practice of yoga.

PAIN SYNDROMES

Because many pain medications can cause unhealthy side effects and even addiction, yoga can be used as a potent natural pain control method. The effective use of yoga and yoga-related techniques in pain management have been documented.[48]

One method of pain relief is to influence the "spinal gate" mechanism. The input of stimuli is prevented from reaching the brain by using mental concentration (meditation) and relaxation techniques.

Breathing techniques can also be used to manage pain, because the breath is directly linked to the pain stimulus. For instance, when one is in great pain, the breath tends to be tense, shallow, and irregular. When one is at ease the breath is relaxed, slow, and rhythmic. Therefore using slow regulated yogic breathing can manage pain by bringing it under the patient's own willful control. Moreover, breathing helps to relax the system. Whenever there is pain in a certain area of the body, the muscles surrounding that area can tense and go into contraction, which further exacerbates the pain. Simple yogic stretching and postures can help relax the muscles in the entire area, decreasing the spasms and thereby decreasing the pain.

In addition, Julius Richmond, MD, professor emeritus of health policy at Harvard's Department of Social Medicine, supports previous information in saying that "many relaxation techniques can help slow heart rate, lower blood pressure and relax large muscle groups—all of which can diminish the perception of pain."

Postures
Balancing postures, such as the tree, to increase concentration
Stretching to discourage tension buildup
Relaxation postures, such as the child posture and relaxation pose

Breathing
Three-part yogic breath
2-to-1 breath
Alternate nostril breathing
Ocean-sounding breath
Meditation on the breath/visualization

Additional Readings

Lasatar J: *Relax and renew, restful yoga for stressful times,* Berkeley, Calif., 1995, Rodmell Press.
Nespor K: Pain management and yoga, *Int J Psychosom* 38(1-4): 76-81, 1991.
Weller S: *Yoga therapy,* Hammersmith, London, 1995, HarperCollins.

SUMMARY

With the increasing emphasis on preventative medicine and the greater awareness of the effects of lifestyle on health, yoga could be an important adjunctive complementary treatment for patients. Stephen Sinatra, MD, author of *Optimal Health* said, "The doctors who are willing to incorporate the disciplines of nutritional, emotional, and spiritual healing will become our most effective healers as we move into the next millennium." The future of health care will be the integration of standard allopathic treatments with an-

cient therapies, such as yoga. Numerous scientific studies have shown that yoga shows great potential in modifying certain neurologic impairments and disorders. Yoga techniques merit further study under controlled situations that could help lead to new approaches for treating a variety of disabilities.

B.K.S. Iyengar, one of the founding fathers who brought yoga to this country put it this way, "Words fail to convey the total value of yoga, it has to be experienced."

APPENDIXES

Costs

Costs for group classes range from $5 a class in hospital- or school-sponsored programs to $15 a class in a small private yoga studio in New York City. Private session costs range from $30 to more than $100, depending upon the location and the training and expertise of the practitioner.

A number of safe videotapes and audiotapes are sold for reasonable prices. Although it is possible to learn yoga from books and/or tapes, the safest way to begin yoga is with a qualified teacher.

Finding a Yoga Teacher

Hatha Yoga in its basic form is a series of postures, breath, and meditation. It is important to understand that the approach to *Hatha Yoga* comes in various styles, levels, and systems.

The type of yoga discussed in this chapter is a therapeutic form of yoga. Not all schools of yoga nor all YTs are equipped to handle vulnerable patients. Therefore it is imperative to research teachers and their credentials to make sure they have skill, experience, and knowledge about the illness being treated. It is best to make an appointment with the YT and experience his or her teaching personally.

Standards of yoga teaching can vary greatly. The recent rise in popularity of yoga created a need for a national organization for yoga. The National Yoga Alliance was formed and is creating standards for yoga certification and eligibility requirements for the National Registry of YTs. It is important to make sure that the YT's qualifications meet these standards because there are no state licensers at this time. Clients should ask the teachers about their qualifications, their philosophy of yoga, their certification, and their teaching style. Their teacher-training curriculum should include a strong background in anatomy and physiology, teaching methodology, philosophy, ethics, yogic lifestyle, and training in the various yoga techniques and practices.

The following yoga associations may provide names of teachers in your area:

Kripalu Yoga Teachers Association	413-448-3202
Integral Yoga Teachers Association	804-969-3121 x137
Integrative Yoga Therapy	800-750-9642
International Association of Yoga Therapists	707-928-9898
B.K.S. Iyengar Yoga National Association of the United States	800-889-9642
Himalayan Institute Teachers Association	570-253-5551 x1305
Prana Yoga Teachers	413-448-3446
Yoga International's Guide to Yoga Teachers	800-253-6243
Yoga Journal's Yoga Teacher Directory	800-436-9642

Hatha Yoga is the most familiar type of yoga in the United States. There are many different approaches or schools to the classic *Hatha Yoga,* based on the work or traditions of particular teachers. Following are but a few of the different approaches: *Kripalu Yoga* is a gentle flowing style focusing on improving awareness of mind, body, and spirit. *Integral Yoga* focuses mainly on breathing and meditation, with a standard routine of postures. *Iyengar Yoga* focuses primarily on alignment of the body, using props to aid the postures. *Kundalini* aims to release dormant bodily energy, which focuses on purification. *Ashtanga,* or power yoga, is more strenuous, involving *vinyasa,* a connection of every asana. *Sivananda Yoga* focuses on proper lifestyle with a vigorous form of yoga. *Viniyoga* also emphasizes the flow of the movements while coordinating breathing; it is a gentler form of *Ashtanga Yoga.*

References

1. Upupa KN, Singh RH: The scientific basis of yoga, *JAMA* 5;220(10):1365, 1972.
2. Hoenig J: Medical research of yoga, *Confin Psychiatr* 11(2):69-89, 1968.
3. La Forge R: Mind-body fitness: encouraging prospects for primary and secondary prevention, *J Cardiovasc Nurs* 11(3):53-65, 1997.
4. Gimbel MA: Yoga, meditation and imagery: clinical application, *Nurs Pract Forum* 9(4):243-255, 1998.
5. http://yogaworld.com.
6. Feuerstein G: *The shambhala enclyclopedia of yoga,* 1997 Shambhala.
7. Feuerstein G: *The yoga sutra of pantanjali,* Rochester, VT , 1979, Inner Traditions.
8. Telles S, Naveen KV: Yoga for rehabilitation: an overview, *Indian J Med Sci* 51(4):123-127, 1997.
9. Winterholler M, Erbguth F, Neundorfer B: The use of alternative medicine by multiple sclerosis patients—patient characteristics and patterns of use, *Fortschr Neurol Psychiatr* 65(12):555-561, 1997.
10. Bhargava R, Gogate MG, Mascarenhas JF: Autonomic responses to breath holding and its variations following pranayama, *Indian J Physiol Pharmacol* 32(4):257-264, 1988.
11. Sundar S et al: Role of yoga in management of essential hypertension, *Acta Cardiol* 39(3):203-208, 1984.
12. Raju PS et al: Influence of intensive yoga training on physiological changes in 6 adult women: a case report, *J Altern Complement Med* 3(3):291, 1997.
13. Schell FJ, Allolio B, Schonecke OW: Physiological and psychological effects of Hatha-Yoga exercise on healthy women, *Int J Psychosom* 41(1-4):46-52, 1994.
14. Chohan IS et al: Influence of yoga on blood coagulation, *Thromb Haemost* 30:51(2):196-197, 1984.
15. Brownstein AH, Dembert ML: Treatment of essential hypertension with yoga relaxation therapy in a USAF aviator: a case report, *Aviat Space Environ Med* 60(7):684-687, 1989.
16. Jamiel A: *Exercise physiologist and yoga teacher,* Unpublished manuscript, 1999.
17. Rama S, Ballentine R, Hymes A: *Science of breath,* Honesdale, Penn., 1979, Himalayan Institute.
18. Judith A: *Wheels of Life,* St Paul, Minn. 1987, Llewellyn.
19. Mohan SM: Svara (nostril dominance) and bilateral volvar GSR, *Indian J Physiol Pharmacol* 40 (1):58-64, 1996.
20. Telles S, Nagarathna R, Nagendra HR: Physiological measures of right nostril breathing, *J Altern Complement Med* 2(4):479-484, 1996.
21. Clark J: Slowing down, the practice of 2-to-1 breathing, 8-10, *Yoga International Magazine,* Reprint Series, "Breathing Lessons" 1994.
22. Davis S: Breathing, *Am Health* 16(9): 54-57, Nov 1997.
23. Stancak A Jr, Kuna M: EEG changes during forced alternate nostril breathing, *Int J Psychophysiol* 18(1):75-79, 1994.
24. Telles S, Nagarathna R, Nagendra HR: Breathing through a particular nostril can alter metabolism and

autonomic activities, *Indian J Physiol Pharmacol* 38(2):133-137, 1994.

25. Shannahoff-Khalsa DS, Kennedy B: The effects of unilateral forced nostril breathing on the heart, *Int J Neurosci* 73(1-2):47-60, 1993.

26. Khalsa DS: *Brain longevity*, New York, 1997, Warner.

27. Jain SC, Talukdar B: Evaluation of yoga therapy programme for patients of bronchial asthma, *Singapore Med J* 34(4): 306-308, 1993.

28. Migdow J, Loehr JE: *Breath in, breath out*, New York, 1999, Time Life.

29. Ornish D: *Dr. Dean Ornish's program for reversing heart disease*, New York, 1996, Ballantine.

30. Benson H: *The relaxation response*, New York, 1975, Avon Books.

31. Telles S et al: Plasticity of motor control system demonstrated by yoga training, *Indian J Pharmacol* 38(2):143-144, 1994.

32. Graham J: *MS: a self-help guide to its management*, Rochester, VT, 1989, Healing Arts Press.

33. Despres L: Yoga and MS, *Yoga Journal Magazine* 135, pp. 94-103 July/August, 1997.

34. Garfinkel MS et al: Yoga-based intervention for carpal tunnel syndrome, *JAMA* 280(18):1601-1603, Nov. 11, 1998.

35. Brody JE: Carpal tunnel syndrome: some new treatment, *New York Times*, Feb. 28, 1996.

36. Freedman M, Hankes J: *Yoga at work*, Rockport, Mass., 1996, Element.

37. Anderson B: *Stretching at your computer or desk*, Bolinas, Calif., 1997, Shelter.

38. Lusk JT: *Desk top yoga*, New York , 1998, Berkley.

39. Schatz MP: *Back care basics*, Berkeley, Calif., 1992, Rodmell.

40. Weller S: *The yoga back book*, Hammersmith, London, 1993, HarperCollins.

41. Goyeche JR: Yoga as therapy in psychosomatic medicine, *Psychother Psychosom* 31(1-4):373-381, 1979.

42. Platania-Solazzo A et al: Relaxation therapy reduces anxiety in child and adolescent psychiatric patients, *Acta Paedopsychiatr* 55(2):115-120, 1992.

43. Weller S: *Yoga therapy*, Hammersmith, London, 1995, HarperCollins.

44. Munro R, Nagarathna, Nagendra HR, R. Nagarathna: *Yoga for common ailments*, New York, 1990, Fireside.

45. Kandel J, Suddert DB: *Migraine-what works!*, 1996, Prima.

46. Reilly R: Acute and prophylactic treatment of migraine, *Nurs Times* 90(29):20-26; 35-36, 1994.

47. Vogel CM et al: Lotus footdrop: sciatic neuropathy in the thigh, *Neurology* 41(4):605-606, 1991.

48. Nespor K: Pain management and yoga, *Int J Psychosom* 38(1-4): 76-81, 1991.

49. Lasatar J: *Relax and renew, restful yoga for stressful times*, Berkeley, Calif., 1995, Rodmell Press.

50. Dr. Jeff Migdow, a holistic physician in private practice in Lenox, Massachusetts. He is the director of the Prana Yoga Teacher Training in New York City and co-author of *Breath In, Breath Out*.[28] He is also the holistic medical editor for the *Alternative Medical Advisor* published by Time Life Books. Dr. Migdow has reviewed this chapter.

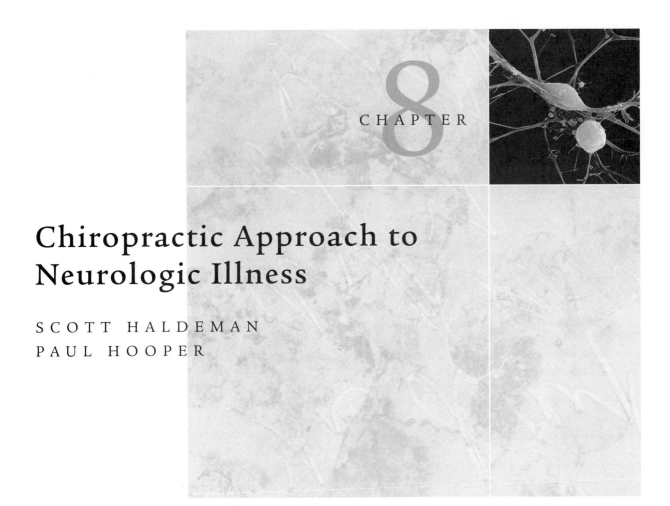

Chiropractic Approach to Neurologic Illness

SCOTT HALDEMAN
PAUL HOOPER

𝒩eurologists in North America can assume that a significant number of their patients will be seeing, have recently been treated by, or are likely to seek the services of a chiropractor during the course of their neurologic care. For example, Schwartz et al.[1] found that one third of patients with multiple sclerosis had used alternative health services in the previous 6 months. This trend appears to be increasing every year along with the growing use of all alternative medicine providers.

A recent survey by Eisenberg et al.[2] demonstrated that the use of alternative therapies increased from 33.8% in 1990 to 42.1% in 1997 and the probability of visiting an alternative medicine practitioner increased from 36.3% to 46.3%. Extrapolations to the population of the United States suggest a 47.3% increase in total visits to alternative medicine practitioners dur-ing the study period. This figure exceeds the total number of visits to all U.S. primary care physicians. According to the authors, estimated expenditures for alternative medicine services increased 45.2% and were conservatively estimated at $27 billion in 1997. This amount is comparable to the projected out-of-pocket expenditures for all U.S. physician services.

Chiropractors appear to be one of the most popular of the alternative medicine providers. The number of individuals who use chiropractors and the number of chiropractic visits per capita have nearly doubled in the past 15 to 20 years. In 1980 the U.S. Department of Health, Education, and Welfare reported that only 3.6% of the population used chiropractic services each year, or 62 visits per 100 person years.[3] Other authors have found similar numbers.[4-6] A more recent survey reported that 7% of the population had used a chiropractor during the previous year,[7] and estimates now place the number of visits at 100 per 100 person years.[8]

THE STATUS OF CHIROPRACTIC

Among the alternative health care providers, chiropractors enjoy the greatest recognition, use, and integration into the health care system. Chiropractors are licensed as a primary contact health care profession in every state in the United States; every province in Canada; and in multiple countries around the world, including England, most of the Scandinavian countries, New Zealand, Australia, South Africa, and Hong Kong. The level of recognition is due in part to an advanced and accredited educational system. The Council on Chiropractic Education requires all chiropractic students to have a minimum of 2 years of preprofessional training, and, increasingly, colleges are requiring a bachelors degree for acceptance. Chiropractic training consists of 4 academic years in the basic and clinical sciences. A National Board of Chiropractic Examiners provides an examination that is required by most states to obtain a license to practice.

An increasing research database that includes a number of randomized clinical trials and outcome-based epidemiologic studies supports a positive effect for spinal manipulation. This research more than anything explains the growing integration of chiropractic into the mainline health care system. The emergence of "evidence-based" health care that focuses attention on patient satisfaction and cost containment has further increased the interest in chiropractic as an accepted treatment for a number of conditions. Reimbursement for manipulative therapy is now provided by workers' compensation systems throughout the United States, Canada, and much of Western Europe. The inclusion of spinal manipulative therapy in treatment guidelines published by government agencies of the United States,[9] Canada,[10] and Great Britain[11] has increased the integration of chiropractic or spinal manipulation in most recommended treatment protocols and treatment pathways.

Along with an increasing interest in manipulative therapy has come a dramatic increase in the number of chiropractors who are primary providers of this treatment approach. In 1970 the number of licensed chiropractors in the United States was estimated to be 13,000. By 1990 the number had tripled to 40,000, and in 1994 estimates placed the number at approximately 50,000. This represents one chiropractor for every 5000 residents in the United States. A recent study estimated that the number of chiropractors will double again by the year 2010 to more than 100,000.[12] Contrast this trend to a projected increase of 16% in the number of physicians and it appears that chiropractors will constitute an ever-larger segment of the health care system in the near future. Furthermore, chiropractic, which at one time was largely confined to North America, is spreading throughout the world, with the establishment of colleges in Europe, Australia, South Africa, Asia, and South America. The World Federation of Chiropractic (WFC), a nongovernmental organization within the World Health Organization (WHO), has representation from 80 countries. The WFC is also a member of the Council of International Organizations of Medical Sciences of the WHO. Since 1993 the WHO has cosponsored the academic program at the biannual congress of the WFC.

The primary sources of payment for chiropractic services are private insurance and direct payments from the patient. Together these account for nearly 60% of chiropractic payments. Workers' compensation and automobile accident insurance account for an additional 10% to 15% each, and Medicare represents another 8%. Other forms of payment, including Medicaid and managed care, contribute the remaining 10%. However, with the growing integration of chiropractic services into managed care, this portion is expected to change.[13]

ALTERNATIVE, COMPLEMENTARY, OR MAINSTREAM

There has been considerable debate regarding what role chiropractors should play in the health care delivery system. It appears there are three choices:
1. Limited musculoskeletal specialists serving on interdisciplinary teams
2. Primary health care gatekeepers focusing on ambulatory musculoskeletal conditions
3. General primary (alternative/complementary) health care providers not limited to musculoskeletal conditions[14,15]

Chiropractic has become so widely accepted and used that it has been debated whether it is still an alternative or complementary health care profession or whether it has now entered the health care mainstream.[13,16-18] There are now a number of places where chiropractors have been fully integrated into spinal clinics and health maintenance organizations (HMOs). Chiropractic care is also being integrated into the military and is being considered in the Veterans Administration system.

Many neurology patients with musculoskeletal complaints can be expected to use chiropractic services in addition to traditional medical care or in combination with it. This has led to an increasingly more common description of chiropractic as complementary care. This definition suggests that chiropractic is being used at the same time and in conjunction with the overall care of a patient.[19-21] As might be expected, the majority of patients seeking care from a chiropractor have a musculoskeletal problem, with approximately two thirds of these presenting with low back pain.[22]

Certain chiropractors, however, continue to treat patients with a variety of nonmusculoskeletal disorders. Although only 10% of chiropractic office visits are for nonmusculoskeletal conditions, this has kept the profession from fully integrating with mainline health care and has kept it in the realm of alternative medicine. The three most frequently diagnosed nonmusculoskeletal complaints treated by chiropractors are asthma, otitis media, and migraine headaches (Table 8-1). However, these conditions accounted for only 1 in 200 patients, and no nonmusculoskeletal symptom accounted for more than 1% of patient symptoms.[8]

At this time, chiropractors practice in all three of the capacities mentioned previously. In formal interprofessional clinics and in practices treating primary

TABLE 8-1

Frequency of Presenting and Concurrent Patient Conditions Seen by Chiropractors

Frequency	Condition	Frequency	Condition
Routine	Spinal subluxation/joint dysfunction	Sometimes— cont'd	TMJ syndrome
	Headaches		Thoracic outlet syndrome
Often	Muscular strain/tear		Systemic rheumatoid arthritis or gout
	Osteoarthritis/degenerative joint disease		Occupational or environmental disorder
	Peripheral neuritis or neuralgia		Muscular atrophy
	Tendinitis/tenosynovitis		Nutritional disorders
	Radiculitis or radiculopathy		Menstrual disorders
	Vertebral facet syndrome		Asthma, emphysema or COPD
	Intervertebral disc syndrome		Upper respiratory or ear infection
	Sprain or dislocation of any joint		Pregnancy
	Extremity subluxation/joint dysfunction		Respiratory viral or bacterial infection
	Hyperlordosis of cervical or lumbar spine		Acne, dermatitis or psoriasis
	Scoliosis		Loss of equilibrium
	Bursitis or synovitis		Diabetes
	High or low blood pressure		Psychological disorders
	Allergies		Eating disorders
	Obesity		Ear or hearing disorders
Sometimes	Kyphosis of thoracic spine		Eye or vision disorders
	Osteoporosis/osteomalacia		Hiatus or inguinal hernia
	Carpal or tarsal tunnel syndrome		Gastrointestinal bacterial or viral infection
	Skeletal congenital/developmental anomaly		Infection of kidney or urinary tract
	Articular joint congenital/developmental anomaly		Colitis or diverticulitis
			Thyroid or parathyroid disorder
			Hemorrhoids

From Mootz and Shekelle, 1998.

spinal disorders, chiropractors are part of the mainstream health care system. Their services are paid for by insurance agencies, and they determine disability and refer to other practitioners and specialists when indicated. In many neurologic settings they are complementary to standard health care for musculoskeletal conditions that patients may experience in conjunction with a neurologic disorder. They sometimes practice in cooperation with a neurologist and at other times independent of the neurologist. When chiropractors treat patients with nonmusculoskeletal conditions for which there is minimal, if any, clinical research support, they practice as true alternative health care practitioners.

TREATMENT APPROACHES USED BY CHIROPRACTORS

Throughout the slightly more than 100 years the chiropractic profession has been in existence, the predominant treatment tool has been the chiropractic adjustment or spinal manipulative therapy (SMT). In a review of office records of 1310 patients who sought chiropractic care for low back pain, 1088 (83%) received spinal manipulation.[23] Although other practitioners, such as osteopaths and physical therapists, have used this method of treatment, the majority of spinal manipulations in North America are provided by chiropractors.

Spinal manipulation, however, is not the only form of treatment provided by chiropractors. Contemporary chiropractors incorporate many physical modalities, such as heat, cold, ultrasound, electrical stimulation, and traction. These are usually used in conjunction with the spinal adjustment. Many chiropractors also include therapeutic exercise as a regular part of the treatment regimen, often incorporating full rehabilitation programs. In addition, chiropractors often counsel their patients on nutrition and sometimes provide vitamins and supplements as a regular part of the treatment regimen. The variation in chiropractic treatment approaches has made it difficult to assess the effectiveness. This variation has led to the common extrapolation of manipulation research to reflect the anticipated chiropractic outcomes.

The manual therapies commonly used by chiropractors include mobilization, manipulation, and massage. Mobilization techniques are rhythmic, repetitive movements that are performed within the patient's normal range of motion. The movements are not associated with any rapid movements or thrusts. Spinal manipulation or adjustments, on the other hand, are performed with a speed and force that the patient cannot resist and are often accompanied by an audible pop or release. Table 8-2 compares the features of mobilization and manipulation. The manipulation or adjustment is usually characterized by the use of a manual thrust. Ideally this thrust uses controlled forces in a specific direction with careful patient positioning. One hand delivers the adjustive thrust through contact with a short lever, such as the transverse or spinous process of a vertebra. The re-

TABLE 8-2

Comparison of the Essential Features of Mobilization and Manipulation

	Mobilization	Manipulation
Techniques	Passive	Passive
	Gentle rhythmic oscillatory	High velocity thrust
	Within range of joint	At limit of joint range
	Better patient control	Greater force
Advantages	May be safer if doubtful	Quicker response
	Greater patient comfort	Fewer treatments required
	Wide variety of techniques	
Disadvantages	Slower response	Higher skill level required
	More treatments required	May aggravate some spinal problems
	Not as effective as manipulation	

Adapted from Kenna C, Murtagh J: Back pain and spinal manipulation: a practical guide, London, Butterworths, 1989.

mainder of the spine is stabilized by the other hand and/or the chiropractor's body (Figures 8-1 and 8-2.)

The goal of a manipulation is to restore maximal, pain-free movement of the spinal segments. Early chiropractic theory suggested that misalignments of spinal vertebrae, or subluxation, interfered with nerve function, resulting in changes in physiologic processes. These changes were thought to lead to pain and disease. Chiropractic theories have since evolved and today focus on the restoration of joint mobility, relaxation of muscle spasm, modulation of spinal reflexes, and the soothing or psychosocial effects of manual therapy. It is now widely believed that immobility of spinal joints is one factor that can lead to joint inflammation, formation of adhesions, and degenerative joint disease. Spinal manipulation is thought to improve joint mobility and restore normal joint function, especially when associated with an exercise and rehabilitation program.

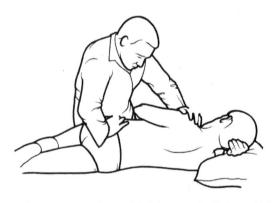

Figure 8-1 Long lever side-lying manipulation. (Adapted from Kenna and Murtaugh: *Back pain and spinal manipulation,* Newton, Mass., 1989, Butterworth-Heinemann.)

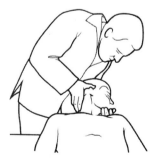

Figure 8-2 Cervical manipulation. (Adapted from Kenna and Murtaugh: *Back pain and spinal manipulation,* Newton, Mass., 1989, Butterworth-Heinemann.)

SPECIFIC NEUROLOGIC CONDITIONS

Most people who seek the care of chiropractors do so primarily for relief of pain, muscle spasm, tension, or stiffness affecting the musculoskeletal system. These conditions are similar to the problems for which individuals are likely to seek other practitioners of alternative treatments, that is, chronic conditions such as back pain, headaches, osteoarthritis, and rheumatoid arthritis.[21,24] The success rates reported for manipulation in case series and in comparative trials are between 60% and 100%.[25-27] In the case of spinal pain the problem of the different populations of patients and the different pathologic conditions that cause pain makes it difficult to compare studies and determine the success of treatment.

There are, however, a growing number of controlled clinical trials that have looked at the effectiveness or efficacy of spinal manipulation or chiropractic. In a review of the literature, 29 clinical trials on low back pain were listed by Shekelle et al.[28] Bronfort[27] reviewed 47 randomized, comparative trials on the treatment of back pain, neck pain, and headaches using manipulation. With sufficient numbers of well-designed trials, these and other authors[29] have performed meta-analyses and have sorted the trials into subgroups of patients. This has made it possible to discuss the effectiveness of manipulation for specific conditions or diagnoses and to establish expected outcome measures.

ACUTE UNCOMPLICATED LOW BACK PAIN

Following a review of the literature by Assendelft et al.,[30] Waddell[31] has stated that the evidence in favor of manipulation in the treatment of low back pain is stronger than that for most orthodox medical treatments. This is consistent with the fact that the most common reason for seeking chiropractic care is pain in the lower back. Between 30% and 50% of all spinal manipulations delivered each year are for low back pain.[32,33] The majority of controlled clinical trials on manipulation have been performed on patients with a recent onset of symptoms (within 2 to 4 weeks) of acute low back pain. Typically these studies have looked at patients with uncomplicated low back pain and have excluded patients with systemic or metabolic diseases. Many of these studies have also excluded patients with leg pain, disk herniation, workers' compensation, or a variety of psychosocial factors.

The interpretation of the results of these studies can be difficult. Jayson,[34] for example, demonstrated that the setting in which manipulation is provided seems to influence the response. In this study, manipulation was found to be superior to controls when given in an outpatient clinic but did not have a similar effect in patients who were hospitalized with back pain. Glover et al.[35,36] found that manipulation had a significant positive effect in patients with acute pain when assessed immediately after treatment but not in later assessments. Berquist-Ullman and Larsson[37] found that manipulation was more effective than a placebo treatment but was no better than a comprehensive education program. Doran and Newell,[38] Coxhead et al.,[39] and Sloop et al.[40] each showed non-statistically significant trends toward improvement in their manipulation groups when compared to controls. To further complicate matters, Greenland et al.[41] found that, if a different statistical analysis of Doran and Newell's data were performed, manipulation would be found significantly more effective than controls.

Some trials have reported manipulation to be definitely more effective than comparative treatments. Even in these studies, however, the picture is not clear. Separate studies by Coyer and Curwen[42] and by Lewith and Turner[43] reported positive benefits for manipulation. Unfortunately, neither of these studies were blinded or statistically analyzed. Other well-controlled studies have shown only short-term changes with no long-lasting results from manipulation.[44-48]

Similar positive responses to manipulation have been found in patients with subacute low back pain within 4 to 12 weeks. A prospective, randomized trial[49] compared SMT with transcutaneous muscle stimulation, massage, and corset use in patients with subacute low back pain. At 3 weeks, the manipulation group showed the greatest improvement in lumbar flexion and pain scores. Patient confidence was also greatest in the group receiving SMT. In another randomized trial, patients with acute and subacute low back pain were assigned to one of two treatment groups: manual therapy (manipulation, specific mobilization, and muscle stretching) or steroid injection.[50] The manual therapy group had significantly less disability and pain in the early phase of treatment and at 90 days. They also had a faster recovery rate and lower overall drug consumption.

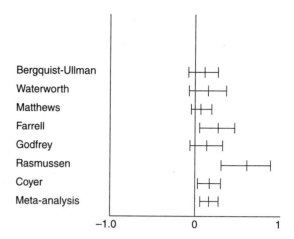

Figure 8-3 Difference in probability of recovery. Adapted from Shekelle PG: Spinal manipulation for low-back pain *Ann Intern Med* 117(7):590-598, 1992.

There are now sufficient trials on the effectiveness of manipulation on acute low back pain to perform meta-analyses and critical reviews. In a comprehensive review in 1992, Shekelle et al.[28] analyzed the controlled trials on manipulation that had been published up to that date and assigned quality scores on the research designs. Of the 58 articles retrieved, 7 papers that had used single outcome measures or had assessed outcome measures independently were selected. Table 8-3 provides a list of these papers, the outcome measures used, and the number of patients who recovered. Based on their analysis, the authors developed differences in probability of recovery for each of the 7 studies (Figure 8-3). Manipulation increased the probability of recovery at 2 or 3 weeks after start of treatment by 0.17 (95% probability limits, 0.07 to 0.28), indicating that the data support the conclusion that manipulation hastens recovery from acute uncomplicated low back pain. To date, none of the published trials have shown that any other conservative treatment is superior to manipulation.[51] It is worth noting that none of the trials have reported any complications from the application of manipulation.

Although most authors agree that SMT may hasten the recovery of patients with acute, noncomplicated low back pain, it is not known what long-term effects it might have. Most of the studies of SMT have not included any long-term follow-up of patients with back pain. Only two studies have specifically attempted to look at the long-term effects of SMT. In a comparison of the effects of hospital-based, outpatient, physical-therapy department treatment and office-based chiro-

TABLE 8-3

Outcome Measures Combined in Meta-analyses of Acute Low Back Pain Studies

Author (reference)	Outcome measure	When assessed	Number of patients recovered in manipulation group	Number of patients recovered in comparison group
Coyer & Curwen 1955	'Well' (relief of symptoms)	3 wk	58 of 76	36 of 60
Bergquist-Ullman & Larsson 1997	Return to work	3 wk	30 of 61	25 of 56
Farrell & Twomey 1982	'Symptom free,' very low pain score, can do all functional activity without difficulty, and objective lumbar movements are without pain	3 wk	22 of 24	15 of 24
Godfrey et al. 1984	1-5 point scale of 'general symptoma-tology' dichotomized by the original authors into 'marked improve-ment' or not	Mean, 2 wk	14 of 39	7 of 33
Rasmussen 1979	'Fully restored,' no pain, normal function, no sign of disease, fit to work	2 wk	11 of 12	3 of 12
Matthews et al. 1987	6-point scale divided into 'recovered' and 'not recovered'	2 wk	116 of 152	73 of 108
Waterworth & Hunder 1985	'Excellent overall improvement' by patient self-report	12 d	23 of 38	15 of 36

Shekelle PG: Spinal manipulation for low-back pain *Ann Intern Med* 117(7):590-598, 1992.

practic treatment, Meade et al.[52] noted a small but detectable (7%) long-term effect on Oswestry scores over a 2-year period. A follow-up study by the same authors compared the effects of hospital outpatient management with chiropractic treatment at 3 years. In this study, based on Oswestry scores, improvement was 29% greater in the chiropractic group.[53] Similarly, Waagen et al.[54] demonstrated a long-term (2 year) higher satisfaction rate with chiropractic care than with care received in a family physician's office. The meta-analyses have not been able to detect a long-term effect of manipulation in patients, but these studies at least raise the possibility that manipulation has benefits beyond simple acute pain relief.

CHRONIC LOW BACK PAIN

In contrast to the relatively large number of studies on the effects of SMT in patients with acute low back pain, a limited number of studies have examined the effect in patients with chronic low back pain (CLBP). Gibson[55] failed to show any significant effect in patients undergoing osteopathic manipulation, but Waagen et al.[56] showed a statistical benefit from manipulation at 2 weeks in patients with recurrent or CLBP. In a crossover-designed clinical trial using patients as their own controls, Evans[57] showed diminished codeine use in patients undergoing manipulation. Ongley[58] demonstrated that a group of patients receiving both rotational manipulation and prolifer-ent injections showed significant improvement com-pared with controls.

In a study to compare the efficacy of physical ther-apy and manipulative therapy,[59] 256 patients with nonspecific back and neck complaints of at least 6 weeks' duration were randomized into one of four groups: physiotherapy, manipulative therapy, treat-ment by general practitioner, or placebo. After 12 months' follow-up, improvement in the main com-plaint was greater with manipulative therapy than with physiotherapy. Manipulative therapy also re-sulted in greater improvements in physical function-ing. The authors concluded that manipulative ther-apy and physiotherapy are more effective than general practitioner and placebo treatment and that manipu-lative therapy is slightly better than physiotherapy af-ter 12 months. In a similar study, Koes et al.[60] found that for patients with chronic conditions of 1 year or longer duration, improvement was greater in those treated with manual therapy.

Several other studies have reported benefits from SMT when compared with other treatments for pa-tients with CLBP. Triano et al.[61] compared the use of SMT to a back education program and noted greater improvement in pain and activity tolerance in the ma-nipulation group. Bronfort et al.[62] studied the relative efficacy of 5 weeks of SMT or non-steroidal anti-inflammatory (NSAID) therapy in combination with supervised trunk exercise, followed by an additional 6 weeks of supervised exercise alone for both groups. Each of the three therapeutic regimens was associated with similar and clinically important improvement. There appeared to be a sustained reduction in med-ication use at the 1-year follow-up in the SMT and therapeutic strengthening exercise group.

Not all studies, however, have found SMT to be su-perior to other treatment. In a comparison of joint manipulation, low-tech exercise, and high-tech exer-cise on objective measures of CLBP, the author con-cluded that both exercise techniques were superior to joint manipulation for CLBP. Low-tech exercise pro-duced the longest period of relief and was the most cost-effective form of treatment for CLBP.[63] In a com-parison of osteopathic manipulation and shortwave diathermy, Gibson[55] also failed to show any signifi-cant difference between these treatments.

The choice between alternative treatments for spinal pain has been studied by Giles and Muller,[64] who compared the use of needle acupuncture, NSAID medication, and chiropractic spinal manipulation for chronic spinal pain syndromes of more than 13-weeks' duration. Seventy-seven patients, without contraindi-cation to manipulation or medication, were recruited. The main outcome measures were changes from ini-tial visit to 4 weeks in the scores of the Oswestry Back Pain Disability Index, Neck Disability Index, and three visual analogue scales of local pain intensity. Af-ter a median intervention period of 30 days, spinal manipulation was the only intervention that achieved significant improvements with a reduction on the Os-westry scale of 30.7%; an improvement of 25% on the neck disability index; and reductions on the visual analogue scale of 50% for low back pain, 46% for up-per back pain, and 33% for neck pain. The authors concluded that in spite of several shortcomings of this study, there is evidence that spinal manipulation re-sults in greater improvement than acupuncture or commonly used medication in patients with chronic spinal pain syndromes.

Many literature reviews on the effectiveness of ma-nipulation have identified a number of controlled trials of sufficient quality to conclude that SMT has a posi-tive effect.[65,66] As a result, there is increasing confi-dence that SMT can be a useful tool in the treatment of CLBP, particularly when combined with other modali-ties, such as exercise and education. In addition to any physical or mechanical effect it may have, it is likely that the support of a physician and the relief following ma-nipulation, even when temporary, helps the patients tolerate their pain and thereby reduce pain scores.[67]

SCIATICA

Currently, insufficient data exist to accurately deter-mine the benefit of SMT in patients with sciatica and disk herniations. Although no good controlled trials have looked specifically at patients with sciatica and disk herniations, a number of case studies and reports suggest that SMT may be useful for such patients. A number of authors have reported improvement in pa-tients with sciatica[39,68,69]; however, they did not in-clude very strict controls so the significance of these studies is not clear. As might be expected, patients with demonstrated disk herniation and sciatica ap-pear to do less well following manipulation than pa-tients with uncomplicated back pain.[70,71]

In a review of data from a back pain clinic at the Royal University Hospital in Saskatoon, the use of side-lying SMT (high-velocity, low-amplitude thrust techniques) was reported to be both safe and effective for the treatment of lumbar disk herniations.[72] In another case series, 59 patients with low back pain and radiating leg pain who were diagnosed with lumbar disk herniations were studied.[73] Fifty three (90%) of the patients who received a course of treatment reported subjective improvement. Improvements were also seen in range of motion and nerve root tension signs. The authors concluded that SMT may be a safe, nonsurgical treatment for low back and radiating leg pain. In a study of 27 patients with symptomatic cervical or lumbar disk herniations that had been verified by magnetic resonance imaging, Ben-Eliyahu[74] demonstrated a good clinical outcome in 22 patients (81%). In addition, either a reduction or complete resorption of the disk was seen in 17 patients (63%). However, the lack of a control group makes it impossible to determine whether the improvement can be directly attributed to the manipulation.

Many clinicians who use SMT for patients with disk herniation and sciatica modify their manipulative technique in the treatment of disk herniations. One of the most popular of these modifications is the use of a flexion-distraction technique combined with side-lying manipulation.[75-77] The flexion-distraction procedure could be considered a mobilization technique because it uses a low-amplitude, rhythmic, repetitive movement. In practice, it is common to provide a few treatments with this procedure during the course of the first few days of care, followed by the addition of side-lying SMT as the pain subsides and the patient permits. Another alternative to manual SMT used by a number of chiropractors is a mechanical activator adjusting instrument that delivers a light force to a vertebra. At least one study has reported positive results from using such a device on patients with disk herniations.[78]

Although the absence of controlled clinical trials makes it difficult to conclude that SMT is a safe and effective treatment for patients with disk herniation and sciatica, no study has suggested that the presence of these conditions is a contraindication to manipulation.

NECK PAIN

The second most common reason for patients to seek chiropractic care is neck pain. A number of studies have evaluated the effectiveness of SMT for these complaints. Much of the evidence has been based on descriptive clinical studies and large case series.[27] Although these reports have been generally enthusiastic, they suffer from a lack of controls and proper research protocols.

Rather than focusing on specific conditions, the few controlled clinical trials that have been performed in patients with head and/or neck pain have covered a wide variety of conditions. However, there have been two reports of an increase in cervical rotation and a decrease in neck pain following manipulation when compared with analgesics or no treatment.[79,80] In addition, there are a few case reports of patients with cervical disk herniations that have responded to manipulation of the cervical spine.[78,81] In contrast, Sloop et al.[40] failed to show any change in neck pain following a single cervical manipulation.

Cassidy et al.[82] compared the immediate results of manipulation with mobilization in 150 consecutive outpatients who suffered from unilateral neck pain with referral into the trapezius muscle. Fifty-two subjects were manipulated, and 48 subjects were mobilized. Sixteen of the subjects had neck pain for less than 1 week, 34 subjects had pain for 1 week to 6 months, and 50 subjects had pain for more than 6 months before treatment. There were no significant differences between the two treatment groups with respect to history of neck pain or level of disability as measured by the Pain Disability Index. The patients received either a single rotational manipulation (high-velocity, low-amplitude thrust) or mobilization in the form of muscle energy technique. Both treatments increased range of motion, but manipulation had a significantly greater effect on pain intensity. Eighty-five percent of the manipulated patients and 69% of the mobilized patients reported pain improvement immediately after treatment. The decrease in pain intensity was more than 1½ times greater in the manipulated group, leading the authors to conclude that a single manipulation was more effective than mobilization in decreasing pain in patients with mechanical neck pain.

A randomized clinical study that included 119 patients with chronic neck pain of greater than 3 months' duration compared the relative effectiveness of intensive training of the cervical musculature, a physiotherapy treatment regimen, and chiropractic treatment.[83] All three interventions demonstrated meaningful improvement in all primary effect parameters, with improvement maintained at both 4- and 12-month follow-up. The authors caution, however, that it could not be determined whether this was a result of the treatments or simply a result of time.

Recently, several authors have attempted to analyze the literature regarding the use of SMT for patients with neck pain. Hurwitz et al.[84] assessed the evidence for the efficacy of cervical spine manipulation and mobilization for the treatment of neck pain and headache. The study involved a structured search of four computerized bibliographic databases. Data were summarized, and randomized controlled trials were critically appraised for study quality. Two of three randomized controlled trials showed a short-term benefit for cervical mobilization for acute neck pain. A combination of three of the randomized controlled trials compared spinal manipulation with other therapies for patients with subacute or chronic neck pain. Subjects showed an improvement of pain at 3 weeks for manipulation compared with muscle relaxants or usual medical care. The authors concluded that cervical spine manipulation and mobilization probably provide at least short-term benefits for some patients with neck pain and headaches. A meta-analysis performed by Aker et al.[85] reached a similar conclusion (Figure 8-4).

Gross et al.[86] investigated reports of the efficacy of conservative treatments, such as drug therapy, manual therapy, patient education, and physical medicine modalities, in reducing pain in adults with mechanical neck disorders. Twenty-four RCTs and eight before-after studies met the investigators' selection criteria. Of these, 20 RCTs rated moderately strong or better in terms of methodologic quality. The authors concluded that, within the limits of methodologic quality, the best available evidence supports the use of manual therapies in combination with other treatments for short-term relief of neck pain. In a similar study to determine the efficacy of physiotherapy or chiropractic treatment for patients with neck pain, Kjellman et al.[87] reviewed 27 randomized clinical trials published between 1986 and 1995. Although the quality of most of the studies was low, with only one third scoring 50 or more of a possible 100 points, positive outcomes were noted for 18 of the investigations. Pooling data and calculating effect size showed that treatments used in the studies were effective for pain, range of motion, and activities of daily living. The authors suggest that broader outcome assessments might have revealed relationships between treatment effect and impairment, functional limitation, and disability.

As mentioned earlier, the study by Giles and Muller[64] comparing SMT with needle acupuncture and NSAID medication demonstrated that spinal manipulation was the only intervention that achieved statistically significant improvements in patients with chronic spinal pain syndromes. In addition to the improvement seen in low back pain, the authors reported an improvement of 25% on the Neck Disability Index, and a 33% reduction for neck pain was reported on the visual analogue scale.

HEADACHES

Approximately 35% of all patients presenting to a chiropractor have complaints of headaches, often in conjunction with back or neck pain.[32] Several recent studies have focused on the efficacy of SMT in some common headache syndromes. These clinical trials have, for the most part, reported improvement in headache severity and frequency when compared with controls.[88,89] It would appear, however, that SMT might have a greater potential effect on some types of headaches than it does on others. In a systematic review of the literature by Hurwitz et al.,[84] 5 RCTs, 10 case series, and 19 case reports specifically addressed the use of SMT for headache. In one RCT and two of

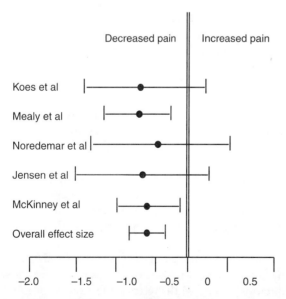

Figure 8-4 Cervical spine manipulation and mobilization provide at least short-term effects. Adapted from Aker PD et al.: Conservative management of mechanical neck pain: systemic overview and meta-analysis, *BMJ* 313:1291-1296, 1996.

the case reports describing positive outcomes, the headaches were classified as migraine. The overall quality of the RCTs was low, ranging from 36 to 77 out of a possible 100 points. The highest quality RCT did demonstrate that spinal manipulation provided short-term relief for patients with tension-type headache.

In one recent study, the relative efficacy of amitriptyline, spinal manipulation, and a combination of both therapies was compared for the prophylaxis of migraine headache.[90] A total of 218 patients with the diagnosis of migraine headache were randomly assigned to 8 weeks of treatment and a 4-week follow-up period. Clinically important improvement was observed in all three study groups over time. The authors reported that SMT seemed to be as effective as amitriptyline and was considered a treatment option for patients with frequent migraine headaches. They also noted that there was no advantage to combining amitriptyline and spinal manipulation.

Bove and Nilsson[91] attempted to determine which form of manual treatment is most effective. They designed an RCT in which 26 men and 49 women aged 20 to 59 years who met the diagnostic criteria for episodic tension-type headache were randomized into two groups. One group received soft tissue therapy and SMT, and the control group received soft tissue therapy and a placebo laser treatment. All participants received eight treatments over 4 weeks, and all treatments were performed by the same chiropractor. By week seven, each group experienced significant reductions in mean daily headache hours and mean number of analgesics per day. These changes were maintained throughout the observation period, but headache pain intensity was unchanged for the duration of the trial. Over the course of 19 weeks, no significant differences were noted in any of the three outcome measures when SMT was added to soft tissue manual therapy.

Headache is one of the most common reasons for seeking care from practitioners of alternative medicine.[2] Currently, it appears that manipulative therapy may be a promising alternative for some patients with certain types of headaches. Interest is growing in the use of SMT for patients presenting with head pain. However, more controlled trials need to be performed to identify which manual procedures offer the most effective treatment and which type of headache is most likely to respond.

CARPAL TUNNEL SYNDROME

In the past, chiropractic manipulation has traditionally focused on spinal disorders. There has been recent interest in the application of manipulative therapy for problems that affect the extremities. One such condition is carpal tunnel syndrome (CTS). Several studies have suggested that a conservative, nonsurgical approach that includes manipulation and other manual procedures may be beneficial in the management of CTS.[92-95] Although the majority of these publications have not had controls, a number of positive outcomes have been reported in case series. Improvements have been reported in range of motion, grip strength, pain, and stress levels. Improvements in electromyographic findings have also been reported. A recent cadaver study demonstrated that a "guywire" manipulation combined with direct transverse extension increased the length of the transverse carpal ligament (TCL). The authors of this study suggest that there is at least some theoretic basis for the use of manipulation in the relief of pressure on the median nerve.[96]

One promising randomized, controlled trial looked at the effect of chiropractic in the treatment of CTS. Davis et al.[97] randomized 91 patients into one of two treatment groups—chiropractic care and medical care. The chiropractic group received manipulation of the soft tissues and bony joints of the upper extremities and spine (three treatments/week for 2 weeks, two treatments/week for 3 weeks, and one treatment/week for 4 weeks), ultrasound over the carpal tunnel, and nocturnal wrist supports. The patients in the medical treatment group received ibuprofen (800 mg three times a day for 1 week, 800 mg twice a day for 1 week, or 800 mg as needed to a maximum daily dose of 2400 mg for 7 weeks), as well as nocturnal wrist supports. Outcome measures included preassessments and postassessments of self-reported physical and mental distress, nerve conduction studies, and vibrometry. The authors reported significant improvement in perceived comfort and function, nerve conduction, and finger sensation overall but no significant differences between the groups. The authors also caution that, because a control group was not included, it is not clear whether either treatment is more effective than doing nothing. It was in the complication rate that manipulation offered an advantage. Ten patients (22%) receiving ibuprofen reported some intolerance within the first 2 weeks; five of these (11%) experienced marked intolerance and had to discontinue the medication. In contrast, only one patient in the chiropractic group complained of a temporary sore neck due to manipulation.

The utility of spinal manipulation and other conservative treatment approaches is gaining some official recognition. Treatment guidelines from the Industrial Medical Council in California[98] recognize that the use of conservative, nonsurgical procedures, including manipulation, may be effective in the initial phase of treatment for CTS. According to these guidelines, manipulation may be continued for several months on the condition that consistent documentation of improvement is provided. The guidelines point out, however, that manipulation is to address joint dysfunction, not nerve entrapment.

OTHER NEUROLOGIC DISORDERS

Most patients commonly seen by neurologists who seek care from a chiropractor do so for musculoskeletal disorders, especially back and neck pain. However, there are a number of case reports of success in other neurologic conditions. Many of these case reports are from the osteopathic and manual medicine literature. These case reports by no means suggest that chiropractic care is effective in these conditions, but they remain intriguing and require mention simply to complete the picture of the scope of certain chiropractic claims. This is the type of anecdotal case report that maintains skepticism of the motives and claims of chiropractors among neurologists. These case reports fall into two categories of patients—those with peripheral neuromuscular symptoms and those with true neurologic diseases.

The case reports on chiropractic treatment of patients with true neurologic disorders are difficult to explain and poorly described. Alcantara et al.[99] report on the chiropractic management of a 63-year-old patient with myasthenia gravis. The authors report that after a series of high-velocity, low-amplitude manipulative treatments, the patient was medication free and had resumed a "normal life." In another case study by the same authors, a patient with low back pain and epileptic seizures presented to a chiropractor.[100] The authors describe improvement in the patient's low back complaints as anticipated. They also, however, report a reduction in seizure frequency, which continued at 18-month follow-up. In addition, Wells et al.[101]

suggest a role for spinal manipulative therapy in the management of movement deficits in patients with Parkinson's disease, but they do not describe how this could have occurred. Stephens and Gorman[102] describe a case of a 22-year-old man who sought chiropractic care for a painful neck. Visual fields were evaluated before and after a manipulative treatment of the spine, and the authors reported a measurable rise in "visual sensitivity" in both eyes posttreatment. Gorman[103] also described a 9-year-old girl who suffered loss of vision following spinal injuries that improved after treatment with spinal manipulation. The same author[104] described recovery of loss of vision in a 44-year-old housewife following spinal manipulation.

The relief of vaguely defined neurologic symptoms associated with peripheral pain syndromes can at least be explained on the basis of simple pain relief or placebo. Duncan et al.[105] describe 20 patients with reflex sympathetic dystrophy involving the upper extremity that improved following chiropractic care. Directed at the intertarsal and mortise joints, manipulative therapy has also been described in the management of diabetic polyneuropathy.[106] Manipulative therapy has potential value in a variety of entrapment neuropathies, such as thoracic outlet syndrome[107-109] and double crush syndrome. According to Sanders,[110] manual therapy is used to manipulate, mobilize, and relax the first rib and the clavicular, scapular, scalene, pectoral, and periscapular muscles. Chiropractic treatment has also been proposed, without an adequate explanation, in the treatment of torticollis,[111] cervical "dysphonia,"[112] fibromyalgia,[113] and Erb's palsy.[114]

SUMMARY

In the past, chiropractic has been considered a marginal profession practicing independently of the other health care professions. Now, at the beginning of the twenty-first century, it is being integrated into the mainstream health care system. This has been largely due to the development of a defined and regulated chiropractic educational process, universal licensure, and insurance recognition in the United States, Canada, and a number of other Western countries. These privileges have come about primarily because of a strong demand from the public and a commitment on the part of chiropractic academic institutions to outcomes-based research as the basis for clinical claims.

The exact role of chiropractors in the treatment of neurologic disorders remains controversial. Although there is a reasonable body of controlled clinical research to support a role for chiropractors in the treatment of low back pain, neck pain, and possibly certain types of headaches, it is not yet easy to isolate the patient most likely to respond to manipulative treatment. The exact mechanism by which manipulation obtains its success is not yet fully developed, but it has become a major area of investigation in the field. The problem of claims based on anecdotal experience and case reports remains a source of contention between chiropractors and neurologists. These issues are being addressed slowly, one at a time. It can be expected that the next century will bring greater clarity in understanding the role, if any, of chiropractic in the care of patients with neurologic disorders. Just as in the past, this is most likely to happen if there are increased levels of communication and cooperation between neurologists and chiropractors. Whether this cooperation takes place or not, it can be anticipated that patients under the care of neurologists will continue to seek the care of chiropractors in ever-greater numbers. Increasing cooperation and understanding of the role of all alternative and complementary practices, especially chiropractic, should be considered in the best interest of the patient.

References

1. Schwartz CE et al.: Utilization of unconventional treatments by persons with MS: is it alternative or complementary? *Neurology* 52(3):626-629, 1999.
2. Eisenberg DM et al: Trends in alternative medicine use in the United States, 1990-1997: results of a follow-up national survey, *JAMA* 280(18):1569-1575, 1998.
3. Von Kuster T Jr: *Chiropractic health care: a national study of cost of education, service, utilization, number of practicing doctors of chiropractic and other key policy issues,* Washington, DC, 1980, The Foundation for the Advancement of Chiropractic Tenets and Science.
4. Mugge RH: *Persons receiving care from selected health care practitioners, United States, 1980.* National Center for Health Statistics, Public Health Service, National Medical Care Utilization and Expenditure Survey, Series B, Descriptive Report No. 6. DHHS Pub No 84-20206, Washington, DC, 1984, US Government Printing Office.
5. Mugge RH: *Utilization of chiropractic services in the United States,* National Center for Health Statistics. Paper presented at the meeting of the American Public Health Association, Las Vegas, Oct 1, 1986.
6. Shekelle PG et al.: The appropriateness of spinal manipulation for low back pain: indications and ratings by a multidisciplinary expert panel, 1991, *N Engl J Med* 328(4):246-252, 1993.
7. DM et al.: Unconventional medicine in the US, *N Engl J Med* 328(4):246-252, 1993.
8. Hurwitz EL et al.: Use of chiropractic services from 1985 through 1991 in the United States and Canada, *Am J Public Health* 88(5):771-776, 1998.
9. Bigos SJ: Acute low back problems in adults. Rockville, Md., U.S. Department of Health and Human Services, Agency for Health Care Policy and Research, 1994.
10. Spitzer WO et al.: Scientific approach to the assessment and management of activity related spinal disorders, *Spine* 12 (7 Suppl): s1-s59, 1987.
11. Waddell G: *Clinical guidelines for the management of acute low back pain: clinical guidelines and evidence review,* London, 1996, Royal College of General Practitioners.
12. Cooper RA, Stoflet SJ: Trends in the education and practice of alternative medicine clinicians, *Health Affairs* 15:226-238, 1996.
13. Coile RC: Chiropractic health care: the second century begins, *Top Clin Chiropr* 2(2):23-30, 1995.
14. Hawk C: Chiropractic and primary care. In Lawrence D et al., editors: *Advances in chiropractic,* vol 3, St Louis, 1996, Mosby.
15. Wardwell WI: *Chiropractic: history and evolution of a new profession,* St Louis, 1992, Mosby.
16. Coile RC: Revolution: the new health care system takes shape, Knoxville, Tenn., 1993, Whittle Communications.
17. Stano M, Ehrhart J, Allenburg T: The growing role of chiropractic in health care delivery, *J Amer Health Policy,* 2(6): 39-45, Nov-Dec 1992.
18. Wardwell WI: Chiropractors: evolution to acceptance, In Norman L, editor: *Other healers: unorthodox medicine in America,* 1988, Baltimore, Johns Hopkins University.
19. Sommer JH, Burgi M, Theiss R: A randomized experiment of the effects of including alternative medicine in the mandatory benefit package of health insurance funds in Switzerland, *Complement Ther Med* 7(2):54-61, 1999.
20. Druss BG, Rosenheck RA: Association between use of unconventional therapies and conventional medical services, *JAMA* 282(7):651-656, 1999.
21. Rao JK et al.: Use of complementary therapies for arthritis among patients of rheumatologists, *Ann Intern Med* 131(6):409-416, 1999.
22. Christensen M, Morgan D, editors: *Job analysis of chiropractic: a project report, survey analysis and summary of the practice of chiropractic within the United States,* Greely, Colo., 1993, NBCE.
23. Shekelle PG et al.: Congruence between decisions to initiate chiropractic spinal manipulations for low back pain and appropriateness in North America, *Ann Intern Med* 129(1):9-17, 1998.

24. Kitai E et al.: Use of complementary and alternative medicine among primary care patients *Fam Pract* 15(5):411-414, 1998.

25. Haldeman S: The clinical basis for discussion of mechanisms of manipulative therapy. In Korr IM, editor: *The neurobiologic mechanisms in manipulative therapy*, New York, 1978, Plenum.

26. Brunarski DJ: Clinical trials of spinal manipulation: a critical appraisal and review of the literature, *J Manipulative Physiol Ther* 7:243-249, 1984.

27. Bronfort G: *Effectiveness of spinal manipulation and adjustment*. In Haldeman S, editor: *Principles and practice of chiropractic*, Norwalk, Conn., 1992, Appleton and Lange.

28. Shekelle PG: Spinal manipulation for low-back pain *Ann Intern Med* 117(7):590-598, 1992.

29. Ottenbacher K, DiFabio RP: Efficiency of spinal manipulation/mobilization therapy: a meta-analysis, *Spine* 10:833-837, 1985.

30. Assendelft WJ, Lankhorst GJ: Effectiveness of manipulative therapy in low back pain: systematic literature reviews and guidelines are inconclusive, *Ned Tijdschr Geneeskd* 142(13):684-687, 1998.

31. Waddell G: Chiropractic for low back pain: evidence for manipulation is stronger than that for most orthodox medical treatments, *BMJ* 318(7178):262, 1999.

32. Breen AC: Chiropractors and the treatment of back pain, *Rheum Rehabil* 16:46-53, 1977.

33. Nyiendo J et al.: A comparison of patients and patient complaints at six chiropractic college teaching clinics, *J Manipulative Physiol Ther* 12:79-85, 1989.

34. Jayson M V: A limited role for manipulation, *BMJ* 293:1454-1455, 1986.

35. Glover JR, Morris JG, Khosla T: Back pain: a randomized clinical trial of rotational manipulation of the trunk, *Br J Ind Med* 31:59-64, 1974.

36. Glover JR, Morris JG, Khosla T: A randomized clinical trial of rotational manipulation of the trunk. In Buerger AA, Tobis JS, editors: *Approaches to the validation of manipulation therapy*, Springfield, Ill., 1977, Charles C Thomas.

37. Berquist-Ullman M, Larsson U: Acute low back pain in industry, *Acta Ortho Scand (Suppl)* 170:1-117, 1977.

38. Doran DML, Newell DJ: Manipulation in treatment of low back pain: a multicentre study, *BMJ* 2:161-164, 1975.

39. Coxhead CE: Multicentre trial of physiotherapy in the management of sciatic symptoms, *Lancet* 1:1065-1068, 1981.

40. Sloop PR et al.: Manipulation for chronic neck pain: a double-blind controlled study, *Spine* 7:532-535, 1982.

41. Greenland S et al.: Controlled clinical trials of manipulation: a review and proposal, *J Occup Med* 22:670-676, 1980.

42. Coyer AB, Curwen IHM: Low back pain treated by manipulation: a controlled series, *BMJ* 19:705-707, 1955.

43. Lewith GT, Turner GMT: Retrospective analysis of the management of acute low back pain, *The Practitioner* 226:1614-1618, 1982.

44. Sims-Williams H: Controlled trial of mobilization and manipulation for patients with low back pain in general practice, *BMJ* 2:1338-1340, 1978.

45. Sims-Williams H: Controlled trial of mobilization and manipulation for patients with low back pain: hospital patients, *BMJ* 2:1318-1320, 1979.

46. Buerger AA: A clinical trial of rotational manipulation, *Pain Abstracts* 1:248, 1978.

47. Buerger AA: A clinical trial of spinal manipulation, *Federation Proceedings* 38:1250, 1979.

48. Hoehler FK, Tobis JS, Buerger AA: Spinal manipulation for low back pain, *JAMA* 245:1835-1838, 1981.

49. Hsieh CY: Functional outcomes of low back pain: comparison of four treatment groups in a randomized controlled trial, *J Manipulative Physiol Ther* 15:4-9, 1992.

50. Blomberg S, Svardsuud K, Tibblin G.: A randomized study of manual therapy with steroid injections in low back pain: telephone interview follow-up of pain, disability, recovery and drug consumption, *Eur Spine J* 3:246-254, 1994.

51. Haldeman S, Hooper PD: Manipulative therapy for postacute occupational musculoskeletal disorders. In Mayer TG, Gatchel RJ, Polatin PB, editors: *Occupational musculoskeletal disorders*, Philadelphia, 1999, Lippincott Williams & Wilkins.

52. Meade TW et al.: Low back pain of mechanical origin: randomized comparison of chiropractic and hospital outpatient treatment, *BMJ* 300:1431-1437, 1990.

53. Meade TW et al.: Randomised comparison of chiropractic and hospital outpatient management for low back pain: results from extended follow-up, *BMJ* 311:349-351, 1995.

54. Waagen GN et al.: *A prospective comparative trial of general practice medical care, chiropractic manipulative therapy and sham manipulation in the management of patients with chronic or repetitive low back pain*, Boston, 1990, International Society for the Study of the Lumbar spine (abstract).

55. Gibson T et al.: Controlled comparison of short-wave diathermy with osteopathic treatment in non-specific low back pain, *Lancet* 1:1258-1260, 1985.

56. Waagen GN et al.: Short term trial of chiropractic adjustments for the relief of chronic low back pain, *Manual Medicine* 2:63-67, 1986.

57. Evans DP et al.: Lumbar spinal manipulation on trial: part 1—clinical assessment, *Rheum Rehabil* 17:46-53, 1978.

58. Ongley MJ et al.: A new approach to the treatment of low back pain, *Lancet* 2:143-146, 1987.

59. Koes B et al.: A blinded randomized clinical trial of manual therapy and physiotherapy for chronic back and neck complaints: physical outcome measures, *J Manipulative Physiol Ther* 15(1):16-23, 1992.

60. Koes BW et al.: A randomized clinical trial of manual therapy and physiotherapy for persistent back and neck complaints: subgroup analysis and relationship between outcome measures, *J Manipulative Physiol Ther* 16(4):211-219, 1993.

61. Triano JJ et al.: Manipulative therapy versus education programs in chronic low back pain, *Spine* 20(8):948-955, 1995.

62. Bronfort G et al.: Trunk exercise combined with spinal manipulative or NSAID therapy for chronic low back pain: a randomized, observer-blinded clinical trial, *J Manipulative Physiol Ther* 19(9):570-582, 1996.

63. Timm KE: A randomized-control study of active and passive treatments for chronic low back pain following L5 laminectomy, *J Orthop Sports Phys Ther* 20(6):276-286, 1994.

64. Giles LG, Muller R: Chronic spinal pain syndromes: a clinical pilot trial comparing acupuncture, a nonsteroidal anti-inflammatory drug, and spinal manipulation, *J Manipulative Physiol Ther* 22(6):376-381, 1999.

65. Koes BW et al.: Spinal manipulation for low back pain: an updated systematic review of randomized clinical trials, *Spine* 21(24):2860-2871, 1996.

66. van Tulder MW, Koes BW, Bouter LM: Conservative treatment of acute and chronic nonspecific low back pain: a systematic review of randomized controlled trials of the most common interventions, *Spine* 22(18):2128-2156, 1997.

67. Haldeman S, Hooper PD: Mobilization, manipulation, massage and exercise for the relief of musculoskeletal pain. In Melzack R, Wall PD, editors: *Textbook of pain,* ed 4, Edinburgh, 1999, Churchill-Livingstone.

68. Nwuga VCB: Relative therapeutic efficacy of vertebral manipulation and conventional treatment in back pain management, *Am J Phys Med Rehabil* 61:273-278, 1982.

69. Edwards BC: Low back pain resulting from lumbar spine conditions: a comparison of treatment results, *Aust J Physioth* 15:104-110, 1969.

70. Chrisman OD, Mittnacht A, Snook GA: A study of the results following rotatory manipulation in the lumbar intervertebral disk syndrome, *J Bone Joint Surg* 46A:517-524, 1964.

71. Cassidy JD, Kirkaldy-Willis WH: Spinal manipulation for the treatment of chronic low back and leg pain: an observational study. In Buerger AA, Greenman PE, editors: *Empirical approaches to the validation of spinal manipulation,* Springfield, Ill., 1985, Charles C Thomas.

72. Cassidy JD, Thiel HW, Kirkaldy-Willis WH: Side posture manipulation for lumbar intervertebral disk herniation, *J Manipulative Physiol Ther* 16(2):96-103, 1993.

73. Stern PJ, Cote P, Cassidy JD: A series of consecutive cases of low back pain with radiating leg pain treated by chiropractors, *J Manipulative Physiol Ther* 18(6):335-342, 1995.

74. Ben-Eliyahu DJ: Magnetic resonance imaging and clinical follow-up: study of 27 patients receiving chiropractic care for cervical and lumbar disk herniations, *J Manipulative Physiol Ther* 19(9):597-606, 1996.

75. Bergmann TF, Jongeward BV: Manipulative therapy in lower back pain with leg pain and neurological deficit, *J Manipulative Physiol Ther* 21(4):288-294, 1998.

76. Cox JM, Hazen LJ, Mungovan M: Distraction manipulation reduction of an L5-S1 disk herniation, *J Manipulative Physiol Ther* 16(5):342-346, 1993.

77. Hession EF, Donald GD: Treatment of multiple lumbar disc herniations in an adolescent athlete utilizing flexion distraction and rotational manipulation, *J Manipulative Physiol Ther* 16(3):185-192, 1993.

78. Polkinghorn BS, Colloca CJ: Treatment of symptomatic lumbar disc herniation using activator methods chiropractic technique, *J Manipulative Physiol Ther* 21(3):187-196, 1998.

79. Brodin H: Cervical pain and mobilization, *Manual Medicine* 20:90-94, 1982.

80. Howe DH, Newcombe RG, Wade MT: Manipulation of the cervical spine—a pilot study, *J R Coll Gen Pract* 33:574-579, 1983.

81. Ben-Eliyahu DJ: Chiropractic management and manipulative therapy for MRI documented cervical disc herniation, *J Manipulative Physiol Ther* 17(3):177-185, 1994.

82. Cassidy JD, Lopes AA, Yong-Hing K: The immediate effect of manipulation versus mobilization on pain and range of motion in the cervical spine: a randomized controlled trial, *J Manipulative Physiol Ther* 15(9):570-575, 1992.

83. Jordan A: Intensive training, physiotherapy, or manipulation for patients with chronic neck pain: a prospective, single-blinded, randomized clinical trial, *Spine* 23(3):311-318, 1998.

84. Hurwitz EL et al.: Manipulation and mobilization of the cervical spine: a systematic review of the literature, *Spine* 21(15):1746-1759, 1996.

85. Aker PD et al.: Conservative management of mechanical neck pain: systemic overview and meta-analysis, *BMJ* 313:1291-1296, 1996.

86. Gross AR, Aker PD, Quartly C: Manual therapy in the treatment of neck pain, *Rheum Dis Clin North Am* 22(3):579-598, 1996.

87. Kjellman GV, Skargren EI, Oberg BE: A critical analysis of randomised clinical trials on neck pain and treatment efficacy: a review of the literature, *Scand J Rehabil Med* 31(3):139-152, 1999.

88. Parker GB, Tupling H, Pryor DS: A controlled trial of cervical manipulation for migraine, *Aust N Z J Med* 8:589-593, 1978.

89. Hoyt WH, Schafter F, Bard DA: Osteopathic manipulation in the treatment of muscle contraction headache, *J Am Osteopath Assoc* 78:325-332, 1979.

90. Nelson BW: The clinical effects of intensive, specific exercise on chronic low back pain: a controlled study of 895 consecutive patients with 1-year follow up, *Orthopedics* 18(10):971-981, 1995.

91. Bove G, Nilsson N: Spinal manipulation in the treatment of episodic tension-type headache: a randomized controlled trial, *JAMA* 280(18):1576-1579, 1998.

92. Bonebrake AR: A treatment for carpal tunnel syndrome: evaluation of objective and subjective measures, *J Manip Physiol Ther* 1(9):507-520, 1990.

93. Brzovic Z: Nerve compression syndromes of the arm, *Acta Med Iugosl* 43(5):373-395, 1989.

94. Sucher BM: Myofascial release of carpal tunnel syndrome, *J Am Osteopath Assoc* 93(1):92-94, 1993.

95. Mariano EC et al.: Thoracic outlet syndrome: proposed protocol for diagnosis and treatment, *Ital J Orthop Traumatol* 13(3):379-386, 1987.

96. Sucher BM, Hinrichs RN: Manipulative treatment of carpal tunnel syndrome: biomechanical and osteopathic intervention to increase the length of the transverse carpal ligament, *J Am Osteopath Assoc* 98(12):679-686, 1998.

97. Davis PT et al.: Comparative efficacy of conservative medical and chiropractic treatments for carpal tunnel syndrome: a randomized clnical trial, *J Manip Physiol Ther* 21:317-326, 1998.

98. *Hand and Wrist Guidelines,* Industrial Medical Council, State of California, San Francisco, May 15, 1997.

99. Alcantara et al.: Comparative efficacy of conservative medical and chiropractic treatments for carpal tunnel syndrome: a randomized clinical trial, *J Manip Physiol Ther* 21:317-326, 1998.

100. Alcantara J et al.: Chiropractic management of a patient with subluxations, low back pain and epileptic seizures, *J Manip Physiol Ther* 21(6):410-418, 1998.

101. Wells MR et al.: A standard osteopathic manipulative treatment acutely improves gait performance in patients with Parkinson's disease, *J Am Osteopath Assoc* 99(2):92-98, 1999.

102. Stephens D, Gorman RF: Does 'normal' vision improve with spinal manipulation? *J Manip Physiol Ther* 19(6):415-418, 1996.

103. Gorman RF: Monocular visual loss after closed head trauma: immediate resolution associated with spinal manipulation, *J Manip Physiol Ther* 18(5):308-314, 1995.

104. Gorman RF: Automated static perimetry in chiropractic, *J Manip Physiol Ther* 16(7):481-487, 1993.

105. Duncan KH et al.: Treatment of upper extremity reflex sympathetic dystrophy with joint stiffness using sympatholytic Bier blocks and manipulation, *Orthopedics* 11(6):883-886, 1988.

106. Murphy DR: Diagnosis and manipulative treatment in diabetic polyneuropathy and its relation to intertarsal joint dysfunction, *J Manip Physiol Ther* 17(1):29-37, 1994.

107. Sucher BM: Thoracic outlet syndrome—a myofascial variant: part 2 treatment, *J Am Osteopath Assoc* 90(9):810-812, 817-823, 1990.

108. Sucher BM, Heath DM: Thoracic outlet syndrome—a myofascial variant: part 3, structural and postural considerations (published erratum appears in *J Am Osteopath*) *J Am Osteopath Assoc* 93(3):334-340, 1993.

109. Dobrusin R: An osteopathic approach to conservative management of thoracic outlet syndrome, *J Am Osteopath Assoc* 89(8):1046-1050, 1053-1057, 1989.

110. Sanders RJ: *Thoracic outlet syndrome—a common sequelae of neck injuries,* 1991, Philadelphia, JB Lippincott.

111. Toto BJ: Chiropractic correction of congenital muscular torticollis, *J Manip Physiol Ther* 16(8):556-559, 1993.

112. Hulse M: Cervical dysphonia, *Folia Phoniatr* (Basel, Switzerland) 43(4):181-196, 1991.

113. Blunt KL, Rajwani MH, Guerriero RC: The effectiveness of chiropractic management of fibromyalgia patients: a pilot study, *J Manip Physiol Ther* 20(6):389-399, 1997.

114. Harris SL, Wood KW: Resolution of infantile Erb's palsy utilizing chiropractic treatment, *J Manip Physiol Ther* 16(6):415-418, 1993.

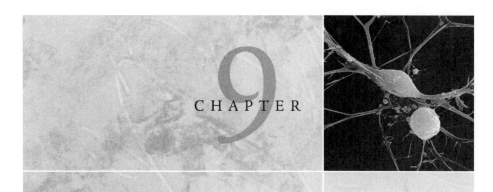

CHAPTER 9

Osteopathy: Alternative Medicine in Neurologic Disease

GLENN N. WAGNER

Osteopathy was founded in 1874 by Andrew Taylor Still (1828-1917), a frontier physician in Kansas and Missouri. Osteopathic medicine celebrated its centennial in 1992, considering as its origins the founding of the American School of Osteopathy in Kirksville, Missouri, in 1892. Today there are 19 osteopathic schools graduating an average of 1600 students per year. Approximately 32,000 doctors of osteopathy (DOs) provide care to some 20 million Americans, or about 10% of the population. Vermont was the first state to license DOs in 1896, and Mississippi was the last of the 50 states to do so in 1973. Osteopathic physicians are recognized by all major insurance carriers and are commissioned in the military and public health services.[1-3]

Still developed his osteopathic philosophy by observing nature and living organisms, performing physical examinations of patients, and carrying out anatomic dissections of cadavers. The philosophy is focused on four primary precepts or principles:

- The body as a unit
- The reciprocal relationship of structure to function
- The body's self-regulatory ability
- The inherent ability of the body to defend and heal itself[4,5]

Greenman describes five useful concepts in manipulative medicine, an important tenet of osteopathic philosophy, that illustrate these precepts. He relates the precepts to the hand and manual medicine to each of the five digits representing the following:

- Holistic man
- Neurologic man
- Circulatory man
- Energy-spending man
- Self-regulating man[3]

Still became frustrated with orthodox medical therapy after his first wife died in 1859, leaving him with three small children. He remarried in 1860 and had four more children. The deaths of three of his children in 1864 from spinal meningitis and the loss of three more children soon after birth encouraged him to explore other options. To what degree Still's military service during the Civil War contributed to his philosophy is uncertain.[6,7] Still published four books: *The Autobiography of Andrew T. Still* in 1897, *Philosophy of Osteopathy* in 1899, *Philosophy and Mechanical Principles of Osteopathy* in 1902, and *Osteopathy Research and Practice* in 1910.

PRECEPTS

Osteopathy is most noted for its emphasis on the neuromusculoskeletal system and its role in body homeostasis. The uniqueness of osteopathic medicine lies in the application of the following evolving osteopathic concepts:

1. The body is a unit.
2. Structure and function are reciprocally related.
3. The body possesses self-regulatory mechanisms.
4. The body has the inherent capacity to defend itself and repair itself.
5. When normal adaptability is disrupted, or when environmental changes overcome the body's capacity for self-maintenance, disease may ensue.
6. Movement of body fluids is essential to the maintenance of health.
7. The nerves play a crucial role in controlling the fluids of the body.
8. There are somatic components to disease that are not only manifestations of disease but also factors that contribute to maintenance of the diseased state.[4,8-12]

Osteopathic medicine is a therapeutic system based on the belief that the body, in normal structural relationship and with adequate nutrition, is capable of mounting its own defenses against most pathologic conditions. DOs follow accepted methods of physical and surgical diagnosis and treatment but are primarily interested in the achievement of normal body mechanics as central to good health. Osteopathic medicine recognizes the neuromusculoskeletal system as fundamental to the expression of life. The manual therapies commonly used in osteopathic manipulation are craniosacral; functional positional release; high-velocity, low-amplitude (thrust); low-velocity, high-amplitude (articular); muscle energy; myofascial; strain-counterstrain; torque unwind; and visceral release.[12-17]

The federal government, state governments, and private and public health agencies recognize osteopathic medicine as a separate but equal part of health care. Therefore osteopathic physicians have the same rights and professional obligations as allopathic physicians (MDs).

LICENSURE

DOs, like MDs, must be licensed by a state licensing board in order to practice. State boards issue licenses to practice in their own states according to the requirements of that state. The boards in 25 states and the District of Columbia are composed of both MDs and DOs. In 11 states, licensing boards are made up entirely of MDs, and in 14 states the boards are made up of only DOs. Requirements for licensure for DOs and MDs are very similar, and in all states licensure allows DOs to provide the same range of professional services as MDs.

OSTEOPATHIC HOSPITALS

Although many DOs practice in allopathic medical institutions, joint University Medical Centers, the Armed Services, and U.S. Public Health Service, more than 190 osteopathic hospitals in 28 states provide more than 31,000 beds for treatment of the sick and injured. An estimated 916,000 patients are admitted to osteopathic hospitals each year, resulting in 5.9 million patient-days of care. About 7.3 million people are treated annually in osteopathic hospital outpatient departments for emergency and other ambulatory care. The American Osteopathic Association (AOA) is designated as the official accrediting agency for osteopathic hospitals that are participating in Medicare and Medicaid programs. Internship, specialty, and subspecialty training for osteopathic physicians is available in both allopathic and osteopathic graduate medical education programs, each leading to eligibility for board certification by the respective certifying board.

BASIS FOR UNDERSTANDING OSTEOPATHIC TREATMENT MODALITIES

An understanding of anatomy (structure) and physiology (function) is fundamental to the practice of medicine. Structure governs function; pathology is altered structure and function. There are seven applied rules of anatomy:

- Proximity: spatial relationships
- Function
- Supply: vascular and neuroendocrine requirements
- Drainage: venous and lymphatic systems
- Pain: direct and referred
- Connectedness: body as a complex unit
- Difference: variation in structure from developmental and historic causes[18]

These basic principles are the guiding basis for medical diagnosis and therapy as reflected in the patient's history, physical examination, and supporting radiographic and laboratory studies. Signs, symptoms, and physical examination provide the examining physician with the means to develop differential diagnosis and, through further examination including appropriate laboratory studies, arrive at a diagnosis and a therapeutic approach.

Approximately 60% of the human body is musculoskeletal, the functional units of which are the synovial joint, muscle-tendon complex, and fascial elements that support skeletal muscles and their neurovascular supply. The embryologic segmental organization of the body is represented in the axial skeleton. The arrangement of nerve and arterial supply, as well as venous and lymphatic drainage, is repeated segmentally throughout the axial skeleton. The appendicular skeleton is modified for upper and lower extremity function based on myofascial continuity affecting posture, balance, and stability. It is this musculoskeletal organization of the body that forms the basis for the response to osteopathic manipulative therapy and the basis for osteopathic philosophy.[3,19-24]

Somatic dysfunction or the osteopathic lesion is an impaired or altered function of related components of the somatic (body framework) system: the skeletal, arthrodial, and myofascial structures, and related vascular, lymphatic, and neural elements. F. Mitchell Sr. states that not all somatic lesions (fractures, degenerative processes, inflammatory processes) are somatic dysfunctions, "implicit in the term 'somatic dysfunc-

tion' is the notion that manipulation is appropriate, effective, and sufficient treatment for it."[25] A somatic dysfunction is a change in the normal functioning of a joint and is diagnosed by using specific criteria. These criteria include tenderness, asymmetry, restriction of motion, and tissue texture changes (TART); neurologic factors including somatic manifestation and reflex manifestations; and circulatory factors including macroscopic and microscopic changes. Temperature, texture, moisture, tension, tenderness, edema, and erythema are criteria for distinguishing acute from chronic soft tissue manifestations of somatic dysfunction. One of the tenets of osteopathic medicine is that visceral reflexes to the soma are an important cause of somatic dysfunction and are of major diagnostic significance.[17,26-30]

Somatic dysfunctions are classified as Type I, II, or III and are named for the freedom of motion. For example C3 FSl Rl refers to C3 vertebra, flexed, side-bent to left, rotated to the left on C4. Type I dysfunctions follow Fryette's first principle of physiologic motion on group curves involving more than one vertebra where rotation is opposite to side bending. Type II coupled dysfunctions follow Fryette's second principle of physiologic motion. Rotation and side bending are in the same direction, and lesions are often traumatic in origin. Predisposing factors to these somatic dysfunctions include posture (habitual or occupational), gravity, anomalies (size/shape, abnormal facets, fusion or lack of fusion, lumbarization, or sacralization), transitional areas (occipito-atlantal, C7-T1, T12-L1, L5-S1), muscle hyperirritability, physiologic locking of a joint, adaptation to stressors, and compensation for other structural deficits. Type III movement, a relatively new classification, refers to the observation that motion introduced within the vertebral column in one direction reduces motion in all other directions. This observation has therapeutic significance.[31-35]

Neurophysiologic mechanisms related to osteopathic diagnosis and treatment are assessed relative to the autonomic nervous system (ANS) and its divisions: the sympathetic and parasympathetic nervous systems. The sympathetic chains of ganglia are ergotropic and are bilaterally oriented in a cephalad-caudad direction at the levels of the first thoracic segment to the second or third lumbar segment with fibers exiting the spinal cord along with the somatic motor neurons as the ventral roots. These preganglionic fibers exit the root along the white ramus and move into the ganglia where they synapse with postganglionic nerves at various levels of the chain and return to the spinal nerve via the gray ramus. There is an important relationship of the sympathetic chain with the ribs. The ganglia lie inferior to the junction between the head and neck of the ribs posterior to the pleura. The parasympathetic system is known as the craniosacral portion of the ANS and is trophotropic, protecting the internal environment. The cranial portion has ganglia associated with the third, seventh, ninth, and tenth cranial nerves. Spinal cord segments S2, S3, and S4 make up the sacral portion. A viscerosomatic reflex is one in which disruption, irritation, or disease of an internal organ or tissue results in reflex dysfunction of a segmentally related musculoskeletal region. Musculoskeletal pain related to visceral dysfunction may be the sole presenting symptom of a viscerosomatic reflex. Somatovisceral reflexes are neuromusculoskeletal disturbances known as somatic dysfunctions.[36-40] Three significant points emerge from studying this autonomic organization:

1. All tissues receive some kind of sympathetic innervation with its primary origin in the spinal cord and a secondary origin in the ganglia, most of them aligned in the paravertebral pair of chains.
2. Parasympathetic influence is limited entirely to the visceral organs, in accordance with the endophylactic and trophotropic function of the parasympathetic nervous system.
3. The sympathetic nervous system is the vasomotor system of the body.[40]

The principles and techniques of manual medicine that constitute the foundation for osteopathic diagnosis and treatment are based on this neuromusculoskeletal relationship of the somatic dysfunction and the neuroendocrine systems. These osteopathic manipulative treatments (OMT) include myofascial release techniques, muscle energy techniques, strain-counterstrain, thrusting techniques, functional (indirect) techniques, exercise therapy, rib-raising techniques, Spencer stretching techniques for upper extremity lesions, lymphatic pump, craniosacral technique, and alternative modalities as indicated. Alternative modality treatments include trigger point therapy, acupuncture, neural therapy, sclerotherapy, homeopathy, herbal medicine, and chapman reflexes (neurolymphatic gangliaform contractures).[17,18,32,34,35,41-48] Manipulative procedures alleviate painful and distressing symptoms of disease and injury by mechanically displacing

fluids and removing toxic substances inducing neurovascular and neuromuscular effects, thus producing metabolic, biochemical, and circulatory changes.

Manual medicine therapy is based on the location, nature, and type of somatic dysfunction, and three cardinal rules for the practitioner: control, balance, and localization. There are six relative contraindications to manual medicine procedures according to Greenman:

- The vertebral artery in the cervical spine
- Primary joint disease (rheumatoid arthritis, infectious arthritis)
- Metabolic bone disease (osteoporosis)
- Primary or metastatic malignant bone disease
- Genetic disease
- Hypermobility in the involved segments[32]

Adverse effects from manipulative medicine are attributed to judgment errors, trauma, excessive relaxation or stimulation, and subjective reactions.[23] According to DiGiovanna, most of the iatrogenic complications from manipulation result from high-velocity, low-amplitude thrusting techniques, especially to the cervical spine. In contrast, muscle energy treatment, strain-counterstrain techniques, craniosacral treatment, and myofacial release are atraumatic.[49] When selecting manipulative procedures, age, acuteness of the lesion(s), degree of inflammation, presence of degenerative processes, amount and type of articular or periarticular change, presence of deformities or anomalies, target structure therapies, and the emotional state of the patient are key considerations.[12]

APPLICATIONS TO NEUROLOGIC SYMPTOMS AND DISEASES

Migraine Vascular Headaches

A migraine vascular headache is a periodic disorder that comprises paroxysmal and blinding, often lateralizing hemicranial pain, vomiting, and photophobia. The headaches recur at regular intervals and are relieved by darkness and sleep. Migraine is more common in women. Those affected have a hereditary predisposition, and the cranial circulatory phenomena appear to be due to a primary brain stem disorder. There are several clinical subtypes of migraine, including classic (with aura), common (without aura), migraine equivalents or accompaniments (focal neurologic symptoms without headache or vomiting), and complicated migraine. Four specific types of classic migraine are usually described:

1. Basilar migraine includes vertigo, dysarthria, and diplopia and is often accompanied by sensorial alterations (confusion), total blindness, ataxia, tinnitus, and distal or perioral paresthesia. Symptoms last about 30 minutes and are followed by a throbbing occipital headache. Basilar migraines are most commonly seen in adolescent women, but sometimes in children or in adults more than 50 years old. Sensorial alterations may last up to 5 days.

2. Carotidynia (facial migraine) has pain localized in the jaw or neck and sometimes periorbital or maxillary. It is often continuous, deep, dull, and aching and becomes throbbing episodically. Attacks occur several times weekly, lasting from minutes to hours. Dental trauma is common, and carotid artery tenderness and palpable pulsations are common at several points homolateral to the cranial side involved. Carotidynia is common in older patients, age 30 to 69 years.

3. Hemiplegic migraine is an occasional prodromal hemiparesis resolving in 20 to 30 minutes followed by contralateral head pain. Hemiplegia, often affecting the same side, may persist for weeks after the headache subsides. There is a clear autosomal dominant pattern (chromosome 19). Dysarthria and aphasia may occur in more than 50% of patients.

4. Ophthalmoplegic migraine involves infrequent periorbital pain accompanied by vomiting for 1 to 4 days. Ipsilateral ptosis appears followed by complete third nerve palsy, often with pupillary dilatation. Ophthalmoplegic migraine usually begins in childhood. The Tolosa-Hunt syndrome is a condition of adults.

Pathogenesis is partitioned into three phases:
- Brain stem generation
- Vasomotor activation
- Trigeminal nucleus caudalis activation

Treatment is primarily pharmacologic with serotonin (5 HT) agonists (Sumatriptan, Zolmitriptan, Naratriptan, Dihydroergotamine), aspirin or acetaminophen with or without butabarbital and caffeine, NSAIDs, and occasionally phenothiazines administered parenterally. Phenelizine and methysergide are reserved for recalcitrant headaches.[50-52] OMT is directed towards the up-per cervical segments, the lower cervical and upper thoracic vertebral segments, associated ribs, and myofascial structures. Look for musculoskeletal triggers or prodromes. Craniosacral therapy is helpful, especially focused on the occipitomastoid junction.[44,53-56,58]

Cluster Headache

Cluster headaches are also known as Raeder syndrome, histamine cephalgia, and sphenopalatine neuralgia. The episodic type is the most common, characterized by 1 to 3 days of short-lived attacks of periorbital or temporal pain, or occasionally forehead, jaw, or teeth pain each day for 4 to 8 weeks without warning. This period is followed by a pain-free interval of variable duration. The chronic form may begin de novo or appear after an episodic attack. Pain is unilateral, intense, deep, nonfluctuating, and explosive in quality, but rarely pulsatile. Cluster headaches are neuronal with secondary vascular changes characterized by three P's: pain, pattern, and parasympathetic phenomenon. Attacks last from 30 minutes to 2 hours, with associated symptoms of homolateral lacrimation, reddening of the eye, nasal stuffiness, lid ptosis, and nausea. The attacks are often provoked by alcohol, histamine, or nitroglycerin. Most patients describe a periodicity of attacks, especially at night during sleep. Men are affected more than women (8:1) and often present with distinguishing facial, body, and psychologic features. Hereditary factors are usually absent. Attacks usually begin in the second decade to the fifth decade. Variants include temporomandibular disorders, myofascial pain syndromes, and spinally mediated headache.[52,57,58]

Pathogenesis appears to point to a central mechanism based on periodicity and the bilateral autonomic symptoms accompanying the pain that are more severe on the affected side. The hypothalmus may be the activation site. Treatment is primarily pharmacologic with prednisone, lithium, methysergide, ergotamine, and verapamil. Lithium is particularly effective in the chronic form. Oxygen inhalation (9L/min by mask) is effective during an attack, and intranasal lidocaine to the inferior nasal turbinate is also effective. Sumatriptan or other second generation serotonin agonists are useful for shortening an attack.[52] OMT is directed to the upper ribs, cervicothoracic spine, relevant soft tissues, and craniofacial structures.[44,54]

Tension Headache

This benign headache may be episodic or chronic, often involving the pericranial muscles. It is usually familial, affecting women more than men, and is also called common migraine. It is periodic, often triggered by tension, and lasts from several hours to days, weeks, or months. The pain is bilateral 90% of the time and described as a pressure or a band-like sensation around the head. Dull, steady, and characteristically worsening throughout the day, the headache is sometimes accompanied by occipital or nuchal tenderness. Evidence of vasoconstriction is suggested by nausea and throbbing pain. Polypharmacy is common in such patients. Posttraumatic headache, cervical spine dysfunction (cervical spondylosis), vascular disorders, temporomandibular dysfunction (TMJ), and nonvascular intracranial disorders should be excluded. Potential triggers include teeth, jaw, sinuses, cranial and cervical bones, joints, ligaments, and myofascial structures. Less specific symptoms suggest need for further evaluation for other neurologic or systemic disorders through cerebral imaging (magnetic resonance imaging [MRI], computerized tomography [CT], angiography), electroencephalogram (EEG), blood/CSF analysis, and neurologic consultation.

Pathogenesis is attributed to activation of the trigeminal nucleus caudalis that relays pain to the head and neck and that has both excitatory and inhibitory outputs and myofascial nociceptors. Biofeedback and acupuncture are both effective. Aerobic exercise reduces adverse effects of stress and can often relieve an acute attack. Pharmacologic agents useful in attacks include NSAIDs, hydrocodone, aspirin or acetaminophen with caffeine and butalbital, and isometheptene with dichloralphenazone. Severe persistent headaches frequently respond to nortriptyline or other tricyclic antidepressant (TCA). Selective serotonin re-uptake inhibitors (SSRIs) such as fluoxetine, sertraline, and paroxetine are effective antidepressants with fewer side effects than TCAs, but they lack the analgesic effect of tricyclics. OMT is symptomatic and is directed at upper cervical vertebral segments and suboccipital triangle, lower cervical and upper thoracic vertebral segments, associated ribs, and myofascial structures. Craniosacral therapy and the Jones strain-counterstrain techniques are helpful.[44,54,59,60] Mauskop indicates that acupuncture can provide fast relief.[61]

Syncope and Fainting

Syncope or postural hypotension is usually a transient, self-limiting interruption of cardiac output resulting in generalized cerebral ischemia, usually with flaccidity. Classified as an autonomic dysfunction, it is relatively common in the general population and more common in the elderly where it is often recurrent. Manifestations range from nonspecific dizziness or a variety of sensory disturbances, including paresthesias and alterations of vision, to loss of consciousness with or without convulsions. Blood donors often show syncopal features and 12% have convulsive features. Important causes include cardiac (arrhythmias, heart block, aortic stenosis, asymmetric septal hypertrophy, primary pulmonary hypertension, atrial myxoma, and prolapsed mitral valve), vascular reflex (neurocardiogenic, orthostatic hypotension, carotid sinus hypersensitivity, cerebral vascular disease, subclavian steal syndrome, posttussive syncope, valsava maneuver, and postmicturition syncope), psychologic-neurologic (seizures and hysteria), and metabolic (hyperventilation, hypoxia, and hypoglycemia). A comprehensive history and physical examination supported by appropriate laboratory and radiographic studies is mandatory. Laboratory studies include ECG, Holter monitoring, exercise stress testing, echocardiography, intracardiac electrophysiologic study (EPS), upright tilt-testing, EEG, radiographic, and serum chemistries. Additional diagnostic studies depending on presentation include digital blood flow, cold pressor test, norepinephrine and tyramine responses, and sweat tests.[62-64]

Pathogenesis is dependent on underlying etiology. Cardiac causes may be from acquired heart disease affecting blood flow (aortic stenosis, mitral prolapse, atrial myxoma, or thrombus), cardiac dysrhythmias due to pathology in the sinoatrial or atrioventricular pathways, or ventricular dysrhythmias including the long Q-T interval syndrome, which is congenital and familial and often associated with deafness. Focal symptoms are rare with cardiac dysrhythmias. Neurocardiogenic syncope or vasovagal syncope accounts for a large number of cases and is marked by bradycardia and vasodilation. The normal compensatory responses to standing up are vasoconstriction, tachycardia, withdrawal of vagal tone, and release of vasoconstricting and volume-retaining hormones (renin and vasopressin). In neurocardiogenic syncope, there is interruption of these sympathetic reflex responses and an increase in vagal activity. Explanations for this manifestation include excessive vagal tone, excessive initial sympathetic stimulation overstimulating intracardiac parasympathetic mechanoreceptors, and hypersensitivity of these receptors. Treatment is symptomatic and directed towards underlying etiology. Pharmacologic treatment includes fluorocortisone, indomethacin, sympathomimetic drugs, beta blockers (propranolol, pindolol), and experimental treatments (vasopressin, dihydroergotamine, yohimbe, milodrine, and clonidine). Cardiac pacing may be indicated. OMT is directed to the site or sites of somatic dysfunction and is determined by the analysis of the physical examination and underlying physiologic responses. Craniosacral therapy and strain-counterstrain techniques should be considered.[65-68,69,70]

Convulsions and Epilepsy

A seizure is a paroxysmal alteration in consciousness or other cerebral cortical function that results from a synchronous activation of a population of neurons either in one focal area or throughout the brain. Epilepsy involves recurrent, unprovoked seizures. Epileptic seizures can result from many types of diseases ranging from hereditary etiologies to vascular, traumatic, and neoplastic causes. Seizures can be classified as partial or generalized (bilateral symmetric and without focal onset). Important precipitants include fever, stroke, alcohol, drug use, and head trauma. Mimicking conditions include transient ischemic attacks, migraine, and local pathology such as nerve compression. Psychotic episodes may resemble complex partial seizures. Differential diagnosis is based on a comprehensive history and physical examination, the age at the time of the first seizure, and the type of seizure. Primary or idiopathic epilepsy is the most common cause of recurrent seizures in children. Secondary epilepsy (after age 30) suggests an underlying cause, such as alcohol, drugs, neoplasm, trauma, or cerebrovascular disease. A nonepileptic convulsion may result from a transient metabolic disturbance such as cerebral hypoperfusion, hypoglycemia, a hyperosmolar state, or hyponatremia.[50,71,72]

Pathogenesis is dependent on underlying etiology based on a comprehensive neurologic assessment. Todd's paralysis (paralysis of one arm) suggests a focal onset. Postural hypotension, abnormalities of heart rate and rhythm, head trauma, carotid disease, cardiac disease, systemic disease, and signs of drug or alcohol abuse should be excluded. Laboratory studies include EEG, MRI (with and without contrast), positron-emission tomography (PET), single photon emission computed tomography (SPECT), and possibly lumbar puncture. Temporal lobe syndromes should be excluded in psychiatric presentation cases. Treatment is primarily pharmacologic with a single substance including phenytoin, carbamazepine, phenobarbital, primidone, valproic acid, ethosuximide, clonazepam, and felbamate directed at the underlying cause. OMT literature on epilepsy is limited; however, craniosacral therapy would appear to be beneficial.[32,54,73-75] Selected seizure disorders like Rasmussen's syndrome (chronic focal encephalitis), which affects children, may respond to radical experimental neurosurgery.

Cerebral Ischemic Attacks

Cerebral ischemic attacks (TIAs) are episodes of temporary, focal cerebral dysfunction due to vascular disease that last less than 24 hours and usually less than 10 minutes. TIA is part of a spectrum that includes ischemic events lasting more than 24 hours and partial, reversible, nondisabling strokes. Differential diagnosis includes focal seizures, migraine, hyperventilation, focal disorders such as carpal tunnel syndrome, and cervical disk disease.

Pathogenesis is attributed to two mechanisms: (1) emboli of platelets and fibrin or atheroscleromatous material transiently occluding the cerebral or ophthalmic artery or one of its branches; or (2) cardiac lesions such as mitral stenosis, mitral valve prolapse, calcified mitral annulus, ventricular aneurysm or dyskinesia, atrial or ventricular clot, valvular vegetations, and interatrial shunts. Atrial fibrillations exacerbate the risk of TIA. Occasionally, intracranial arteries are the source of emboli. Subclavian steal syndrome or hyperviscosity states such as polycythemia should be excluded. The TIA may have a basis in the carotid circulation or vertebrobasilar territory. Carotid-based disease manifests as a transient monoocular blindness, clumsiness, weakness, numbness of the hand, or disturbed speech. Vertebrobasilar symptoms include binocular visual disturbance, vertigo, paresthesias, diplopia, ataxia, dysarthria, light headedness, generalized weakness, loss of consciousness, and transient global amnesia. A comprehensive history and physical examination with supporting laboratory studies such as transcranial doppler, B mode ultrasound, MRI angiography, Holter monitoring, transesophageal echocardiography, a coagulopathy workup, and arteriography provide a basis for diagnosis. Treatment is directed towards reducing risk of emboli with aspirin therapy or, if indicated, warfarin for cardioembolic disease. OMT, if used, is supportive and directed towards focal residual somatic dysfunctions.[76,77]

Stroke with Paralysis and/or Aphasia

Stroke with paralysis and/or aphasia is the most common neurologic disorder in the United States and the fourth most common cause of death. More often disabling than fatal, stroke and its complications have an enormous impact from an economic and quality-of-life perspective. Stroke is defined as the abrupt or ictal onset of focal or global neurologic symptoms caused by ischemia or hemorrhage within or around the brain resulting from diseases of the cerebral blood vessels. Stroke is classified by duration and by the type of underlying disorder, either infarction or hemorrhage. Intracranial hemorrhage is either subarachnoid or intracerebral. The cardinal feature is the sudden onset of neurologic symptoms, and premonitory symptoms are infrequent. Headache, vomiting, seizures, or coma suggest hemorrhage rather than infarction.

Pathogenesis is brain infarction from multiple mechanisms resulting in local vasodilatation and stasis of the blood column with red cell segmentation, followed by edema and necrosis of brain tissue. Types of infarction include atherosclerotic, cardiac embolism, small-vessel lacunar infarction, and cryptogenic infarction. Hemorrhage is intracerebral or subarachnoid. Modifiable risk factors include hypertension,[78] cardiac disease, atrial fibrillation, coronary artery disease, cardiac failure, diabetes, cigarette smoking, TIAs, and asymptomatic carotid artery disease. A comprehensive neurologic examination is mandatory, including laboratory radiologic imaging studies (CT, MRI, MR angiogram/MR venogram, ultrasound of carotid, vertebral, transcranial, echocardiogram, nuclear medicine, SPECT), serum blood and urine studies, CSF chemistries and cell count, EEG, and PPD (for moyamoya). Treatment is directed at underlying etiology and is supportive. Medical therapy is antithrombotic, thrombolytic, and neuroprotective. Acute surgical stroke therapy includes intraarterial thrombolysis, suboccipital craniectomy, craniotomy and temporal lobectomy, and strokectomy. Stroke prevention includes carotid endarterectomy, carotid angioplasty, and stenting. OMT is supportive and directed towards medical complications arising from the stroke, particularly residual shoulder pain. Pharmacologic therapies include aspirin, ticlopidine, dipyridamole-ASA, clopidogrel, warfarin, heparin, and r-TPA.[79-82]

Peripheral Neuropathy

The syndromes resulting from diffuse lesions of peripheral nerves manifested by weakness, sensory loss, and autonomic dysfunction are peripheral neuropathy and polyneuropathy. Mononeuropathy indicates a disorder of a single nerve often due to trauma or entrapment. Mononeuropathy multiplex signifies focal involvement of two or more nerves, usually as a result of a generalized disorder such as diabetes mellitus or vasculitis. Neuritis is an inflammatory disorder of nerves from infection or autoimmunity.

Pathogenesis is divided into hereditary and acquired etiologies. Hereditary conditions include Marie-Charcot-Tooth diseases, hereditary sensory neuropathies, and familial amyloid polyneuropathy. Acquired etiologies include Guillain-Barre syndrome and variants; inflammatory demyelinating polyneuropathy; idiopathic sensory neuropathy or ganglioneuritis; idiopathic autonomic neuropathy; vasculitic and cryoglobulinemic neuropathies; neuropathies associated with myeloma and nonmalignant IgG or IgA monoclonal gammopathies; motor, sensory, and sensorimotor neuropathies associated with IgM monoclonal or polyclonal autoantibodies to peripheral nerve; amyloid neuropathy; neuropathy associated with carcinoma (paraneoplastic); hypothyroid neuropathy; acromegalic neuropathy; uremic neuropathy; hepatic disease neuropathy; leprosy; diptheria; HIV-related neuropathies; herpes zoster; bacterial endocarditis; tick paralysis; sarcoid neuropathy; dietary polyneuropathy; critical illness polyneuropathy; metal and therapeutic agent neuropathy; diabetes; brachial plexitis; radiation neuropathy; and Lyme neuropathy. A detailed family, social, and medical history; neurologic examination; and electrodiagnostic laboratory and nerve biopsy are necessary for diagnosis. Treatment is in two phases: (1) removal or treatment of responsible condition and (2) symptomatic therapy. Symptomatic treatment of polyneuropathy consists of general supportive measures, amelioration of pain, and physiotherapy. OMT is directed towards diagnosed somatic dysfunction. The neurologic examination should identify upper motor neuron (UMN) or lower motor neuron (LMN) lesions. Fasciculations, flaccidity, and lack of reflexes indicate an LMN lesion of the anterior horn cell or peripheral nerve. Spasticity and increased reflexes indicate a UMN above the anterior horn cell that supplies the involved musculature. If the nerve dysfunction is confined to one root or dermatome or to one peripheral nerve, it suggests a compression neuropathy. Diffuse peripheral neuropathy is suggested by more generalized dysfunction, diffusely decreased deep tendon reflexes, absent vibration sense at the ankles, and a stocking-glove pattern of sensory loss. Weakness may be due to nerve or muscle disease. Muscle disease is suggested with preserved reflexes and normal sensation. Characteristic patterns of muscle weakness occur in genetically determined muscular dystrophies. EMG and nerve conduction studies can distinguish primary muscle disease from neuropathic processes. Evidence of acute spinal cord compression is an indication for neurosurgical consultation and hospitalization.[83-91]

Paresthesias and Cramps

Pain syndromes often include sensory aberration, paresthesia, or a spontaneous and abnormal sensation. The problem or lesion may arise anywhere along the sensory pathway from the peripheral nerves to the sensory cortex. Paresthesias are often described as a pins-and-needles sensation. CNS disorders cause paresthesia-focal sensory seizures with cortical lesions, spontaneous pain in the thalamic syndrome, or bursts of paresthesia down the back or into the arms on neck flexion (Lhermitte syndrome) in patients with multiple sclerosis or other cervical spinal cord lesions. Level lesions of the spinal cord create a "band or girdle" sensation or a sensory level. Nerve root lesions or isolated peripheral nerve lesions may also cause paresthesias. Polyneuropathies cause the most intense paresthesias. If paresthesias do not persist, they are probably not due to a neurologic lesion. If paresthesias do persist and a corresponding abnormality cannot be defined, the patient should be reexamined

for a sensory lesion, nerve root compression. Paresthesias are described with chronic Lyme disease from *B. burgdorferi* and tick exposure. Disorders of nerve roots and peripheral nerves in the upper and lower extremities are common. The nerves are usually injured by mechanical means or are vulnerable to specific anatomic variants or degenerative disease.

Pathogenesis is related to underlying etiology. Upper extremity syndromes include cervical radiculopathy and melopathy that is usually age-related, brachial plexus neuritis, thoracic outlet syndrome, long thoracic nerve entrapment, carpal tunnel syndrome, ulnar nerve entrapment, and radial nerve injuries. Lower extremity syndromes include lateral femoral cutaneous nerve compression (meralgia paresthetica), femoral neuropathy, sciatic nerve syndromes, lumbar disk syndromes, and peripheral polyneuropathy. Diagnosis and therapy is directed at the underlying etiology supported by imaging modalities, EMG, nerve conduction studies, and clinical laboratory blood studies to exclude visceral pathology. OMT is particularly valuable in focal segmental lesions.[92-94,95a,b&c,96]

Tinnitus

Tinnitus is an auditory sensation described as a "ringing, buzzing, or roaring" that arises within the head and is perceived in one or both ears, or inside the head. The sound may be continuous, intermittent, or pulsatile. Objective tinnitus results from intravascular turbulence; increased blood flow; or movement in the eustachian tube, soft palate (myoclonus), or temporomandibular joint (Costen's syndrome). Listen for bruits: their presence is indicative of vascular turbulence and the need for futher evaluation. Subjective tinnitus results from damage or abnormality in the auditory system in the external ear, middle or inner ear, eighth nerve, or central auditory connections. Cochlear injury should be excluded.

Most tinnitus results from the same conditions that cause hearing loss, whether conductive, sensorineural, peripheral, or central. Ototoxic drugs include aminoglycoside antibiotics and salicylates. Meniere's disease results in transient, low-pitched tinnitus that varies with the intensity of the other symptoms. Acoustic neuroma produces a similar set of symptoms but is usually progressive. External and middle ear pathologies are usually clearly defined, such as impacted cerumen, tympanic membrane perforation, or middle ear fluid. Otosclerosis and acute otitis media should be excluded. Pulsatile tinnitus is often found in inflammations, glomus tumors, and arteriovenous fistulas. A comprehensive medical history and a physical examination are necessary. Laboratory studies should include an audiogram and neuroimaging. Referral is expected with a conductive hearing loss because many lesions are correctable. OMT, especially craniosacral therapy, is directed towards the underlying etiology in a supportive role. The use of pharmacologic agents is questionable, but homeopathic therapies have been described as helpful.[64,97-100]

Disequilibrium Syndromes: Vertigo

Dizziness may result from a variety of etiologies ranging from psychiatric disease or cardiovascular disease to peripheral and central defects within the nervous system, such as vestibular dysfunction, metabolic derangement, multiple sensory defects, or cerebellar disease. Vestibular disease includes benign positional vertigo, vestibular neuronitis and ototoxic drugs, Meniere's disease, acoustic neuroma and other tumors of the cerebellopontine angle, basilar insufficiency, and multiple sclerosis. Cardiac and vascular diseases include aortic stenosis, carotid sinus hypersensitivity, volume depletion and severe anemia, autonomic insufficiency (drugs, diabetes), and diminished vascular reflexes in the elderly. Multiple sensory deficits include diabetes mellitus, cataract surgery, multiple sclerosis, cervical spondylosis, and cerebellar vascular disease. Psychiatric disease includes anxiety, depression, and psychosis. Metabolic disturbances include hypoxia, hyperglycemia, and hypo or hypercapnia. Vertigo is usually classified as vestibular, visual, or somatosensory with four recognized types:

• Attacks of rotational vertigo
• Sustained rotational vertigo
• Positional vertigo
• Dizziness with postural imbalance[64,99,101,102]

The medical history and physical examination is fundamental to defining the etiology. Look for diplopia, facial numbness, weakness, hemiplegia, or dysphasia as brainstem symptoms that exclude a peripheral lesion. Peripheral lesions include cochlear versus retrocochlear disease (acoustic neuroma). Vestibular stimulation studies such as the Barany maneuver may trigger vertigo and other symptoms. Laboratory studies include electonystagmography (ENG), audiologic

testing, brainstem auditory evoked response testing, and neuroimaging (CT,MRI). Therapy is directed at the underlying pathophysiology. Pharmacologic treatment includes meclizine, promethazine, dimenhydrinate, and transdermal scopolamine, or antidepressants. OMT is directed towards identified somatic dysfunctions. Vertigo is also common in the posttraumatic head syndrome. Craniosacral therapy is described as helpful.[54]

Dementia

Dementia is defined as the generalized, sustained, and progressive decline in intellectual ability from a previously attained state. Changes are reflected in memory, speech, judgment, and mood changes. Dementia increases in frequency with age. Fifteen percent of patients have conditions that are amenable to therapy. The primary differential diagnosis is between dementia and cortical defects such as aphasia, agnosia, and isolated memory loss. The presenting or developing signs include forgetfulness, attention and concentration deficits, repetitiousness and inconsistencies, impaired judgment, difficulties with attractions, and personality changes (rigidity, perseveration, irritability, and confusion). The signs often manifest with concomitant disorders of the extrapyramidal functions. Primary neurologic conditions causing dementia include the following:

• Alzheimer's
• Vascular dementia (multiinfarct dementia)
• Mixed disease
• Normal pressure hydrocephalus (dementia with gait disturbance and urinary or fecal incontinence)
• Space occupying lesions (chronic subdural hematoma or tumors, especially from frontal and temporal lobes)
• Depression
• Other primary neurologic diseases such as Parkinson's, Wilson's, multiple sclerosis, Jacobs disease, neurosyphilis, and Huntington's disease

Secondary conditions are classified as a result of toxins, infections, metabolic disorders, and nutrition deficits.[103-105]

Diagnosis and therapy is directed at the underlying etiology and pathophysiology. Infections causing dementia include syphilis, HIV, Jacob-Creutzfeld disease, and cryptococcal. Metabolic disorders include hypo- or hyperthyroidism, panhypopituitarism, and high-dose glucocorticosteroids. Nutrition disorders include deficiencies of vitamin B_{12}, thiamine, and niacin. Chemical toxins include alcohol, metals, and aniline dyes. Drugs include barbiturates, opiates, lithium, bromides, haloperidol, antihypertensives, and anticholinergics. Workup in addition to the history and physical examination should include standardized mental status tests, neuroimaging (CT, MRI), lumbar puncture and CSF analysis, EEGs, psychiatric assessment, clinical laboratory blood analysis, and toxicology as indicated. Treatment is supportive with pharmacologic regimens for symptoms, such as haloperidol or thioridazine for extreme agitation, delusions, and hallucinations; experimental drugs causing acetylcholine release to improve mental function; acetylcholinesterase inhibitors and cholinergic receptor agonists; restorative therapy with nerve growth factor; protective therapy with antioxidants; and preventive therapy inhibiting amyloid formation. OMT is supportive and is a valuable adjunct to physical therapy.[106-108]

Tremors

Tremors are regular oscillations of a body part described as shakiness. The onset is often insidious with steady progression. Tremors can be present during postural maintenance, at rest, or during an action (intention tremor). Tremors need to be distinguished from tics (repetitive, coordinated , usually stereotyped movements often triggered by stress); hemifacial spasm (oscillating movement beginning in middle age and localized to facial muscles from a degenerative lesion of the facial nucleus or peripheral nerve); asterixis (irregular, skeletal muscle contractions with hand flapping); chorea (irregular, jerking movements usually involving the fingers and often accompanied by athetosis, or writhing movements); epilepsy partialis continuens (focal seizure with continuous seizure activity resulting in a rhythmic jerking with sudden onset); dyskinesias (rhythmic, involuntary orofacial muscular contractions with tongue protrusion and chewing movements often from use of phenothiazines and tranquilizers).[109]

Postural or physiologic tremors have a frequency of 8 to 12 Hz with no symptoms. The tremors are often exaggerated by anxiety, coffee ingestion, hyperthyroidism, and some drugs including lithium and tricyclic antidepressants. These tremors are unaffected by propanolol or alcohol.

Intention tremors are classified as essential, familial or cerebellar, and senile; 50% are autosomal dominant and 50% are sporadic and involve the hands, head, voice, legs, or trunk. The tremors are most prominent when the hands or head are outstretched and least noticeable at rest. Precision movements may accentuate the tremor. Cerebellar disease with progressive amplitude of the tremor as the patient brings the limb towards the target suggests multiple sclerosis in young people, cerebellar infarction, degenerative disorders of the spinocerebellar pathways, or chronic relapsing steroid-sensitive polyneuropathy.

Rest tremors are characteristic of Parkinson's disease, usually beginning in the fingers and possibly involving the arms and legs. Flexion and extension of the fingers, abduction and adduction of the thumb, and pronation and supination of the wrist produce characteristic "pill-rolling" movements. These tremors are followed by bradykinesia and postural difficulties. The tremors are slow, 3 to 8 Hz. EMGs show alternating discharge in antagonistic muscle groups. An essential tremor may be worsened by L dopa, and phenothiazines and haloperidol worsen the tremor at rest.

The medical history and physical examination is critical. The history can identify the type of tremor and the physical exam demonstrates movement and response to movement. Neurologic testing is fundamental, and laboratory studies should include EMG, blood chemistries, and neuroimaging (MRI), if indicated. Treatment is supportive with propranolol or primidone with alprazolam or other benzodiazepines often prescribed for essential tremors. Beta blockers are contraindicated in asthmatics, diabetics, heart block patients, and those with congestive heart failure. Physiologic tremors respond well to beta blockers and benzodiazepines but they may be habituating. Cerebellar lesions are generally unresponsive but respond to physical therapy such as wrist weights.

Parkinson's disease is an adult onset neurodegenerative disorder characterized by tremors at rest, rigidity, bradykinesia, masked face, stooped posture, and shuffling gait. There are many etiologies including infection, substance exposure to toxins and drugs, multisystem degenerations (striatonigral degeneration, progressive supranuclear palsy, olivopontocerebellar degeneration, Shy-Drager syndrome), Alzheimer's disease, C-J disease, Binswanger's disease, posttraumatic encephalopathy, hereditary disorders (Wilson's disease, juvenile Huntington's disease), and metabolic (hypoparathyroidism, chronic hepatocerebral degeneration, idiopathic calcification of the basal ganglia) or idiopathic conditions. Parkinson's is responsive to dopaminergic agents (L dopa, bromocriptine, carbidopa/levodopa, amantadine, pergolide mesylate, and selegiline hydrochloride) and anticholinergics (trihexyphenidyl hydrochloride or benztropine mesylate). Combination therapy is often required. Transplantation of fetal brain tissue has been tried with mixed results. Physical therapy, psychological support, and treatment of depression are important supportive adjuncts.[110] OMT is also supportive.

Multiple Sclerosis

Multiple sclerosis (MS) is the most common demyelinating disease of the CNS in young adults. Disease manifestations are protean with a variable clinical course. Etiology remains unknown but research suggests genetic susceptibility, environmental exposures, and defective regulation of the immune response. These factors result in discrete, episodic myelin-specific autoimmune CNS injury, separated in time and space. Chronicity of the inflammatory process results in formation of a plaque or gliotic scar. Lesions occur predominantly in the white matter with the demyelination characteristically focal and some remyelination occurring postattack. Transient sensory deficits are the most common initial presentation. These deficits include paresthesias in the extremities, which may be bilateral and symmetric. Ophthalmic complaints are not uncommon, such as acute monocular visual loss due to optic neuritis. A central scotomata, transient pain on eye movement, and the Marcus-Gunn pupil are characteristic features of optic neuritis. Diplopia due to internuclear ophthalmoplegia or an oculomotor defect is common. Ataxia and intention tremors are manifestations of cerebellar involvement. Motor deficits may be insidious or acute, with legs being affected more often than arms and the deficits often being asymmetric. Cerebral involvement is usually a late finding.[111]

Neuroimaging, particularly MRI, is helpful with the demonstration of multiple periventricular plaques. CSF analysis is abnormal in 95% of MS patients. At present, there is no cure. Treatments are directed at the acute attack with high-dose corticosteroids. Progressive disease is treated with IV cyclophosphamide and ACTH, and experimentally

with beta interferon and copolymer-1. Treatment of complications includes carbamazepine for paroxysmal symptoms, TCAs for emotional lability, baclofen for spasticity, anticholinergics for incontinence, and amantadine for fatigue. OMT is largely limited to muscle-energy and myofascial techniques including myofascial trigger points.[112-116]

Bell's Palsy, or Idiopathic Facial Mononeuropathy

Bell's palsy is an idiopathic paralysis of the facial muscles innervated by the seventh nerve and encompassing 80% of all facial mononeuropathies, presumably from viral infection and ischemia. The condition has an increasing incidence with age; it is more common in the winter; and it is associated with pregnancy, diabetes, and hypothyroidism. In patients under 50 years of age, the condition is more common in women. The onset is acute with unilateral motor deficit. It is usually accompanied by pain in or behind the ear. Fever, tinnitus, and mild hearing loss may be experienced. Voluntary and involuntary motor responses are lost affecting upper and lower facial elements. The majority of patients recover without treatment. Prognosis can be predicted by EMG studies after 72 hours from the clinical nadir. Differential diagnoses include bacterial infections, herpes zoster, diabetes, sarcoidosis, Guillain-Barre syndrome, tumor (acoustic neuroma, pontine glioma, neurofibroma, cholesteatoma), trauma, and Lyme disease.

Laboratory studies are of limited value for a patient with a characteristic history and physical. Neuroimaging is necessary, with a posterior fossa massas being the cause of VII nerve palsy. Lumbar puncture and CSF analysis are indicated if inflammation, granuloma, or malignancy is a consideration. Corticosteroid therapy in a short course regimen is often beneficial. OMT of craniosacral therapy is usually applied.[54,117]

Tic Douloureux, or Trigeminal Neuralgia

Most patients with tic douloureux are middle aged or elderly. About 15,000 new cases occur annually in the United States. The illness is characterized by paroxysms of unilateral lancinating facial pain involving the jaw, gums, lips, or maxillary area. The maxillary and mandibular divisions of the trigeminal nerve are affected more than the ophthalmic division. Attacks are often precipitated by a trigger zone and are unaccompanied by either sensory or motor deficits. The condition can be chronic, and spontaneous remissions are not uncommon. Women are affected more often than men and the incidence increases with age. The etiology remains unknown, and treatment is symptomatic. Carbamazepine is the drug of choice but its effectiveness decreases over time. Side effects are frequent (bone marrow suppression, rash, liver disease), but baclofen offers relief in many. Combination therapy with carbamazepine and baclofen, or either of these drugs combined with phenytoin has helped. If the patient is unresponsive to medical therapy surgical treatments including microvascular decompression or percutaneous radiofrequency rhizotomy may be considered.[109] Craniosacral therapy is also helpful.[16,54]

Nerve Root and Peripheral Nerve Syndromes

Because of their superficial location, peripheral nerves are easily injured mechanically. Syndromes are usually divided into upper and lower extremity by location and motor/sensory deficit. Upper extremity syndromes include cervical radiculopathy and myelopathy from osteophytic cervical spurs encroaching on nerve roots; brachial plexus neuritis often following an immunization; thoracic outlet syndrome from a cervical rib or bony abnormality of the first rib; long thoracic nerve entrapment with winging of the scapula; carpal tunnel syndrome with median nerve entrapment; ulnar nerve entrapment usually at the elbow from fracture deformities, arthritis, repetitive trauma, or surgery; and radial nerve injuries from compression in the axilla or upper arm-wrist drop. Lower extremity syndromes include lateral femoral cutaneous nerve compression often occurring in obesity or pregnancy, especially with diabetics; femoral neuropathy from entrapment in the inguinal region and direct retroperitoneal compression by tumor or hematoma, or diabetic nerve infarction; sciatic nerve syndromes resulting from tumor compression or prolonged sitting or lying on the buttocks, and common peroneal compression usually at the fibular head seen in prolonged bedrest, diabetics, alcoholics, and tight

casts that result in foot drop and a slapping gait; lumbar disk syndromes; and peripheral polyneuropathies.[84,108]

Treatment is directed towards underlying etiology and often involves surgery, physical therapy, and correction of metabolic disturbances. Behavioral modification, especially in occupationally induced injuries, is essential. A comprehensive history, a physical examination, and laboratory studies that include radiographic, EMG, and nerve conduction studies are indicated. OMT is beneficial and usually supportive based on the underlying etiology and evidence of somatic dysfunction. OMT has been helpful in whiplash injuries, scoliosis, thoracic outlet syndrome, lumbar radiculopathies, spondylolisthesis and spondylolysis, coccygodynia, and traumatic brain syndrome.[118-131]

Sleep Disorders

Approximately 10% of the population has chronic and severe insomnia. Sleep disorders are more common with age and in women. About 40% of these patients have major depression or anxiety disorders. Societal and behavioral factors, as well as medication and psychiatric factors are among the etiologies identified. The International Classification of Sleep Disorders divides conditions into four main categories: dyssomnia, parasomnias, sleep disorders associated with medical/psychiatric disorders, and proposed sleep disorders. The last category includes short and long sleepers, subwakefulness syndrome, fragmentary myoclonus, sleep hyperhidrosis, menstrual and pregnancy associated sleep disorders, terrifying hypnagogic hallucinations, sleep related neurogenic tachypnea and laryngospasm, and sleep choking syndrome. The classification is based on clinical signs, symptoms, age of onset, and history. Clinical polysomnography is an important diagnostic tool that provides objective confirmation of the clinical syndromes. This capability comes from understanding sleep physiology. Degenerative neurologic disorders including dementia and Parkinson's disease have associated sleep disturbances. There are a considerable number of medical conditions that can cause insomnia that respond to treatment of the associated pain, respiratory insufficiency, nocturia, and so forth.[132]

Principles of sleep hygiene are directed towards behavioral modification, including schedules, avoidance of certain foods and beverages, and exercise. Medications include benzodiazepines, newer nonbenzodiazepine drugs (zolpidem), and medications directed at the underlying medical or psychiatric disorder. Clonazepam has been useful in the restless legs syndrome as have other antiparkinsonian agents including pergolide, L dopa, carbidopa, and bromocriptine. Narcotic analgesics are very effective, and megadose vitamins have been reported to be effective. OMT is directed at the underlying medical etiologies in cases where a structural component can be identified.[133-135]

Cranial Neuropathies

The peripheral and cranial nerves are subject to trauma, infections, tumors, toxic agents, and vascular and metabolic disorders. Trauma is the most common cause of localized injury in a mononeuropathy. Toxic and metabolic disorders usually affect many nerves (mononeuropathy multiplex or symmetric polyneuropathy). Olfactory nerve and tract disorders result in smell disturbances such as hyposmia, anosmia, and parosmia. Optic nerve and tract disorders can result from a multitude of conditions, many systemic or toxic. Oculomotor, trochlear, and abducen nerve pathologies cause eye muscle paralysis. A trigeminal nerve injury causes paralysis of the muscles of mastication with deviation of the jaw to the side of the lesion, loss of sensory feelings in the face, and loss of the corneal and sneezing (sternutatory) reflexes. Injuries to the facial nerve manifest as Bell's palsy, blepharospasm, myokymia, and hemifacial spasm. Acoustic nerve injuries result in dizziness and hearing loss. Glossopharyngeal nerve injuries cause neuralgia (tic douloureux of the ninth nerve), taste alterations, or signs of compression (jugular foramen syndrome) of the ninth, tenth, and eleventh nerves. Injuries to the tenth (vagus) nerve can cause dysarthria and dysphagia, vocal cord paralysis, and difficulties in swallowing. Eleventh (spinal accessory) nerve injuries cause weakness and atrophy of the trapezius, and winging of the scapula and their sequelae. Myotonic muscular dystrophy, polymyositis, and myasthenia gravis involve these same muscles. The twelfth (hypoglossal) nerve is the motor nerve to the tongue. Injury manifestations include alternating hemiplegia, atrophy and paralysis, dysarthria, homolateral weakness of the tongue, tremors, and apraxia.[84,136]

Treatment is directed to the underlying etiology and includes both medical and surgical interventions.

Because many of these cranial neuropathies are of structural etiologies, they respond well to OMT such as craniosacral therapy, strain-counterstrain treatment, and myofascial release.[15,44,49,54]

Pain Syndromes

All pain sensations are carried by nerves; however, not all pain is relevant to neurologic diagnosis. Pain may occur from a traumatic lesion or a visceral disorder. Most chronic neck pain is caused by bony abnormalities such as cervical osteoarthritis, other forms of arthritis, or local trauma. The most common cause of low back pain is herniated nucleus pulposus. Chronic low back pain is often caused by tumor, lumbar spondylosis with or without stenosis, or arachnoiditis. Local arm pain is usually due to musculoskeletal diseases. Chronic pain may arise from tumors, especially in the lung or breast, and from transient illnesses including brachial plexus neuritis, thoracic outlet syndromes, entrapment neuropathies, causalgia, and reflex sympathetic dystrophy. Leg pain is often due to occlusive vascular disease, especially with diabetes; nutritional neuropathy; intraspinal disease; multiple symmetric peripheral neuropathy; and tumor invasion of the lumbosacral plexus. Chronic pain syndromes are often associated with depression and insomnia, and include the myofascial syndromes of fibromyalgia, myofascial pain syndrome (MPS), and soft tissue lesion/mechanical disorders. Each has distinguishing characteristics.[137,138] Cancer pain is caused by peripheral nerve compression or entrapment, nerve root compression, osseous lesions, abdominal lesions, thoracic lesions, and special pains from a phantom limb, herpes zoster, or hypertrophic pulmonary osteoarthropathy.[139]

Treatment is directed at relief of pain and the underlying etiology, and is medical, surgical, pharmacologic, behavioral, and often manipulative. From an osteopathic perspective, these manifestations reflect the somatic-somatic, somatovisceral, viscerosomatic, and viscerovisceral reflexes that establish the somatic dysfunction amenable to OMT.[140,141-144] The myofascial syndromes respond well to trigger point management and acupuncture as well as osteopathic manipulative treatments.[33,117,138,145,146] Approaches to cancer-related pain include psychological support, tumor control, drug therapy, neurosurgical ablative procedures, and alternative pain management methods such as hypnosis, acupuncture, and behavior modification. Oral analgesics range from aspirin and NSAIDs (level I) to narcotic analgesics (level II, III) often in combination with other adjuvant agents such as tricyclic antidepressants, sympathomimetics, methylprednisolone, and benzodiazepines. Nerve blocks, chemotherapy, and hormonal therapy may also be required. Nonmalignant pain syndromes include myofascial pain, radiculopathy, sympathetically maintained pain (causalgia and RSD), herpes zoster and postherpetic neuralgia, peripheral neuralgias, postamputation pain, spinal joint pain, pancreatitis, facial pain, headache, pelvic pain, and central and post spinal cord injury pain.[147-151]

SUMMARY

Osteopathy embraces all of the concepts of medicine and surgery. In addition, osteopathy provides a special relationship between the neuromusculoskeletal system and somatic dysfunction, and the system's responsiveness to osteopathic manipulative therapy. The osteopathic lesion or somatic dysfunction that can be corrected by manual medicine techniques is well defined. J. Stedman Denslow[152] described the segmental facilitation concept in osteopathic lesions during the 1940s based on EMG studies. I.M. Korr[153] has expanded these observations in his many writings relative to the physiologic basis of osteopathic medicine[154] and emphasized the role of the nervous system as an integrator of function between the various body systems. Relevant to the osteopathic physician is the intimate relationship between the nervous system and manifestations of somatic dysfunction. The subtotal of the nervous system activity is a complex system of electrophysiologic and neurochemical phenomenon.[57,154-156] Treatment is regional and tailored to the observed dysfunction. The practice of osteopathic medicine is the potentiation of the intrinsic health-maintaining and health-restoring resources of the individual. This holistic approach to health and disease prevention is the basis for this unique American medical philosophy.

References

1. Peterson BA: Major events in osteopathic history. In Ward RC, editor: *Foundations for osteopathic medicine*, Baltimore, 1997, Williams & Wilkins.

2. DiGiovanna EL: History of osteopathy. In DiGiovanna EL, Schiowitz S, editors: *An osteopathic approach to diagnosis and treatment*, Hagerstown, Md., 1991, Lippincott.

3. Greenman PE: Structural diagnosis and manipulative medicine. In Greenman, PE, editor: *Principles of manual medicine*, Baltimore, 1989, Williams & Wilkins.

4. Cathie AG: *Textbook of osteopathic philosophy and principles*, Philadelphia, 1969, Philadelphia College of Osteopathic Medicine.

5. Truhlar RE: *Doctor A.T. Still in the living*, Cleveland, 1950 (Published privately).

6. Gevitz N: *The DO's: osteopathic medicine in America*, Baltimore, 1982, Johns Hopkins University Press.

7. Bezilla TA: Traditional osteopathy as an integrated model of holistic medicine, *Alternative & Complementary Therapies* 3(3):140-144, 1997.

8. Still AT: *The philosophy and mechanical principles of osteopathy*, Kansas City, Mo., 1902, Hudson-Kimberly.

9. Hoag JM: Concepts of osteopathic medicine. In Hoag M, Cole WC, Bradford SG, editors: *Osteopathic medicine*, New York, 1969, McGraw-Hill.

10. Martinke DL: Philosophy of osteopathic medicine. In DiGiovanna EL, Schiowitz S, editors: *An osteopathic approach to diagnosis and treatment*, Hagerstown, Md., 1991, Lippincott.

11. Seffinger MA: Development of osteopathic philosophy. In Ward RC, editor: *Foundations for osteopathic medicine*, Baltimore, 1997, Williams & Wilkins.

12. Cathie AG: *1974 yearbook of American academy of osteopathy—selected papers from the writings and lectures of Angus G. Cathie*, reprinted 1983, Colorado Springs, Colo..

13. Steiner C: Osteopathic manipulative treatment: What does it do? *JAOA* 94(1):85-87, 1994.

14. DiGiovanna EL: What is osteopathic medicine? In DiGiovanna EL, Schiowitz S, editors: *An osteopathic approach to diagnosis and treatment*, Hagerstown, Md., 1991, Lippincott.

15. Greenman PE: *Principles of manual medicine*, ed 2, Baltimore, 1996, Williams & Wilkins.

16. Kuchera M, Kuchera W: *Osteopathic principles in practice*, ed 2, Columbus, Ohio, 1994, Greyden.

17. Wagner GN: Osteopathy. In Miccozzi M, editor: *Fundamentals of complementary and alternative medicine*, London, 1996, Churchill-Livingstone.

18. Ward RC, editor: *Foundations for osteopathic medicine*, Baltimore, 1997, Williams & Wilkins.

19. Hewitt WF: Somatic aspects of applied physiology. In Hoag JM, Cole, WC, Bradford, SG: *Osteopathic medicine*, New York, 1969, McGraw-Hill.

20. Cole WV: Physiologic communications and controls. In Hoag JM, Cole WC, Bradford SG, editors: *Osteopathic medicine*, New York, 1969, McGraw-Hill.

21. Thomas PH: Evidences of autonomic mediation between structure and function. In Hoag JM, Cole WC,

Bradford SG, editors: *Osteopathic medicine,* New York, 1969, McGraw-Hill.

22. Heilig D: Pathogenesis of structural disorders related to osteopathic lesions. In Hoag JM, Cole WC, Bradford SG, editors: *Osteopathic medicine,* New York, 1969, McGraw-Hill.

23. Bradford SG: Application of osteopathic manipulative therapy. In Hoag JM, Cole WC, Bradford SG, editors: *Osteopathic medicine,* New York, 1969, McGraw-Hill.

24. Junghanns H: *Clinical implications of normal biomechanical stresses on spinal function,* Gaithersburg, Md., 1990, Aspen.

25. Mitchell FL Sr: 1979.

26. Patterson MM: A model mechanism for spinal segmental facilitation, *JAOA* 76:62-72, 1976.

27. Johnston WL: Segmental behavior during motion: extending behavioral boundaries, *JAOA* 72:462-473, 1973.

28. Korr IM: Proprioceptors and somatic dysfunction, *JAOA* 74:638-650, 1975.

29. Korr IM: Spinal cord as organizer of disease processes: some preliminary perspectives, *JAOA* 76:35-45, 1976.

30. Korr IM: Spinal cord as organizer of disease processes: axonal transport and neurotropic function in relation to somatic dysfunction, *JAOA* 80(7):451-459, 1981.

31. DiGiovanna EL: *Somatic dysfunction.* In *An osteopathic approach to diagnosis and treatment,* Hagerstown, Md., 1991, Lippincott.

32. Greenman PE: *Principles of manual medicine,* Baltimore, 1989, Williams & Wilkins.

33. Kuchera WA et al: *Foundations for osteopathic medicine,* Baltimore, 1997, Williams & Wilkins.

34. Fryette HH: *Principles of osteopathic techniques,* Carmel, Calif., 1994, Academy of Applied Osteopathy.

35. Magoun HI Sr: *Practical osteopathic procedures,* Kirksville, Mo., 1978, Journal Printing.

36. Dowling DJ: Neurophysiological mechanisms related to osteopathic diagnosis and treatment. In DiGiovanna E, Schiowitz S, editors: *An osteopathic approach to diagnosis and treatment,* Hagerstown, Md., 1991, Lippincott.

37. Willard FH: Autonomic nervous system. In Ward RC, editor: *Foundations for osteopathic medicine,* Baltimore, 1997, Williams & Wilkins.

38. Patterson WM, Wurster RD: Neurophysiologic system: integration and disintegration. In Ward RC, editor: *Foundations for osteopathic medicine,* Baltimore, 1997, Williams & Wilkins.

39. Kuchera WA, Kuchera ML: *Osteopathic principles in practice,* ed 2, Columbus Ohio, 1992, Greyden.

40. Korr IM: *Vulnerability of the segmental nervous system to somatic insults,* New York, 1970, Postgraduate Institute of Osteopathic Medicine and Surgery.

41. DiGiovanna EL, Schiowitz S: *An approach to osteopathic diagnosis and treatment,* Hagerstown, Md., 1991, Lippincott.

42. Nicholas NS: *Atlas of osteopathic techniques,* Philadelphia, 1974, Philadelphia College of Osteopathic Medicine.

43. Howard WH III: *Easy OMT,* Siloam Springs, Ark., 1998, Momentum.

44. Jones LH, Kusunose R, Goering E: *Jones strain-counterstrain,* Boise, Idaho, 1995, Jones Strain-Counterstrain.

45. Stoddard A: *Manual of osteopathic technique,* London, 1959, Hutchinson Med.

46. Cyriax J, Russel G: *Textbook of orthopedic medicine, vol 2,* ed 10, London, 1980, Baillere-Tindall.

47. Maigne R: *Diagnosis and treatment of pain of vertebral origin: a manual medicine approach,* Baltimore, 1996, Williams & Wilkins.

48. McM Mennel J: *The musculoskeletal system: differential diagnosis from symptoms and physical signs,* Gaithersburg, Md., 1992, Aspen.

49. DiGiovanna EL: Osteopathic manipulative treatment: contraindications, precautions and side effects. In DiGiovanna EL, Schiowitz S, editors: *An osteopathic approach to diagnosis and treatment,* Hagerstown, Md., 1991, Lippincott.

50. Pruitt AA: Approach to patient with a headache. In Goroll AH, May LA, Mulley AG Jr, editors: *Primary care medicine,* ed 3, Philadelphia, 1995, Lippincott.

51. Raskin NH: Headaches. In Rowland LP, editor: *Merritt's textbook of neurology,* ed 9, Baltimore, 1995, Williams & Wilkins.

52. Mauskop A: Headaches. In Rakel RE, editor: *The nervous system, Conn's current therapy,* Philadelphia, 1999, WB Saunders.

53. Elkis ML, Rentz LE: Neurology. In Ward RC, editor: *Foundations for osteopathic medicine,* Baltimore, 1997, Williams & Wilkins.

54. Magoun HI: *Osteopathy in the cranial field,* ed 3, Kirksville, Mo., 1976, Journal Printing.

55. Lay EM: Cranial field. In Ward RC, editor: *Foundations for osteopathic medicine,* Baltimore, 1997, Williams & Wilkins.

56. Magoun HI: Entrapment neuropathy in the cranium, *JAOA* 67:643-652, 1968.

57. Elkiss ML, Rentz LE: Neurology. In Ward RC, editor: *Foundations for osteopathic medicine,* Baltimore, 1997, Williams & Wilkins.

58. Connors MJ: Cluster headaches: a review, *JAOA* 95(9):533-539, 1995.

59. Hankinson D: Headaches. In DiGiovanna EL, Schiowitz S, editors: *An osteopathic approach to diagnosis and treatment,* Hagerstown, Md., 1991, Lippincott.

60. Jones LH: 1981.

61. Mauskop A: Headaches. In Ward RE, editor: *The nervous system, Conn's current therapy,* Philadelphia, 1999, WB Saunders.

62. Aminoff MJ: Postural hypotension. In Aminoff MJ, editor: *Neurology and general medicine,* ed 2, London, 1995, Churchill-Livingstone.

63. Goroll AH, May LA, Mulley AG Jr: *Evaluation of syncope in primary care medicine,* ed 3, Philadelphia, 1995, Lippincott.

64. Wazen JJ: Dizziness and hearing loss. In Rowland LP, editor: *Merritt's textbook of neurology,* ed 9, Baltimore, 1995, Williams & Wilkins.

65. Johnston WL, Kelso AF, Babcock HB: Changes in presence of a segmental dysfunction pattern associated with hypertension—a short term longitudinal study, *JAOA* 95(4):243-255, 1995.

66. VanBuskirk RL: Nociceptive reflexes and the somatic dysfunction: a model, *JAOA* 90(9):792-808, 1990.

67. Bailey M, Dick L: Nociceptive considerations in treating with counterstrain, *JAOA* 92(3):334-341, 1992.

68. Mitchell FL Jr: Voluntary and involuntary respiration and the craniosacral mechanism, *Osteopathic Annals,* March 1977, pp. 52-59.

69a. Thorpe RG: *Psychodynamics of stress and relationships with the musculoskeletal system: osteopathic medicine—clinical review series,* Acton, Mass., 1975, Publishing Science Group.

69b. Thorpe RG: *The hypothalamic axis and its relationship to the sympathetic nervous system: osteopathic medicine-clinical review series,* Acton, Mass., 1975, Publishing Science Group.

70. Luciani RJ: *The somatic-visceral autonomic reflex: one mechanism in acupuncture therapeutics: osteopathic medicine-clinical review series,* Acton, Mass., 1975, Publishing Science Group.

71. Granner MA: Epilepsy in adolescents and adults. In Rakel RE, editor: *The nervous system, Conn's current therapy,* Philadelphia, 1999, WB Saunders.

72. Holmes GL: Epilepsy in infants and children. In Rakel RE, editor: *The nervous system, Conn's current therapy,* Philadelphia, 1999, WB Saunders, pp. 113-124.

73. Ettinger H, Gintis B: Craniosacral concepts. In DiGiovanna EL, Schiowitz S, editors: *An osteopathic approach to diagnosis and treatment,* Hagerstown, Md., 1991, Lippincott.

74. Sutherland AS: *With thinking fingers,* Kansas City, Mo., 1962, Cranial Academy.

75. Norton JM: A tissue pressure model for palpatory perception of the cranial rhythmic impulse, *JAOA* 91(10):975-994, 1991.

76. Pruitt AA: Approach to the patient with a seizure. In Goroll AH, May LA, Mulley AG Jr, editors: *Primary care medicine,* ed 3, Philadelphia, 1995, JB Lippincott.

77. Johnston WL, Kelso AF, Babcock HB: Changes in presence of a segmental dysfunction pattern associated with hypertension, *JAOA* 95(4):243-255, 1995.

78. Harrison MJC: Neurological complications of hypertension. In Aminoff MJ, editor: *Neurology and general medicine,* ed 2, London, 1995, Churchill-Livingstone.

79. Molov JP: 1995.

80. Fayad PB: Ischemic cerebrovascular disease. In Rakel RD, editor: *The nervous system, Conn's current therapy,* Philadelphia, 1999, WB Saunders.

81. Goldszmidt AJ, Caplan LR: Intracerebral hemorrhage. In Rakel RE, editor: *The nervous system, Conn's current therapy,* Philadelphia, 1999, WB Saunders.

82. Gershkoff AM: Rehabilitation of the stroke victim. In Rakel RE, editor: *The nervous system, Conn's current therapy,* Philadelphia, 1999, WB Saunders.

83. Pruitt AA: Management of the patient with a transient ischemic attack or an asymptomatic carotid bruit. In Goroll AH et al, editors: *Primary care medicine,* ed 3, Philadelphia, 1995, Lippincott.

84. Lange et al: 1995.

85. Lovelace, Rowland: 1995.

86. Vorro J, Johnston WL, Hubbard RP: Clinical biomechanical correlates for cervical function: part I—a kinematic study, *JAOA* 85:429-437, 1985.

87. Vorro J, Johnston WL, Hubbard RP: Clinical biomechanical correlates for cervical function: part II—a myoelectric study, *JAOA* 87:353-367, 1987.

88. Vorro J, Johnston WL, Hubbard RP: Clinical biomechanical correlates for cervical function: part III—intermittent secondary movements, *JAOA* 91(2):145-155, 1991.

89. Goldman SI, Krings MS: Phenobarbital induced fibromyalgia as the cause of bilateral shoulder pain, *JAOA* 95(8):487-490, 1995.

90. Kesler R, Mendizabal JE: Headache in chiari malformation: a distinct clinical entity, *JAOA* 99(3):153-156, 1999.

91. Edmond SL: Manipulation and mobilization: extremity and spinal techniques, St Louis, 1993, Mosby.

92. Thompson HG, Rowland LP:1995.

93. Korr IM: The spinal cord as organizer of disease processes: some preliminary perspectives, *JAOA* 76:35-45, 1976.

94. Korr IM: The spinal cord as organizer of disease processes: axonal transport and neurotropic function in relation to somatic dysfunction, *JAOA* 80(7):451-459, 1981.

95a. Korr IM: Proprioceptors and somatic dysfunction, *JAOA* 74:638-650, 1975.

95b. Korr IM: The facilitated segment: a factor in injury to the body framework. In Stark EH, editor: *Osteopathic medicine—clinical review series,* Acton, Mass., 1975, Publishing Sciences Group.

95c. Korr IM: Proprioceptors and the behavior of lesioned segments. In Stark EH, editor: *Osteopathic medicine—clinical review series,* Acton, Mass., 1975, Publishing Sciences Group.

96. VanBuskirk RL: Nociceptor reflexes and the somatic dysfunction: a model, *JAOA* 90(9):792-808, 1990.

97. Elliot FA: *Tinnitus, in clinical neurology,* Philadelphia, 1971, WB Saunders.

98. DeWeese DD, Saunders WH: *Textbook of otolaryngology,* St Louis, 1968, Mosby.

99. Schuknecht HF: *Pathology of the ear,* ed 2, Philadelphia, 1993, Lea & Febiger.

100. Brookler KH: Tinnitus. In Rakel RE, editor: *Conn's current therapy,* Philadelphia, 1999, WB Saunders.

101. Aminoff MJ: *Neurology and general medicine,* ed 2, London, 1995, Churchill-Livingstone.

102. Fife TD: Episodic vertigo. In Rakel RE, editor: *The Nervous System, Conn's current therapy,* Philadelphia, 1999, WB Saunders.

103. Pruitt AA: Evaluation of dementia. In Goroll AH, May LA, Mulley AG Jr, editors: *Primary care medicine,* ed 3, Philadelphia, 1995, Lippincott.

104. Doody RS: Alzheimer's Disease. In Rakel RE, editor: *The nervous system, Conn's current therapy,* Philadelphia, 1999, WB Saunders.

105. Sackler NC, Mayew L: Delirium and dementia. In Rowland LP, editor: *Merritt's textbook of neurology,* ed 9, Baltimore, 1995, Williams & Wilkins.

106. Rumney IC: Osteopathic manipulative treatment of infectious diseases. In Stark EH, editor: *Osteopathic medicine-a clinical review series,* Acton, Mass., 1975, Publishing Sciences Group.

107. Allen EG: Immunologically mediated enhancement of nonspecific host resistance. In Stark EH, editor: *Osteopathic medicine: a clinical review series,* Acton, Mass., 1975, Publishing Sciences Group.

108. Mitchell FL Jr: Influence of chapman reflexes and the immune reactions. In Stark EH, editor: *Osteopathic medicine: clinical review series,* Acton, Mass., 1975, Publishing Sciences Group.

109. Pruitt AA: Evaluation of tremor. In Goroll AH, May LA, Mulley AG Jr, editors: *Primary care medicine,* ed 3, Philadelphia, 1995, Lippincott.

110. Pruitt AA: Evaluation of tremor. In Goroll AH, May LA, Mulley AG Jr, editors: *Approach to the patient with Parkinson's disease,* ed 3, Philadelphia, 1995, Lippincott.

111. Goroll AH, May LA, Mulley AG Jr: Management of multiple sclerosis. In *Primary care medicine,* ed 3, Philadelphia, 1995, Lippincott.

112. Goodridge JP: Muscle energy technique procedures. In Ward RC, editor: *Foundations for osteopathic medicine,* Baltimore, 1997, Williams & Wilkins.

113. Ward RC: Integrated neuromusculoskeletal techniques for specific areas. In Ward RC, editor: *Foundations for osteopathic medicine,* Baltimore, 1997, Williams & Wilkins.

114. Schiowitz S: Functional anatomy and biomechanics. In DiGiovanna EL, Schiowitz S, editors: *An osteopathic approach to diagnosis and treatment,* Hagerstown, Md., 1991, Lippincott.

115. Kuchera ML, McPartland JM: Myofascial trigger points: an introduction. In Ward RC, editor: *Foundations for osteopathic medicine,* Baltimore, 1997, Williams & Wilkins.

116. Kuchera ML: Travell and Simons' myofascial trigger points. In Ward RC, editor: *Foundations for osteopathic medicine,* Baltimore, 1997, Williams & Wilkins.

117. Patriquin DA: Chapman's reflexes. In Ward RC, editor: *Foundations for osteopathic medicine,* Baltimore, 1997, Williams & Wilkins.

118. Phykitt DE: Whiplash injuries. In DiGiovanna EL, Schiowitz S, editors: *An osteopathic approach to diagnosis and treatment,* Hagerstown, Md., 1991, Lippincott.

119. Yale SD: Scoliosis. In DiGiovanna EL, Schiowitz S, editors: *An osteopathic approach to diagnosis and treatment,* Hagerstown, Md., 1991, Lippincott.

120. Polstein B: Lumbar radiculopathies. In DiGiovanna EL, Schiowitz S, editors: *An osteopathic approach to diagnosis and treatment,* Hagerstown, Md., 1991, JB Lippincott.

121. DiGiovanna EL: Thoracic Outlet Syndrome. In DiGiovanna EL, Schiowitz S, editors: *An osteopathic approach to diagnosis and treatment,* Hagerstown, Md., 1991, Lippincott.

122. Scariati PD: Coccygodynia. In DiGiovanna EL, Schiowitz S, editors: *An osteopathic approach to diagnosis and treatment,* Hagerstown, Md., 1991, Lippincott.

123. Goldman HS: Occupational shoulder injuries, *Osteopathic Annals* 5(7):41-46, 1977.

124. Schnatz P & Steiner C: Tennis elbow: a biomechanical and therapeutic approach, *JAOA* 93(7):778-788, 1993.

125. Sucher BM: Palpatory diagnosis and manipulative management of carpal tunnel syndrome, *JAOA* 94(8):647-663, 1994.

126. Sucher BM: Palpatory diagnosis and manipulative management of carpal tunnel syndrome, part II, *JAOA* 95(8):471-479. 1995.

127. Sucher BM, Heath DM: Thoracic outlet syndrome: a myofascial variant, postural and structural consequences, *JAOA* 93(3):334-345, 1993.

128. Sucher BM: Thoracic outlet syndrome: a myofascial variant—treatment, *JAOA* 90(9):810-823, 1990.

129. Luckenbill-Edds L, Bechill GB: Nerve compression syndromes as models for research on osteopathic manipulative treatment, *JAOA* 95(5):319-326, 1995.

130. Wilkerson LA: Martial arts injuries, *JAOA* 97(4):221-226, 1997.

131. Greenman PE, McPartland JM: Cranial findings and iatrogenesis from craniosacral manipulation in patients with traumatic brain syndrome, *JAOA* 95(3):182-192, 1995.

132. Weilburg JB: Approach to the patient with insomnia. In Goroll AH, May LA, Mulley AG Jr, editors: *Primary care medicine,* ed 3, Philadelphia, 1995, Lippincott.

133. Kaluza CL, Krachman SL, D'Alonzo GE: Obstructive sleep apnea: a multisystem disorder, *JAOA* 95(7):420-426, 1995.

134. Adams RD, Victor M, Ropper AH, editors: Sleep and its abnormalities. In *Principles of neurology,* ed 6, New York, 1997, McGraw-Hill.

135. Kryger MH, Roth T, Dement WC: *Principles and practice of sleep medicine,* Philadelphia, 1989, WB Saunders.

136. Rizzo M, Tranel D: *Head injury and postconcussive syndrome,* London, 1996, Churchill-Livingstone.

137. Travell JG, Simons DG: *Myofascial pain and dysfunction: the trigger point manual,* Baltimore, 1983, Williams & Wilkins.
138. Rachlin ES: *Myofascial pain and fibromyalgia: trigger point management,* St Louis, 1994, Mosby.
139. Rogers JN: Pain. In Rakel RE, editor: *Conn's current therapy,* Philadelphia, 1999, WB Saunders.
140. Jerome JA: 1997.
141. Wilbur WV: Disorders of the nervous system. In Hoag JM, Cole WC, Bradford SG, editors: *Osteopathic medicine,* New York, 1969, McGraw-Hill.
142. Korr IM: Sympathetic nervous system mediation between the somatic and supportive processes. In *Physiological basis of osteopathic medicine,* New York, 1970, Postgraduate Institute of Osteopathic Medicine and Surgery.
143. Hix EL: Visceroviseral and somatovisceral reflex communication. In *Physiological basis of osteopathic medicine,* New York, 1970, Postgraduate Institute of Osteopathic Medicine and Surgery.
144. Luciani RJ: The somatic-visceral autonomic reflex: one mechanism for acupuncture therapeutics. In Stark EH, editor: *Osteopathic medicine: clinical review series,* Acton, Mass., 1975, Publishing Sciences Group.
145. Cantu RI, Groden AJ: *Myofascial manipulation theory and clinical application,* Gaithersburg, Md., 1992, Aspen.
146. Baldry PE: *Acupuncture, trigger points, and musculoskeletal pain,* ed 2, London, 1993, Churchill-Livingstone.
147. Abram SE: *The pain clinic manual,* Philadelphia, 1990, Lippincott.
148. Warfield CA: *Manual of pain management,* Philadelphia, 1991, Lippincott.
149. Patt RB: *Cancer pain,* Philadelphia, 1993, JB Lippincott.
150. Maigne R: *Diagnosis and treatment of pain of vertebral origin: a manual medicine approach,* Baltimore, 1996, Williams & Wilkins.
151. Cousins MJ, Bridenbaugh PO: *Neural blockade pain management,* ed 2, Philadelphia, 1988, Lippincott.
152. Denslow JS: An analysis of the variability of spinal reflex thresholds, *J Neurophysiol* 7:207-216, 1944.
153. Korr IM: *An explication of osteopathic principles, foundations for osteopathic medicine,* Baltimore, 1997, Williams & Wilkins.
154. Still AT: *Autobiography of A.T. Still,* 1897 (Published by author).
155. Truhlar RE: *Doctor A.T. Still in the living,* Cleveland, Ohio, 1950 (Privately published).
156. Downing CH: *Osteopathic principles in disease,* Newark Ohio, 1988, American Academy of Osteopathy (originally published in 1935).

Additional Readings:

Denslow JS, Korr IM, Krems AD: Quantitative studies of chronic facilitation in human motoneuron pools, *Am J Physiol* 105:229-238, 1947.

DiGiovanna EL: Chapman's reflexes. In DiGiovanna EL, Schiowitz S, editors: *An osteopathic approach to diagnosis and treatment,* Hagerstown, Md., 1991, Lippincott.
Ettinger H, Gintis B: Craniosacral conceptsin. In DiGiovanna EL, Schiowitz S, editors: *An osteopathic approach to diagnosis and treatment,* Hagerstown, Md., 1991, Lippincott.
Goldstein R: Acupuncture. In DiGiovanna EL, Schiowitz S, editors: *An osteopathic approach to diagnosis and treatment,* Hagerstown, Md., 1991, Lippincott.
Goodridge JP: Muscle energy technique: definition, explanation, methods of procedure, *JAOA* 81(4):249-254, 1981.
Goodridge JP, Kuchera WA: Muscle energy treatment techniques for specific areas. In Ward RC, editor: *Foundations for osteopathic medicine,* Baltimore, 1997, Williams & Wilkins.
Goroll AH, May LA, Mulley AG Jr: Approach to the patient with sleep apnea. In *Primary care medicine,* ed 3, Philadelphia, 1995, Lippincott.
Goroll AH, May LA, Mulley AG Jr: *Evaluation of dizziness in primary care medicine,* ed 3, Philadelphia, 1995, Lippincott.
Hix EL: The trophic function of visceral nerves. In *Physiological basis of osteopathic medicine,* New York, 1970, Postgraduate Institute of Osteopathic Medicine and Surgery.
Johnson WL, Kelso AF, Babcock HB: Changes in presence of a segmental dysfunction pattern associated with hypertension, *JAOA* 95(4):243-255, 1995.
Korr IM: The neural basis of the osteopathic lesion, *JAOA* 47:191-198, 1947.
Norton JM: A tissue pressure model for palpatory perception of the cranial rhythmic impulse, *JAOA* 91(10):975-994, 1991.
Polstein B: Spondylolisthesis and spondylolysis. In DiGiovanna EL, Schiowitz S, editors: *An osteopathic approach to diagnosis and treatment,* Hagerstown, Md., 1991, Lippincott.
Pruitt AA: Focal neurologic complaints:evaluation of nerve root and peripheral nerve syndromes. In Goroll AH, May AM, Mulley AG Jr, editors: *Primary care medicine,* ed 3, Philadelphia, 1995, Lippincott.
Upledger JE: Integration of acupuncture and manipulation, *Osteopathic Medicine,* 19-111, July 1977.
Van Den Noort S: Parkinson's disease. In Rakel RE, editor: *The nervous system, Conn's current therapy,* Philadelphia, 1999, WB Saunders.
Weiner HI, Stazzone L: Multiple Sclerosis. In Rakel RE, editor: *The nervous system, Conn's current therapy,* Philadelphia, 1999, WB Saunders.
Willard FH, Mokler DJ, Morgane PJ: Neuroendocrine-immune system and homeostasis. In Ward RC, editor: *Foundations for osteopathic medicine,* Baltimore, 1997, Williams & Wilkins.

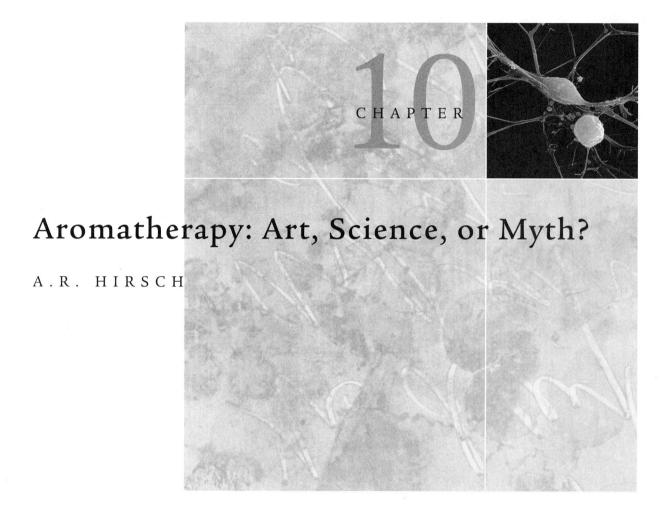

CHAPTER

10

Aromatherapy: Art, Science, or Myth?

A . R .   H I R S C H

$\mathcal{I}$n explaining the persuasive attraction of alternative medicine, Kaptchuk and Eisenberg note, "The fundamental premises are an advocacy of nature, vitalism, science, and spirituality."[1] With this in mind, the science underpinning aromatherapy is explored.

DEFINITIONS

One of the difficulties in understanding aromatherapy is that it means different things to different people. The one part of its definition that is agreed upon is that aromatherapy uses odorous compounds to promote health and healing.[2] Beyond this, opinions differ. Aromachologists speak of using odors not to treat disease, but to promote wellness. Aromatologists believe in ingestion of the substance being used as well as its inhalation.[2] Many aromatherapists believe in using massage coincident with inhalation.[3] In this chapter, aromatherapy is defined as the use of odorants as inhalants to treat underlying medical or psychiatric conditions. This definition excludes any effects of ingestion or percutaneous absorption, although they may be significant depending upon the method of application.[4] As defined, aromatherapy use is also independent of any effects of coincident, noninhalational therapy, such as massage, interpersonal interaction, or bathing.

This definition is consistent with the literature indicating that "real aromatherapy" involves the uptake of fragrant compounds *only* through inhalation, not by other methods.[5]

Many in the aromatherapy community believe that natural or essential oils are effective and that artificial synthesized compounds are not. However, in the treatment of neurologic and psychiatric diseases, literature does not differentiate between them.[6] No distinction is made herein between the use of synthesized as opposed to naturally occurring oils.

BACKGROUND

Why is the concept of aromatherapy under consideration today? One reason is its historicity. Throughout history, odorants have been used to treat various diseases. More than 5000 years ago Egyptians treated disease using odors,[7] and 3500 years ago Babylonians used odors to exorcise demons of disease.[8] Ancient Aztecs also used odors to treat disease. Aromatherapy has known no cultural or geographic boundaries. Virtually all cultures have fumigated the sick.[5]

ANATOMY OF OLFACTION

Neuroscience provides insight into the mechanisms by which odors may impact behavior and neurologic functioning. There is an anatomic basis for the belief that odors can affect the brain and behavior.[9] Once an odor passes through the olfactory epithelium, it must stimulate the olfactory nerve, which consists of unmyelinated olfactory fila. The olfactory nerve has the slowest conduction rate of any nerve in the body. The olfactory fila pass through the cribiform plate of the ethmoid bone and enter the olfactory bulb. During trauma, much damage occurs in this bulb.[10] Different odors localize in different areas of the olfactory bulb.

Inside the olfactory bulb is a conglomeration of neuropil called the *glomeruli*. Approximately 2000 glomeruli reside in the olfactory bulb. Four different cell types make up the glomeruli: processes of receptor cell axons, mitral cells, tufted cells, and second-order neurons that give off collaterals to the granule cells and to cells in the periglomerular and external plexiform layers. The mitral and tufted cells form the lateral olfactory tract and establish a reverberating circuit with the granule cells. The mitral cells stimulate firing of the granule cells, which in turn inhibit firing of the mitral cells.

A reciprocal inhibition exists between the mitral and tufted cells. This results in a sharpening of olfactory acuity. The olfactory bulb receives several efferent projections, including the primary olfactory fibers, the contralateral olfactory bulb and the anterior nucleus, the prepiriform cortex (inhibitory), the diagonal band of Broca (with neurotransmitters acetylcholine and GABA), the locus coeruleus, the dorsal raphe, and the tuberomamillary nucleus of the hypothalamus.

The olfactory bulb's efferent fibers project into the olfactory tract, which divides at the olfactory trigona into the medial and lateral olfactory stria. These project to the anterior olfactory nucleus; the olfactory tubercle; the amygdaloid nucleus (which in turn projects to the ventral medial nucleus of the hypothalamus, a feeding center); the cortex of the piriform lobe; the septal nuclei; and the hypothalamus, in particular the anterolateral regions of the hypothalamus, which are involved in reproduction. The neurotransmitters by which the olfactory bulb conducts its information include glutamate, aspartate, NAAG, CCK, and GABA.

The anterior olfactory nucleus receives afferent fibers from the olfactory tract and projects efferent fibers, which decussate in the anterior commissure and synapse in the contralateral olfactory bulb. Some of the efferent projections from the anterior olfactory nucleus remain ipsilateral, and synapse on internal granular cells of the ipsilateral olfactory bulb.

The olfactory tubercle receives afferent fibers from the olfactory bulb and the anterior olfactory nucleus. Efferent fibers from the olfactory tubercle project to the nucleus accumbens as well as the striatum. Neurotransmitters of the olfactory tubercle include acetylcholine and dopamine.

The area on the cortex where olfaction is localized, that is, the primary olfactory cortex, includes the prepiriform area, the periamygdaloid area, and the entorhinal area. Afferent projections to the primary olfactory cortex include the mitral cells, which enter the lateral olfactory tract and synapse in the prepiriform cortex (lateral olfactory gyrus) and the corticomedial part of the amygdala. Efferent projections from the primary olfactory cortex extend to the entorhinal cortex (area 28), the basal and lateral amygdaloid nuclei, the lateral preoptic area of the hypothalamus, the nucleus of the diagonal band of Broca, the medial forebrain bundle, the dorsal medial nucleus and submedial nucleus of the thalamus, and the nucleus accumbens.

It should be noted that the entorhinal cortex is both a primary and a secondary olfactory cortical area. Efferent fibers from the cortex project via the uncinate fasciculus to the hippocampus, the anterior insular cortex (next to the gustatory cortical area, and the frontal cortex. This may explain why temporal lobe epilepsy that involves the uncinate often produces parageusias of burning rubber, uncinate fits.[11]

Some of the efferent projections of the mitral and tufted cells decussate in the anterior commissure and form the medial olfactory tract. They then synapse in the contralateral parolfactory area and contralateral subcallosal gyrus. The exact function of the medial olfactory stria and tract is not clear. The accessory olfactory bulb receives afferent fibers from the bed nucleus of the accessory olfactory tract and the medial and posterior corticoamygdaloid nuclei. Efferent fibers from the accessory olfactory bulb project through the accessory olfactory tract to the same afferent areas, for example, the bed nucleus of the accessory olfactory tract and the medial and posterior corticoamygdaloid nuclei. It should be noted that the medial and posterior corticoamygdaloid nuclei project secondary fibers to the anterior and medial hypothalamus, the areas associated with reproduction. Therefore the accessory olfactory bulb in humans may be the mediator for human pheromones.[12]

Some unique aspects of the anatomy of the olfactory system are worth mentioning. Smell is the only sensation to reach the cortex before reaching the thalamus. The only sensory system that is primarily ipsilateral in its projection, olfaction does not depend upon the cortex, as has been demonstrated in decorticated cats.

Neurotransmitters of the olfactory cortex are multiple, including glutamate, aspartate cholcystekinin, LHRH, and somatastatin. Furthermore, perception of odors causes modulation of olfactory neurotransmitters within the olfactory bulb and the limbic system. Virtually all known neurotransmitters are present in the olfactory bulb. Thus odorant modulation of neurotransmitter levels in the olfactory bulb, tract, and limbic system intended for transmission of sensory information may have unintended secondary effects on a variety of different behaviors and disease states that are regulated by the same neurotransmitters. For instance, odorant modulation of dopamine in the olfactory bulb/limbic system may affect manifestations of Parkinson's disease. Mesolimbic override to many of the components of Parkinson's disease have been well documented, for example, motoric activation associated with emotional distress and fear of injury in a fire.

EMOTIONAL AND BEHAVIORAL EFFECTS OF ODORS

Odors can affect behavior by acting as alternative sensory stimuli. The phenomenon of visual system mediation of the movements of parkinsonian gait through the visual stimuli of lines placed on the floor[13] is an example of alternative stimuli. Other sensory input, including pain, has been shown to inhibit the jacksonian march in epilepsy.[14] Similarly, odors may act as competing sensory stimuli during an uncinate seizure.[15] It seems possible that other sensory input, including odors, could modify Parkinson's disease as well as other neurologic conditions by acting as competing sensory stimuli.

Using another mechanism of action, odors can affect behavior and mood by producing secondary effects on the emotions of the individual. This is different from a direct neurophysiologic effect of the limbic system. Rather, the odor can change the mood of the individual, which then has secondary neurologic effects. For instance, the mood or level of alertness can affect a variety of neurologic conditions, including the perception of pain. A soldier who is severely wounded in battle may continue to fight and not feel pain until the battle is over. Studies also suggest that persons in a positive state of mind are less bothered by pain.[16]

Substantial evidence exists that odors can affect mood. As early as 1908, Freud[17] stressed the importance of olfaction on emotion in his description of a patient with an obsessional neurosis:

By his own account, when a child, he recognized every one by their smell, like a dog, and even when he was grown up he was more susceptible to sensations of smell than other people . . . and I have come to recognize that a tendency towards osphresiolagnia which has become extinct since childhood may play a part in the genesis of neuroses.

In a general way I should like to raise the question whether the inevitable shunting of the sense of smell as a result of man's turning away from the earth and the organic repression of smell pleasure produced by it does not largely share in his predisposition to nervous diseases. It would thus furnish an explanation for the fact that with the advance of civilization it is precisely the sexual life which must become the victim of repression. For we have long known what an intimate relation exists in the animal organization between the sexual impulse and the function of the olfactory organs.

Of all the sensations, olfaction is the one most intertwined with limbic system functioning.[18] The profuse anatomic and physiologic interconnections through the olfactory bulb, stria, and nuclei to the olfactory tubercle, and from there to the prepiriform cortex, the amygdala, and numerous other limbic system structures support this.[19]

Smells are described differently from other sensory modalities, adding credence to their connection to emotion. Other sensory modalities are first described cognitively; a picture, for instance, is identified as being of a ship, a woman, or a house and only secondarily is it described affectively: "I like it," or "I dislike it."[20] But odors are first and foremost described affectively: "I like it," or "I dislike it."

The olfactory/limbic/hippocampal connections help to explain olfactory-evoked nostalgia, the phenomenon whereby an odor induces a vivid recall of a scene from the distant past.[21] In 86% of 989 subjects queried, certain odors triggered vivid associations analogous to a flashbulb memory. Classically an event must induce strong emotions for deposition of such memories to occur.[22,23] By directly stimulating the limbic system, odors likewise can act as the inducing agent. This phenomenon was vividly described by Proust,[24] who wrote that the aroma of madeleine dipped in tea evoked his flood of memories and nostalgic feelings. Olfactory-evoked recall is usually a positive experience, but it can be negative, as in the olfactory flashbacks of post-traumatic stress disorder.[25] Hence, it seems possible that olfactory-evoked nostalgia may affect behavior because approximately 90% of these memories are associated with strong affective tones.[26]

The facts bring to the forefront the question of how odors impact on behavior or mood. The answer can be represented by either of two constructs: the lock and key theory or the general affective theory of odors.

THE LOCK AND KEY THEORY OF ODORS

The lock and key theory of odors (also called the *systemic effect theory*)[5] suggests that odor acts very much like a specific neurotransmitter, a drug, or an enzyme. In this paradigm, an odorant has a specific effect on behavior or emotion—one odor for one emotion or one odor for, at most, a few emotions. Thus an odor could be viewed like a medication in the pharma-copeia. For instance, in the world of neurology, propranolol is used for modulation of essential tremor, migraine headache, and anxiety. However, one would not use propranolol as a treatment for insomnia, dementia, or multiple sclerosis. The lock and key theory suggests that specific odors have specific effects. This theory has been proposed in virtually every book about aromatherapy in which specific odors are recommended for specific health effects.[2,27-32]

An argument supporting the lock and key theory is that odorants exert central nervous system (CNS) effects outside a subject's conscious awareness. In test animals, the more lipophilic an odor is, the greater its sedative effect. In addition, steric differences in odors create different effects despite similarities in perceived odor and volatility.[5,33]

According to the lock and key theory, odors act as a drug[34] with a potentially pharmacologic mechanism of action. The odorants are integrated in the membrane of the cells, causing an increase in membrane volume due to disruption of the membrane lipids. This leads to electrical stabilization of the membrane, thus blocking the inflow of calcium ions and suppressing permeability for sodium ions. As a result, action potential production is inhibited, which induces narcosis or local anesthesia. At higher concentrations of odorant, the conductivity of potassium ions is reduced. It is also possible that the odorants act on protein kinase C, which could impact upon the spontaneous rhythm of nerve cells.[5]

This mechanism of action is further supported by established physiology for the action of an odor on the target organ—in this case the brain. Inhalation of an odorant would have to produce measurable levels in the blood, sufficient to pass through the blood brain barrier. Stimpfl[35] demonstrated that this does occur. One subject inhaled 1,8-cineol for 20 minutes, which produced a linear increase of 1,8-cineol in the blood, up to 275ng/ml, a level high enough to allow penetration of the blood brain barrier.[35]

THE GENERAL AFFECTIVE THEORY OF ODORS

An alternative theory, the general affective theory of odors, also called the *reflectorial effect theory*,[5] holds that an odor experienced as hedonically positive induces a positive, happy mood and when in a happy mood, an individual does almost everything better.

For instance, when a person feels happy, it is easier to learn and to sleep, and headaches are less frequent. According to the general affective theory, a single odor could have a multitude of diverse effects, thus affecting virtually all behaviors.

The major premise that hedonically positive odors induce happier moods was demonstrated by Alaoui-Ismaili.[36] Forty-four subjects inhaled five odorants, namely, vanillin, menthol, eugenol, methyl methacrylate, and propionic acid. Six autonomic nervous system parameters were recorded: skin potential, skin resistance, skin temperature, skin blood flow, instantaneous respiratory frequency, and instantaneous heart rate. Evaluation of these parameters demonstrated a pattern consistent with known emotional states. Hedonically pleasant odors evoked mainly happiness and surprise, and unpleasant ones induced mainly disgust and anger.[36]

Milter also showed that exposure to odors could change emotions in the same direction as the hedonic valence of the odor.[37] Using the startle reflex amplitude as a physiologic indicator of emotional valence, he found that the odor of hydrogen sulfide (H_2S) increased the startle reflex amplitude and the odor of vanillin reduced it.

Aromatherapists recognize the affective impact of odors as the mechanism of action. Buchbauer notes, "A pleasant odor has always been, and still is, an important factor for people to feel good, and feeling well is synonymous with good health. Therefore we can conclude that all substances which are able to create a certain amount of well-being and well-feeling possess therapeutic properties and, therefore, can be called therapeutic agents."[38] The general affective theory of odors might be extended to include nonodorants in the pharmacologic arena, such as Valium. Valium may be useful for virtually all medical conditions because reducing anxiety makes conditions such as chronic pain, movement disorders, or insomnia less bothersome. Hence an entire branch of medicine could be built around Valium: "Valiotherapy." If one ascribes aromatherapeutic results to the general affective theory as the mechanism of action, it follows that any odor that one likes induces a happier state and hence would have a positive effect on any disease. Again, the concept could be expanded beyond odors to any environmental stimuli, for example, a bird singing or a pretty landscape. A *Star Wars* movie might induce happiness in some observers and could be seen as inducing a positive mood state. The positive mood might lead to a reduction in pain, anxiety, and negative feelings. One could then categorize this as a form of alternative therapy: "Lucastherapy."

Reliance on the general affective theory of odors implies that virtually any sensory stimulus could be used as a therapeutic tool. This largely trivializes the definition of therapy.

Another problem with the general affective theory of odors is that the same odor, in different contexts, may induce opposite emotional tones.[39] In *The Invalid's Story*, Mark Twain compares the disgust at the odor of a rotting corpse to the delight at the smell of cheese. The odors were the same but perceived to be from different sources. This suggests that an odor that is contextually appropriate in one situation might be considered totally inappropriate in another. Smelled in a positive context, it would be appreciated as hedonically positive and would enhance a positive affective state; smelled in a negative context, it would be perceived as hedonically negative and would, thus, induce a negative affective state. Therefore the same odor could produce opposite mood states and opposite effects.

A variant of the general affective theory is that odors may induce a mood more congruent with the demands of the external environment. For instance, if the external environment requires that the individual be alert, the odor induces awareness of this. Therefore the individual responds by becoming more alert. Alternatively, if the external environment is such that it is more appropriate to be relaxed, the odor induces that awareness and the individual responds by becoming more relaxed. Evidence for the validity of this variant comes from studies of muguet odor. Where the external demand is for a greater degree of relaxation, individuals do become more relaxed, and in an environment where they are required to be more alert and vigilant, they become more alert. Warm et al.,[40] demonstrated this effect of odorant-induced recognition of affective demands. Forty subjects underwent vigilance tasks for 40 minutes during which they received periodic 30-second whiffs of air or one of two hedonically positive fragrances: muguet (independently judged as relaxing) or peppermint (independently judged as alerting). Those who received either the relaxing or alerting fragrance detected more signals during the vigilance task than the unscented air controls ($p = .05$).

This odorant-induced congruence of mood may also be applied to the pharmacologic agent Valium.

Valium can induce opposite mood states in the same individual at different times. It can reduce anxiety to enhance concentration on a test, or it can reduce concentration to act as a soporific when the same individual is suffering with insomnia.

A corollary to the general affective theory is that hedonically negative odors or malodors have a negative effect on mood. If this is true, the simple elimination or masking of malodors with neutral or hedonically positive odors would induce positive effects.

Literature supports the negative effects of hedonically negative odors. In 1980, Miner[41] described some effects of exposure to the odor of livestock waste. They included annoyance, depression, nausea, vomiting, headache, shallow breathing, coughing, insomnia, and impaired appetite.

One of the malodorous pollutants that has been studied, trichloroethylene, a universally present air pollutant, can cause cephalgia.[42] Acute exposure to nitrogen tetroxide can cause cephalgia[43] and chronic neurotoxicity.[44] Acute exposure to chlorine gas can cause neurotoxicity.[45] In 1991, Neutra[46] reported that people living near hazardous waste sites suffer more physical symptoms during times when they can detect malodors than when they are unaware of them. Shusterman[47] demonstrated that even at levels considered nontoxic, chemical effluviums can cause physical symptoms.

HEALTH EFFECTS OF MALODORS

Health effects of malodors can be divided into six categories: respiratory, chemosensory, cardiovascular, immune, neurologic, and psychologic.

Respiratory. Asthmatics are especially affected by malodors. Any strong odor may induce an attack in persons with unstable asthma and, even in nonasthmatics, malodors have been demonstrated to affect the cardiorespiratory system. Increased ambient oxidant levels correlate with slower cross-country running times in high school students.[48]

Chemosensory. Chronic exposure to malodors from pulp mills can cause permanent olfactory loss.[49]

Cardiovascular. Certain malodors can induce an adrenocortic and adrenomedullary response leading to elevated blood pressure and a subsequent increase in stroke and heart disease.[50]

Immune. Immune function may be compromised either directly, as a result of olfactory/neural projections to lymphoid tissue,[50] or indirectly, as a result of malodor-induced depression or other negative mood states.[51]

Neurologic. Chronic exposure to intermittent malodors from a U.S. Navy dump site in Port Orchard, Washington, induced cortical and subcortical dysfunction, which was manifested by encephalopathy: limbic encephalopathy and cephalgia.[52] Both ambient NO_2 and SO_2 impair visual adaptation to darkness and sensitivity to brightness, and increase alpha wave desynchronization on EEG.[53]

Psychologic. Recognized for centuries and noted by Freud and others, psychologic effects of odors vary widely among individuals. Persons under major stress are particularly vulnerable to the psychologic effects of ambient malodors.[50] Persons with a distorted or impaired olfactory sense may be annoyed by odors that other persons usually consider pleasant.[50]

Certain bad odors irritate nasal passages. Resultant trigeminal stimulation releases adrenaline, leading to a tense and angry state. Thus bad odors can trigger aggression that may then be covertly expressed. For example, in one experiment college men were instructed to apply electric shocks of varying intensity to their colleagues, supposedly for the purpose of training them. When bad odors were present, the subjects chose to inflict greater degrees of pain upon their colleagues.[54] Another example involves air pollution. On days when malodorous air pollution is high, the number of motor vehicle accidents increase, indicating that people drive more aggressively in a polluted environment.[55]

Various studies show how mood and well being suffer in the presence of malodors. Residents exposed to the effluvium from nearby commercial swine operations reported that they suffered increased tension, fatigue, confusion, depression, and anger and that their vigor decreased.[56] According to one study[57] ambient pollutants decreased personal attraction. In a German urban area, the moods of young adults fluctuated in synchrony with the daily fluctuations in quality of environmental air, a pattern especially marked among more emotionally unstable individuals.[58] Further, daily diary entries of women in Bavaria showed that variations in their psychologic well being coincided with variations in ambient air quality. The correlation was particularly marked among women suffering from chronic diseases, such as diabetes.[59,60] In Israel negative health effects were significantly associated with levels of urban pollution.[61]

The number of family disturbances and the number of 911 emergency psychiatric calls were also linked to malodors in the environment, as determined by ozone levels.[62] In several cities the number of psychiatric admissions paralleled the quality of environmental air.[63]

In a study of the malodorous emanations from a mulching site southeast of Chicago, it was found that on days when the miasma wafted from the site to the school across the street, children at the school demonstrated increased behavioral problems.[64]

Malodorous ambient SO_2 levels correlate with psychiatric admissions, child psychiatric emergencies,[65] and behavioral difficulties with decreased cooperation.[66] Ambient NO_2 levels covary with psychiatric emergency room visits.[67] In nonsmokers the odor of cigarette smoke has been demonstrated to exacerbate aggressive behavior.[68]

The fatigue and annoyance caused by ambient malodors undoubtedly reduce individuals' capacities to function normally. Their abilities to tolerate frustration, to learn, and to cope with other stressors are impaired. In one laboratory study, subjects exposed to unpleasant odors experienced increased feelings of helplessness.[69]

CONTRADICTORY THEORIES

If the general affective theory of odors is true, a single odor can induce a positive mood in one person and a negative mood in another. This negates the lock and key theory in which odors' effects are produced outside of conscious awareness. Robin et al. demonstrated this using eugenol.[70] Eugenol, which is often associated with the smell of dental cement, was rated pleasant by nonfearful dental subjects and unpleasant by fearful subjects ($p=0.036$). Changes in subjects' autonomic nervous system measurements were consistent with their emotional states.[70,71] Nineteen subjects were exposed to eugenol while recording six autonomic nervous system parameters, including two electrodermal, two thermovascular, and two cardiorespiratory. The results of 7 subjects with high dental fear were compared with those of 12 without

such fear. Those with dental fear had a stronger electrodermal response ($p=0.006$), suggesting that eugenol triggered different emotional responses depending upon the unpleasantness of the subject's past dental experiences. Thus the same odor can have different effects depending upon the past experience of the individual.[71]

On the other hand, if the lock and key theory is true, and an odors' behavioral effects are produced outside of awareness and independent of affective reaction, this negates the general affective theory of odors. Ludvigson and Rottman do just that, demonstrating that the scent of lavender enhances mood state while impairing arithmetic reasoning ($p=0.01$).[72]

Given the previous information, several factors must be taken into account in reviewing the literature regarding efficacy of aromatherapy in the treatment of neurologic disease. Can odors elevate mood as the general affective theory maintains or do they act in lock and key fashion? Were the odors tested considered hedonically positive by each subject? This question is essential because what is hedonically positive for one person can be hedonically negative for another, and an odor that is hedonically positive at one concentration may be hedonically negative at another.[73] Was an associated change in mood independent of the desired effect? Was there a control group? Was the procedure single blinded or double blinded? Was the subject size sufficient to obviate falsely positive test results? Did the subjects of the experiment have a normal or near-normal sense of smell?

Could suggestion have an effect? This is particularly relevant because various studies suggest that, as in traditional pharmacologic intervention,[74] odors have both placebo and nocebo effects as demonstrated by Knasko et al.[75] Knasko subjected 90 subjects to water vapor sprayed in a room; 30 subjects were told that the water vapor odor was pleasant, 30 that it was unpleasant, and 30 that it was neutral. Those who had been told that the odorant was pleasant reported being in a better mood than did the other two groups ($p=0.05$). Subjects who been told the odor was unpleasant, reported having more health symptoms ($p<0.0003$).

Were the experiments controlled not only for the effect of suggestion, but also for the effect of expectation of outcome? It seems possible that persons with a positive view of aromatherapy who believe that odors can have a positive effect will experience a positive effect because of their bias.

The effect of expectation has been demonstrated neurophysiologically by Lorig and Roberts[76] who measured the contingent negative variation (CNV) of the EEG in 18 subjects presented with a mixed odor of lavender, jasmine, and galbanium. They found CNV amplitude for the mixed odors varied depending on what the subjects were told about it ($p=0.05$).

Did the experimenter consider the effect of social desirability whereby subjects try to please the examiner by biasing their answers?[77]

In light of such questions, one must be circumspect regarding articles touting aromatherapeutic efficacy in the treatment of neurologic disease. Because the basic physiologic mechanism of aromatherapy intervention has not been fully established, skepticism seems all the more appropriate.

AROMATHERAPY FOR VARIOUS NEUROLOGIC DISEASES

As a general rule, neurologic diseases can be positively influenced by improving the patient's mood or allaying anxiety. Virtually all neurologic diseases are made worse with depression and/or high anxiety. If moods can be ameliorated by aromatherapy, it would suggest that aromatherapy could have a positive role in treating neurologic disease.

With this in mind, let us review the literature discussing the effects of aromatherapy in specific neurologic complaints and diseases.

Headache

Nontraditional therapies are frequently used in the management of headache, such as acupuncture, massage, and biofeedback.

Historically, odors have been recognized to have analgesic effects. When Roman soldiers returned from battle, they placed bay leaves in their baths to reduce their pains.[78] In ancient Greece, the Corinthian physician, Philonides, recommended pressing cool, scented flowers against the temples to relieve headaches.[78]

In contemporary lay literature, a multitude of unsupported claims are made for headache and pain reduction using specific odorants. These claims do not indicate whether the mechanism of action is primarily analgesic, soporific, or anxiolytic. Suggested odorants include cloves for dental pain;[2] wintergreen for muscle pain;[2,79] menthol, ginger, lemon grass, rosewood, clary sage,[27] cajeput, tea tree, juniper, pepper, and[80] for headaches;[2] lavender,[81] lavandula angustifoia, chamaemelum mobile, ocimium basilicum, origanum majorala, rosmarinus officinalis,[82] eucalyptus,[27] and true melissa[30] for migraine; mentha x piperila for "headache caused by digestive disorder";[82] peppermint and eucalyptus for tension headache.[83]

Experimental studies of odors for pain management are few. Hirsch and Kang[84] studied 50 chronic sufferers whose headaches met International Headache Society criteria. Upon olfactory testing, only 31 demonstrated normal olfactory ability. Green apple odor was given in an aromatherapy inhaler. Only 15 subjects found the odor hedonically pleasant. In this open-label, nonblinded study, subjects served as their own controls. The control condition consisted of resting in a dark, quiet room, and the experimental condition involved inhaling the green apple odor while resting in the same dark, quiet room. Results indicated that green apple odor produced *no* statistically significant improvement over simple resting in a dark, quiet room. However, in the subgroup of 15 subjects who liked the odor, there was a statistically significant reduction in the severity of the headache ($p<0.03$). Therefore the efficacy of the green apple odor was hedonically dependent. Subjects who liked the smell experienced a statistically significant reduction in the severity of the headaches, but patients who disliked the smell experienced no significant improvement.

The mechanism of the odor's action in reducing headaches in these 15 patients is subject to speculation. The odor may have induced a variety of psychologic effects. The therapeutic result may have been mediated through pavlovian conditioning. For example, the respondents may have consciously or unconsciously associated[85] the green apple odor with past anxiolytic or pain-alleviating experiences so that the association reproduced this same effect during the headache episodes. The odor might also have worked through olfactory-evoked recall, because olfactory-evoked recall is usually pleasant and associated with a positive mood state. The green apple scent, by inducing a positive mood state in the 15 patients, could thus have reduced perception of pain.[16] This corresponds with the general affective theory of odors described previously.

The lack of response in those who found the green apple scent unpleasant indicates that hedonics were more important than the particular odor used. This does not preclude the possibility of a neurophysiologic effect of the odor, inducing a change in serotonin, dopamine, acetylcholine, norepinephrine, GABA, gastrin, beta endorphin, or substance P, all of which are known to be modulators of headache, including migraine. Because these neurotransmitters exist within the olfactory bulb, they could, theoretically, be influenced by odors.[86-101]

Green apple odor may have worked somewhat like pharmacologic agents used in the treatment of headache, for example, amitriptyline or propranolol, by modifying the neurotransmitters in the pain pathway. In the patients who disliked the odor, a strong negative mood state may have been induced that overwhelmed the odor's neurophysiologic effect. Therefore their pain was not alleviated.

Gobel also studied the effects of odors on headaches.[79,102] In that study, 32 healthy subjects underwent a double-blind, placebo-controlled, randomized crossover study of the effects of peppermint oil, eucalyptus, and ethanol. The odors were used in different combinations on various measures of headache pain, including the relaxation of pericranial muscles and contingent negative variation. In this study, three applications of odorant were placed on the skin of the forehead and temples at 15-minute intervals using a small sponge. After 45 minutes, parameters were assessed. To avoid factors of circadian rhythm, all testing took place between 3 PM and 6 PM. To prevent subjects from recognizing the presence versus the absence of odors and thereby breaking the double-blind nature of the study, "traces" of peppermint oil and eucalyptus oil were added to all applications.

Eucalyptus had no effect. Peppermint combined with eucalyptus and ethanol relaxed pericranial muscles ($p<0.05$) as did a combination of peppermint and ethanol. The most reduction of pain sensitivity as measured by algesimetry was from a combination of peppermint oil and ethanol. Regulation of pericranial muscles was a postulated mechanism of action of the peppermint.

This study has several potential problems. Because the "traces" of peppermint and eucalyptus were sufficient to cause olfactory response, they may also have been sufficient to produce an effect, although they were described as inert. Hence the authors may not have tested the particular odors they thought they tested. Furthermore, no parameter was measured to determine whether the effect was based on hedonics, to eliminate any influence of the general affective theory of odors. No assessment was made of subjects' olfactory abilities, nor was the anticipation effect (belief versus nonbelief in aromatherapy) addressed.

The author postulated that the odors, through a peripheral mechanism in the gate control theory of pain, acted by segmental inhibition of the posterior horn.[79] However, this same pathway could have been activated totally independently of the odors. The experimental procedure of applying the odors by rubbing cold oils on the skin may, in and of itself, have influenced the pain pathway. The cold stimuli could have induced firing of A delta fibers, which would have increased blood flow in the skin and created a counterstimulus to reduce the headache pain. Alternatively, the inhalation of odors may have affected central serotonergic systems, leading to a change in mood state and thus a reduction in pain (general affective theory of odors).

In another study, Gobel et al. found aromatherapy with peppermint oil was effective in treating tension headaches meeting IHS classification.[103] Peppermint oil was applied locally in a randomized, placebo-controlled, double-blind, crossover fashion. Ten grams of peppermint oil and 90% ethanol was used. Placebo was 90% ethanol solution to which "traces" of peppermint oil were added for blinding purposes. During their headache attacks, peppermint oil was applied across the forehead and temples of 41 patients. The application was repeated after 15 and 30 minutes. Compared with the placebo, peppermint oil significantly reduced headache intensity after 15 minutes ($p<0.01$). The analgesic effect equaled that of 1000 mg of acetaminophen. Very few studies that claim to have demonstrated efficacy of aromatherapy have been as carefully performed.[104]

Another possible mechanism by which peppermint may relieve headache is by noncompetitive inhibition of serotonin and substance P.[83]

Odors may inhibit headaches by acting as calcium channel blockers. *Romarinus officinalis,* for example, has been demonstrated to relax tracheal smooth muscle by way of its calcium antagonistic property.[105]

Other Chronic Pain

Opinion regarding relief of nonheadache pain is mixed. In a blinded study by Dale[106] of 635 postpartum women, use of lavender in the daily bath was compared with an aromatic placebo consisting of 2-methyl-3-isobutyl tyrosine diluted in distilled water. Of the women, 217 received lavender, 213 synthetic, and 205 control. This study demonstrated no statistically significant effect of using lavender in treating peroneal pain. In a study that was not randomized, not double blinded, and not age controlled, Woolfson and Huet gave aromatherapy and massage in 20-minute sessions twice a week to 12 patients. Another 12 patients received massage only. The aromatherapy patients were massaged with lavender oil in an almond oil base. The other patients were massaged with almond oil only. Observations were recorded at the beginning and end of each 20-minute session and 30 minutes after treatment. All sessions were conducted in midafternoon. Approximately 50% of the patients were in the coronary care unit and the others were in intensive-care units. Fifty percent of the patients were artificially ventilated. The authors state that 50% of the aromatherapy patients and 41% of massage-only patients reported a decrease in pain. This could be misleading, however. That six patients responded to aromatherapy and five patients responded to massage without aromatherapy is clearly not a statistically significant difference. If anything, these results indicate that aromatherapy was no better than massage alone. Given their selection of patients, however, one would not anticipate that aromatherapy would be effective, because the pathway for olfactory input was compromised by artificial ventilation.

In a study by Burns and Blamey[107] of 585 women, no statistically significant effects were described, but analgesia was noted in 4 women who inhaled lavender, 1 who inhaled eucalyptus, 3 who inhaled clary sage, 1 who inhaled jasmine, 2 who inhaled chamomile, and 1 who inhaled lemon.

In 100 patients with pain of the periarticular system,[108] treatment of from 10 to 20 days compared the efficacy of mint oil with that of hydroxyethylsalicylate gel. The mint oil was put into a gel and applied topically. Of the patients and physicians, 78% thought that mint therapy was highly effective and 50% of patients and 34% of physicians thought that hydroxyethylsalicylate gel was highly effective. None of the confounding parameters previously mentioned, such as olfactory ability, expectation, and hedonics, were addressed in this study.

Multiple Sclerosis

Of 848 patients with clinically definite multiple sclerosis (MS) who responded to a mail survey in British Columbia, 52 (6.1%) admitted to using aromatherapy to help manage their conditions.[109] Yet no scientific studies support the use of aromatherapy in the treatment of MS and because 23% of MS patients experience olfactory deficit,[110] the efficacy of aromatherapy for this condition would be questionable.

Epilepsy

Aromatherapists suggest the use of a variety of odorants as anticonvulsants, including chamomile, clary sage, and lavender,[3] but few studies have been performed.

Yamada et al.[111] found that inhaling lavender oil vapor blocked pentatetrazol and nicotine-induced convulsions in mice. Gowers noted that the olfactory and trigeminal countermeasures—ammonia and amyl nitrite—inhibit seizure induction, especially in patients with olfactory auras.[14] Efron[15] described a patient with uncinate fits that were inhibited within 8 seconds of inhaling dimercaprol (Bal). Other odorants found to be effective seizure abortants included hydrogen sulfide, n-ethyl butyrate, skatole, the haptenes, and pure jasmine. All were strong and unpleasant, an indication that their effect may have been based on their trigeminal stimulating properties.

More recently, Betts et al.[112] described the inhalation of aromatherapy oil as a countermeasure against epileptic seizures. This was an open-label study of 30 patients but neither the percent success, nor the exact odors used, were described.

Movement Disorders

Several odorants have been advocated for the treatment of movement disorders, including bergamot, chamomile, clary sage, fennel, marjoram,[113] white birch, rosemary,[29] and mandarin[30] for muscle spasms; lavender for leg cramps;[29] and marjoram for tics.[3] These must be viewed skeptically because no scientific studies have been performed, and many movement disorders, including Parkinson's disease[114] and Huntington's disease,[115] are associated with olfactory impairment, which would render any odorant superfluous.

Alcoholism

Many odorants have been suggested for use in alcohol recovery to help alleviate both the physical and emotional problems associated with the desire to drink[116]

BOX 10-1

Oils Used in Aromatherapy Treatment of Alcohol Recovery

Rose otto	Clary sage	Mytrle
Ginger	Myrrh	Niaouli
Grapefruit	Pimento	Pine
Chamomile,	berry	Rosewood
Roman	Spruce	Sandalwood
Neroli	Thyme	Turmeric
Juniper	linalool	Verbena
Lavender	Yarrow	lemon
Rosemary	Carrot	Almond
Frankincense	Coriander	Cinnamon
Marjoram	Hyssop	leaf
Peppermint	Kanuka	Cypress
Lavandin	Linden	Fennel
Lemon	absolute	Hyacinth
Angelica	Manuka	absolute
Cedarwood,	Orange,	Immortelle
Atlas	sweet	Jasmin
Lemongrass	Patchouli	Sambac
Mandarin	Petitgrain	(Abs)
May chang	Rose	Palmarosa
Nutmeg	absolute	Spikenard
Black pepper	Ylang-ylang	Tea tree
Geranium	Cardamon	Tea tree,
Benzoin	Chamomile,	lemon
Melissa	German	Valerian
Ravensara	Eucalyptus	Vetiver
Thyme	citriodora	Violet leaf
thujanol	Eucalyptus	absolute
Bergamot	globulus	

(Box 10-1). However, both acute intoxication[117] and chronic alcoholism[118] are associated with olfactory loss, and no formal studies have been performed. Therefore aromatherapy for alcoholism cannot be recommended at this time.

Insomnia

A multitude of odorants have been touted for use as hypnotics in the treatment of insomnia, including valerian,[119] asafetida,[119] musk,[119] lavender,[27,29,119,120] basil, chamomile, clary sage, everlasting, mandarin, marjoram, neroli, sandalwood, ylang-ylang,[27] berg-

amot, celery, hops, hyacinth, jasmine,[121] camphor, cypress, frankincense, geranium, lemon, melissa, myrrh, nutmeg, patchouly, petitgrain, rose, sage,[32] and orange.[80]

Animal studies support the use of odorants as hypnotics. Decreased motility, an indication of sedation, was produced in mice after inhalation of the essential oils of lime- blossoms and Herba Passiflora.[120] In young albino rats, inhalation of valerian and asafetida induced sedation, compared with control conditions.[119] Odorants that were not found to be significantly sedating included musk, lavender, violets, oil of roses, incense, gum olibanum, gum galbanum, Hinode, and sandalwood. Due to the low levels used, the mechanism of action was postulated to be due not to systemic absorption, but rather to the olfactory sensation with secondary effects from olfactory CNS projections.[119]

Sedation was produced in Swiss mice by inhalation of lavender oil and its components linalool and linalyl acetate.[120] Based on studies with rats, Elisabetsky et al. postulated that linalool's hypnotic properties are mediated through inhibition of glutamatergic transmission in the CNS.[122,123]

Buchbauer et al.[33] exposed Swiss mice to more than 40 odorants. In general, the more lipophilic, the greater the biologic effect (Table 10-1). It was suggested that the sedative effect of these essential oils was due to their interactions with lipids of the neural cell membranes in the cortex.

Experiments with humans have also been performed to assess the soporific effects of odors, with mixed results. Hudson[124] evaluated nine older patients, many with dementia, in a hospital setting. Her assumption was that lavender inhalation would promote sleep and that, secondarily, it would reduce confusion and enhance alertness the next day. The effects of the application of one drop of lavender oil on the pillow each night for 1 week were compared with a 1-week baseline period with no odor. Nocturnal sleep improved 2% and daytime wakefulness increased 3% with lavender. The conclusion, that all elderly patients would benefit from nocturnal inhalation of essential oil of lavender, must be viewed with some reservation for the following reasons:

- No statistical analysis was performed on the results.
- It would be expected that with time, patients would adjust to the hospital surroundings and their sleeping patterns would improve.
- No tests for hedonics or olfactory ability were performed. Being elderly,[125] on medication,[126] and

TABLE 10-1

*Effects of Fragrance Compounds and Essential Oils on the Motility of Mice after
a 1-h Inhalation Period*

Compound	Effect on Motility after		Compound	Effect on Motility after	
	Motility %	Caffeine, %		Motility %	Caffeine, %
Anethole	−10.81	−1.26	Isoeugenol	+30.05	−74.34
Anthranillic acid			Beta-Ionone	+14.20	−27.97
methyl ester	+17.70	+38.22	Lavender oil		
Balm leaves oil (Austria)	−5.21	+16.29	(Mont Blanc)	−78.40	−91.67
Benzaldehyde	−43.69	−34.28	Lime blossoms oil		
Benzyl alcohol	−11.21	−23.68	(France)	−34.34	+30.41
Borneol	−3.05	−1.88	Linaloof	−73.00	−56.67
Bornyl acetate	−7.79	+2.27	Linalyl acetate	−69.10	−46.67
Bornyl salicylate	−17.29	−2.99	Maitol	+13.74	−50.04
Carvone	−2.46	−47.51	Methyl salicylate	+16.64	−49.88
Citral	−1.43	+17.24	Nerol	+12.93	+29.31
Citronellal	−49.82	−37.40	Neroli oil	−65.27	+1.87
Citronellol	−3.56	−13.71	Orange flower oil (Spain)	−4.64	−14.62
Coumarin	−15.00	−13.75	Orange terpenes	+35.25	−33.19
Dimethyl vinyl carbinol	+5.36	−2.11	Passion flower oil (USA)	+8.15	−27.93
Ethylmaltol	+9.73	+2.09	2-Phenyl ethanol	+2.67	−30.61
Eugenol	+2.10	−38.73	2-Phenylethyl acetate	−45.04	+12.42
Farnesol	+5.76	+36.34	Alpha-Pinene	+13.77	+4.73
Farnesyl acetate	+4.62	−30.71	Rose oil (Bulgaria)	−9.50	+4.31
Furfural	+3.04	−4.51	Sandalwood oil		
Geraniol	+20.56	+1.20	(East India)	−40.00	−20.70
Geranyl acetate	−29.18	−7.46	Alpha-Terpineol	−45.00	−12.50
Isoborneol	+46.90	−11.23	Thymol	+33.02	+19.05
Isobornyl acetate	+3.16	−22.35	Valerian root oil (China)	−2.70	−12.01

demented[127] is apt to impair olfactory ability, bringing into question whether these subjects could even detect an odor.

- The nurse observers were not blinded to the intent of the study and, hence, may have been inadvertently biased in their observations. This bias has been demonstrated to occur in other aromatherapy studies.[77]

Because changes of only 2% to 3% were observed, a more accurate interpretation of this study might be that the lavender did *not* promote sedation.

However, other investigators also believe that odorants have a soporific effect on humans. Karamat et al.[128] evaluated the effects of inhaling lavender oil on 24 subjects undergoing vigilance tasks. A significant increase in their reaction time was found, consistent with a sedative effect. But, no *p* value was noted for significance, nor were hedonics, blinding, or olfactory ability assessed.

Miyake et al.[129] used EEGs to assess sleep latency of subjects who inhaled spike lavender, sweet fennel, bitter orange, linden, valerian, and marjoram compared with those given no odors. The one odor found to significantly reduce sleep latency was bitter orange. Neither the number of subjects nor further details regarding blinding, subjects' expectations, hedonics, or olfactory ability were provided.

Aromatherapy must be tried judiciously in patients with insomnia because of the huge comorbidity of insomnia and respiratory disease. Insomnia is present in 53% of patients with chronic bronchitis and

55% of those with primary emphysema.[130] The inhalation of odorants by these patients could worsen their respiratory status and thus exacerbate, rather than relieve, their insomnia.

Aggression

Just as malodors increase aggressive feelings, evidence also exists that odors can reduce aggressive behavior. Although aromatherapists advocate using a variety of pleasant odors to reduce aggression and hostility, including chamomile, cypress lavender, marjoram, and ylang-ylang,[27] studies suggest very different odors act to reduce aggression. In a double-blinded study of 18 undergraduate women, Benton[131] found that inhalation of 5-alpha-androst-16-en-3 alpha-ol (a potential human pheromone, androstenol) reduced aggression and increased submission ($p<0.01$) compared with inhalation of the 70% ethanol control.

Hirsch[132] studied the effects of the odor of garlic bread on family interactions at dinner. Among the 50 families in this single-blinded, randomized, crossover study, there were 22.7% fewer negative remarks per family member per minute ($p=0.05$) and 7.4% more positive comments per family member per minute ($p=0.04$) when the aroma of garlic bread was present. The decrease in negative remarks was more pronounced among older rather than younger family members, among male rather than female members, among those who liked the aroma, and among those who had nostalgic feelings evoked by the aroma.

For family members who liked garlic bread, the aroma of garlic bread enhanced their mood so they became more positive and less critical of others and therefore made fewer negative comments. This supports Baron's demonstration that a positive mood can cause reduced critical appraisals both of products and of people.[133,134] The garlic bread aroma may have evoked nostalgic feelings that are usually associated with happy memories of childhood. Happy family members have more positive interactions.[135] The appetizing aroma and satisfying taste of garlic bread may induce generous feelings so family members reduce critical comments and increase pleasant and positive ones.[136] Just as a bad odor can cause aggressive feelings,[64] a pleasant aroma of garlic bread can enhance harmonious and agreeable feelings among family members, leading to more positive and fewer negative interactions.

In clinical practice, treatment with aversion aromas have been used to reduce both aggressive behavior[137] and deviate sexual behavior.[138] Tanner and Zeiler[139] describe the use of an odorant to treat for pathologic aggression in a 20-year-old autistic woman. In a nonblinded, open-label, single-case study, treatment with aromatic ammonia was found to reduce her self-injurious behavior from a baseline of 36.2 slaps per minute to 1.3 slaps per minute. Whenever self-injurious behavior was noted, the ammonia was thrust under the patient's nose and then withdrawn at cessation of the aggressive behavior. Statistical significance of the odor was not determined. When the routine application of aversive stimuli was discontinued, self-injurious behavior recurred. Moreover, frequent use of the odorant caused nasal irritation and scabbing at the tip of the nose.

Suppression of aggressive self-injurious behavior using aromatherapy was reported also by Baumeister and Baumeister.[140] Two severely retarded children, 4 and 7 years of age, demonstrated a reduction of their self-injurious behavior contingent with inhalation of aromatic ammonia, which persisted for at least 6 months after discontinuation of the inhalation.

In another experiment, four severely demented geriatric inpatients inhaled lavender with and without massage, to reduce agitated and self-aggressive behavior.[141] On individualized agitation scales, no benefits were demonstrated from the combined massage and aromatherapy as opposed to aromatherapy alone. One patient benefited from the aromatherapy, whereas for two, agitated behavior actually worsened as compared with the no-treatment control periods.

The staff providing care, blinded to the objectives measures, thought that aromatherapy reduced agitation and self-injurious behavior in all four patients. This experiment demonstrates the importance of scientific methods and techniques for objective measurements and the need to consider the examiners' preexisting bias and the effects of social desirability.[77]

Anxiety

Patients with DSM-III-R generalized anxiety disorder are known to have impaired olfactory ability.[142] Still, aromatherapists recommend numerous odors, including chamomile, cypress, orange blossom, lavender, marjoram, rose, sandalwood, clary sage,[3] basil, bergamot, cedarwood, geranium, jasmine, juniper, neroli, petitgrain, ylang-ylang,[27] melissa,[29] benzoin, camphor, cardamon, fennel, frankincense, nutmeg, patchouly, peppermint, pine, rosemary, rosewood,[32] mandarin, lemon verbena,[31] neroli, and juniper berry.[30]

Studies of the effects of odorants on anxiety have relied primarily on individuals' self-appraisals of their feeling state. In one instance, apple/nutmeg odor associated with the task of performing certain mathematical calculations led to an attenuated increase in anxiety as determined by subjects' self-reports and blood pressure measurements.[143]

The odor of green apple eased the anxiety of being in a space-deprivation booth for six normosmic subjects as demonstrated in a double-blind, controlled, randomized experiment.[144]

Physiologic evidence is less conclusive regarding the potential of odorants on anxiolytics. Lavender odor was found to reduce the CNV among perfumers, and the lavender correlated with a more relaxed state.[145] This change on the CNV, however, may also indicate a distracting effect of the odorant.[143] Mild reduction in systolic blood pressure, an indicator of anxiolysis,[146] with inhaled odors was assessed in a double-blind, controlled, randomized fashion in normosmic and anosmic, awake and anesthetized adults.[147] No significant effect was noted with inhalation of hedonically positive odors, but inhalation of an irritant (ammonia) caused an increase in blood pressure.

Studies have also addressed the anxiolytic effects of aromatherapy in the clinical setting with, at best, ambiguous results. In a case-controlled study of 36 men with public speaking anxiety, jasmine and apple spice were no more effective than the odorless control condition in reducing speech anxiety.[148]

Likewise, no clear efficacy has been demonstrated for aromatherapy for anxiety reduction in patients confined to the hospital. Aromas of marjoram, lavender, rose, eucalyptus, geranium, chamomile, and neroli were used in combination with massage and music therapy to treat 69 terminally ill patients.[149] An 80% rate of success, defined as "deriving benefit in some way," was found, but this must be viewed critically for the following reasons:

- Statistical significance was not determined.
- Treatments ancillary to the aromatherapy including talking, massage, or music may have been the true agents.
- Concomitant medical treatment, for example, to decrease pain, may have been the agent of beneficial effects ascribed to aromatherapy.

- Different odors were used for each subject.
- No consideration was given to hedonics, anosmia, a control group, expectation bias, or examiner bias.

In 122 intensive-care patients, aromatherapy with massage was no more effective than either massage alone or no treatment (the control subgroup) in either subjective perception of aromas ($p > 0.05$) or physiologic parameters of anxiety (systolic blood pressure, respiratory rate, and heart rate).[150,151]

Similarly, a randomized, double-blind trial of aromatherapy with two different species of lavender and massage was performed on 24 postoperative intensive-care cardiac patients. No statistically significant self-perceived anxiolytic effect for either species of lavender was found ($p = 0.09$).[152]

The same results were documented with inhaled neroli aroma combined with massage in 100 1-day postoperative intensive-care cardiac patients.[153] In this randomized, controlled study, again, no statistical significance was found in physiologic parameters of anxiety (heart rate, systolic blood pressure) or subjects' self-perceptions of anxiety as reported in a modified Spielberger State-Trait Anxiety Inventory (STAI) State Self-Evaluation Questionnaire.

Wilkinson[154] also used the STAI and the psychologic scale of the Rotterdam Symptom Checklist (RSCL) to assess anxiolytic effects of aromatherapy. Fifty-one cancer patients receiving palliative care were randomly assigned to receive three sessions of either full body massage with carrier oil only or full body massage with carrier oil and 1% Roman Chamomile essential oil. Upon completion of the sessions, there was no statistically significant effect ($p = 0.8$) of aromatherapy with massage as opposed to massage alone on the psychologic scale of the RSCL or the STAI. Definitive evidence validating aromatherapy in anxiolysis remains to be seen.

Depression

A variety of odorants, including basil, bergamot, chamomile, frankincense, geranium, jasmine, lavender, neroli, patchouly, peppermint, rose, sandalwood, ylang-ylang,[155] clary sage, grapefruit, lemon, mandarin orange,[27] camphor, hyssop, melissa, petitgrain, pine, thyme,[29] coriander, helichrysum, rosewood, vetivert,[32] marjoram, and thyme,[80] have been advocated for the treatment of depression.[3] However, scientific studies have yielded disappointing results. Citrus odor (a combination of lemon oil, orange oil, bergamot oil, and cis-4-hexenol) was applied to the ambient air for 4 to 11 weeks in the rooms where 12 men were hospitalized for DSM-III-R major depression.[156] During this time, antidepressant medications were reduced or eliminated for 11 of the 12 men and kept constant for another 8 control patients whose rooms were not perfumed. The criteria for medication tapering was apparently nonformal on a clinical basis. Comparing effects of odorant and antidepressant treatment versus antidepressant treatment alone, the odorant had no statistically significant effect on objective measures of depression including the Hamilton Rating Scale for Depression, the Self-Rating Depression Scale, and number of days of hospital treatment. Despite this, the results of the study are difficult to interpret because levels of antidepressant were not kept constant. Furthermore, olfactory ability was never assessed and because many antidepressants impair olfactory ability, this is particularly important.[157] Also, depression itself is associated with olfactory impairment.[142]

Kite et al.[158] suggested that aromatherapy significantly improved depression as determined by the Hospital Anxiety-Depression Scale ($p<0.001$) and reduced parameters consistent with adjustment disorders or major depressive disorders. These results must be viewed critically for the following reasons:

- Of 89 entrants, only 58 (65%) completed the study, an indication that the dropouts may have been treatment failures.
- The majority of subjects (74%) had breast cancer and were receiving oncologic therapy including radiation therapy or surgery. Olfactory ability was not assessed, yet chemotherapy, radiation therapy, and simply having breast cancer (estrogen receptor positive type)[159] are associated with olfactory impairment. Thus any positive results could be spurious and unrelated to the aromatherapy. The experimental design supports that this may be the case.
- No control group was provided, therefore mood improvement could have been due to coincident improvement of the underlying disease state.
- Aromatherapy was not provided alone, but along with massage and empathic therapeutic sessions, either of which might have been effective.

- One-third of the patients concomitantly received counseling and some were on antidepressants, both of which could improve depression.
- Twenty different essential oils were used, alone or in various combinations. The odors were different for each subject and changed during the course of treatment in more than one-third of the cases. Thus even though relief of depression was reported, the effects of the odorants are indeterminate.

At this time, the use of odorants to treat major depression cannot be advocated.

Learning Disabilities, Mild Cognitive Impairment, and Dementia

The odorants that aromatherapists suggest can improve memory, mental function, and learning ability include vanilla,[78] rosemary, basil, cardamon, bergamot, cedarwood, grapefruit, lemon, peppermint, rosemary,[29] clove, coriander, lily of the valley, sage,[160] bay, melissa, ylang-ylang,[32] and juniper.[80] The combined odor of lavender and orange essential oil has been recommended in the management of dementia.[161]

Animal studies support the concept that odorants can improve learning and cognition. Following the logic that if odors improve learning, their lack would impair learning, Sitaras et al. induced peripheral anosmia in rats with intranasal infusion of $ZnSO_4$. They found that this markedly impaired the rats conditioned avoidance response ($p<0.05$).[162] Furthermore, the fact that odors may improve normal learning indicates they may prove therapeutic in disorders of cognition.

Ludvigson and Rottman[72] evaluated the odors of lavender and cloves for their possible impact on learning, using as paradigms the group-embedded figure, word recall, multiple-choice vocabulary, analogies, and arithmetic tasks. They found that these odors did not affect memory or cognition;[164] in fact, the odor of lavender significantly impaired performance of arithmetic tasks ($p=0.01$).

On the other hand, odors of peppermint and muguet (lily of the valley) improved the performance of stressful visual tasks.[163] Among subjects who found them hedonically positive, these odors improved creativity scores on the remote associates test[193] and increased efficiency in work situations.[165]

Hirsch and Johnston,[166] in a double-blind, controlled, crossover study found that the presence of a mixed floral odor improved speed of learning on the Halsted-Reitan Test Battery by 17% as compared with an odorless control condition for 10 normosmic adults who found the odor hedonically pleasant ($p=0.05$). The odors of oriental spice, baked goods, lavender, citrus, parsley, and spearmint, which were tested in a similar manner, showed no effect on learning time even though subjects considered them hedonically positive. Thus positive hedonics alone appear to be insufficient, which argues against the general affective theory of odor.

The neurophysiologic mechanism by which the floral odor mediated the improvement in learning is unclear. The odor may have facilitated deposition of short-term memory, the processing of newly learned material, or the access of these memories for subsequent tasks. Or it could have facilitated the creation of new strategies for solving problems. Because a degree of alertness is necessary for learning, the mixed floral odor may have acted by stimulating the reticular activating system. This system has been shown to be affected by other odors, for example, jasmine and smelling salts.[167,168] The activating effects of inhalation of 1,8-cineol have been demonstrated physiologically through an increase in global cerebral blood flow.[169]

An odor might increase motivation through a classic pavlovian conditioned response in which a stimulus, in this case the odor, induces recall of a past behavior.[170]

Odors may have a direct physiologic impact on the brain.[171] The anatomy of learning involves multiple structures: two that are essential are the hippocampus and cortex. These areas are directly influenced by anatomic projections from the olfactory system.

Many of the same neurotransmitters are involved in the processes of learning and of olfaction; modulation of these might explain how an odor enhanced the learning process. The neurotransmitters include the classic norepinephrine, dopamine, serotonin, acetylcholine, and GABA,[172-174] as well as the hypophyseal neuropeptides and nonhypophyseal hormones. Examples of the hypophyseal hormones are methionine-enkephalin and beta endorphin. Examples of the nonhypophyseal hormones include substance P, neurotensin, and cholecystokinin.[172, 175]

The floral odor could have induced a positive feeling, which secondarily enhanced cognition. Odors experienced as hedonically positive produce a positive affective state,[165] and positive mood states may directly improve learning. The floral odor may also have acted as an anxiolytic, decreasing anxiety, which inhibits learning. By removing this inhibiting factor, it facilitated learning.

The trail-making test is a paradigm for the learning tasks of spatial analyses, motor control, attention shifting, alertness, concentration, and number sense.[176] Brain damage at any of various locations can impair trail making, so it is logical that intervention at these locations could improve performance. The floral odor may have acted at any of these sites to improve learning. Although the odor may have affected any of these tasks, its effect on improved spatial analysis/orientation is of particular interest. This cognitive process is localized in the nondominant right hemisphere.[177,178] Olfaction also is predominantly processed in the right, nondominant hemisphere.[179] This anatomic overlap may be of such significance that the results of Hirsch and Johnston are not generalizable to learning paradigms that do not involve the right hemisphere.[166]

Possibly the floral odor did not directly affect learning but acted on noncognitive variables mentioned previously to improve hand-eye coordination, cerebellar and basal-ganglia function for coordination of movements, or pyramidal-system function for motor integration of fine movements.

The subjects could have experienced a placebo effect based on preconceived notions that the odor would affect their learning. Another difficulty in generalizing this study is that it was conducted in a relatively isolated environment, unlike a normal classroom where a cacophony of sensory stimuli may be so compelling as to lessen any positive effects of odors on learning.

Inhalation of the essential oils of peppermint, rosemary, and lemon was reported to enhance memory in normosmic 15- and 16-year-old high school students.[180]

Parasuraman et al.[181] and Nelson et al.[182] reported that peppermint odor enhanced cognition as measured by inhibition of vigilance decrement, especially in subjects with attention-maintenance difficulties[182] and head injuries.[183] The mechanism of peppermint-enhanced cognition may be that it more efficiently allocates attention. This was demonstrated neurophysiologically; no reduction of amplitude of N160-evoked brain potential occurred in response to peppermint.[181]

This seems anatomically reasonable because, as has been demonstrated in PET imaging, odors increase cerebral blood flow to the juncture of the inferior frontal and temporal lobes bilaterally and unilaterally activate the right orbitofrontal cortex.[183] These same areas are essential for vigilance task performance.[183]

On the other hand, Heuberger[184] found that inhalation of 1,8-cineol and linalool had no effect on human vigilance performance.

Aromatherapy has been advocated for treatment of learning disabilities.[185] Using a counterbalanced, crossover design, eight adults with profound learning disabilities underwent simple concentration tasks after a combination of massage and aromatherapy with orange flower, lemon grass, and lavender.[7] When compared with the baseline no-treatment condition, aromatherapy demonstrated no effect on concentration.

Shakespeare may have been the first to recommend rosemary for improving the memory: "There's rosemary, that's for rememberance; . . ."[186] Because it contains Cineole, an acetylcholinesterase inhibitor,[187] rosemary has been recommended for treatment of senile dementia of the Alzheimer's type. Rodent studies demonstrated that inhalation of cineole or rosemary enhanced ability to traverse a maze. In human studies, rosemary shortens reaction time.

Common Susceptibilities

Before using aromatherapy in neurologic conditions, consideration must be given to the potential risks of the treatment. Adverse reactions can occur among patients with diseases that predispose them to the development of side effects, and among the population as a whole as well.

Certain diseases make their sufferers particularly susceptible to adverse effects of aromatherapy. Approximately 40% of migraineurs report osmophobia, whereby an odorant induces a migraine headache.[188] A wide range of odorants can act as such triggers, depending on the individual. These triggers include perfume, cigarette smoke, and food odors.[189]

Asthmatics, upon exposure to common odors, can suffer a worsening of their respiratory status independent of their olfactory ability. In a survey of 60 asthmatic patients, 57 (95%) described respiratory symptoms upon exposure to common odors, including insecticide (85%), household cleaning agents (78%), perfume and cologne (72%), cigarette smoke (75%), fresh paint (73%), automobile exhaust or gas fumes (60%), and cooking aromas (37%). Room deodorant and mint candy also could cause respiratory distress.[190] Four subjects who underwent an odor challenge with 4 squirts of a popular cologne all had an immediate decline in 1-second forced expiratory volume (18% to 58% reduction).[190]

Among persons who suffer complaints consistent with multiple chemical sensitivities, 24% of the men and 39% of the women note that odors precipitate their complaints.[191] However, double-blind studies fail to demonstrate odorant-induced multiple chemical sensitivity symptoms.[192]

Inhalation of odorants can produce measurable levels in the blood.[35] And because many common fragrances contain naphthalene-related compounds (including menthol and camphor), persons with G6PD deficiency may be at risk from aromatherapeutic exposures.[193] In neonates, dermal application has demonstrated this, but in adults it remains only a theoretic risk for inhalational aromatherapy.

A variety of essential oils is said to be able to precipitate seizures in epileptics. Whether these effects can occur by inhalation alone as opposed to ingestion or by percutaneous absorption is unclear. Proconvulsant odorants include rosemary,[3,194] fennel, hyssop, sage, and wormwood.[3]

Because aromatherapeutic inhalation of essential oils can produce detectable levels of the oils in the blood, these compounds, like any pharmacologic agents, could induce adverse drug-drug interactions in persons on medication. Such interactions could enhance metabolism of anticonvulsants or pain medications, for example, thus predisposing an epileptic to have a seizure or a chronic pain patient to withdraw from medication. Jori et al.[195] demonstrated this potential. Inhalation of eucalyptol by rats increased microsomal enzyme systems, thus decreasing the effect of pentobarbital.

Odorants can produce harmful side effects not only among persons predisposed to disease but among the healthy population as well. Airborne-induced allergic contact dermatitis is a recognized result of aromatherapeutic inhalation of tea tree oil (melaleuca oil).[196] Examples of common melaleuca oil allergens include d-limonene, aromadendrene, alpha-terpinene, 1,8-cineole (eucalyptol), terpinen-4-ol, p-cymene, and alpha-phellandrene. Because of the highly volatile nature of essential oils, their common constituents and cross-sensitization, DeGroot postulated that the same airborne-induced contact dermatitis could occur with several other essential oils, including lavender and a mixture of eucalyptus, pine, and peppermint.[196] Bridges suggested that if odorants can sensitize the respiratory system as they do the skin, they might not only exacerbate asthma, but might actually precipitate asthma.[197]

SUMMARY

With aromatherapy, just as with any therapeutic tool, practitioners must weigh the relative risk/benefit ratio in deciding upon its use in the treatment of neurologic disease.

Having spent the last decade and a half investigating the scientific basis of aromatherapy and having published more than 100 peer-reviewed articles in this area, the author does not believe that scientific literature supports or that the risk/benefit ratio justifies use of aromatherapy in neurologic conditions at present. This is a fluid position, and as more studies are performed delineating the efficacy of aromatherapy, the author expects to endorse and use aromatherapy as part of the therapeutic armamentarium. Until such time, this form of alternative medicine in the treatment of neurologic disease cannot be recommended.

References

1. Kaptchuk TJ, Eisenberg DM: The persuasive appeal of alternative medicine, *Ann Intern Med* 129:1061-1065, 1998
2. Price S, Price L: *Aromatherapy for health professionals,* New York, 1995, Churchill-Livingstone.
3. Tisserand RB: *The art of aromatherapy,* Rochester, Vt., 1977, Healing Arts.
4. Weyers W, Brodbeck R: Hautdurchdringung atherischer ole (Skin absorption of volatile oils), *Pharmazie in Unserer Zeit* 18(3):82-86, 1989.
5. Buchbauer G: Biological effects of fragrances and essential oils, *Perfumer & Flavorist* 18:19-24, 1993.
6. King JR: Scientific status of aromatherapy, *Perspect Biol Med* 37(3):409-415, 1994.
7. Lindsay WR, Pitcaithly D, Geelen N: A comparison of the effects of four therapy procedures on concentration and responsiveness in people with profound learning disabilities, *J Intellect Disabil Res* 41(3):201-207, 1997.
8. Roebuck A: Aromatherapy: fact or fiction, *Perfumer & Flavorist* 13:43-45, 1988.
9. Brodal A: *Neurological anatomy in relation to clinical medicine,* ed 3, vol 10, New York, 1969, Oxford University Press.
10. Hirsch AR, Wyse JP: Posttraumatic dysosmia: central vs peripheral, *J Neurol Orthop Med Surg* 14:152-155, 1993.
11. Acharya V, Acharya J, Luders H: Olfactory epileptic auras, *Neurology* 46:A446, 1996.
12. Hirsch AR: *Scentsational sex,* Boston, 1998, Element Books.
13. Dietz MA, Goetz CJ, Steddings GT: Evaluation of visual cues as a modified inverted walking stick in the treatment of Parkinson's disease freezing episodes, *Mov Disord* 5:243-247, 1990.
14. Gowers WR: Epilepsy and other chronic convulsive diseases. In Efron R: The effect of olfactory stimuli in arresting uncinate fits, *Brain* 79:267-281, 1957.
15. Efron R: The effect of olfaction stimuli in arresting uncinate fits, *Brain* 79:267-281, 1957.
16. Fields H: *Pain,* New York, 1967, McGraw-Hill.
17. Freud S: Bemerkungen uber einen Fall von Zwangs Neurosa, *Ges Schr* VIII:350, 1908.
18. MacLean PD: *Triune concept of the brain and behavior,* Toronto, 1973, University of Toronto Press.
19. Brodal A: Neurological anatomy in relation to clinical medicine, ed 3, New York, 1981, Oxford University Press.
20. Ehrlichman H, Halpern JN: Affect and memory: effects of pleasant and unpleasant odors on retrieval of happy and unhappy memories, *J Pers Soc Psychol* 55:769-779, 1988.
21. Hirsch AR: Nostalgia: neuropsychiatric understanding, *Adv Consumer Res* 19:390-395, 1992.
22. Squire LR: *Memory and brain,* New York, 1987, Oxford University Press.
23. Brown R, Kulik J: Flashbulb memories, *Cognition* 5:73-99, 1977.
24. Proust M: Remembrance of things past, vol 1, New York, 1934, Random House (Translated by CK Scott Moncrieff).
25. Kline N, Rausch J: Olfactory precipitants of flashbacks in post traumatic stress disorders: case reports, *J Clin Psychiatr* 46:383-384, 1985.
26. Laird DA: What can you do with your nose? *Scientific Monthly.*
27. Damian P, Damian K: *Aromatherapy scent and psyche,* Rochester, Vt., 1995, Healing Arts.
28. Cunningham S: *Magical aromatherapy: the power of scent,* St Paul, Minn., 1995, Llewellyn Publications.
29. Feller RM: *Practical aromatherapy: understanding and using essential oils to heal the mind and body,* New York, 1997, Berkley Books.
30. Price S: *Aromatherapy for common ailments,* New York, 1991, Fireside Books.
31. Schnaubelt K: *Advanced aromatherapy: the science of essential oil therapy,* Rochester, Vt., 1995, Healing Arts.
32. Keville K, Green M: *Aromatherapy: a complete guide to the healing art,* Freedom, Calif., 1995, Crossing Press.

33. Buchbauer G et al.: Fragrance compounds and essential oils with sedative effects upon inhalation, *J Pharm Sci* 82(6):660-664, 1993.

34. Buchbauer G: Biological effects of fragrances and essential oils, *Perfumer & Flavorist* 18:20, 1993.

35. Stimpfl T et al.: Concentration of 1,8- cineol in human blood during prolonged inhalation, *Chem Senses* 20(3):349-350, 1995.

36. Alaoui-Ismaili O et al.: Basic emotions evoked by odorants: comparison between autonomic responses and self-evaluation, *Physiol Behav* 62:713-720, 1997.

37. Miltner W et al.: Emotional qualities of odorants and their influence on the startle reflex in humans, *Psychophysiology* 31:107-110, 1994.

38. Buchbauer G: Aromatherapy: do essential oils have therapeutic properties? *Perfumer & Flavorist* 15:47-50, 1990.

39. Sugawara Y, Hino Y, Kawasaki M: Alteration of perceived fragrance of essential oils in relation to type of work: a simple screening test for efficacy of aroma, *Chem Senses* 24:415-421, 1999.

40. Warm JS, Dember WN, Parasuraman R: Effects of olfactory stimulation on performance and stress in a visual sustained attention task, *J Soc Cosmet Chem* 42:199-210, 1991.

41. Miner JR: Controlling odors from livestock production facilities: state-of-the-art. In *Livestock waste: renewable resource*, St Joseph, Mich., 1980, American Society of Agricultural Engineers.

42. Hirsch AR, Rankin KM: Trichloroethylene exposure and headache, *Headache* 33:275, 1993.

43. Hirsch AR: Cephalgia as a result of acute nitrogen tetroxide exposure, *Headache* 35:310, 1995.

44. Hirsch AR: *Neurotoxicity as a result of acute nitrogen tetroxide exposure*. International Congress on Hazardous Waste: impact on human and ecological health, Atlanta, 1995, U.S. Department of Health and Human Services: Public Health Agency for Toxic Substances and Disease Registry.

45. Hirsch AR: *Chronic neurotoxicity of acute chlorine gas exposure.* Thirteenth International Neurotoxicity Conference, Hot Springs, Ark., 1995.

46. Neutra R et al.: Hypotheses to explain the higher symptom rates observed around hazardous waste sites, *Environ Health Perspectt* 94:31-38, 1991.

47. Shusterman D: Critical review: health significance of environmental odor pollution, *Arch Environ Health* 47:76-87, 1992.

48. Wayne W, Wehrle P, Carroll R: Oxidant air pollution and athletic performance, *JAMA* 199:901-904, 1967.

49. Maruniak JA: Deprivation and the olfactory system. In Doty RL, editor: *Handbook of olfaction and gustation,* New York, 1995, Marcel Dekker.

50. Evans GW: Psychological costs of chronic exposure to ambient air pollution. In Isaacson RI, Jensen KF, editors: *The vulnerable brain and environmental risks,* vol 3, New York, 1994, Plenum Press.

51. Weisse CS: Depression and immunocompetence: review of the literature, *Psychol Bull* 111:475-489, 1992.

52. Hirsch AR: *Chronic neurotoxicity as a result of landfill exposure in Port Orchard, Washington, international Congress on Hazardous Waste—Impact on human and ecological health,* Atlanta, 1995, U.S. Department of Health and Human Services: Public Health Agency for Toxic Substances and Disease Registry.

53. Izmerov N: Establishment of air quality standards, *Arch Environ Health* 22:711-719, 1971.

54. Rotton J et al.: Air pollution experience and physical aggression, *J Appl Soc Psychol* 9:347-412, 1979.

55. Ury HK, Perkins MA, Goldsmith JR: Motor vehicle accidents and vehicular pollution in Los Angeles, *Arch Environ Health* 25:314-322, 1972.

56. Shiffman SS et al.: The effect of environmental odors emanating from commercial swine operations on the mood of nearby residents, *Brain Res Bull* 37:369-375, 1995.

57. Rotton J et al: Air pollution and interpersonal attraction, *J Appl Soc Psychol* 8:57-71, 1978.

58. Brandstatter H, Furhwirth M, Kitchler E: Effects of weather and air pollution on mood: individual difference approach. In Canter D et al., editors: *NATO advanced research workshop on social and environmental psychology in the European context: environmental social psychology,* Boston, 1988, G Kluwer.

59. Bullinger M: Psychological effects of air pollution on healthy residents: a time series approach, *J Environ Psychol* 9:103-118, 1989.

60. Bullinger M: Relationships between air-pollution and well-being, *Z Sozial Praventivmed* 34:231-238, 1989.

61. Zeidner M, Schechter M: Psychological responses to air pollution: some personality and demographic correlates, *J Environ Psychol* 8:191-208, 1988.

62. Rotton J, Frey J: Air pollution, weather, and violent crimes: concomitant time series analysis of archival data, *J Pers Social Psychol* 49:1207-1220, 1985.

63. Briere J, Downes A, Spensley J: Summer in the city: urban weather conditions and psychiatric-emergency room visits, *J Abnorm Psychol* 92:77-80, 1983.

64. Hirsch AR: Negative health effects of malodors in the environment: a brief review, *J Neurol Orthop Med Surg* 18:43-45, 1998.

65. Valentine JH et al.: Human crises and the physical environment, *Man-Environ Sys* 5(1):23-28, 1975.

66. Cunningham M: Weather, mood, and helping behavior: quasi-experiments with the sunshine samaritan, *J Personal Soc Psychol* 37:1947-1956, 1979.

67. Strahilevitz M, Strahilevitz A, Miller JE: Air pollutants and the admission rate of psychiatric patients, *Amer J Psychiatry* 136(2):205-207, 1979.

68. Jones JW, Bogat GA: Air pollution and human aggression, *Psychol Rep* 43:721-722, 1978.

69. Rotton J: Affective and cognitive consequences of malodorous pollution, *Basic Appl Soc Psychol* 4:171-191, 1983.

70. Robin O et al.: Basic emotions evoked by eugenol odor differ according to the dental experience.: a neurovegetative analysis, *Chem Senses* 24:327-335, 1999.

71. Robin O et al.: Emotional responses evoked by dental odors: an evaluation from autonomic parameters, *J Dent Res* 77(8):1638-1646, 1998.

72. Ludvigson HW, Rottman TR: Effects of ambient odors of lavender and cloves on cognition, memory, affect and mood, *Chem Senses* 14:525-536, 1989.

73. Distel H et al.: Perception of everyday odors—correlation between intensity, familiarity and strength of hedonic judgement, *Chem Senses* 24:191-199, 1999.

74. Flaten MA, Simonsen T, Olsen H: Drug-related information generates placebo and nocebo responses that modify the drug response, *Psychosom Med* 61:250-255, 1999.

75. Knasko SC, Gilbert AN, Sabini J: Emotional state, physical well-being, and performance in the presence of feigned ambient odor, *J Appl Soc Psychol* 20(16):1345-1357, 1990.

76. Lorig TS, Roberts M: Odor and cognitive alteration of the contingent negative variation, *Chem Senses* 15(5):537-545, 1990.

77. Visser A: Social desirability in health research, *Psychosom Med* 61:106, 1999.

78. Genders R: *Perfume through the ages,* New York, 1972, G Putnam and Sons.

79. Gobel H et al.: Essential plant oils and headache mechanisms, *Phytomed* 2(2):93-102, 1995.

80. Walji H: *The healing power of aromatherapy,* Rocklin, Calif., 1996, Prima Publishing.

81. Passant H: A holistic approach in the ward, *Nursing Times* 86(4):26-28, 1990.

82. Price S, Price L: *Aromatherapy for health professionals,* New York, 199, Churchill-Livingstone.

83. Saller R, Hellstein A, Hellenbrecht D: Klinische Pharmakologie und therapeutische Anwendung von Cineol (Eukalyptus) und Menthol als Bestandteil atherischer Ole, *Internistiche Praxis* 28/2: 355-364, 1988. In Gobel H et al.: Essential plant oils and headache mechanisms, *Phytomedicine* 2(2):93-102, 1995.

84. Hirsch AR, Kang C: The effect of inhaling green apple fragrance to reduce the severity of migraine: a pilot study, *Headache Q* 9:159-163, 1998.

85. Kirk-Smith MD, Van Toller C, Dodd GH: Unconscious odour conditioning in human subjects, *Biol Psychol* 17:221-231, 1983.

86. Halasz N, Shepherd GM: Neurochemistry of the vertebrate olfactory bulb, *Neurosci* 10:578-579, 1983.

87. Macrides F, Davis BJ: Olfactory bulb. In Emson PC, editor: *Chem neuroana,* New York, 1983, Raven Press.

88. Haberly LB, Price JL: Association and commissural fiber systems of the olfactory cortex in the rat. II. Systems originating in the olfactory peduncle, *J Comp Neurol* 178:781-808, 1978.

89. Mair RG, Harrison LM: Influence of drugs on smell function. In Laing DG, Doty RL, Briephol W, editors: *Human sense of smell,* Berlin, 1991, Springer-Verlag.

90. Zaborsky L et al.: Cholinergic and GABA-ergic projections to the olfactory bulb in the rat, *J Comp Neurol* 243:468-509, 1985.

91. Sjaastad O: Cluster headaches. In Vinken PJ, Bruyn GW, Klawans HL, editors: *Handbook of clinical neurology: headache,* vol 48, New York, 1986, Elsevier Science.

92. Gall CM et al.: Events for co-existence of GABA and dopamine in neurons of the rat olfactory bulb, *J Comp Neurol* 266:307-318, 1987.

93. Leston J et al.: Free and conjugated plasma catecholamines in cluster headache, *Cephalalgia* 7(6):331, 1987.

94. Foote S, Bloom F, Aston-Jones G: Nucleus locus coeruleus: new evidence of anatomical and physiological specificity, *Physiol Rev* 86:844-914, 1983.

95. Shipley M, Halloran F, Torre J: Surprisingly rich projection from locus coeruleus to the olfactory bulb in the rat, *Brain Res* 329:294-299, 1985.

96. Igarashi H et al.: Cerebrovascular sympathetic nervous activity during cluster headaches, *Handbook Clin Neurol* 7(6):87-89, 1987.

97. Anselmi B et al.: Endogenous opioids in cerebrospinal fluid and blood in idiopathic headache sufferers, *Headache* 20:294-299, 1980.

98. Nattero G et al.: Serum gastrin levels in cluster headache and migraine attacks. In Pfaffenrath V, Lundberg PO, Sjaastad O, editors: *Updating in headache,* Berlin, 1985, Springer-Verlag.

99. Appenzeller O, Atkinson RA, Standefer JC: Serum beta endorphin in cluster headache and common migraine. In Rose FC, Zikha E, editors: *Progress in migraine,* London, 1981, Pitman.

100. Hardebo JE et al.: CSF opioid levels in cluster headache. In Rose FC, editor: *Migraine,* Basel, 1985, Karger.

101. Moskowitz MA: Neurobiology of vascular head pain, *Ann Neurol* 16:157-158, 1984.

102. Gobel H, Schmidt G, Soyka D: Effect of peppermint and eucalyptus oil preparations on neurophysiological and experimental algesimetric headache parameters, *Cephalalgia* 14:228-234, 1994.

103. Gobel H et al.: Effectiveness of peppermint oil and paracetamol in the treatment of tension headache, *Nervenarzt* 67:672-681, 1996.

104. Woolfson A, Hewitt D: Intensive aromacare, *Intl J Aromather* 4(2):12-13, 1992.

105. Aqel MB: Relaxant effect of the volatile oil of *Romarinus officinalis* on tracheal smooth muscle, *J Ethnopharmacol* 33:57-62, 1991.

106. Dale A, Cornwell S: The role of lavender oil in relieving perineal discomfort following childbirth: a blind randomized clinical trial, *J Adv Nurs* 19:89-96, 1994.

107. Burns E, Blamey C: Using aromatherapy in childbirth, *Nurs Times* 90(9):54-60, 1994.

108. Krall B, Krause W: *Efficacy intolerance of mentha arvensis aetheroleum*. Program abstracts, Twenty-fourth International Symposium of Essential Oils, 1993.

109. Wang Y et al.: A pilot study of the use of alternative medicine in multiple sclerosis patients with special focus on acupuncture, *Neurology* 52(2):A550, 1999.

110. Doty RL, Shaman P, Dann M: Development of the University of Pennsylvania smell identification test: a standardized microencapsulated test of olfactory function, *Physiol Behav* 32:489-502, 1984.

111. Yamada K, Mimaki Y, Sashida Y: Anticonvulsive effects of inhaling lavender oil vapour, *Biol Pharm Bull* 17(2):359-360, 1994.

112. Betts T et al.: An olfactory countermeasure treatment for epileptic seizures using a conditioned arousal response to specific aromatherapy oils, *Epilepsia* 36(3):S130-S131, 1995.

113. Davies P: Aromatherapy: an A-Z. Saffron Walden, 1989, C.W. Daniel. As referenced in Mantle F: Moving experiences, *Nurs Times* 92(14):46-48, 1996.

114. Markopoulou K et al.: Olfactory dysfunction in familial parkinsonism, *Neurology* 49:1262-1267, 1977.

115. Mobert RJ, Doty RL: Olfactory function in Huntington's disease patients and at-risk offspring, *Int J Neurosci* 89:133-139, 1997.

116. Plum V: Working with alcoholism, *Intl J Aromather* 9(1):9-11, 1998.

117. Schiffman SS: Taste and smell in disease, *N Engl J Med* 308:1275-1279, 1983.

118. Getchell T, Bartoschuk L, Doty R: *Smell and taste in health and disease*, New York, 1991, Raven Press.

119. Macht DI, Ting GC: Experimental inquiry into the sedative properties of some aromatic drugs and fumes, *J Pharmacol Exp Ther* 18:361-372, 1921.

120. Buchbauer G et al.: Aromatherapy: evidence for sedative effects of the essential oil of lavender after inhalation, *J Biosci (Zeitschrift fur Naturforschung)* Sect C, 46(11-12):1067-1072, 1991.

121. Cunningham S: *Magical aromatherapy: the power of scent*, St Paul, Minn., 1995, Llewellyn.

122. Buchbauer G, Jirovetz L, Jager W: Passiflora and lime-blossoms: motility effects after inhalation of the essential oils and of some of the main constituents in animal experiment, *Arch Pharm (Weinheim)* 325:247-248, 1992.

123. Elisabetsky E, Marschner J, Souza DO: Effects of linalool on glutamatergic system in the rat cerebral cortex, *Neurochem Res* 20(4):461-465, 1995.

124. Hudson R: The value of lavender for rest and activity in the elderly patient, *Compl Ther Med* 4:5257, 1996.

125. Hirsch AR: Olfaction and aging, *Ann Clin Lab Sci* 25(1):100, 1995.

126. Scott AE: Clinical characteristics of taste and smell disorders, *Ear Nose Throat J* 68:297-298, 1989.

127. Doty R, Reyes P, Gregor T: Presence of both odor identification and detection deficits in Alzheimer's disease, *Brain Res Bull* 18:598, 1987.

128. Karamat E et al.: Excitatory and sedative effects of essential oils on human reaction time performance, Ecro X: Abstracts, *Chem Senses* 17:847, 1992.

129. Miyake Y, Nakagawa M, Asakura: Effects of odors on humans: effects on sleep latency, Abstract, *JASTS* XXIV:183, 1990.

130. Klink M, Quan SF: Prevalence of reported sleep disturbances in a general adult population and their relationship to obstructive airways diseases, *Chest* 91:540-546, 1987.

131. Benton D: The influence of androstenol—a putative human pheromone—on mood throughout the menstrual cycle, *Biol Psychol* 15:249-256, 1982.

132. Hirsch AR: Garlic therapy, Harper's Magazine 298(1788):32, 1999.

133. Baron RA: The sweet smell of . . . helping: effects of pleasant ambient odors on prosocial behavior in shopping malls, *Per Soc Psychol Bull* 23:498-504, 1997.

134. Baron RA, Kalsher MJ: Effects of a pleasant ambient fragrance on simulated driving performance: the sweet smell of . . . safety? *Environ Behav* 30:535-552, 1998.

135. Hirsch AR: Nostalgia, the odors of childhood and society, *Psychiatr Times* 9(8):29, 1992.

136. Baron RA, Thomley J: A whiff of reality: positive affect as a potential mediator of the effects of pleasant fragrance on task performance and helping, *Environ Behav* 26:766-784, 1994.

137. Dixon JM, Helsel WJ, Rojahn J: Aversive conditioning of visual screening with aromatic ammonia for treating aggressive and disruptive behavior in a developmentally disabled child, *Behav Modif* 13:91-107, 1989.

138. Earls CM, Castonguay LG: The evaluation of olfactory aversion for a bisexual pedophile with a single-case multiple baseline design, *Behav Ther* 20:137-146, 1989. As referenced in Spector IP et al.: Cue-controlled relaxation and "aromatherapy" in the treatment of speech anxiety, *Behav Cogn Psychother* 21:239-253, 1993.

139. Tanner BA, Zeiler M: Punishment of self-injurious behavior using aromatic ammonia as the aversive stimulus, *J Appl Behav An* 8:53-57, 1975.

140. Baumeister AA, Baumeister AA: Suppression of repetitive self-injurious behavior by contingent inhalation of aromatic ammonia, *J Autism Childhood Schizophr* 8(1):71-77, 1978.

141. Brooker DJR, Snape M, Johnson E: Single case evaluation of the effects of aromatherapy and massage on disturbed behaviour in severe dementia, *Brit J Clin Psychol* 36:287-296, 1997.

142. Hirsch AR, Trannel TJ: Chemosensory disorders and psychiatric diagnoses, *J Neurol Orthop Med Surg* 17:25-30, 1996.

143. Warren C, Warrenburg S: Mood benefits of fragrance, *Perfumer & Flavorist* 18:9-16, 1993.

144. Hirsch AR, Gruss, JJ: Ambient odors in the treatment of claustrophobia: a pilot study, *J Neurol Orthop Med Surg* 18:98-103, 1998.

145. Torii S et al.: Contingent negative variation (CNV) and the psychological effects of odour. In Van Toller S, Dodd G, editors: *Perfumery: the psychology and biology of fragrance,* New York, 1988, Chapman and Hall.

146. Langewitz W, Ruddel H, Von Eiff AW: Influence of perceived level of stress upon ambulatory blood pressure, heart rate, and respiratory frequency, *J Clin Hypertens* 3:743-748, 1987.

147. Allen WF: Effect of various inhaled vapors on respiration and blood pressure in anesthetized, unanesthetized, sleeping and anosmic subjects, *Am J Physiol* 1988:620-632, 1929.

148. Spector IP et al.: Cue-controlled relaxation and "aromatherapy" in the treatment of speech anxiety, *Behav Cogn Psychother* 21:239–253, 1993.

149. Evans B: An audit into the effects of aromatherapy massage and the cancer patient in palliative and terminal care, *Compl Ther Med* 3:239-241, 1995.

150. Dunn C: A report on a randomised controlled trial to evaluate the use of massage and aromatherapy in an intensive care unit, bachelor's thesis, 1992, as referenced in Waldman CS et al.: Aromatherapy in the intensive care unit, *Care of the Critically Ill* 9(4):170-174, 1993.

151. Dunn C, Sleep J, Collett D: Sensing an improvement: an experimental study to evaluate the use of aromatherapy, massage and periods of rest in an intensive care unit, *J Adv Nurs* 21:34-40, 1995.

152. Buckle J: Aromatherapy, *Nurs Times* 89(20):32-35, 1993.

153. Stevensen CJ: The psychophysiological effects of aromatherapy massage following cardiac surgery, *Compl Ther Med* 2:27-35, 1994.

154. Wilkinson S: Aromatherapy and massage in palliative care, *Intl J Palliat Nurs* 1(1):21-30, 1995.

155. DeGroot AC: Airborne allergic contact dermatitis from tea tree oil, *Contact Dermatitis* 35:101, 1996.

156. Komori T, Fujiwara R, Tanida M: Effects of citrus fragrance on immune function and depressive states, *Neuroimmunomodulation* 2:174-180, 1995.

157. Estrem SA, Renner G: Disorders of smell and taste, *Otolaryngol Clin North Am* 20:133-147, 1987.

158. Kite SM et al.: Development of an aromatherapy service on a cancer centre, *Palliat Med* 12:171-180, 1998.

159. Lehrer S, Levine E, Bloomer W: Abnormally diminished sense of smell in women with oestrogen receptor positive breast cancer, *Lancet* 2:333, 1985.

160. Cunningham S: *Magical aromatherapy: the power of scent,* St Paul, Minn., 1995, elewellyn.

161. Tobin P: Aromatherapy and its application in the management of people with dementia, *Lamp* 52(5):34, 1995,

162. Sitaras N et al.: Olfactory involvement in learning processes, *Rhinology* 21:273-280, 1983.

163. Ehrlichman H, Bastone L: Olfaction and emotion. In Serby MJ, Chobor KL, editors: *Science of olfaction,* New York, 1992, Springer-Verlag.

164. Ehrlichman H, Bastone L: Odor experience as an affective state: effects of odor pleasantness on cognition, *Perfume & Flavorist* 16:11-12, 1991.

165. Baron RA: Environmentally-induced positive affect: its impact on self-efficacy, task performance, negotiation, and conflict, *J Appl Soc Psychol* 20:368-384, 1990.

166. Hirsch AR, Johnston LH: Odors and learning, *J Neurol Orthop Med Surg* 17(1):119-126, 1996.

167. Sugano H: Effects of odors on mental function (abstract), *JASTS* XXII:8, 1988.

168. Arnold MB: *Memory and the brain,* Hillsdale, NJ, 1984, Lawrence Erlbaum Associates.

169. Nasel C et al.: Functional imaging of effects of fragrances on the human brain after prolonged inhalation, *Chem Senses* 19(4):359-364, 1994.

170. Piaget J: Contributions of the psychosocial sciences to human behavior. In Kaplan HI, Sadock BJ, editors: *Synopsis of psychiatry, behavioral sciences, clinical psychiatry,* ed 5, Baltimore, Williams & Wilkins.

171. Long TS et al.: EEG and behavioral responses to low-level galaxolide administration. (Abstract) Associations of Chemoreception Science Annual Meeting, Sarasota, Fla, 1989.

172. Halasz N, Shepherd GM: Neurochemistry of the vertebrate olfactory bulb, *Neurosci* 10:579-619, 1983.

173. Macrides F, Davis BJ: Olfactory bulb. In Emso PC, editor: *Chemical Neuroanalysis,* New York, 1983, Raven Press.

174. Squire LR: *Memory and the brain,* New York, 1987, Oxford University Press.

175. Koob GF: Neuropeptides and memory. In Iversen LL, Iversen SD, Snyder SH, editors: *Handbook of psychopharmacology,* New York, 1987, Plenum Press.

176. Lishman WA: *Organic psychiatry: psychological consequences of cerebral disorder,* Oxford, 1978, Blackwell Scientific Publications.

177. Smith ML, Milner B: Role of the right hippocampus in the recall of spatial location, *Neuropsychologia* 19:781-793, 1981.

178. Richardson JTE, Zucco GM: Cognition and olfaction: a review, *Psychol Bull* 105(3):352-360, 1989.

179. Hirsch AR: Demography of olfaction, *Pro Inst Med Chgo* 45:6, 1992.

180. Perala BT: Do specific ambient odors enhance long-term memory? (Abstract) *Ohio J Sci* 94(2):11, 1994.

181. Parasuraman R, Warm JS, Dember WN: *Effects of olfactory stimulation on skin conductance and event-related brain potentials during visual sustained attention.* Progress Report No. 6. Submitted to the Fragrance Research Fund, Ltd., 1992. As referenced in Sullivan TE et al.: Recent advances in the neuropsychology of human olfaction and anosmia, *Brain Inj* 641-646, 1995.

182. Nelson WT et al.: *The effects of fragrance administration and attentiveness on vigilance performance.* Paper presented at the meeting of the Southern Society for Philosophy and Psychology, Memphis, Tennessee, 1992. As referenced in Sullivan TE et al.: *Brain Inj* 9(6):641-646, 1995.

183. Sullivan TE et al.: Recent advances in the neuropsychology of human olfaction and anosmia, *Brain Inj* 9(6):643, 1995.

184. Heuberger E, Ilmberger J, Buchbauer G: *Fragrance compounds and their influence on human attentional processing.* ECRO Abstracts, p. 76.

185. Sanderson H, Carter A: Healing hands, *Nurs Times* 90(11):46-48, 1994.

186. Shakespeare W: *Hamlet,* Act IV, Scene VI.

187. Duke J: Can rosemary save your memory? *Organic Gardening* 44(8):52, 1997.

188. Blau JN, Solomon F: Smell and other sensory disturbances in migraine, *J Neurol* 232:275-276, 1985.

189. Hirsch AR, Kang C: The effect of inhaling green apple fragrance to reduce the severity of migraine: a pilot study, *Headache Q* 9:159-163, 1998.

190. Shim C, Williams MH Jr: Effect of odors in asthma, *Am J Med* 80:18-22, 1986.

191. Miller CS: Chemical sensitivity: symptom, syndrome or mechanism for disease? *Toxicology* 111:69-86, 1996.

192. Ross PM et al.: Olfaction and symptoms in the multiple chemical sensitivities syndrome, *Prev Med* 28:467-480, 1999.

193. Olowe SA, Ransome-Kuti O: The risk of jaundice in glucose-6-phosphate dehydrogenase deficient babies exposed to menthol, *Acta Paediatr Scand* 69:341-345, 1980.

194. Betts T: Sniffing the breeze, *Aromather Quar* p. 19-22. 1994.

195. Jori A, Bianchetti A, Prestini PE: Effect of essential oils on drug metabolism, *Biochem Pharmacol* 18(9):2081-2085, 1969.

196. DeGroot AC: Airborne allergic contact dermatitis from tea tree oil, *Contact Dermatitis* 35:304-305, 1996.

197. Bridges B: Fragrances and health, *Environ Health Perspect* 107(7):A340, 1999.

CHAPTER 11

The Placebo Effect and Alternative Medicine: Reimagining the Relationship

ANNE HARRINGTON

The growing popularity of alternative medicine among the industrialized Western countries has the so-called *mainstream* medical community scrambling to assert a stance. In two separate recent surveys, it was found that about half of all Americans and two-thirds of all Germans admitted to making use of at least one form of nontraditional therapy within the past year.[1,2] Dr. Anthony S. Luder's comments concerning complementary medicine are typical of one reaction to this phenomenon:[3]

A characteristic of high technology in the late 20th century is the loss of control felt by the common citizen, who does not understand it and feels alienated. This explains in large degree the incredible phenomenon of the rush to non-medical therapy when modern scientific medicine has made remarkable advances in all fields and continues to do so. No doubt the impersonal and, at times insensi-

tive, medical system . . . is in no small measure to blame. Nevertheless, pandering to superstition, rumor, ignorance, prejudice and other emotional extremes is no way to develop medicine. It should be clearly stated and has been by the Israel Medical Association and others; there is only one medicine—scientific medicine. All the rest, valid though it may be as a psychological prop or placebo, is not medicine, either "integrated," "alternative," "complementary" or any other title given to it.

Others—perhaps driven more by a sense of necessity than preference—appear to take a more conciliatory stance. We will not refuse you entry to our ranks, they seem to say, but first you must pass our ritual rite of passage: the subjection of your treatment to a placebo-controlled trial. Set up a situation, they say, in which all outcome effects that are plausibly due to psychologic props can be sifted out, and we'll then be persuaded you have something more here than a palliative that panders to public superstition, rumor, ignorance, and prejudice.

What, if anything, is wrong with this demand? To answer this, it is necessary to begin less with a direct answer than with a probe of the assumptions that structure the demand itself. The most fundamental assumption underlying the idea of a placebo-controlled trial is that the placebo control group provides a baseline against which the effectiveness of the real treatment can be measured. Any effects seen in the control group are assumed to be due to a nonspecific effect that ultimately does not have an enduring or measurable impact on the course of the specific disorder in question.

The great question facing both mainstream and alternative medicine is whether this way of thinking about the placebo effect makes sense. Of course, alternative medicine, with its insecure status, has perhaps the most to gain from tackling this question. Serious study of the placebo effect is still in its infancy, but already enough is known to say with some confidence that the placebo effect is far more than a mere psychologic prop. How much more, or in what ways it can be much more, is still a source of controversy and investigation. At the same time, there are some resources and reference points to guide further investigations. The past 20 years have seen the growth of both laboratory and clinical, behavioral and neurobiologic research into the placebo effect. Collectively, this research already stands as a formidable challenge to the complacency of those who would call placebos a mere nothing. Following is some of what that literature shows.[4]

The initial attempts to refer the placebo response to a specific kind of probably unstable personality have largely failed.[5,6] Instead, situational factors and environmental cues—the visible signs and symbols of healing—matter more than any personality traits an individual brings to the situation. Under the right circumstances, virtually anyone can become responsive to placebo influences.

At least some of the ways that people respond to some of these environmental cues can be modeled using a standard conditioning paradigm.[7] According to conditioning theory, previous benefits from taking pills or interacting with a white-coated physician serve as the conditioning stimulus. This conditioning is comparable to the bell stimulus in Pavlov's famous experiments. At the same time, that conditioning cannot be the whole story, at least in human beings. Other studies have shown that expectation of a certain outcome can influence experience, even if that expectation countermands the effects one would expect to see if the effect were simply conditioned. Kirsch showed, for example, that people get drunk on placebo alcohol in the way that their culture has scripted the drama of getting drunk. This may or may not have much to do with the actual sedative effects of alcohol.[8] There is even evidence that expectation can sometimes override the actual pharmacology of an active substance. A case was reported some decades ago of a severely nauseated pregnant woman who was given an emetic, ipecac. Although ipecac is actually given to induce vomiting, the patient was assured that this medication would help her. She believed her physician, and within minutes her nausea went away and a balloon in her stomach showed that her stomach had begun contracting normally.[9]

One of the most potent placebogenic cues we can encounter in any environment is another human being. The placebo effect has a powerful and complex relationship with individuals' functioning as incorrigibly social beings, highly susceptible to influence by specific kinds of human interactions. Simply stated, this means that the physician might be a potent placebo in his or her own right. In particular, if a physician seems confident or enthusiastic about a treatment, this predicts a good placebo response. Conversely, there is evidence that recovery can be undermined by physicians who appear to be indifferent or dubious about the patient and the treatment, even in the case of interventions we tend to think of as wholly skill-based, such as surgery.[10]

The placebo effect is not just a product of cognition. The modulation of emotional experience also facilitates some kinds of placebogenic processes. It is known, for example, that the experience of physical pain is increased by anxiety. Therefore, any intervention that influences anxiety levels is also likely to contribute to a more general experience of bodily relief. The story may go deeper into the body than that, however. It is known that high stress can increase cortisol output, which in turn can depress the immune system, though no one has yet measured changes in cortisol output in response to a placebo intervention.[11]

The biologic mediator of at least one frequent form of placebo response, placebo-induced analgesia, has been identified. The now-classic studies from the late 1970s by Levine and colleagues[12] were the first to show that placebo-induced analgesia can be reversed by naloxone, an opioid antagonist. Since then, these studies have been probed, challenged, modified, and basically confirmed in multiple followups. For many, they serve as a model for how to proceed with the task of identifying other biologic mediators of placebo-genic processes.

Many forms of placebo response that are mediated by real biology are also modulated by real culture. For example, group beliefs shape tacit convictions of what an illness is and how individuals will feel and behave when they get one. Daniel Moerman's work comparing placebo effects across various national cultural contexts is one empirical reference point for this claim, although its full meaning remains unclear. Moerman found that in 117 studies of treatments for ulcers, Germans responded to placebos at a rate of about 63%, other countries averaged about 36%, and Brazilians checked in at a mere 7%.[13,14]

None of the research directions and insights cited in the current literature are comprehensive enough to serve on their own as a framework for doing full justice to the placebo effect. Therefore, it is useful to note that beyond the accumulated insights from literature written by card-carrying placebo researchers are various studies that are not flagged in the literature as being about this effect. In spite of that, these studies may help enrich the sense of all that may be contained by the placebo effect. Following are examples of the types of studies that may be useful:

1. **Lessons from orphanages** Studies of orphans undertaken during World War II first called attention to the phenomenon of children whose material needs are all met, but whose emotional needs are not. These children were physically stunted and suffered from a measurable deficit of growth-hormone secretion. The children lacked a secure bond with a loving caretaker, or were otherwise growing up in an emotionally impoverished or insecure environment. Known technically as reversible somatotropin deficiency, and more informally as psychosocial dwarfism, the standard treatment is to remove the child from the toxic environment and put him or her into a home setting that is loving and secure.[15]

2. **Postponement of death** A number of epidemiologic studies have shown that mortality in coherent groups dips below expected levels just before a symbolically meaningful occasion, such as a major cultural or religious holiday,

and then peaks in the weeks just afterward. The finding has been established for a large population of Chinese before the Harvest Moon Festival, and in a large population of Jewish men, but not women, before the Jewish Passover holiday. Other studies have shown that there is a statisically significant tendency for people, especially famous people, to survive through a last birthday. And of course the clinical world is filled with anecdotal reports of dying patients who hang on until they can be reconciled with an absent child or complete some other unfinished business.[16]

3. **They "cried until they could not see"** In California, some 200 cases of blindness have been reported and investigated among Cambodian refugee women who were forced by the Khmer Rouge to witness the torture and slaughter of those close to them, particularly the men in their families. Examination of these women has repeatedly confirmed that there is nothing physically wrong with their eyes. However, having been made to bear witness to the unbearable, they "cried until they could not see," as the title of a *New York Times* article put it.[17] A case like this opens up the broad arena of so-called hysterical physical symptoms, which were encountered frequently and studied intensively in European neurology during the prepsychoanalytic era. Observations concerning these symptoms might well be harvested and looked at afresh within the framework of our own explanatory models.

4. **The physiology of social stigma** A whole range of literature from the past 40 years drives home the point that a patient's capacity to rally in the face of illness is irretrievably intertwined with the sick person's sense that loved ones and the community wish for and support that survival. The phenomenon of voodoo death has perhaps served as the most dramatic example of this phenomenon. Voodoo death is a rare cause of death in which a person feels so isolated from the community, that he or she already feels dead. In the words of pioneering physiologist Walter Bradford Cannon: "All people who stand in kinship relation with him withdraw their sustaining support. . . . The organization of his social life has collapsed and, no longer a member of a group, he is alone and

isolated. The doomed man is in a situation from which the only escape is by death."[18]

For many years, voodoo death seemed like an exotic, even esoteric kind of phenomenon associated with the cultural life of primitives but not relevant to the Western world. In the late 1980s, Sanford Cohen said that "Voodoo death, the stress response and AIDS" picked up the theme and brought it squarely into our own world. Cohen was interested in a range of situations in which death seemed to be hastened by experiences of extreme hopelessness and isolation; for example, displaced refugees trying to come to terms with an isolating and alienating new culture. The most poignant evidence that Cohen explored came from the clinical literature on the apparent physiologic effects of familial rejection and social stigma associated with AIDS. Cohen reported the case of a mother who "learned on the same day that her son was gay and had AIDS. She reacted to this with hostility and openly maintained a prayer vigil outside the intensive-care unit, praying that her son would die because of the shame he had caused her. The patient could hear his mother praying. One hour later the patient died, much to the surprise of his physician, since he did not appear to be terminal."[19]

5. **Bearing the marks of Christ's Passion** A recent MGM film, *Stigmata*, introduced the general public to a phenomenon that has long existed on the margins of ecstatic Christian, and especially Catholic, religious practice. This phenomenon is visible stigmata, or the spontaneous appearance of bloody wounds in places on the experiencer's body, especially the hands or wrists, where Jesus is believed to have been wounded during his torture and crucifixion. Investigators of this controversial phenomenon have called attention to "the extraordinary precision of conformity" between the manifestation of the wounds themselves and the specific visualization or point of doctrine that the researchers believe somehow trigger them. Some wounds take on the shape of the sufferer's favorite crucifix; other wounds only bleed on Good Friday.[20,21]

Other examples could be added, but the point is surely clear. To renegotiate the relationship with the placebo effect requires the courage to examine the periphery of human phenomena that may be relevant to its elu-

dication. Researchers cannot be limited by definitions that have their origins in the artefactual world of clinical trials. At the same time, generosity of scope must be accompanied by an equally stalwart commitment to methodological rigor and self-criticism. Our understanding of the placebo effect must be put on a far richer empirical and theoretical basis than it is now. Only then will it be possible to return to a dialogue with the gatekeepers of mainstream modern medicine and to look again at their demand that all alternative treatments demonstrate their efficacy by passing the rigors imposed by a placebo-controlled trial.

At that point, the basic premise underlying the current "gold standard" of clinical trial work may be questioned. That premise is that all treatment must demonstrate efficacy beyond the placebo effect because it is understood that the effect is a mere additive, with no relevance to understanding the working of the real treatment being tested. One of the most intriguing possibilities that may emerge from a future robust research program into the placebo effect is a different vision of the relationship between the placebo effect and the specific biological treatments that are being compared. Rather than the placebo effect happening on top of a specific effect of a treatment, it can be concluded that it has a direct modulating effect on the treatment itself. If so, this would mean that a specific biologic or skill-based treatment that has taken pains to eliminate the placebo effect is not purifying itself of all psychological noise, but actually altering the magnitude and specific nature of its own efficacy.

If it does turn out that the placebo effect is not a mere additive to specific biological treatments, but an active modulator of them, then clearly better ways would need to be devised to test the efficacy of drugs and other specific treatments. A virologist or bacteriologist would not look at the effects of a microorganism on biological functioning without paying attention to the preexisting state of the particular host it has invaded. Those studying placebo effect must be at least as vigilant in their work.

Why might this issue matter particularly to alternative medicine? Both critics and sometimes apologists claim that alternative medicine has a certain edge over much of modern mainstream medical care in its ability to create sets and settings that are placebogenic. If this is the case, then alternative medicine has a particular stake in determining to what extent these factors are not simply incidental additives to a treatment, but integral modulators of it. Otherwise, alternative medicine might say that any study that asks alternative medical practitioners to cook up their effects using an impoverished repertoire of ingredients might deprive them of a key leaven or spice.

The stakes here go beyond those of pragmatic self-interest. Much of alternative medical therapy has historic roots in a clinical ethos. This ethos largely declined to sign on to the project in biomedicine to eradicate subjective (placebo-inducing) factors in treatment. Because of this, alternative medicine is in a particularly strong position to ask questions about the larger costs of this project, both for patient care and for deeper scientific understanding of how humans really function psychobiologically. If alternative medicine can find a way to set itself up as a responsible critic on behalf of all medicine on this front, it will have helped itself to secure better conditions for negotiating its relationship to the mainstream. In addition, it may contribute to a larger future effort to reinvent the sciences that study human functioning and begin to make room for all of what humans are.

References

1. Eisenberg D et al: Trends in alternative medicine use in the United States, 1990-1997, *JAMA* 280:1569-1575, 1998.
2. Häusermann D: Wachsendes Vertrauen in Naturheilmittel, *Dtsch Ärzteblatt* 94:1857-1858, 1997.
3. Luder AS: *Complementary medicine,* Jerusalem Post, www.jpost.com, Nov. 22, 1996.
4. Harrington A: *The placebo effect: an interdisciplinary exploration,* Cambridge, Mass., 1997, Harvard University Press.
5. Roberts AH et al: The power of nonspecific effects in healing: implications for psychosocial and biological treatments, *Clin Psychol Rev* 13:375-391, 1993.
6. Swartzman LC, Burkell J: Expectations and the placebo effect in clinical drug trials: why we should not turn a blind eye to unblinding, and other cautionary notes, *Clin Pharmacol Ther* 64:1-7, 1998.
7. Ader R: The role of conditioning in pharmacotherapy. In Harrington A, editor: *The placebo effect: an interdisciplinary exploration,* Cambridge, Mass. 1997, Harvard University Press.
8. Kirsch I: Specifying nonspecifics: psychological mechanisms of placebo effects. In Harrington A: *The placebo effect: an interdisciplinary exploration,* Cambridge, Mass., 1997, Harvard University Press.
9. Frank JD: *Persuasion and healing: a comparative study of psychotherapy,* Baltimore, 1961, Johns Hopkins Press.
10. Talbot M: The placebo prescription, *The New York Times* Sunday Magazine, p. 34, Jan 9, 2000.
11. Kiecolt-Glaser JK, Glaser R: Stress and immune function in humans. In Ader R, Felten DL, Cohen N, editors: *Psychoneuroimmunology,* ed 2, New York, 1991, Academic Press.
12. Levine JD, Gordon, NC, Fields HL: The mechanism of placebo analgesia, *Lancet* 2:654-657, 1978.
13. Bennett R: The power of placebos: shaking off their image as "inert substances," placebos are finding new respect, *The Oregonian,* July 28, 1999 (http://oregonlive.com/news/99/07/st072820.html).
14. Moerman D: General medical effectiveness and human biology: placebo effects in the treatment of ulcer disease, *Med Anthropol Q* 14:3, 14-16, 1983.
15. Mouridsen SE, Nielsen S: Reversible somatotropin deficiency (psychosocial dwarfism) presenting as conduct disorder and growth hormone deficiency, *Dev Med Child Neurol* 32(12):1093-1098, 1990.
16. Phillips DP, Smith DG: Postponement of death until symbolically meaningful occasions, *JAMA* 263(14): 1947-1951, 1990.
17. Cooke P: They cried until they could not see, *New York Times Magazine,* pp. 24-25, 45-47, June 23, 1991.
18. Cannon WB: Voodoo death, *Am Anthropol* 44:169-181, 1942.
19. Cohen S: Voodoo death, the stress response, and AIDs. In Bridge TP, Mirsky AF, Goodwin FK, editors: *Psychological, neuropsychiatric, and substance abuse aspects of AIDS,* New York, 1988, Raven Press.
20. Wilson I: *The bleeding mind: an investigation into the mysterious phenomenon of stigmata,* London, 1988, Weidenfeld and Nicolson.
21. Harrison T: *Stigmata: a medieval mystery in a modern age,* Fount, 1994, London.

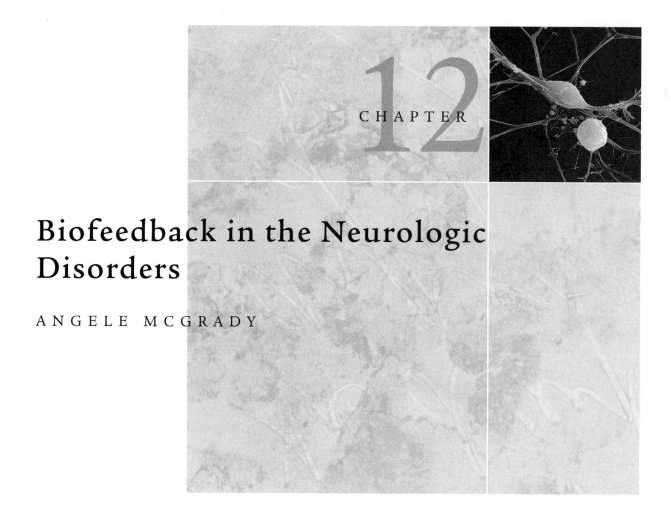

CHAPTER 12

Biofeedback in the Neurologic Disorders

ANGELE MCGRADY

iofeedback (BF) is a therapeutic technique by which a person learns, through the guidance of a health care provider, to be aware of and to control a specific physiological parameter. For example, muscle tension or heart rate is monitored by surface sensors and the output is converted to a recognizable visual or auditory signal, which is made available to the patient. Integral components of treatment include becoming aware of the level of activity of the physiological function and acquiring control of that function through operant conditioning. BF requires monitoring and displaying accurate and meaningful information from a body site in an easily recognizable form. Knowing which muscles are tense or relaxed allows the person to learn to self-regulate the physiological process. Undesirable internal states are associated with increased levels of sound or light, and reinforce-

ment is provided for desired responses, such as relaxed muscles.[1] The goals of BF treatment fall into three broad categories: lower arousal, retraining of poorly functioning muscles, and brain wave training.

MODALITIES

Electromyograph (EMG), thermal, skin conductance, blood pressure (BP), brain wave, and heart rate are the most common types of feedback. The signal from the EMG indicates the levels of skeletal muscle contraction and is accessed via surface or needle electrodes. For disorders in which overarousal is associated with symptoms and lowered responsiveness is the goal, surface monitoring is most appropriate. However, when the objective is to increase motor unit potentials, needle technique is often used. Thermal biofeedback (TBF) provides information about the temperature of the skin, which is correlated with blood flow in the small arterioles underlying the skin. The most common placement is on the index or middle finger of either hand, with occasional placement on the underside of the toes. Skin conductance feedback monitors the activity of the sweat glands directly beneath the sensors. Brain wave (electroencephalogram, or EEG) feedback reflects the activity of certain areas of the brain and specific patterns of activity there. Neurofeedback is linked to the frequency, duration, or amplitude of the electrical activity of the brain. Heart rate and BP feedback provide information about dysregulation of the cardiovascular system. Examples of cardiovascular disorders treated with biofeedback include essential hypertension, white-coat hypertension, tachycardia, and atrial fibrillation.[1]

MULTICOMPONENT TREATMENT INCORPORATING BIOFEEDBACK

BF is coupled with relaxation therapy (RT), patient education, psychotherapy, and medical management, particularly pharmacotherapy. Relaxation is of two basic types: passive or active. Active relaxation is defined as producing lower arousal by voluntarily tensing and releasing tension from specific muscle groups. Appreciation of the contrast between tension and relaxation is emphasized, with the goal being to consciously lower tension.[2] Passive relaxation consists of deep breathing or self-relaxation with words, phrases, or imagery. Autogenic relaxation uses specific phrases dealing with sensations of heaviness in the muscles and warmth in the hands.[3] The key to effective relaxation is repetition of phrases or behavior (such as breathing) on a daily basis until a reliable relaxation response can be produced quickly when needed.[4] Home practice of relaxation with or without portable feedback devices is critical to learning. The relaxation response must be generalized to conditions of daily living and practiced when the stressful situation occurs. The experience of decreasing the severity of a stress response or blocking the response with relaxation rather than relying solely on medication increases the patients' confidence in their ability to use the technique.[5] Because different relaxation techniques have specific effects, the patient must learn to

differentiate among maladaptive psychophysiological signals and to match each signal to breathing, passive and active relaxation, or imagery.[6]

Symptom monitoring and logging by the patient serves several purposes:
1. The patient becomes fully engaged in the therapeutic process.
2. The baseline (pre-treatment) average symptom severity and frequency is established.
3. Progress can be easily monitored during therapy and used as a reinforcement for continuation.
4. A summary of treatment efficacy for each patient can be produced by comparing end-of-therapy averages with baseline values. Other information relevant to therapy, such as medication usage or frequency of relaxation practice, is also appropriately noted on the log sheet.

Patient education provides easy-to-understand explanations of the rationale for BF based on physiological principles. The use of EMG feedback for disorders of excess muscle tension is logical and quickly grasped; the relationship between a high-pitched or high-frequency sound and high tension is intuitively obvious. Other symptom-feedback pairs are less so, necessitating greater efforts to make the required tasks comprehensible to patients. For example, a patient who is going to learn to warm her hands with TBF might be told the following: "When you are in a stressful situation, your body gets ready to react. This reaction includes tensing your muscles, increasing your pulse rate, and sending blood to your muscles. Thus blood is diverted away from nonessential tissues, like your digestive system and your hands and feet. When there is less warm blood in your fingers, they get cold. With feedback, you will learn to warm your hands consciously. This is part of learning how to decrease overresponding to stress."

Psychotherapy is combined with BF for patients who have comorbid conditions such as mood or anxiety disorders. For example, patients with headache may also have generalized anxiety disorder or adjustment disorder with anxiety. Clinical depression is often prominent in chronic pain patients. Cognitive-behavioral therapy (CBT) is a type of psychotherapy commonly used in conjunction with BF in anxiety and mood disorders. CBT explores negative thoughts, and dysfunctional attitudes and behaviors. The therapy emphasizes generating more positive thinking patterns and acquiring effective coping skills.[7]

It is best but not always possible for the same practitioner to provide both psychotherapy and BF. When a clinical psychologist, clinical counselor, social worker, or psychiatric nurse is also trained in BF, single sessions can integrate psychotherapy, hypnosis, or imagery with BF. For example, the patient might spend the first 30 minutes of a 50-minute session engaged in psychotherapy, and the last 20 minutes practicing BF. On the other hand, the session might consist of 20 minutes of guided imagery-assisted BF to create an atmosphere of trust between patient and practitioner followed by 30 minutes of psychotherapy.

TYPES OF BIOFEEDBACK TREATMENT PROTOCOLS

The number and structure of sessions should be matched to the patients' conditions and the severity of the disorders for which they are seeking treatment. Three basic formats are used in the lower arousal applications of BF: standard, brief, and psychotherapy based. After the clinical interview, and before beginning any BF treatment, a psychophysiological assessment should be carried out. This profile consists of measuring muscle tension, cutaneous temperature, heart rate, and skin conductance under various conditions. First, the patient is asked to sit quietly with eyes closed and then with eyes open. Then, stressful mental imagery or mental arithmetic is used to determine which physiological system responds most acutely. Finally, the patient is then asked to attempt to relax in any familiar way. Data collected during the latter phase of the assessment suggests the extent of past experience that the patient brings to the therapeutic setting.

The standard format of BF therapy consists of 8 to 12, 50-minute sessions of BF, RT, and stress management-oriented counseling.[8,9] The limited contact protocol includes 3 to 4 sessions of BF and emphasizes home practice of relaxation. This is appropriate for patients who are highly motivated, can follow directions, and have no diagnosed psychopathology.[10,11] An intensive protocol is one in which BF and RT are used as adjuncts to psychotherapy, as is common in treating chronic low back pain.[12] This format is recommended for patients who have long-standing severe symptoms, who are poorly motivated, whose lives are focused on pain, or who need in-depth psychotherapy to explore emotional conflicts or interpersonal difficulties.

It is important to note that BF and RT are not contraindicated in patients who are also medically managed by physicians. In fact, if pain or disability is severe, the BF practitioner may request that the patient return to the physician for medication to facilitate the relaxation process. As symptoms improve, the need for some types of medicine, particularly analgesics or antianxiety agents, may decrease. When log sheets indicate steadily decreasing medication use, the patient is encouraged to talk to the physician about decreasing the dosage of preventative drugs. The joint management of patients by physicians and BF practitioners is more the norm than the exception.

HEADACHE

The literature on BF and RT treatment of headache is rich and consistent. It demonstrates that EMG BF combined with RT is effective in tension-type headache and that TBF assists patients with migraine headache. Two reviews[13,14] serve as summaries of the data on EMG BF for tension-type headache. The efficacy of behavioral treatments for chronic pain was assessed through an extensive literature review and analysis by a panel of experts. In the case of chronic pain, there was strong evidence to support relaxation techniques and hypnosis, and moderately strong evidence for BF and CBT. BF worked best with tension-type headaches and CBT was most effective for lower back pain and arthritis.[13] A meta-analysis of 78 publications that included 2866 participants found that EMG BF alone or combined with RT was superior to no treatment and to pseudo-placebo therapy in tension-type headache.[14]

A typical 8- to 12-session treatment protocol for tension-type headache includes the following: EMG BF with sensors placed on the forehead or back of the neck, active and then passive RT, home practice of relaxation, daily symptom logging, and psychotherapy or stress management as appropriate. Patients are trained to decrease tension levels and to produce a general relaxation response. Sensors placed on the forehead detect a wide range of EMG activity. Recognizing the influence of grimacing, frowning, and teeth clenching helps patients to regulate muscle tension and decrease pain.[12] The relaxation process is then generalized to situations where patients feel their muscles tensing or notice the early signs of headache.

Migraine headache is treated with TBF accompanied by RT. Efficacy has been demonstrated for TBF in the reduction of headache frequency, intensity, duration, and medication use.[15] Rigorous evaluation criteria have been used to evaluate controlled studies of psychosocial interventions in migraine. Conclusions were that "thermal biofeedback plus relaxation . . . qualifies as an efficacious treatment for migraine headaches."[16] BF has also been compared with medical therapy in migraine.[17] Abortive ergotamine tartrate was associated with a 30% decrease in headache index in the first month of treatment and an additional 11% decrease later. TBF resulted in an early reduction of 25% and an additional 26% at posttreatment. Seventy-eight percent of the BF group and 40% of the medication group decreased analgesic use by a minimum of 50%.[11] In a meta-analysis involving 2445 patients with migraine, BF was found to be equivalent to propranolol; both resulted in a 43% improvement in headaches according to patients' diaries. Placebo yielded a 14% improvement, and monitoring alone produced no changes.[18] The treatment regimen used in the author's clinic for patients with migraine consists of four sessions of EMG BF and six to eight sessions of TBF combined with passive relaxation, home practice of relaxation, symptom logging, and stress management or psychotherapy as appropriate.[19,20]

Posttraumatic headache and high medication consumption headache are two problems that pose special therapy challenges for practitioners of BF. Forty subjects with posttraumatic head pain were treated with EMG BF, TBF, and RT. Of the subjects, 53% reported at least moderate improvement in the number of headaches, and 80% found that the therapy increased their ability to relax and cope with the pain. In general, chronicity of posttraumatic pain is a poor prognostic indicator for improvement mediated by BF.[21] Another difficult population of headache patients is the group who use high doses of multiple classes of medication. Withdrawal of medication, which can be accomplished on an outpatient basis, should precede treatment in this group. In a small study, progressive relaxation and BF were found to be helpful in six of the ten patients who were treated. Pain levels and medication use were reduced. However, the involvement of the therapist who provided the CBT was critically important to success.[22]

Children and the elderly are also appropriate candidates for BF therapy. Children and adolescents are often intrigued by the BF equipment and adapt to the treatment setting quite easily. Minimal contact and standard models of treatment have been tested and found to be effective in childhood migraine and tension headache.[23,24,25] On the other hand, elderly persons often require additional sessions and learning may be somewhat slower. Nonetheless, EMG BF has been found to help decrease total headache activity and increase headache-free days in elderly persons.[26] Long-term maintenance of headache improvement mediated by BF and RT therapy is good if patients are able to generalize the relaxation response to stressful situations and continue to use the adaptive coping techniques learned during therapy.[27]

MUSCULOSKELETAL PAIN

Treating patients with chronic low back pain requires a multimodal approach that combines BF with other modalities such as physical therapy, exercise, correction of gait and posture, and CBT. As the following examples demonstrate, though, BF is useful in training general relaxation and in correcting specific muscle tension abnormalities.[12] Fifty-seven patients with chronic back pain were provided with EMG BF from the site of the pain and were taught tension-reduction exercises. The EMG BF group did better than either the CBT group or the patients who continued medical treatment alone. At 6- and 24-month followup in the BF group, there were significant reductions in pain severity and fewer visits to the health care system. In this population, follow-up sessions are strongly recommended because continued relaxation practice is a key component in maintaining improvement. Relapse can occur after patients have learned the basic skills, particularly if lifestyle and posture have not changed.[28] Advanced age does not contraindicate BF treatment of patients with chronic pain.

A 12- to 16-session EMG BF and RT protocol integrated in a multidisciplinary pain program was used to treat an elderly group of patients with cervical pain. The older adults did as well as the younger adults in acquiring self-regulation skills and achieving reduction of pain.[29]

EMG BF is provided to the patient in the sitting and standing positions. It is important to monitor tension when the patient is in postures other than reclining in a chair because muscles automatically relax if the head is supported by a head rest. Poor posture, bracing, insomnia, and depression are often contributory or perpetuating factors in the long-term pain patient. Although EMG BF is used to help relax specific muscle groups, TBF combined with deep breathing training facilitates the general relaxation response. CBT may be necessary to modify maladaptive thoughts and behaviors.[30]

ANXIETY AND PANIC

Anxiety and mood disorders are common psychiatric conditions as well as frequent accompaniments to medical complaints, such as chronic pain. Appropriate candidates for BF include patients with psychiatric illnesses who can learn to modify specific physiological or psychological responses associated with their disorder.[31] Anxiety disorder may present as cognitive symptoms such as fear of losing control, dying, or going crazy, or as somatic symptoms such as racing heart, sweating, or shortness of breath. Subclinical anxiety syndromes often cause sufficient distress and functional impairment to merit therapy.[7] In one study of school-age children, teachers identified 150 students as "anxious," although the children were not diagnosed with a specific disorder by a mental health provider. Twelve sessions (six EMG and six TBF) were provided during a 6-week period. Significant reductions in situational and trait anxiety were reported.[32] Learning facial relaxation with EMG BF promotes lower central and autonomic nervous system activity and can be effective in managing both the somatic and cognitive components of anxiety.[33] Generalized anxiety disorder was treated in 38 adults diagnosed with the condition and in an additional 7 subjects with subclinical symptoms. Fifteen sessions of EEG feedback resulted in decreased self-reported and observer-rated anxiety and in improved quality of life.[34] The effects of eight sessions of frontal EMG-BF or EEG feedback to increase or to decrease alpha wave activity, or pseudo-meditation control, were compared. Based on the results of a validated paper and pencil anxiety inventory, all treated subjects reported significantly decreased anxiety symptoms, which were maintained at 6-weeks followup. The authors suggest that the effects of BF may be nonspecific in anxiety.[35] Behavioral treatment consisting of TBF and skin conductance BF with CBT was compared with CBT alone in a group of anxious patients treated with the antianxiety drug Alprazolam. The time necessary to discontinue drug therapy was shorter in the group who received combined BF and CBT. At the 6-month follow-up session, the improvements in anxiety and lower drug use obtained during active treatment were maintained.[36]

With phobic patients, RT is integral to systematic desensitization therapy; gradual exposure to the phobic stimulus is combined with guided relaxation. Psychophysiological approaches including BF and RT are suggested as a first step in management, to be followed by medication if necessary. BF can shorten the time required to learn relaxation under conditions of exposure to the phobic stimulus.[37] Syncope can also be symptomatic of simple phobia. For example, the sight of blood or injury can result in loss of consciousness in susceptible individuals. In a single case study, EMG and TBF were combined with systematic desensitization to treat an individual with longstanding blood injury phobia. With therapy, the individual learned to identify presyncopal cues and used BF and RT to block syncope when confronted with the phobic stimulus.[38]

AUTONOMIC NERVOUS SYSTEM DISORDERS

Syncope, near syncope, and dizziness are symptomatic of many primary and secondary autonomic disorders. Neurocardiogenic syncope is associated with hypotension and bradycardia; dysautonomia is characterized by progressive and gradual loss of consciousness, which commonly occurs during walking or standing. The rate and magnitude of fall in BP varies among autonomic disorders, but the disorders share the common feature of postural hypotension. Diagnosis is made by tilt table testing, and treatment usually combines pharmacotherapy and behavioral therapy.[39,40] A case series of ten patients who were tilt positive and diagnosed with one of the autonomic disorders used BF as part of overall management. Patients had headache, lightheadedness, dizziness, near syncope, or true syncope. Therapy consisted of 10 to 12 sessions of EMG, TBF, and RT. Active relaxation and EMG BF were introduced initially, followed by TBF and passive relaxation. Five of the ten patients obtained clinically significant improvement in each of their symptoms. Six of the seven with syncope had none at posttreatment.[41] Similar behavioral techniques have been applied to individuals who demonstrate orthostatic intolerance after exposure to microgravity in space. Pilots were trained with BP BF to increase BP under supine and head-up tilt conditions.[42] Autogenic therapy and BF were applied to control motion sickness in otherwise healthy and well conditioned astronauts. The protocol comprised training multiple physiological responses simultaneously for a total of 6 hours. Transfer of the responses learned in the laboratory to a variety of stimulus conditions, such as rotary chair, flight, and shuttle missions, was accomplished.[43]

SLEEP DISORDERS

Categories of disturbed sleep relevant to this chapter include primary insomnia and insomnia related to an anxiety disorder. Patients report difficulties in initiating and maintaining sleep, which are sometimes associated with racing thoughts and preoccupation.[7] The best evidence favoring BF and RT shows decreased sleep latency and fewer awakenings during sleep.[44] However, more recent findings do not support the superiority of BF over pseudofeedback.[45] In summary, sleep hygiene is always important and should be tried first. BF facilitates low levels of facial tension and RT promotes general relaxation. The associated lower arousal and decreased emotional and cognitive responsiveness are corollaries of drowsiness and sleep.[33] It is unlikely, however, that BF will be effective as sole or primary therapy for sleep disorders.[13]

EPILEPSY

EEG BF has helped individuals with epilepsy to decrease the frequency of seizures and improve performance on neuropsychologic testing.[46] Animal studies formed the scientific foundation for the use of EEG BF as a clinical tool, as reviewed recently.[47] Currently, the BF paradigm is configured to provide reinforcement for the control of slow cortical potentials (SCP). Positive SCPs are associated with reduction in seizure frequency.[48] Twenty-five patients with focal seizures and intractable epilepsy were offered 35 sessions of SCP BF and 20 sessions of behavioral self-control training. Patients were able to discriminate between cortical negativity and positivity. Successful patients, those who evidenced fewer seizures at 1-year post-treatment compared with the 3-month baseline, evidenced less negative SCPs.[49] Eighteen of 25 patients learned to control their SCPs with 29 one-hour sessions and obtained improvement in seizure frequency.

At one year, six were free of seizures.[50] Pervasive negativity may reflect cortical hyperexcitability. Patients with epilepsy may have an impaired capacity to self-regulate cortical potentials. Control can be enhanced with BF, but patients need to be able to transfer or generalize the training in order to use the technique without feedback. Successful patients were younger than age 35, were motivated, had sufficient hours of training, and were not on large doses of antiepileptic medications.[51] Long-term maintenance of benefits achieved during treatment is supported, though the evidence is not conclusive.[52]

REHABILITATION

EMG BF provided to patients undergoing rehabilitation increases the effectiveness of the standard therapies, but is rarely used as sole treatment. Using an operant conditioning paradigm, patients learn to discriminate between different levels of muscle tension. With accurate and rapid information from the BF device, high levels of activity in specific muscles can be reinforced, while relaxation of other muscles is promoted.[53] In the rehabilitation hospital, BF equipment can be transported to the patient's bedside to avoid the counterproductive effects of transporting patients to the physical therapy clinic. Several examples of the use of BF in rehabilitation are discussed here; more extensive coverage of this topic may be found elsewhere.[54-56] One-hundred patients with spinal cord injury at C 6 or higher for longer than one year were offered EMG BF. The goal was to increase voluntary responses from the triceps muscles. After one to four BF sessions, a significant increase in EMG activity from the triceps muscle was observed.[57]

Patients with paretic muscles can be trained to recruit motor units and to produce a stronger voluntary contraction. In this context, BF protocols are designed to complement and build on naturally occurring sensory feedback. A three-stage process of neuromuscular reeducation is suggested. In stage one, the patient learns to contract and relax muscles voluntarily. Stage two comprises joint movement and posture. The third stage focuses on generalization of learning to the complex functions which are necessary for daily living. Improvements in stage three skills do not occur after training directed only to stage one.[30] A group of 10 patients with hand dystonia were provided with EMG BF emanating from the proximal large limb muscles that manifested maximum tension and over-activity during writing. After a minimum of four sessions, 9 of the 10 patients reported improvement in handwriting and lessening of pain.[58]

For stroke patients in the rehabilitation setting, BF can be used to enhance the effects of exercise, to strengthen weakened muscles, and to return to more normal posture and gait. Despite reports of clinical efficacy and improvements in motor function of small groups of post-stroke patients, meta-analyses have produced inconsistent results. These range from evidence that EMG-BF is an effective tool for muscle re-education[59] to negative findings, that is, no advantage of biofeedback over physical therapy in upper extremity function in patients following stroke.[60] A recent meta-analysis was performed on data from eight studies in which EMG BF was compared to physiotherapy to improve lower extremity function in post-stroke patients.

The findings pointed to EMG-BF as more effective than conventional physiotherapy alone for improving ankle dorsiflexion muscle strength.[61] Differences in training protocols may explain some of these inconsistencies. Nonetheless, based on the known impact of psychological factors in patients undergoing rehabilitation, the clinician should enhance patients' motivation, reinforce positive psychological and physical change, and foster adaptation to lingering disability.

ATTENTION DEFICIT/ HYPERACTIVITY DISORDER

Treatment of children, adolescents, and adults with attention deficit/hyperactivity disorder (ADHD) is not founded on the lower arousal principle of BF. Rather, treatment is based on individuals learning to regulate brain wave activity in a manner similar to EEG training in epilepsy. If ADHD and ADD are associated with neurologic dysfunction in cortical and prefrontal lobe areas, then learned control of brain wave activity can translate into improved attention, better task completion, reduced impulsiveness, and mild hyperactivity. Amelioration of symptoms is proposed to occur after multisession (n = 20-40) BF therapy to increase beta activity (14 hertz) and to inhibit theta (4-8 hertz).[62,63] The beta/theta ratio was used as feedback in a 6-month training paradigm. Compared with controls, the experimental group reduced inattentive behaviors and improved composite IQ scores.

Therapists always remained in the room with the patients, providing additional encouragement and helping the children stay on task.[64,65]

EEG BF training has traditionally been used in therapists' offices and clinics. However, the large number of sessions required to learn the skill suggests that the school setting might be a practical alternative. Small numbers of students could be provided with daily EEG training sessions as part of the school day.[66] Home EEG equipment may be available in the future, so the required daily training sessions can be provided at home under the guidance of motivated, trained parents. Much like the limited therapist protocols for the lower arousal applications of BF, motivation and the ability to understand and follow instructions become critical factors influencing success.[67]

URINARY INCONTINENCE

Training the muscles of the pelvic floor with EMG BF has been successful in patients with stress and mixed incontinence. After 6 months of home BF training, the number of pads, number of incontinent episodes, and frequency of voiding decreased significantly. Eighty-five percent of the participants reported that they were cured or significantly improved.[68] In a similar manner, BF training was provided to home-bound older adults. A 75% reduction in incontinent episodes was reported in the trained group compared with the controls. Following their participation as controls, these individuals achieved a 74% reduction in incontinent episodes after completing the same EMG BF training protocol.[69] Patients with urge incontinence who had urodynamic evidence of bladder dysfunction were treated behaviorally. An 80% reduction in symptoms was observed in the treated group compared with 68.5% improvement with drug therapy and 40% with placebo. The reduction was most rapid early in treatment, followed by a more gradual improvement later.[70] EMG BF should be considered as first line therapy in urinary incontinence because there are no known side effects and no evidence exists for paradoxical worsening of symptoms.

SUMMARY

There is strong scientific evidence for the efficacy of BF as treatment for several neurologic disorders. Understanding the mechanisms underlying success and the subtypes of patients for which BF is most beneficial continues to be challenging. The effects of BF may be specific, nonspecific, or both. Nonspecific positive effects are mediated by gaining confidence, improving concentration, and developing more effective coping strategies. The primary effects of BF, in which control of individual physiological processes such as brain waves or muscle tension is learned, may also be specific. BF actively involves the patient in the therapeutic process; therapy is a partnership between provider and patient. Immediacy and accuracy of the BF information are critical, but the relationship between the practitioner and the patient remains important in all but a few of the treatment protocols. Patients with stress-related disorders have acquired maladaptive response patterns that have led to dysfunctional coping and oversensitivity to stress. Even neutral stimuli are perceived as threats so that, over time, risk for somatic manifestations of psychological conflict increases dramatically.[71] The patient who reacts maladaptively needs new skills, but skills may not be enough. The ability to self-regulate entails more than simply learning a technique. Self-regulation requires a conceptual shift towards the realization that control of physiological and psychological responses is possible. As the patient learns to self-regulate, sensory information is processed differently. For example, pain is interpreted as a message from the body, not as an inevitable prelude to an incapacitating migraine. The reply to the message involves skills in part, but cognitive adjustments and positive psychological responses are also necessary. The challenges of future research are to expand the applications of BF, to develop an understanding of mechanisms, and to differentiate the subtypes of patients and disorders that are most appropriate for BF therapy.

References

1. Schwartz M: *Biofeedback: a practitioners guide,* New York, 1995, Guilford Press.
2. Bernstein DA, Carlson CR: Progressive relaxation: abbreviated methods. In Lehrer P, Woolfolk P, editors: *Principles and practice of stress management,* ed 2, New York, 1993, Guilford Press.
3. Norris PA, Fahrion SL: Autogenic biofeedback in psychophysiological therapy and stress management. In Lehrer P, Woolfolk P, editors: *Principles and practice of stress management,* ed 2, New York, 1993, Guilford Press.
4. Davis M, Eshelman E, McKay M: *The relaxation and stress reduction workbook,* ed 4, Oakland, 1995, New Harbinger.
5. Blanchard EB et al: The role of home practice in thermal biofeedback, *J Consult Clin Psychol* 59:507-512, 1991.
6. Lehrer P et al: Stress management techniques: are they all equivalent or do they have specific effects? *Biofeedback Self Regul* 19(4):353-402, 1994.
7. Kaplan HI, Sadock BJ: *Synopsis of psychiatry,* ed 8, Baltimore, 1997, Williams & Wilkins.
8. McGrady A et al: Psychophysiologic therapy for chronic headache in primary care companion, *J Clin Psychiatry* 1(4):96-102, 1999.
9. Penzien DB, Holroyd KA: Psychosocial interventions in the management of recurrent headache disorders 2: description of treatment techniques, *Behav Med* 20:64-73, 1994.
10. Rowan AB, Andrasik F: Efficacy and cost-effectiveness of minimal therapist contact treatments of chronic headaches: a review, *Behav Ther* 27:207-234, 1996.
11. Holroyd KA et al: Recurrent vascular headache home-based treatment versus abortive pharmacological treatment, *J Consult Clin Psychol* 56(2):281-223, 1988.
12. Arena J, Blanchard B: Biofeedback and relaxation therapy for chronic pain disorders. In Gatchel R, Turk D, editors: *Psychological approaches to pain management: a practitioner's handbook,* New York, 1996, Guilford Press.
13. NIH Technology Assessment Panel: Integration of behavioral and relaxation approaches into the treatment of chronic pain and insomnia, *JAMA* 276(4):313-318, 1996.
14. Bogaard MC, ter Kuile MM: Treatment of recurrent tension headache: a meta analytic review, *Clin J Pain* 10:174-190, 1994.
15. Blanchard EB: Psychological treatment of benign headache disorders, *J Consult Clin Psychol* 60:537-551, 1992.
16. Compas BE et al: Sampling of empirically supported psychological treatments from health psychology: smoking, chronic pain, cancer and bulimia nervosa, *J Consult Clin Psychol* 66(1):89-112, 1998.
17. Holroyd K, Penzien D: Pharmacological versus non-pharmacological prophylaxis of recurrent migraine headache: meta-analytic review of clinical trials, *Pain* 42:1-13, 1990.
18. Holroyd KA et al: Enhancing the effectiveness of relaxation-thermal biofeedback training with propranolol hydrochloride, *J Consult Clin Psychol* 63:327-330, 1995.
19. McGrady A et al: Effect of biofeedback assisted relaxation on migraine headache and changes in cerebral blood flow velocity in the middle cerebral artery, *Headache* 34(7):424-428, 1994.
20. Wauquier A et al: Changes in cerebral blood flow velocity associated with biofeedback-assisted relaxation treatment of migraine headaches are specific for the middle cerebral artery, *Headache* 35:358-362, 1995.
21. Ham LP, Packard RC: A retrospective, follow-up study of biofeedback-assisted relaxation therapy in patients

with posttraumatic headache, *Biofeedback Self Regul* 21(2):93-104, 1996.

22. Blanchard EB, Taylor AE, Dentinger MP: Preliminary results from the self-regulatory treatment of high-medication-consumption headache, *Biofeedback Self Regul* 17(3):179-202, 1992.

23. Grazzi L et al: A therapeutic alternative for tension headache in children: treatment and 1-year follow-up results, *Biofeedback Self Regul* 15(1):1-6, 1990.

24. Allen KD, Shriver MD: Role of parent-mediated pain behavior management strategies in biofeedback treatment of childhood migraines, *Behav Ther* 29(3):447-490, 1998.

25. Bussone G et al: Biofeedback-assisted relaxation training for young adolescents with tension-type headache: a controlled study, *Cephalalgia* 18:463-467, 1998.

26. Arena J et al: Electromyographic biofeedback training for tension headache in the elderly: a prospective study, *Biofeedback Self Regul* 16(4):379-390, 1991.

27. Cott A et al: Long-term efficacy of combined relaxation: biofeedback treatments for chronic headache, *Pain* 51:49-56, 1992.

28. Flor H, Fydrich T, Tutk DC: Long term efficacy of EMG biofeedback for chronic rheumatic back pain, *Pain* 49:221-230, 1992.

29. Middaugh S et al: Biofeedback assisted relaxation training for the aging chronic pain patient, *Biofeedback Self Regul* 16(4):361-377, 1991.

30. Middaugh SJ: On clinical efficacy: why biofeedback does and does not work, *Biofeedback Self Regul* 15(3):191-208, 1990.

31. Futterman AD, Shapiro D: A review of biofeedback for mental disorders, *Hosp Community Psychiatry* 37(1):27-33, 1986.

32. Wenck LS, Leu PW, D'Amato RC: Evaluating the efficacy of a biofeedback intervention to reduce children's anxiety, *J Clin Psychol* 52(4):469-473, 1996.

33. Stoyva J, Thomas B: Biofeedback methods in the treatment of anxiety and stress disorders. In Lehrer P, Woolfolk P, editors: *Principles and practice of stress management,* ed 2, New York, 1993, Guilford Press.

34. Vanathy S, Sharma PSVN, Kumar KB: The efficacy of alpha and theta neurofeedback training in treatment of generalized anxiety disorder, *Indian J Clin Psychol* 25(2):136-143, 1998.

35. Rice KM, Blanchard EB, Purcell M: Biofeedback treatments of generalized anxiety disorder: preliminary results, *Biofeedback Self Regul* 18(2):93-105, 1993.

36. Scherzer BR: Biofeedback-assisted cognitive-behavioral therapy in the reduction of Alprazolam dependence after panic attacks with cardiophobia, doctoral dissertation, Cinncinati, 1997, Union Institute.

37. Barlow D: *Anxiety and its disorders: the nature and treatment of anxiety and panic,* New York, 1988, Guilford Press.

38. McGrady A, Bernal GAA: Relaxation based treatment of stress induced syncope, *J Behav Ther Exp Psychiatry* 17:23-27, 1986.

39. Grubb BP, Karas B: Clinical disorders of the autonomic nervous system associated with orthostatic intolerance: an overview of classification, clinical evaluation, and management, *PACE* 22:798-810, 1999.

40. Kosinski DJ, Wolfe DA, Grubb BP: Neurocardiogenic syncope: a review of pathophysiology, diagnosis and treatment, *Cardiovasc Rev Rep* 14:22-29, 1993.

41. McGrady A, Bush EG, Grubb BP: Outcome of biofeedback-assisted relaxation for neurocardiogenic syncope and headaches: a clinical replication series, *Appl Psychophysiol Biofeedback* 22:63-72, 1997.

42. Cowings PS et al: Autogenic-feedback training: a potential treatment for orthostatic intolerance in aerospace crews, *Pharmacology* 34:599-608, 1994.

43. Toscano WB, Cowlings PS: Reducing motion sickness: a comparison of autogenic-feedback training and an alternative cognitive task, *Aviat Space Environ Med* 53(5):449-453, 1982.

44. Turner RM: Behavioral self-control procedures for disorders of initiating and maintaining sleep (DIMS), *Clin Psychol Rev* 6(1):27-38, 1986.

45. VanderPlate CE, Eno EN: Electromyograph biofeedback and sleep onset insomnia: comparison of treatment and placebo, *Behav Eng* 8(4):146-153, 1983.

46. Lantz D, Sterman MB: Neuropsychological assessment of subjects with uncontrolled epilepsy: effects of EEG feedback training, *Epilepsia* 29:163-171, 1988.

47. Sterman MB: Physiological origins and functional correlates of EEG rhythmic activities: implications for self-regulation, *Biofeedback Self Regul* 21(1):3-33, 1996.

48. Kotchoubey B et al: Negative potential shifts and the prediction of the outcome of neurofeedback therapy in epilepsy, *Clin Neurophysiol* 110(4):683-686, 1999.

49. Strehl U, Kotchoubey B: A psychophysiological treatment of epilepsy, *Appl Psychophysiol Biofeedback* 224(2):138, 1999.

50. Rockstroh B et al: Cortical self regulation in patients with epilepsies, *Epilepsy Res* 14:63-72, 1993.

51. Kotchoubey B et al: Self regulation of slow cortical potentials in epilepsy: a retrial with analysis of influencing factors, *Epilepsy Res* 25(3):269-276, 1996.

52. Kotchoubey B et al: Stability of cortical self-regulation in epilepsy patients, *Neuroreport* 8(8):1867-1870, 1997.

53. Barton LA, Wolf SL: Is EMG feedback a successful adjunct to neuromuscular rehabilitation? *Phys Ther Pract* 2(2):41-49, 1992.

54. Sherman RJ, Arena JG: Biofeedback in the assessment and treatment of low back pain. In Basmajian J, Nyberg R, editors: *Spinal manipulative therapies,* Baltimore, 1992, Williams & Wilkins.

55. Krebs DE: Biofeedback in neuromuscular re-education and gait training. In Schwartz M, editor: *Biofeedback: a practitioners guide,* ed 2, New York, 1995, Guilford Press.

56. Wolf SL, Binder-Macleod SA: Electromyographic biofeedback in the physical therapy clinic. In Basmajian JV, editor: *Biofeedback: principles and practice for clinicians,* ed 3, Baltimore, 1989, Williams & Wilkins.

57. Brucker B, Bulaeva N: Biofeedback effect on electromyography responses in patients with spinal cord injury, *Arch Phys Med Rehabil* 77:133-137, 1996.

58. Deepak KK, Behari M: Specific muscle EMG biofeedback for hand dystonia, *Appl Psychophysiol Biofeedback* 24(4):267-280, 1999.

59. Schleenbaker RE, Mainous AG III: Electromyographic biofeedback for neuromuscular reeducation in the hemiplegic stroke patient: a meta-analysis, *Arch Phys Med Rehabil* 74:1301-1304, 1993.

60. Moreland JD, Thomson MA: Efficacy of electromyographic biofeedback compared with conventional physical therapy for upper-extremity function in patients following stroke: a research overview and meta-analysis, *Physical Therapy* 74:534-543, 1994.

61. Moreland JD, Thomson MA, Fuoco AR: Electromyographic biofeedback to improve lower extremity function after stroke: a meta-analysis, *Arch Phys Med Rehabil* 79: 134-140, 1998.

62. Lubar JF: Neurofeedback for the management of attention-deficit/hyperactivity disorders. In Schwartz, M, editor: *Biofeedback: a practitioner's guide,* ed 2, New York, 1995, Guilford Press.

63. Patrick GJ: Improved neuronal regulation of ADHD: an application of fifteen sessions of photic-driven EEG neurotherapy, *J Neurotherapy* 1(4):27-36, 1996.

64. Lubar JF et al: Evaluation of the effectiveness of EEG neurofeedback training for ADHD in a clinical setting as measured by changes in TOVA scores, behavioral ratings, and WISC-R performance, *Biofeedback Self Regul* 20(1):83-99, 1995.

65. Linden M, Habib T, Radojevic V: A controlled study of the effects of EEG biofeedback and cognition and behavior of children with attention deficit disorder and learning disabilities, *Biofeedback Self Regul* 21(1):35-49, 1996.

66. Boyd WD, Campbell SE: EEG biofeedback in the schools: the use of EEG biofeedback to treat ADHD in a school setting, *J Neurotherapy* 2(4):65-71, 1998.

67. Rossiter TR: Patient-directed neurofeedback for AD/HD, *J Neurotherapy* 2(4):54-63, 1998.

68. Hirsch A et al: Treatment of female urinary incontinence with EMG-controlled biofeedback home training, *Int Urogynecol J Pelvic Floor Dysfunct* 10(1):7-10, 1999.

69. McDowell BJ et al: Effectiveness of behavioral therapy to treat incontinence in homebound older adults, *J Am Geriatr Soc* 47(3):309-318, 1999.

70. Burgio KL et al: Behavioral vs drug treatment for urge urinary incontinence in older women: a randomized controlled trial, *JAMA* 280(23):1995-2000, 1998.

71. Wickramasekera I: Somatization: concepts, data, and predictions from the high risk model of threat perception, *J Nerv Ment Dis* 183:15-23, 1995.

CHAPTER

13

Mind-Body Theory and Application

SIDNEY J. KURN
R. LEA BORDEN

An impressive body of evidence has already been accumulated which demonstrates our capacity to use mind-body approaches to alter virtually every aspect of our physiological functioning. The ability to create the states necessary for this process and to bring about desirable changes is easily taught and relatively inexpensive. It should be a cornerstone of, not an adjunct to, all health care.

JAMES S. GORDON, M.D., CLINICAL PROFESSOR AT GEORGETOWN UNIVERSITY
SCHOOL OF MEDICINE, IN TESTIMONY TO THE U.S. CONGRESS, NOVEMBER 1997.

The seamless unity of body and mind is salient in ancient healing systems. These systems are vitalistic in the best sense of the word; our humanity and our health are not reducible to substance, to molecular interactions. In Chinese medicine, thousands of years old, the heart is the residence of the mind, including both mental activity and consciousness. "If the Heart is strong and Blood abundant, there will be normal mental activity, a balanced emotional life, a clear consciousness, a good memory, keen thinking and good sleep."[1] The ancient names of acupuncture points clearly reflect this unitarian view. Some of these points, called Spirit points, include shen men or Spirit Gate, the seventh heart meridian point; shen rang or Spirit Hall, the forty-fourth bladder meridian point; and shen cang or Spirit Storehouse, the twenty-fifth kidney meridian point.

Tibetan medicine, another holistic system, dates back 2600 years to the time of the historic Buddha, Siddhartha Gautama. Based on canonical texts, Tibetan medicine interweaves physical, emotional, and spiritual dimensions. *The Quintessence Tantras of Tibetan Medicine* says, "Thus with regard to the sixty-three disorders to be healed, attachment, hatred and closed [-mindedness] are the three causes which in turn give rise to wind, bile and phlegm [disorders]."[2] In the ancient texts of the original canonical Buddhist Pali Canon, " . . . healing is discussed from three points of view: (1) the cure of disease through healing agents (herbs and foods), surgery, and other physical means; (2) spiritual causes and cures of disease; and (3) the healing process as a metaphor for spiritual growth, with the Buddha named as Supreme Physician and the Buddhist teachings termed the King of Medicines."[3]

With some exceptions, Western medicine evolved into a nonvitalistic system, particularly during the twentieth century. This condition existed until the past few decades when scientific discoveries belied the validity of the dualistic approach to health. This chapter lays the current scientific foundation for mind-body theory, which restores vitalism to Western medicine. Solid scientific evidence now supports the known efficacy of mind-body practices.

HISTORIC DEVELOPMENTS

The history of Western mind-body thought started with the early Greek philosophers, Heraclitus and Empedocles. Life, and health in particular, were conceived as a dynamic balance of constituent elements whose imbalance resulted in disease. These ideas were iterated later in the thinking of Hippocrates and Epicurus, who also separated the natural from the supernatural elements, with the natural elements counterbalancing one another. The ensuing history of mind-body theory consists of a continual refinement of vitalistic—and a parallel lineage in which the concept of substance assumes an inordinate priority. Paracelsus, the great physician-alchemist born in 1494, opened the door to a reductionist, nonvitalist approach to human health. Paracelsus' given name was Philippus Theophrastus Bombastus von Hohenheim. He had a great passion for healing, wrote 14 large volumes, and was an outspoken prophet of truth as he saw it, to the

outrage of his contemporaries. A highly effective herbalist, Paracelsus was also a pioneer in the use of chemicals and an advocate of the concept of an "active principle" in plants. This interest in extracting an *active principle* or active substance from plants together with his interest in chemicals made him a progenitor of the modern pharmacologist and the "patron saint of the pharmaceutical industry."[4] As a master alchemist, however, he believed in the unitary quality of life. Alchemists believed that the "prima materia,"the chaos, was to be divided into the active principle, or soul, and the passive principle, or body. These were then reunited in personified form in the coniunctio or "chymical" marriage.[5] The objective and subjective reflected each other. The spiritual evolution of the individual from copper to silver and then to gold was mirrored in the experimental attempts to transmute the baser metals into gold. In sum, the thinking of Paracelsus remains paradoxical, moving toward both a materialistic and vitalistic paradigm at the same time.

The clearest expression of the priority of substance and the separation of mind from body is articulated in the writings of René Descartes. In his *Principles of Philosophy,* published in 1644, he wrote the following:

But I recognize only two ultimate classes of things: first, intellectual or thinking things, i.e. those which pertain to mind or thinking substance; and secondly, material things, i.e. those which pertain to extended substance or body. Perception, volition and all the modes both of perceiving and of willing are referred to thinking substance; while to extended substance belong size (that is, extension in length, breadth and depth), shape, motion, position, divisibility of component parts and the like.

Although this postulate of two classes of substances certainly sets the stage for medical thought during the next three centuries, Descartes does go on to say the following in the same essay:

But we also experience within ourselves certain other things which must not be referred either to the mind alone or to the body alone. These arise from the close and intimate union of our mind with the body. This list includes, first, appetites like hunger and thirst; secondly, the emotions or passions of the mind which do not consist of thought alone, such as the emotions of anger, joy, sadness and love."[6]

The long tradition of herbal healing, while not so important in the history of ideas, maintained a unitary approach to health and healing. Culpepper, a distinguished British herbalist of the seventeenth century writes in his famous *Herbal* about the herb balm, "It promotes digestion and opens obstructions of the brain, and hath so much purging quality in it . . . as to expel those melancholy vapours from the spirits and blood which are in the heart and arteries. . . ."[7]

During the nineteenth century, the Greek ideas of health were once again embraced. The balance of constituent elements were redefined as the dynamic equilibrium of forces by Thomas Sydenham, a Renaissance physician, and Claude Bernard, a nineteenth-century professor at the University of Paris. During the 1920s, Walter Bradford Cannon, a physiology professor at Harvard, described the concept of equilibrium as homeostasis. In addition, he connected this dynamic equilibrium to the autonomic nervous system and to biochemicals called catecholamines secreted by that system. During the 1930s, Hans Selye made the conceptual advance of describing the primary perturbation of this equilibrium as *stress,* a term he borrowed from physics. He also recognized that dissimilar stresses resulted in the same series of physiologic changes. In fact, he identified the General Adaptation Syndrome (GAS) as the clinical manifestation of any type of stress. Like Cannon before him, he was able to connect this syndrome to physical and biochemical elements of the body. In particular, he hypothesized that the adrenal glands and their secretions, the adrenal hormones, were the mediators of the more delayed psychophysiologic manifestations of stress.

The deconstruction of mind-body duality evolved rapidly with the recent work of George Solomon, at Stanford; Robert Ader at University of Rochester; Candace Pert at Johns Hopkins; and numerous other investigators. Before their work, only a few chemicals, the sympathoamines, acetylcholine, and pituitary hormones crossed the great mind-body divide. Thanks to their work, dozens of chemicals, mainly peptides, were found to mediate information reciprocally between the mind and body. The classic neurotransmitters and hormones are now understood to be only a few of the many information molecules that mediate information between the mind-brain and all other parts of the body, including the immune system. As will be shown, the Cartesian postulate of two separate substances, mental and physical, is no longer tenable. A flood of data over the past 20 to 30 years

has firmly established a biochemical intimacy between mind and body, which was only intuited in Western medicine by astute clinicians such as Sir William Osler, who noted that "In the medicine of the future" the interdependence of mind and body would be fully realized and that the influence of the one over the other "will be asserted in a manner which is not now thought possible."[8]

MIND-BODY ANATOMY

A simple, direct observation confirms the mind-body connection. A person thinks of moving a limb and it moves, unless that region of the brain is damaged. The pyramidal pathways from the cerebral cortex, subservient to consciousness, innervate all the somatic musculature. In addition, the autonomic pathways have long been known to extensively innervate somatic tissues including the heart, gut, and vasculature. Recently, neuroimmunomodulating autonomic pathways have been discovered that innervate the immune system. The autonomic pathways originate in a number of brainstem autonomic nuclei, including sympathetic, parasympathetic, and non-adrenergic non-cholinergic nuclei (NANC). These nuclei include the locus ceruleus, periaqueductal gray matter, parabrachial nucleus, parasympathetic preganglionic nucleus of the medulla, and the nucleus of the tractus solitarius.[9]

Fibers from the autonomic nuclei innervate the bone marrow and thymus, the secondary lymphoid organs, and the tertiary lymphoid tissues of the airway and intestines, that is, the gut-associated lymphoid tissue. Not only do the sympathetic nerves release sympathoamines, they also release a peptide known as neuropeptide Y. The parasympathetic nerves can release acetylcholine or nitric oxide, and a peptide known as vasointestinal polypeptide (VIP). A single nerve population can release several neuropeptides and a single neuropeptide can be released from sympathetic, parasympathetic, or NANC nerves.[9]

Studies of lymphoid tissue reveal that in the thymus, noradrenergic (NA) fibers are found in the thymic cortex. Thymocytes possess beta-adrenoceptors and respond to catecholamines. Multiple parts of lymph nodes are innervated by NA fibers. NA innervation in the spleen is distributed with the vascular and trabecular system, mainly with the central artery and its branches. There are several regions of contact between the nerves and the lymphocytes or macrophages. Cholinergic receptors exist on thymic epithelial cells and might be on thymocytes as well. Bone marrow stem cells also possess cholinergic receptors.[10]

The autonomic effects of these pathways depend on the specific neuropeptide that is released and the specific cells that are innervated. Specific systems may inhibit one another. For example, the tachykinins released by excitatory NANC nerves might interfere with inhibitory NANC or adrenergic nerves. Both positive and negative feedback loops occur, including some neuropeptides stimulating their own release from their cell of origin or from inflammatory cells.[9]

Several cortical areas, including portions of the limbic system, regulate autonomic output. This regulation suggests that the autonomic nuclei are not as autonomous as was once thought. These cortical areas include the insular cortex, the medial prefrontal cortex, and the sensory-motor cortex. They integrate autonomic responses with more conscious experience. Based on its anatomic connections, the insular cortex appears to integrate emotional and autonomic responses. The medial prefrontal/infralimbic areas specifically integrate visceral-motor responses with emotional stressful stimuli. Finally, the sensori-motor cortex appears to control cardiovascular responses to exercise.[9]

The cortical innervation of autonomic nuclei, and in turn their innervation of lymphoid and other bodily tissues, provides an anatomical basis for mind-body interactions. Threatening or sexual mental images are rapidly transduced into changes in sympathetic tone. Physiological changes start within a second, culminating within 5 to 30 seconds. The sympathetic system can alter widely disparate somatic functions simultaneously, including pupillary and bronchial dilation, increased cardiac rate and muscular blood supply, depressed gastrointestinal function, and increased adrenal secretion of epinephrine. The four F's of behavior—referred to by Sapolsky—flight, fight, fright, and "sex," are mediated by the sympathetic system[11] and the vegetative activities—including growth, gastrointestinal activity, and energy storage—are mediated by the parasympathetic system. As will be discussed later, these rapid autonomic changes are supplemented in rapid succession by the hypothalamic-pituitary axis' release of neuropeptides that, again, have wide-ranging effects on the body.

MIND-BODY CHEMISTRY

In addition to the pyramidal and autonomic nervous systems, studies during the past two decades have revealed numerous messenger substances that are secreted by both brain and other visceral cells, as well as the widespread occurrence of receptors to these ligands.[12] Following is a discussion of this new information in terms of a bidirectional communication among cells of the immune system, visceral organs, and central nervous system (CNS). It was observed first that leukocytes produced adrenocorticotropic hormone (ACTH) and endorphins, which are traditional CNS information substances, in response to viral infection. Subsequently, a long series of CNS substances including thyrotropin-stimulating hormone (TSH), endogenous opioid peptides, chorionic gonadotropin (CG), growth hormone, prolactin, tyrosine, vasoactive intestinal peptide, somatostatin, substance P, oxytocin, neurophysin,[13] and glucocorticoids[14] were found to be produced and secreted by leukocytes. Not only do these substances secreted by leukocytes appear to mediate functions within the immune system, they also act on neural and non-neural receptors. In terms of direct immune action, substance P and somatostatin affect immunoglobulin synthesis by the spleen, growth hormone increases superoxide anion concentration in macrophages, and the endogenous opioid peptides affect a number of different immune functions.[13]

In addition to producing traditional CNS peptides, receptors for neuropeptides have been discovered on leukocytes. For example, opioid, ACTH, substance P, oxytocin, bombesin, cholecystokinin, vasoactive intestinal peptide, and growth hormone receptors on leukocytes have been demonstrated. The existence of these receptors substantiates the role these traditional CNS peptides play in immune function.

Furthermore, substances secreted by lymphocytes, called cytokines or lymphokines, were found to influence cells of the CNS. For example, interleuken 1(IL-1), a particular type of cytokine secreted by lymphocytes, stimulates the hypothalamic-pituitary-adrenal (HPA) axis, causing increased levels of corticotropin-releasing hormone (CRH), ACTH, endorphin, vasopressin, and somatostatin. IL-6 also acts on the hypothalamus to promote release of CRH, with subsequent release of ACTH. IL-11 stimulates the proliferation of hippocampal neuronal progenitor cell lines. Tumor necrosis factor (TNF) also activates the

HPA axis and causes fever and anorexia by a central mechanism of action. Transforming Growth Factor-Beta (TGF-beta) promotes proliferation of Schwann cells.[15] Interferon gamma and IL-2 also significantly affect the hypothalamic-pituitary axis.[16]

In addition to secretion by lymphocytes, neural cells also produce cytokines. TNF is produced by astrocytes and microglial cells that then act on multiple tissues, causing joint tissue inflammation, insulin resistance of somatic cells, and increases in airway responsiveness and sputum production in lung tissue. A recent study using in situ hybridization and immunochemistry demonstrated the induction of IL-1, IL-4, IL-6, IL-10, TNF-beta, interferon gamma, and TGF-beta in human embryonic forebrain cells.[17] This study confirms that glial cells can be a major source of cytokines and that they play a role in brain development. IL-6 is also produced by CNS cells and appears to play a role in antibody production in multiple sclerosis and in the generation of amyloid protein in Alzheimer's disease. The cells of the CNS and lymphocytes appear then to produce the same messenger substances.

Work by Candace Pert and others have demonstrated that in addition to receptors for cytokines, there are neural receptors for many other peptides such as insulin, angiotensin, vasoactive intestinal peptide, and bombesin, making the CNS sensitive to peptides secreted by other organs of the body.[18] In fact, Pert points out that most peptides traditionally found in the body are also found in the brain. Receptors for these peptides are found in the brain as well. These peptides are found not only in the hypothalamus but also in unanticipated parts of the brain such as the cortex and limbic system.

In summary, bidirectional communication exists among cells of the immune system, other visceral organs, and the CNS. The immune system acts as an additional sensory system, sensing noncognitive stimuli such as bacteria, viruses, tumors, and antigens. The recognition of these stimuli causes the production of cytokines, which then act on the CNS. In turn, information from the classic five senses processed in the CNS produces informational substances that act on the immune system.[19] There appears to be a common chemical language for the neuroendocrine and immune systems that includes an immunoregulator role for the CNS and a sensory function for the immune system.[20] Information theory has also been used to explain the complex dynamic changes of endocrine and peptide molecules.[21,22] As noted by Mayer and Baldi, regulatory peptides may be regarded as "signals in a universal structured code for biological communication."[21] Individual cytokines may be thought of as words and combinations of cytokines as sentences.

The information from peptide signals is integrated by complex mechanisms and ultimately affects gene activity. The resultant alterations in gene transcription affects, in turn, protein synthesis and receptor membrane structure.[23] Transduction mechanisms that ultimately transduce the messenger signals into secretory and structural changes vary depending upon the particular information substance. Glucocorticoids appear to directly modulate the transcription of specific sets of genes,[24] whereas other ligands act through intracellular signaling molecules. Cellular information transduction may result in alteration of cell receptors through a change in function or in the density of the receptors.[25] A change in receptor function or density changes the sensitivity of the receptor so that it will be further sensitized to the same ligand that caused the change in the first place. This occurs in all tissues of the body including the brain and would appear to be the biochemical basis for memory, both neural and somatic. In fact, peptide information theory would easily explain state-dependent memory, learning, and behavior as developed by Ernest Lawrence Rossi.[26] The theory would also explain Candace Pert's reference to Freud's notion that "the body is the unconscious mind."[18] Peptide information theory explains the surprisingly intimate connection between the mind and the very genes themselves, and provides a basis for understanding the observed clinical effects of mind-body techniques.

BIOCHEMICAL ANATOMY OF STRESS

As mentioned previously, stress is the cardinal perturbation or disturbance in the complex mind-body system. It is a universal experience and probably the substrate for the efficacy of mind-body techniques. Stress not only results in acute cognitive and physical changes, but may play a role in a number of neurodegenerative conditions as well.

The stress system of the CNS is complex, involving multiple neuronal centers and chemical mediators. An emotional event is relayed through the sensory thalamus up to the sensory cortex. The event can also be relayed directly from the thalamus to the amygdala, the pathway for fear-conditioned unconscious memories. The event that reaches the cortex is then relayed to the hippocampus, the basis for conscious memories. Cortical information can also be relayed back through the amygdala and to the hippocampus. Both structures then relay information to the paraventricular nucleus of the hypothalamus (PVN), where the information is transduced into hormonal information. The amygdala stimulates the PVN to secrete CRH, whereas the hippocampus inhibits CRH secretion from the hypothalamus. These two systems create a modulated balance of input into the hypothalamus for the hormonal transduction of the stressor.[27]

The other major neuronal system involved in stress is the locus ceruleus-norepinephrine/sympathetic system in the brainstem. Information transfer between the hypothalamus and the locus ceruleus (LC) results in a positive feedback system. CRH activates the LC and norepinephrine (NE) causes CRH release. Anatomic connections occur between the two neuronal centers, the hypothalamus and the LG. Arginine vasopressin, serotonin, and acetylcholine stimulate both centers whereas gamma aminobutyric acid (GABA), endogenous opioids, and glucocorticoids inhibit both centers.[28] Because of this sensitivity to multiple information molecules, the stress system is sensitive to the general activity of the mind-body system.

During stress, the mesocortical (pathways from the midbrain to the cortex) and mesolimbic (pathways from the midbrain to the limbic system) dopamine systems are activated by the LC system. The mesocortical system activates the prefrontal cortex involved in anticipation and cognition. The mesolimbic system, linked to the nucleus accumbens, involves states of motivation, reinforcement, and reward. These are elements of the healthy, constructive aspects of stress—the adaptation to the changing contingencies of life.

Selye recognized three phases to the stress response or GAS: the alarm, adaptive, and exhaustive phases. Recent work has defined the biochemical attributes of these phases. CRH secreted by the hypothalamus is a 41 amino acid peptide that mediates early endocrine and behavioral aspects of the stress reaction and, via the LC system, the autonomic responses to stress. CRH plays a role in increasing vigilance and arousal during stress and suppresses appetite. CRH goes up within seconds of a stressful stimulus. After about 15 seconds, ACTH is released

from the pituitary via CRH stimulation. Many minutes later, the adrenal gland secretes increased amounts of glucocorticoids secondary to ACTH stimulation.[11] CRH suppresses appetite, the reproductive and growth axes, and thyroid function. The glucocorticoids, increased secondary to CRH, have profound immunosuppressive effects. All of these changes conserve energy for a life-saving response to an acute event. However, these changes can cause disease when there is prolonged stress.

The stages of Selye's GAS can be applied to other biochemical changes occurring with stress, such as the body's free-radical-antioxidant status (redox state). In 1980, Russian investigator Meerson reported that, with severe emotional-painful stress (EPS), the increase in catecholamines results in lipid peroxidation in the myocardium. Changes in the myocellular membranes affect calcium transport, resulting in local necrobiosis and changes in myocardial contractility. Another study of the alarm stage was reported in 1982 by Shredova et al. EPS in rats inhibited the electrical activity (ERG) of the retina with an accumulation of the products of lipid peroxidation and a decrease in the anti-oxidant alpha-tocopherol.[29]

The alarm phase may also affect mast cells. In 1995, Theoharides et al. at Tufts demonstrated that atraumatic stress (EPS) resulted in degranulation of 70% of rat dura mast cells within 30 minutes of stress. This response could be inhibited by substance P depletion with capsaicin, and polyclonal antiserum to CRH. This depletion implies that sensory neuropeptides and CRH mediate mast cell degranulation. These findings provide a biochemical basis for the relationship of stress to migraine, which is hypothesized to occur in part by the release of vasoactive, nociceptive, and proinflammatory mediators by mast cells.[30]

In the adaptive phase, the body attempts to limit myocardial injury by an increase in Gaba-ergic tone. A study by Meerson in animals revealed that in brain tissue EPS caused activation of GABA. Also noted was an inhibition of FAD-dependent oxidation of succinate in the tricarboxylic acid cycle. This oxidation might lead to increased gamma-hydroxybutyric acid (GHB), an inhibitory molecule of the stress reaction. GHB is derived from GABA via the enzyme succinic semialdehyde reductase. It appears to reduce energy substrate consumption in brain and peripheral tissues, and functions as an endogenous protective agent in these tissues.[31] This suggests that GHB might have a role in limiting the metabolic consequences of the stress reaction. In the heart muscle, an increase of GABA was associated with an increase in FAD-dependent oxidation of succinate. This metabolic change ultimately leads to increased ATP and NADPH formation, which is necessary for energy and biosynthesis.[32]

In the early adaptation to stress, studies by Guliaeva et al.[33] revealed an increase in superoxide dismutase activity in the brain, an increase in superoxide-scavenging blood serum activity, a reduction in lipid peroxidation, and a decrease in brain lipid cholesterol. This early one-week phase is described as the transition from urgent to long-lasting adaptation with a predominance of fear reactions and suppression of search behavior. The second phase (second week of stress) involves normalization of behavior and maximum anti-free-radical brain activity with a low level of lipid peroxidation. Guliaeva describes a third stage (third week) as a transition from long-lasting adaptation to exhaustion with lower blood pressures, disturbed regulation of vegetative functions, increased open field behavior, increased lipid peroxidation, and decreased brain phospholipid content.

The third exhaustive phase of the GAS is disputed, with evidence for persistent adrenocortical activity with ongoing stress.[11] The persistence of elevated adrenocortical activity with chronic stress does not support the idea of adrenal exhaustion originally put forward by Selye. In fact, the persistent elevated cortisol levels are responsible for many facets of stress-related illness. These Russian studies, in animals, do suggest an exhaustion of the body's capacity to maintain a normal redox state with ongoing stress, a condition that may mediate stress-related illness.

In addition to the brain and heart, stress affects the liver biochemically with a significant decrease in clearance of xenobiotics secondary to diminished hepatic oxidation. Other hepatic functions, including uptake, storage, and clearance, are also diminished after atraumatic stress.[34]

It is interesting to note that animals adapted to short-term stressors do not clearly demonstrate the alarm and adaptive phases of the stress reaction. In particular, they do not demonstrate the excessive activation of the adrenergic and HPA system. They also do not have the impairments of oxidation and phosphorylation in heart muscle mitochondria with its associated impairment in myocardial contractility that occurs after long-duration EPS.[35] These findings were confirmed in a report by Sazontova in 1987 describing an increase in antioxidant enzyme activities, par-

ticularly catalase with adaptation to short-term EPS. Nonadapted rats showed a drop in catalase activity with subsequent stress but adapted animals showed an actual increase over baseline levels. Lipid peroxidation in heart homogenates increased threefold in nonadapted rats with a 1% decrease in adapted animals.[36] These findings all point to the importance of mind-body techniques that help cultivate adaptation to stress. Adaptation prevents the biochemical consequences of acute stressors, particularly emotionally painful stressors.

Finally, there may be sufficient biochemical evidence to link stress to neurodegenerative disorders and cancer. It is known that increased glutamate levels are associated with trauma, epilepsy, stroke, Alzheimer's disease, multiple sclerosis,[37] and other brain injuries. Several studies have confirmed that stress leads to increased concentrations of glutamate in brain tissue.[38,39] Increased glutamate levels cause an intracellular influx of calcium with activation of calcium-dependent enzymes such as nitric oxide synthase. This, in turn, leads to increased nitric oxide (NO) levels. NO reacts with the superoxide anion, forming an extremely potent free radical, peroxynitrite. Peroxynitrite causes DNA injury as well as mitochondrial injury. Mitochondrial injury affects energy metabolism. Furthermore, any impairment in cellular energy metabolism increases neuronal vulnerability to glutamate by attenuating the Mg^{++} blockage of the N-methyl-D-aspartate receptor[40] which is the receptor for glutamate. Environmental toxins play a role here because coexposure of neurons to glutamate and environmental toxins, such as lead, greatly amplifies glutamate exitotoxicity and cell death via apoptosis (programmed cell death) or necrosis.[41] Stress also affects gene expression. DNA transcription factors, NF-kappaB and AP-1, are regulated by the intracellular redox potential and may be involved in gene induction. This induction includes the elevated expression of genes encoding cyclo-oxygenase-2 involved in the apoptotic or necrotic processes of cells. The intracellular redox potential is definitely affected by the peroxynitrite free radical. Experimentally, a report by Adachi et al. in 1993 revealed that psychological stress in rats caused oxidative damage to nuclear DNA,[42] perhaps via the mechanism discussed previously. This evidence suggests that unmitigated stress alters gene function and structure and ultimately contributes to the development of degenerative and neoplastic diseases.

THE HPA-HIPPOCAMPAL SYSTEM

A particularly salient aspect of stress is the relationship between the HPA axis and the hippocampus. It was noted in the early 1980's that the hippocampus had the highest concentration of glucocorticoid receptors in the brain. In addition, as noted previously, the hippocampus exerts an inhibitory influence over adrenocortical activity by inhibiting CRH secretion from the hypothalamus. This action by the hippocampus responds to glucocorticoid feedback. A study by Sapolsky et al.[43] published in 1984 demonstrated that depletion of glucocorticoid receptors in the hippocampus of rats resulted in corticosterone (CORT) hypersecretion. Subsequent correction of the receptor population resulted in normal CORT secretion. Frank loss of hippocampal neurons was not necessary for this alteration in the feedback loop. This study revealed the plasticity of the hippocampal glucocorticoid receptor system, which is controlled by CORT as well as vasopressin. Given this finding, in 1985, Sapolsky et al., studied the effects of CORT and its implication for aging. Rats exposed to daily CORT had significant depletion of CORT receptors in the hippocampus, which did not reappear when daily CORT injections were stopped. Further analysis revealed that the loss of receptors was secondary to the actual loss of neuronal cells and that there was, in addition, an increase in glial cells. These findings in the experimental group resembled the histological findings in control-aged rats. The authors concluded that a lifetime exposure to endogenous CORT might contribute to hippocampal neuronal loss and that prolonged stress or treatment with CORT might accelerate these hippocampal changes.[44] Given the role of the hippocampus in memory, these findings have significant implications for the relationship of stress to memory loss. The issue is slightly more complex in that studies with experimental elimination of corticosteroids also results in loss of hippocampal dentate neurons. Sapolsky confirmed this in a study in 1991[45] in rats undergoing adrenalectomy. It appears that severe underexposure or overexposure to CORT can result in the loss of a number of hippocampal neuronal cell types.

Part of the mechanism of hippocampal neuronal injury appears to be related to the accumulation of glutamate with increased CORT levels. In 1994, researchers demonstrated in rats that an increase of CORT from circadian trough to peak levels doubled the concentration of hippocampal extracellular glutamate. An increase of CORT into the stress range caused a fourfold increase in glutamate. Because glutamate, an excitotoxic neurotransmitter, can damage neurons, this information may explain how sustained stress might damage the hippocampus.[46] In addition, this relationship between CORT and glutamate may substantiate the role of stress in multiple neurodegenerative diseases in which the excitotoxin, glutamate, appears to play a significant role.

It is common knowledge that stress affects cognitive ability. In a review article by McEwen and Sapolsky[47] it is noted that stress affects cognition quickly via catecholamines and more slowly via glucocorticoids. Catecholamines act on CNS beta-adrenergic receptors and affect glucose availability. CORT modulates synaptic plasticity over hours and affects dendritic structures for weeks. Although CORT affects declarative memory via the hippocampus, catecholamines may affect emotionally laden and stressful memories via the amygdala. Epidemiological studies in humans correlate well with these experimental findings. Increased cortisol levels with acute/chronic stress may be important in the occurrence of memory loss in aged populations.[48] Hippocampal atrophy and hippocampus-dependent memory loss in humans occurs with prolonged cortisol elevation. The degree of atrophy correlates strongly with both the level of cortisol increase and the basal level.[49] Lupien et al. reported in 1994 that the slope of change of cortisol over time in elderly individuals predicted the cognitive impairment they would eventually suffer. Individuals with high basal cortisol levels and a significant increase in cortisol were eventually impaired in measures of explicit memory and selective attention. Subjects with decreasing cortisol levels performed as well as healthy young subjects.[50]

As noted, stress causes rapid changes in memory. One study examined declarative and nondeclarative memory versus salivary cortisol levels in a nonstressful (attentional task) and stressful (public speaking) condition. The stressful condition significantly decreased declarative but not nondeclarative memory, and the nonstressful condition did not affect either. Salivary CORT levels clustered into two groups; responders had increased cortisol 60 minutes before the stressful event and nonresponders had an increase 25 minutes before the event. The responders showed a comparative decrease in declarative memory before and after the stressful event. Anticipation of stress may have played a significant role in the decline of declarative memory in the responder group.[51]

This concludes a brief review of mind-body theory. It is anticipated that the pace of scientific research into mind-body theory and its implication for neurologic conditions will continue to increase. For example, the National Institutes of Health National Center for Complementary and Alternative Medicine provides funding for 11 academic specialty research centers to conduct ongoing scientific research on complementary and alternative medicine practices. Of the 11, the research agendas at the following four institutions are of particular interest for neurology:

- Stroke and Neurologic Conditions: Center for Research in Complementary and Alternative Medicine at the Kessler Institute for Rehabilitation of the University of Medicine and Dentistry at New Jersey
- Aging: Complementary and Alternative Medicine Program at Stanford University
- Pain: University of Maryland School of Medicine, Division of Complementary Medicine
- Pain: University of Virginia Center for the Study of Complementary and Alternative Therapies at the University of Virginia School of Nursing

MIND-BODY PRACTICES

Extensive clinical and experimental data support the concept that information is widely dispersed throughout the body and not confined solely to the CNS. Information from the senses and fleeting images of the mind are transduced into neuronal and peptidergic signals to all parts of the body. The limbic-hypothalamic system plays a key role in this transduction. In reciprocal fashion, stimuli to the body, including the immune system, are transduced into molecular information that acts on receptors in the CNS. These stimuli may be from the gut, or they may be microbial, antigenic, or neoplastic in nature. Through second messengers and gene transcription factors, information alters gene activity and is ultimately stored at both the genetic and membrane receptor levels. Homeostasis may be maintained through feedback loops such as the HPA-hippocampal system or possibly through neuropeptide-cytokine interactions.

The information field of the body has characteristics of an energy or fluid system with levels of intensity, flow patterns, and states of equilibrium. Stress would represent a state of disequilibrium in this fluid system. In a sense, all nurturing clinical modalities are mind-body in nature, given this fluid or energetic structure of the mind-body field. Practices such as yoga, tai chi, qigong, and acupuncture simply enter the mind-body field differently than do the more traditional mind-body techniques such as meditation, mantra, or imagery. One technique might address an imbalance more directly than another and be more appropriate for a particular individual.

Mind-body practices are particularly important for individuals with neurological disorders. Because our neurological ability is closely aligned with our identity and our core sense of self, the diagnosis of a neurological disorder can be extremely alarming. Fear, anxiety, grief, and depression may arise along with uncertainties about longevity, physical function, dependency, existential meaning, and finances. The illness will impact the patient's relationship with his or her family and with others. From a systems theory point of view, mind, body, spirit, and environment are parts of an interdependent, complex whole. Health and well being arise from a harmonious balance of the component parts of this unified whole. Such a view recognizes that a problem on a spiritual, mental, or even an environmental level may ultimately express itself in the body's physiology. Likewise, a physiological disorder may manifest itself in the mind or spirit. This insight leads to an appreciation of therapeutic modalities that help recapture a state of balance.

As has been discussed, the unmitigated stress response bathes the body in biochemicals that, under some circumstances, can be neurotoxic. There is strong clinical evidence, then, for the efficacy of mind-body approaches in stress reduction, leading to a more internalized locus of control, enhanced coping skills, and improved mood. The ability to actively take part in self-care helps patients minimize the helpless-hopeless state associated with deteriorating health. Reducing stress may also help the individual succeed in behavior modifications such as giving up smoking, reducing alcohol intake, and increasing exercise. The body has a broad range of innate healing mechanisms. Mind-body practices help recruit and mobilize inner resources that directly enhance the healing process. This has the added benefit of reducing health care costs. People with complex, chronic conditions are underserved by current models of health care delivery. The system's inability to meet the real needs of these individuals results in increased visits to physicians for support, and more expensive emergency room visits and hospitalizations. Studies have linked untreated depression with twice the medical costs compared to non-depressed people even after controlling for general medical comorbidity.[52] Health care services are used by depressed persons at a rate that is three times that of nondepressed individuals.[53] Programs using a combination of complementary and behavioral medicine interventions appear to reduce the cost of health care.[54] These practices are also helpful for members of a patient's family. Caretaker strain results in the increased risk of multiple physical disorders. Mind-body practices can help address these risk factors and reduce stress-related physical disorders in family members. Caregivers also improve their coping mechanisms, which enables them to continue taking an active role in the care of their loved one.

Mind-body practices that are useful for patients with neurologic conditions include deep relaxation, music therapy, multimodal surgical support, journaling, psychosocial support, meditation, imagery, hypnosis, self-hypnosis, and breathing techniques.

Deep Relaxation

The state of profound relaxation is related to and found within several mind-body techniques, including meditation, imagery, hypnosis, and self-hypnosis practices. However it is reached, it is well documented that the state of deep relaxation decreases heart and respiratory rate, reduces anxiety, normalizes blood pressure, increases peripheral vasodilation, slows metabolism, decreases muscle tension, alters brainwave activity, increases perceived self-efficacy and control, reduces chronic pain, and improves some aspects of sleep.[55,56] In this quiescent state, the body more efficiently metabolizes toxins, repairs micro-injuries, and regulates catecholamines and other stress-related biochemicals.

Music Therapy

The value of music for relaxation and anxiety reduction is common knowledge. Its pervasive personal and cultural value suggests making cassette players and taped music as available as oxygen outlets in every hospital. Multiple studies in medical settings, including critical care units, correlate music with all the measures indicative of the relaxation response.[57-61] In addition, programs using active music therapy are effective for patients with dementia, stroke, head trauma, coma, aphasia, Alzheimer's disease, migraine, and pain syndromes.[62-65]

Multimodal Surgical Support

Multiple studies have established the efficacy of mind-body techniques for individuals preparing for surgery. The outcomes have shown less overall distress and optimal recovery. People undergoing neurosurgery can draw on psychosocial support and imagery techniques to enhance comfort and confidence while reducing postoperative pain and depression, stress-related immune system suppression, time to normalization of gastrointestinal function, length of hospitalization, and cost.[66-73]

Psychosocial Support

For a person encountering a serious illness or disability, psychosocial interventions can have a substantial impact on the progression of the disease process. Such support may offer active emotive approaches, including grief work, and expressive methods such as dance therapy, authentic movement, art therapy, as well as development of communication skills, family systems counseling, and other methods. Offered in an individual or group context, the patient is helped to process emotions associated with negative health outcomes such as anxiety, depression, anger, fear, and isolation. Also supported are psychophysiological elements associated with a tendency towards a more positive prognosis, including self-efficacy, optimism, and a passionate engagement with life. This is particularly critical if the individual carries the added burden of a childhood characterized by abuse or neglect. For such individuals, the stress response is particularly well conditioned and hyperresponsive. In addition, persistent and profound neural changes in cortical brain development have been demonstrated among abused and neglected children.[74-76] This circumstance appears to increase the risk of later drug and behavioral addictions, complicating recovery from any physical disorder.

One psychologic technique called cognitive restructuring offers alternatives to automatic negative thought patterns that may contribute to anxiety and depression. This increased consciousness allows the individual to have greater autonomy in relation to his or her thoughts or beliefs. When cognitive approaches are not taught in a wooden formalistic way, they bear some similarities to aspects of the psychology of Buddhism and other Eastern traditions.

Psychosocial support for the individual's work with the illness and related emotions may well contribute to positive changes in the physical disorder itself. A profound opening of spiritual life may be experienced in the wake of this deep exploration of illness, and the energy used for repression of difficult feelings may be released for the healing process.

Journaling

Although studies are lacking for neurological patients, individuals with other physical conditions definitely benefit from writing about stressful events. Well-replicated studies indicate that the simple act of writing about such experiences for 20 minutes a day on 3 consecutive days decreases physical and emotional distress. Among 70 people with rheumatoid arthritis or asthma, almost half discovered a reduction in physical discomfort.[78] Similar studies have found a decrease in health service use or positive immunologic responses[79-81] related to writing about personal difficulties or traumatic events.

Meditation

Meditation is an ancient technique for calming and focusing the mind. Sogyal Rinpoche, a Tibetan lama, makes the analogy of the mind "to a jar of muddy water. The more we leave the water without interfering or stirring it, the more the particles of dirt will sink to the bottom, letting the natural clarity of the water shine through."[82] There are a number of meditation techniques including focus on the breath, repetitive sound or mantra, or a visual image gently moving attention from the unrelenting mental chatter. As the attention inevitably wanders back to the ever-present thoughts, it is gently drawn back to the chosen object. Although meditation may be completely detached from any religion, all of the world's great spiritual traditions include forms of meditation. Meditation can be accomplished either seated or in motion. In moving meditation, such as tai chi, walking meditation, or yoga, the intention is also to gently bring the attention back to the physical sensation or simply into moment to moment awareness. Regular, daily practice yields the greatest benefits.

A number of studies exist on the biochemical effects of meditation.[83] The results are somewhat inconsistent, but in general meditation is associated with a reduction in serum cortisol[84,85] and catecholamines.[85] One study showed an increase in DHEA sulfate and 5-HIAA in meditators[86] and another showed a significant reduction in lipid peroxide levels.[87] A study at the All India Institute of Medical Sciences in New Delhi revealed a significant lowering of seizure frequency in individuals with epilepsy who practiced meditation.[88]

Of interest is a hypothesis by Elias and Wilson about meditation. In a report in 1995, they noted that the hormonal changes seen with transcendental meditation (TM) resemble the effects of GABA. They hypothesized that TM increases hypothalamic Gaba-ergic tone, resulting in changes of pituitary function. They also hypothesized that meditation reduces anxiety as a result of other localized CNS increases in GABA concentration.[89]

Regarding clinical efficacy, J. J. Kabat-Zinn reported in 1982 on the effects of mindfulness meditation in chronic pain patients. He notes that this practice promotes "detached observation" and an "uncoupling of the sensory dimension of the pain experience from the affective/evaluative alarm reaction." The pain disorders being studied included low back, neck, shoulder, headache, facial, angina pectoris, noncoronary chest, and gastrointestinal (GI) pain. At 10 weeks, 50% of the patients reported pain reduction of 50% or more. Significant improvement in mood and psychiatric symptoms accompanied the reduction in pain.[90] In 1989, four groups of elderly patients with an average age of 81 were studied. Each of the groups received either no treatment, TM training, mindfulness training in active distinction making (MF), or relaxation (low mindfulness) training. The TM group improved the most, followed by the mindfulness training group. Improvement was measured on paired associate learning, measures of cognitive flexibility, mental health, systolic BP, behavioral flexibility, aging, and treatment efficacy. The MF group improved the most followed by the TM group on perceived control and word fluency. After 3 years, the survival rate was 100% for TM, 85% for MF, and lower for the other two groups.[91]

This brief review reveals the need for further studies on the biochemical, physiological, and clinical effects of meditation. In particular, stress parameters including cortisol and catecholamines, levels of glutamate and GABA, and measures of redox potential, such as glutathione levels, lipid peroxides, and DNA status would be of interest. These measures would be particularly salient in patients with degenerative diseases that appear to be directly or indirectly related to oxidation and glutamate-GABA status such as Parkinson's and Alzheimer's disease.

Yoga Breathing Techniques

Yogic breathing exercises called pranayama have ancient roots and continue to be popular therapeutic techniques. The exercises have also been the subject of some recent supportive scientific studies. The well-established ultradian nasal cycle is particularly important in understanding the efficacy of these exercises. The nasal structures have both sympathetic and parasympathetic innervation. There is a well-documented ultradian rhythm known as the nasal cycle that lasts from 25 to 200 minutes. The nasal airway patency alternates between sides, apparently correlating with increased sympathetic activity on one side and parasympathetic activity on the other.[92] The degree of electroencephalographic (EEG) integration in one hemisphere correlates with predominant airflow in the contralateral nostril.[93] In addition, although somewhat counterintuitive, catecholamine levels from the antecubital veins on the right or left side correlate with the nasal cycle; that is, there is an increased level of norepinephrine, epinephrine, and dopamine from the antecubital vein ipsilateral to the patent nostril.[94] Another study at the Salk Institute in 1991 showed that there is greater cognitive ability in the hemisphere contralateral to the patent nostril. This was studied using verbal/performance abilities as measures of left or right hemisphere activity. In addition, cognitive performance ratios can be altered by forcibly altering the breathing pattern.[95] A subsequent study from the Department of Psychiatry at the University of California-Davis studied the effects of forced nostril breathing on cognitive performance in 51 undergraduate psychology students. A verbal analogy test measured left hemisphere performance and a

mental rotation task measured right hemisphere performance. Spatial task ability was significantly enhanced with left nostril breathing. Verbal task performance was increased, but not significantly, with right nostril breathing.[96]

These breathing techniques add another level of refinement to the stress reduction provided by other mind-body techniques. By controlling the ultradian nasal cycle, one can effect cerebral dominance and lateralization of autonomic outflow. This may have application in the use of visual imagery and verbal processes and conceivably in lateralized autonomic dysfunction, such as reflex sympathetic dystrophy. Additionally, the effects on cerebral EEG activity suggest possible application in epilepsy. These potential applications require further study.

Imagery

Like deep relaxation, imagery is at once a therapeutic modality in its own right and a component of several other mind-body techniques, including some forms of meditation, hypnosis, self-hypnosis, and biofeedback. The belief that imagery may evoke both psychological insight and physical change is evidenced by its place in the medicine systems of countless cultures on every continent throughout the centuries. Thoughts and images in the mind are themselves biochemical events that, in turn, elicit widespread physiological responses. The mental image of a dear loved one returning home evokes the same physical responses as does the actual person entering the front door. Physiologist and psychologist Jeanne Achterberg, pioneering researcher and clinician with the use of imagery for over 25 years, points to the newest neurotransmitter research, which is dissolving the wall behind mind and body. She says, "We need to develop a new vocabulary, but that hasn't happened yet. You might think of imagery as the way that what we call the 'mind' and what we call the 'body' communicate. Imagery is the thought process that invokes and uses the senses: vision, auditory senses, smell, taste, the senses of movement, position, and touch. It is the communication mechanism between perception, emotion, and bodily change. The image, the imagination, is the vehicle by which mental processes reach deep into the cellular structure."

Imagery-based approaches are used in a number of therapeutic programs for people with chronic pain, cardiac disorders, cancer, surgery, autoimmune disorders, and other physical challenges.[97-108] In addition to fostering self-efficacy, calmness, behavioral changes, awareness, and psychological insights, imagery may at times allow access to mechanisms of physiological change that support and engage the body's own healing mechanisms.

Imagery is useful for people facing catastrophic conditions. In a study of patients with burns covering an average of 25% of skin surface, imagery techniques were used to "inform, desensitize, reduce anxiety and control pain." The study by Achterberg and Kenner demonstrated improvements across 15 different indices, including vital signs, measures of anxiety and pain, muscle tension, quantities of pain medication required, peripheral temperature, and distance walked.[109]

A study with stroke patients used an imagery technique called *lighthouse strategy,* in which they imagined their eyes to be like horizontal sweeping beams of a lighthouse. While enrolled in a day rehabilitation program, they were instructed to use this technique during therapy training tasks as part of their treatment for visual inattention. By the time of discharge, the experimental group had improved significantly in multiple measures of attention compared with controls.[110]

In 1984, Brown reported on two types of imagery used to treat migraine in two experimental groups versus a control group. The first group imagined pleasant scenes as they engaged in somatic processes including muscular relaxation and deep breathing. The other group was trained to imagine scenes in great detail. Both groups were instructed to use the imagery techniques while experiencing headaches. Both imagery groups were definitely superior to the control group in terms of reducing headache activity. This finding was sustained at a two-month follow-up assessment.[111] However, a follow-up study in 1994 by Ilacqua did not reveal a significant reduction of migraine activity in an imagery group or biofeedback group. The imagery group did, however, report an improved capacity for dealing with the pain, as well as a decreased perception of the pain itself. The imagery appeared to empower the patient into a more active role in dealing with the migraine process.[112]

Smania et al. reported in 1997 on the use of visuomotor imagery in unilateral neglect in two brain-injured patients with large cortical and subcortical right brain lesions. Visual and movement imagery exercises were used in 50-minute intervals during 40 sessions with assessment via neuropsychologic testing. The imagery exercises decreased deficits in performance related to neglect in both patients. All of the outcome measures improved and were stable over a six-month follow-up period.[113]

The benefits of imagery[114] and cognitive therapy[115] in multiple sclerosis have been reported in two recent studies. Using imagery resulted in significant reductions in state anxiety and a stable internal locus of control. The control group shifted to a less internal locus of control in the second study. The use of multimodal cognitive therapy revealed significant improvements in verbal learning, verbal abstraction, and depression, and in some measures of grip strength and tactile sensitivity. This study involved group psychotherapy, visualization techniques, guided imagery, meditation, relaxation, and mental and physical exercises.

Of interest is an event-related potential (ERP) study by Yamamoto and Mukai in subjects performing imagery. The ERPs were recorded while the subjects were visualizing a letter and while changing a presented upper case letter into a lower case form. During the latter task, negative potentials were noted in left frontal, central, and parietal areas approximately 220 ms post stimulus. It was hypothesized that these potentials reflected working memory processes involved in mental image formation.[116]

This brief review suggests the application of imagery in migraine, multiple sclerosis, and stroke. The experimental study discussed previously, in which mast cell degranulation was blocked in experimental animals with inhibition of the effects of substance P and CRH, suggests a pathway of information transduction in the inhibitory effects of imagery in migraine. The pathway in attentional mechanisms, such as benefiting inattention in stroke, would be different. This would be fertile ground for further clinical studies.

SUMMARY

Stress creates constant perturbations in the biochemical field of the mind-body system. These perturbations are experienced quickly as fear, anxiety, or anger and over the long run as changes in the structure and function of our mind and body. Adapting to stress can reduce both its short-term effects and such long-term consequences as accelerated aging and shortened life span. Mind-body practices alter the biochemical indices of stress—indices that also relate to the degenerative diseases of aging. Although much research remains to be done, studies on corticosteroids, glutamate, GABA, and the body's antioxidant system confirm the importance of stress adaptation for health and well being. Implementation of mind-body practices into the health care system offers a natural method of reducing stress, increasing health and longevity, and reducing health care expenditures.

Tenzin Gyatso, the fourteenth Dalai Lama and Nobel Peace Prize winner, put it the following way at a 1998 conference with physicians at Harvard-affiliated Beth Israel Deaconess Hospital: "According to my little experience, the mental attitude is very, very important when you face illness. It's a crucial factor, the interaction between the mind and the body. . . . The West pays so much attention to knowledge, and so little attention to the heart, to affection, to a sense of human caring. . . . Western medicine is very useful. But there are many possibilities in trying new things. One can manipulate physiology through meditation. One can neutralize pain, instead of using drugs. It's also cheaper."

References

1. Maciocia G: *The foundations of Chinese medicine,* New York, 1989, Churchill-Livingstone.
2. Clark B: *The quintessence tantras of Tibetan medicine,* Ithaca, NY, 1995, Snow Lion.
3. Birnbaum R: *The healing Buddha,* Boulder, Colo., 1979, Shambala.
4. Griggs B: *Green pharmacy,* Rochester, Vt., 1997, Healing Arts Press.
5. Jung C: *Alchemical studies,* Princeton, NJ, 1967, Princeton University Press.
6. Descartes R: *The philosophical writings of Descartes,* vol 1, Cambridge, Mass., 1985, Cambridge University Press.
7. Culpepper N: *Complete herbal,* London, 1992, Bloomsbury Books.
8. Gordon JS: Role of the mind in healing, Testimony to the House Appropriations Committee, Porter J, Chairman, Nov. 5, 1997.
9. Watkins A: Mind-body pathways. In Watkins A, editor: *Mind-body medicine,* New York, 1997, Churchill-Livingstone.
10. Khansari DN, Murgo AJ, Faith RE: Effects of stress on immune system, *Immunol Today* 11(5):170-175, 1990.
11. Sapolsky RM: *Why zebras don't get ulcers,* New York, 1998, WH Freeman.
12. Carr DJ, Blalock JE: From the neuroendocrinology of lymphocytes toward a molecular basis of the network theory, *Horm Res* 31(1-2):76-80, 1989.
13. Carr DJ, Blalock JE: *In Neuropeptide hormones and receptors common to the immune and neuroendocrine systems: bidirectional pathway of intersystem communication in psychoneuroimmunology,* San Diego, 1991, Academic Press. R Ader, DL Felten, N Cohen, editors.
14. Dardenne M, Savino W: Interdependence of the endocrine and immune system, *Adv Neuroimmunol* 6(4):297-307, 1996.
15. Vojdani A, Roundtree R: *Lymphocytes: mediators and messengers in health and disease,* Gig Harbor, Wash., 1999, Institute for Functional Medicine.
16. Weigent DA, Blalock JE: Associations between the neuroendocrine and immune systems, *J Leukoc Biol* 58(2):137-150, 1995.
17. Mousa A et al: Human first trimester forebrain cells express genes for inflammatory and anti-inflammatory cytokines, *Cytokine* 11(1):55-60, 1999.
18. Pert CB: *Molecules of emotion,* New York, 1997, Simon and Schuster.
19. Weigent DA, Carr DJ, Blalock JE: Bidirectional communication between the neuroendocrine and immune systems: common hormones and hormone receptors, *Ann N Y Acad Sci* 579:17-27, 1990.
20. Blalock JE: The syntax of immune-neuroendocrine communication, *Immunol Today* 15(11):504-511, 1994.
21. Mayer ES, Baldi JP: Can regulatory peptides be regarded as words of a biological language, *Am J Physiol* 261(2Pt1):G171-184, 1991.
22. Vincent LM: Reflexions on the usage of information theory in biology, *Acta Biotheor* 42(2-3):167-179, 1994.
23. Kushner I: Regulation of the acute phase response by cytokines, *Perspect Biol Med* 36(4):611-622, 1993.
24. Boumpas DT et al: Glucocorticosteroid action on the immune system: molecular and cellular aspects, *Clin Exp Rheumatol* 9(4):413-423, 1991.
25. Ascoli M: Functional consequences of the phosphorylation of the gonadotropin receptors, *Biochem Pharmacol* 52(11):1647-1655, 1996.
26. Rossi EL: *The psychobiology of mind-body healing,* New York, 1993, WW Norton.
27. LeDoux J: *The emotional brain,* New York, 1996, Simon and Schuster.
28. Chrousos GP, Gold PW: Concepts of stress and stress system disorders, *JAMA* 267(9):1244-1252, 1992.
29. Shredova AA et al: Lipid peroxidation and retinal damage in stress, *Biull Eksp Biol Med* 3(4):24-26, 1982.
30. Theoharides TC et al: Stress-induced intracranial mast cell degranulation: a corticotropin-releasing hormone-mediated effect, *Endocrinology* 136(12): 5745-5750, 1995.
31. Mamelak M: Gammahydroxybutyrate: an endogenous regulator of energy metabolism, *Neurosci Biobehav Rev* 13(4):187-198, 1989.

32. Meerson FZ, Lifshits RI, Pavlova VI : Dynamics and physiological significance of GABA-system activation in brain and cardiac muscle during emotional-pain stress, *Vopr Med Khim* 27(1):35-39, 1981.

33. Guliaeva NV, Levshina IP: Characteristics of free-radical oxidation and antiradical protection of the brain in adaptation to chronic stress, *Biull Eksp Biol Med* 106(8):153-156, 1988.

34. Pollack et al: Chronic stress impairs oxidative metabolism and hepatic excretion of model xenobiotic substrates in the rat, *Drug Metab Dispos* 19(1): 130-134, 1991.

35. Meerson FZ et al: Effect of adaptation to brief stress exposure on the realization of the stress reaction, impairment of metabolism and myocardial contraction caused by prolonged emotional-pain stress, *Vopr Med Khim* 32(1):76-81, 1986.

36. Sazontova TG, Arkhipenko IV, Meerson FZ: Increased enzymatic activity of antioxidant protection of the heart in the adaptation of rats to short-term stress exposure, *Biull Eksp Biol Med* 104(10):411-413, 1987.

37. Westfall FC et al: Abnormal glutamic acid metabolism in multiple sclerosis, *J Neurol Sci* 47(3):353-364, 1980.

38. Timmerman W: Effects of handling on extracellular levels of glutamate and other amino acids in various areas of the brain measured by microdialysis, *Brain Res* 833(2):150-160, 1999.

39. Hauser R et al: The concentration of glutamate in cerebral tissue as a factor for the assessment of the emotional state before death: a preliminary report, *Int J Legal Med* 112(3):184-187, 1999.

40. Ikonomidou C, Turski L: Excitotoxicity and neurodegenerative disorders, *Curr Opin Neurol* 8(6):487-497, 1995.

41. Savolainen KM et al: Interactions of excitatory neurotransmitters and xenobiotics in excitotoxicity and oxidative stress: glutamate and lead, *Toxicol Lett* 102-103:363-367, 1998.

42. Adachi S, Kawamura K, Takemotot K: Oxidative damage of nuclear DNA in liver of rats exposed to psychological stress, *Cancer Res* 53(18):4153-4155, 1993.

43. Sapolsky RM, Krey LC, McEwen BS: Glucocorticoid-sensitive hippocampal neurons are involved in terminating the adrenocortical stress response, *Proceedings of the National Academy of Science* 81(19):6174-6177, 1984.

44. Sapolsky RM, Krey LC, McEwen BS: Prolonged glucocorticoid exposure reduces hippocampal neuron number: implication for aging, *J Neurosci* 5(5):1222-1227, 1985.

45. Sapolsky RM, Stein-Behrens BA, Armanini MP: Long-term adrenalectomy causes loss of dentate gyrus and pyramidal neurons in the adult hippocampus, *Exp Neurol* 114(2):246-249, 1991.

46. Stein-Behrens BA, Lin WJ, Sapolsky RM: Physiological elevations of glucocorticoids potentiate glutamate accumulation in the hippocampus, *J Neurochem* 63(2):596-602, 1994.

47. McEwen BS, Sapolsky RM: Stress and cognitive function, *Curr Opin Neurobiol* 5(2):205-216, 1995.

48. Lupien S et al: Basal cortisol levels and cognitive deficits in human aging, *J Neurosci* 4(5Pt1):2893-2903, 1994.

49. Lupien SJ et al: Cortisol levels during human aging predict hippocampal atrophy and memory deficits, *Nat Neurosci* 1(1):69-73, 1998.

50. Lupien SJ et al: Stress-induced declarative memory impairment in healthy elderly subjects: relationship to cortisol reactivity, *J Clin Endocrinol Metab* 82(7):2070-2075, 1997.

51. Lupien SJ et al: Stress-induced declarative memory impairment in healthy elderly subjects: relationship to cortisol reactivity, *J Clin Endocrinol Metab* 82(7):2170-2175, 1997.

52. Simon G et al: Health care costs associated with depressive and anxiety disorders in primary care, *Am J Psychiatry* 152:352-357, 1995.

53. Katon W, Schulberg H: Epidemiology of depression in primary care, *Gen Hosp Psychiatry* 14:237-247, 1992.

54. Friedman R, Sobel D, Myers P, Caudill M, Benson H et al: Behavioral medicine, clinical health psychology, and cost offset, *Health Psychol* 4(6)509-518, 1995.

55. NIH Technology Assessment: Special Communication: Integration of behavioral and relaxation approaches into the treatment of chronic pain and insomnia, *JAMA* 276(4):313-318, 1996.

56. Chilton M: Panel recommends integrating behavioral and relaxation approaches into medical treatment of chronic pain, insomnia, *Altern Ther Health Med* 2(1):18-28, 1996.

57. Guzetta CE: Effects of relaxation and music therapy on patients in a coronary care unit with presumptive acute myocardial infarction, *Heart Lung* 18:609-616, 1989.

58. Guzetta CE et al: Alternative/complementary therapies. In *American Association of Critical Care Nurses' clinical handbook for critical care nursing*, ed 4, St Louis, Mosby, 1998.

59. Updike P: Music therapy results for ICU patients, *Dimens Crit Care Nurs* 9(1):39-45, 1990.

60. Aldridge D: The music of the body: music therapy in medical settings, *Advances* 9(1):17-35, 1993.

61. Zimmerman LM: Effects of music on patient anxiety in coronary care units, *Heart Lung* 17:560-566, 1988.

62. Shoor JA: Music and pattern change in chronic pain, *Adv Nurs Sci* 15(4):27-36, 1993.

63. Lucia CA: Toward development of a model of music therapy intervention in the rehabilitation of head trauma patients, *Music Ther Perspect* 4:34-39, 1987.

64. Aldridge D: An overview of music therapy research, *Compl Ther Med* 2:204-216, 1994.

65. Tyson J: Meeting the needs of dementia, *Nurs Elderly* 1:18-19, 1989.

66. Disbrow EA, Bennett HL, Owings J: Effect of preoperative suggestion on postoperative gastrointestinal motility, *West J Med* 158(5):488-492, 1993.

67. Holden-Lund C: Effects of relaxation with guided imagery on surgical stress and wound healing, *Res Nurs Health* 11:235-244, 1988.

68. Johnson J: Sensory information, instruction in a coping strategy and recovery from surgery, *Res Nurs Health* 1:4-17, 1978.

69. Lawlis GF et al: Reduction of postoperative pain parameters by pre-surgical relaxation instructions for spinal pain patients, *Spine* 10(7):649-651, 1985.

70. Bennett HL, Benson DR, Kuiken DA: Preoperative instructions for decreased bleeding during spinal surgery, *Anesthesiology* 65(3A): 245, Sep 1986.

71. Blankfield RP: Suggestion, relaxation, and hypnosis as adjuncts in the care of surgery patients, *Am J Clin Hypn* 33:172-186, 1991.

72. Borden RL: Preparation for surgery: an imagery-based approach for less distress and optimal recovery. Proceedings of the Sixth International Conference on the Psychology of Health, Immunity and Disease sponsored by the National Institute for the Clinical Application of Behavioral Medicine, Hilton Head, South Carolina, 1994.

73. Rapkin DA, Straubing M, Holroyd JC: Guided imagery, hypnosis and recovery from head and neck cancer surgery: an exploratory study, *Int J Clin Exp Hypnother* 39:215-226, 1991.

74. Anderson CM: Functional asymmetry of the temporal lobes in young adults verbally and sexually abused as children using fMRI, *Abstracts of Developmental Psychobiology* 1997.

75. Teicher MH et al: Preliminary evidence for abnormal cortical development in physically and sexually abused children using EEG coherence and MRI, *NY Acad Sci,* 821:160-175, 1997.

76. Bremner JD: Magnetic resonance imaging-based measurement of hippocampal volume in post-traumatic stress disorder related to childhood physical and sexual abuse: a preliminary report, *Biol Psychiatry* 41 (1):23-32, 1997.

77. Simonsick EM et al: Depressive symptomatology and hypertension-associated morbidity and mortality in older adults, *Psychosom Med* 57:427-435, Sep-Oct 1995.

78. Smyth JM et al: Effects of writing about stressful experiences on symptom reduction in patients with asthma or rheumatoid arthritis: a randomized trial, *JAMA* 281:1304-1309, 1999.

79. Pennebaker JW, Beall SK: Confronting a traumatic event: toward an understanding of inhibition and disease, *J Abnorm Psychol* 95:274-281, 1986.

80. Pennebaker JW, Kiecolt-Glaser JK, Glaser R: Disclosures of traumas and immune function: health implications for psychotherapy, *J Consult Clin Psychol* 56:239-245, 1988.

81. Kiecolt-Glaser JK, Glaser R: Psychoneuroimmunology: can psychological interventions modulate immunity? *J Consult Clin Psychol* 60:569-575, 1992.

82. Rinpoche S: *The Tibetan book of living and dying,* San Francisco, 1992, HarperCollins.

83. Jevning R, Wilson AF, Davidson JM: Adrenocortical activity during meditation, *Horm Behav* 10(1):54-60, 1978.

84. Michaels RR: Renin, cortisol and aldosterone during transcendental meditation, *Psychosom Med* 41(1):50-54, 1979.

85. Gallois P: Hormonal changes during relaxation, *Encephale* 10(2):79-82, 1984.

86. Cooper R: Hormonal and biochemical responses to transcendental meditation, *Postgrad Med J* 61(714):301-304, 1985.

87. Schneider RH et al: Lower lipid peroxide levels in practitioners of the transcendental meditation program, *Psychosom Med* 60(1):38-41, 1998.

88. Depak KK, Manchanda SK, Maheshwari MC: Meditation improves clinicoelectroencephalographic measures in drug-resistant epileptics, *Biofeedback Self Regul* 19(1):25-40, 1994.

89. Elias AN, Wilson AF: Serum hormonal concentrations following transcendental meditation-potential role of gamma aminobutyric acid, *Med Hypotheses* 44(4):287-291, 1995.

90. Kabat-Zinn J: An outpatient program in behavioral medicine for chronic pain patients based on the practice of mindfulness meditation: theoretical considerations and preliminary results, *Gen Hosp Psychiatry* 4(1):33-47, 1982.

91. Alexander CN: Transcendental meditation, mindfulness, and longevity: an experimental study with the elderly, *J Pers Soc Psychol* 57(6):950-964, 1989.

92. Kennedy B, Ziegler MG, Shannahoff-Khalsa DS: Alternating lateralization of plasma catecholamines and nasal patency in humans, *Life Sci* 38(13):1203-1214, 1986.

93. Werntz DA et al: Alternating cerebral hemispheric activity and the lateralization of autonomic nervous function, *Hum Neurobiol* 2(1):39-43, 1983.

94. Kennedy B, Ziegler MG, Shannahoff-Khalsa DS: Alternating lateralization of plasma catecholamines and nasal patency in humans, *Life Sci* 38(13):1203-1214, 1986.

95. Shannahoff-Khalsa DS, Boyle MR, Buebel ME: The effects of unilateral forced nostril breathing on cognition, *Int J Neurosci* 57(3-4):230-249, 1991.

96. Jella SA, Shannahoff-Khalsa DS: The effects of unilateral forced nostril breathing on cognitive performance, *Int J Neurosci* 73(1-2):61-68, 1993.

97. Achterberg J, McGraw P, Lawlis GF: Rheumatoid arthritis: a study of relaxation and temperature biofeedback training, *Biofeedback Self Regul* 6(2):207-223, 1981.

98. Eppley KR, Abrams AI, Shear J: Differential effects of relaxation techniques on trait anxiety: a meta-analysis, *J Clin Psychol* 45:957-974, 1989.

99. Richardson MA et al: Coping, life attitudes, and immune responses to imagery and group support after breast cancer treatment, *Altern Ther Health Med* 3:62-70, 1997.

100. Gruber BL et al: Immune system and psychological changes in metastatic cancer patients using relaxation and guided imagery: a pilot study, *Scand J Behav Ther* 17:25-46, 1988.

101. Gruber BL et al: Immunological responses of breast cancer patients to behavioral interventions, *Biofeedback Self Regul* 18:1-22, 1993.

102. Achterberg J, Lawlis GF: *Bridges of the bodymind: behavioral approaches to health care,* Champaign, Il., 1980, Institute for Personality and Ability Testing.

103. Kiecolt-Glaser J et al: Visions to boost immunity, *Am Health* 6:54-61, 1987.

104. Donovan M: Relaxation with guided imagery: a useful technique, *Cancer Nurs* 3:27-32, 1980.

105. Lyles JN et al: Efficacy of relaxation training and guided imagery in reducing the aversiveness of cancer chemotherapy, *J Consult Clin Psychol* 50:509-524, 1982.

106. Frank J: The effects of music therapy and guided visual imagery on chemotherapy induced nausea and vomiting, *Oncol Nurs Forum* 12:47-52, 1985.

107. Spiegel D, Moore R: Imagery and hypnosis in the treatment of cancer patients, *Oncology* 11:1179-1189, 1997.

108. Dossey BM, Guzzetta CE, Kenner CV: *Critical care nursing: body-mind-spirit,* ed 3, Philadelphia, 1992, Lippincott.

109. Kenner C, Achterberg J: Non-pharmacologic pain relief for burn patients. Presented at the annual meeting of the American Burn Association, New Orleans, 1983.

110. Niemeier JP: The lighthouse strategy: use of a visual imagery technique to treat visual inattention in stroke patients, *Brain Inj* 12(5):399-406, 1998.

111. Brown JM: Imagery coping strategies in the treatment of migraine, *Pain* 18(2):157-167, 1984.

112. Ilacqua GE: Migraine headaches: coping efficacy of guided imagery training, *Headache* 34(2):99-102, 1994.

113. Smania N: Visuomotor imagery and rehabilitation of neglect, *Arch Phys Med Rehabil* 78(4):430-436, 1997.

114. Maguire BL: The effects of imagery on attitudes and moods in multiple sclerosis patients, *Alt Ther* 2(5):75-79, 1996.

115. Rodgers D et al: Cognitive therapy for multiple sclerosis: a preliminary study, *Alt Ther* 2(5):70-74, 1996.

116. Yamamoto S, Mukai H: Event-related potentials during mental imagery, *Neuroreport* 9(15):3359-3362, 1998.

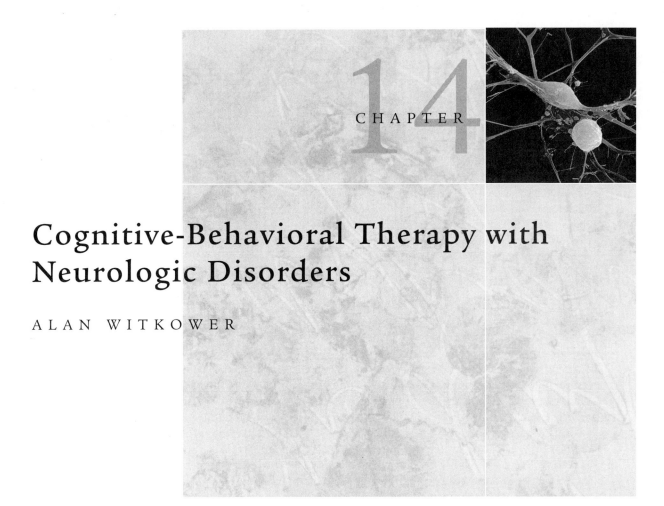

CHAPTER

14

Cognitive-Behavioral Therapy with Neurologic Disorders

ALAN WITKOWER

he goal of this chapter is to provide the reader with a conceptualization of cognitive-
behavioral therapy (CBT) and to review the
literature on its efficacy, specifically its application
to neurologic disease. An overview of the treatment
components of CBT as they pertain to sleep and
headache disorders, two common disorders presenting to a neurologic practice, complete the chapter.
Although CBT is typically conducted by a trained
mental health clinician, when it is viewed as a psy-
choeducational intervention[1] it is appropriate for
the physician to have adequate knowledge and understanding of the procedure to be able to introduce
the concepts to patients.

CONCEPTUALIZATION

CBT is based on a theoretical approach that defines behavior very broadly to encompass thoughts, feelings,
and behaviors, including physiological processes. Early
theorists of CBT conceptualized behavior as reciprocally influenced by emotions and thoughts. These theorists believed that behavior could be unlearned and that
psychological disturbances result from maladaptive
and dysfunctional cognitions.[1-5] Approaches of CBT
encompass many techniques that, despite their differences, share the following assumptions:

- Cognitive mediational processes are involved
  in human learning. Individuals continually

apprise the meaning of their symptoms, using their memories of similar or observed situations and their current knowledge of their experience. From this they develop hypotheses and expectations regarding the possible outcome of their efforts to cope with the symptoms.[6-8] Cognitions, feelings, and behaviors are causally interrelated. Individuals' cognitions may alter their behavior by influencing both emotional and physiological responses. In turn, these cognitions are equally influenced by emotional, physiological, and behavioral events. The emphasis here is that these variables are all interrelated. At any given time a patient's behavior, cognitions, or physiology may contribute to a change in other variables.[6-8]

- Cognitive activities such as expectations, self-statements, and attributions are important in understanding and predicting psychopathology and psychotherapeutic change.[6-8]
- Behaviors may be influenced by the environment and, reciprocally, the individual's behaviors may influence environmental events. A patient who is fearful about his or her prognosis and expresses that anxiety in an angry outburst at the caregiver might receive a response that confirms his or her fears of a negative outcome, for example that the condition is untreatable.[6-8]
- Cognitions and behaviors are compatible; cognitive processes can be integrated into behavioral paradigms, and cognitive techniques can be combined with behavioral procedures. Treatment approaches must address the emotional, cognitive, and behavioral dimensions of individuals' problems if they are to be effective. Individuals can then acquire more adaptive ways of thinking, feeling, and behaving. It is important to note that the cognitive-behavioral (C-B) model is multidimensional and recognizes that a person will need to learn alternative ways of behaving and feeling in addition to modifying cognitions.[6-8]
- The task of the CBT therapist is to collaborate with the patient to assess distorted or deficient cognitive processes and behaviors, and then to design new learning experiences to remediate the dysfunctional or deficient cognitions, behaviors, and affective patterns. This implies that individuals must become active participants in treatment if they are to learn adaptive

methods of responding to their problems. In contrast to the medical model, which reinforces the passive and compliant behavior of patients by expecting them to simply follow a physician's orders, the C-B model maintains that patients can be instrumental in learning adaptive strategies for coping with and managing symptoms.[6-8]

- Finally, an important assumption of CBT is that diagnostically similar patient populations have common dysfunctions and symptom complexes and are therefore similar in their potential to respond to standardized treatment programs.[9]

Based on these assumptions, CBT attempts to achieve a series of outcomes in the course of treatment. The major goals of CBT include the following:[8,10,11]

- Reconceptualizing the patients' view of their medical problems from being overwhelming to being manageable
- Shifting the patients' view of themselves from being passive and powerless to being resourceful and proactive
- Assisting the patients in learning to monitor their thoughts, feelings, and behaviors during activities to highlight the connection between those variables and their symptoms
- Teaching the patients the necessary skills to adaptively manage their physical symptoms
- Encouraging the patients to attribute their successes to their efforts at employing those sets of skills
- Supporting the patients in anticipating and managing future exacerbations of symptoms or changes in their physical status

LITERATURE REVIEW

Cognitive therapy (CT) and CBT have been extensively studied and are widely regarded as the nonpharmacologic treatments of choice for depressive illness.[11] In studies comparing CT and CBT to pharmacologic treatments it was concluded that CT and CBT were as effective as medication in reducing depressive symptoms.[12-15] Some studies also determined that CT and CBT provided a preventative effect in reducing relapse rates when treatment was discontinued.[16,17]

Another set of common psychiatric disturbances, generalized anxiety disorder (GAD) and panic disorder (PD), has also demonstrated a positive response to CT and/or CBT. One large review of the literature on treatments for GAD examined several models of CT and CBT[18] and concluded that these therapies were more effective, in general, than wait-list controls, nondirective therapy, or pill placebo.[19]

CT and CBT were found to surpass an active comparison condition at posttreatment and followup[20,21] and to be significantly more effective than a wait-list or minimal-contact control condition.[22,23]

In a study comparing three of the most widely regarded antipanic treatments with one another and with a wait-list control, CT was found to be superior at posttreatment to applied relaxation, imipramine pharmacotherapy, and the control condition.[24]

The literature shows that CBT has been either studied or used to conceptualize the development or maintenance of a wide range of medical disorders. Clearly the most widespread use of CBT approaches has been with functional somatic or psychophysiological disorders. These are disorders in which psychological factors and stress are considered primary contributors to the initiation, exacerbation, or maintenance of the symptoms of the disorder.[25-27] For example, the application of CBT for treating chronic fatigue syndrome has been studied and reviewed.[28-30] These studies have found CBT to be substantially more effective than both standard medical care[29] and time-matched relaxation therapy.[30]

Similar CBT approaches have been studied and found to be more effective than nonspecific treatment for noncardiac chest pain,[31] irritable bowel syndrome,[32-34] hypochondriasis,[35] and mixed functional somatic symptoms.[36]

CBT has also been applied to medical conditions that are not considered to be functional or that do not have significant psychological contributions to the etiology of the disorder. Motion sickness[37-39] and nausea and vomiting associated with chemotherapy[40,41] are conditions that have responded favorably to the use of CBT, particularly in situations in which traditional medical intervention has failed or is contraindicated. CBT is being used increasingly to assist patients with surgical procedures. CBT can enhance postoperative recovery by directly reducing the patient's preoperative anxiety and fear and by training the patient in strategies to reduce preoperative and postoperative pain and anxiety.[42-44]

Patients with cancer have benefited from the introduction of CBT into their medical treatment regimens to enhance coping efforts and reduce psychological distress.[45-47] In addition, arthritis is a disease that causes considerable suffering and contributes to a significant amount of disability.[48] The use of CBT for patients with rheumatoid arthritis has demonstrated positive benefits, particularly in reducing functional limitations secondary to pain.[49-51]

In the field of cardiac care and rehabilitation, CBT has become increasingly popular in addressing a range of cardiac conditions. CBT for cardiovascular disease has been directed at reducing mortality and morbidity by controlling the risk factors for disease progression, such as smoking, exercise, diet, and Type A behavior, and by reducing emotional distress and enhancing active coping following an acute cardiac event.[52] The Recurrent Coronary Prevention Project[53] compared the effectiveness of group cardiac counseling and cardiac counseling combined with a C-B program to modify Type A behavior. At followup, significantly greater changes in global ratings of Type A behavior were found in the patients from the combined counseling and C-B group. This change translated into a cumulative reinfarction rate in the combined treatment group that was half of that in the counseling only group. Death from myocardial infarction was also reduced significantly in the combined group.[53] Several studies have supported the notion that CBT can improve the psychological distress of patients during and following cardiac rehabilitation. Patients in these studies reported less depression, more vigor,[54] and more confidence in their ability to handle stress,[55] and evidenced more lifestyle changes including reducing cigarette and alcohol consumption.[56] CBT has even been considered as a potentially therapeutic model for patients with ventricular dysrhythmia who require antidysrhythmic therapy or an internal pacemaker.[57] These patients experience a number of psychological symptoms and complaints, including anxiety, depression, insomnia, irritability, helplessness, and loss of control.[58,59]

A search of the literature through Medline, PsycLIT, and APA Psych/INFO resulted in a relative dearth of studies examining the efficacy of CBT with neurologic diseases. Only in the areas of headache and insomnia were there thorough representations of studies and review articles. To a much lesser extent there were case studies and review articles on the use of CBT with epilepsy. This relative paucity of research on CBT and epilepsy is surprising considering the estimate that 5% to 36% of individuals with epilepsy present with pseudo-seizures rather than true epileptic attacks.[61-63] A pseudo-seizure is seizure-like activity that is not accompanied by abnormal EEG patterns.[60] There is also evidence that patients with psychogenic seizures affect a significant proportion of individuals with epilepsy.[63,65] Psychogenic seizures are true seizures that are contingent upon the occurrence of psychologic events.[64] These findings are best summarized by Fenwick:[66]

There is abundant evidence of the close interrelation between the induction and inhibition of seizure activity and the patient's thoughts, feelings, and behavior. The detailed knowledge that we now have of the epileptic focus and the way that it is connected to the surrounding cerebral mechanisms, makes it possible for many patients with focal epilepsy to establish a significant degree of seizure control by altering their thinking and behavior.[66]

The studies that were reviewed all used an approach that focused on aspects of the CBT treatment that included (a) teaching patients how to become more aware of the occurrence of their seizures through self-monitoring[67,68] and (b) training patients in self-management techniques to enable them to cope more successfully with the stimuli associated with their seizure activity.[69,70] The outcome of the studies was mixed with two studies demonstrating efficacy of CBT in reducing seizure behavior[68,69] and two studies reporting improvement in psychological adjustment but no decline in seizure frequency.[70,71]

The category of sleep disturbances characterized by complaints of insufficient or nonrestorative sleep is called *insomnia*.[72] The prevalence of insomnia in the adult population varies across studies from less than 2%[73] to 38%[74] and 45%[74] in adults 65 to 79 years of age. Numerous psychological interventions have been designed to treat insomnia. The most widely studied have been progressive relaxation training,[75] stimulus control,[76] paradoxic intention,[77] sleep hygiene,[78] imagery training,[79] sleep restriction,[80] and cognitive therapy.[81] Each of these procedures has been demonstrated to have efficacy in sleep-onset latency, total sleep time, wake time after sleep onset, and/or sleep efficiency.[82] Meta-analyses of these studies and combined treatment approaches further corroborate the benefits of these CBT strategies.[83-85]

The literature about CBT for the treatment of headache is far more extensive than for CBT and other neurologic disorders. This is not surprising, however,

considering that the overall headache prevalence rate is well above 60%[86,87] and that headache is one of the most frequent complaints encountered in outpatient practices. Headaches account for more than 18 million outpatient visits per year in the United States.[88] The underlying assumption of CBT, as it has been applied to the treatment of headache, is that the way a patient copes with both environmental and headache-related stress contributes to the development and exacerbation of the headache, and influences the course of headache-related disability.[89,90] Therefore, CBT uses cognitive and behavioral strategies to alter maladaptive responses to environmental and interpersonal events that are assumed to mediate the development of headache[91,92] or to modify stress responses to the headache.[93] Several studies have found CBT to be significantly superior to wait-list or self-monitoring control conditions in both migraine[94,95] and tension-type headaches.[96,97] Comparisons between CBT and attention-placebo controls has also demonstrated CBT superiority for both migraine headaches[98,99] and tension-type headaches.[100] Long-term maintenance of these improvements has been supported for CBT as well. In one study, 80% of patients with tension-type headaches still exhibited a 50% improvement in their headaches 2 years after treatment.[97] For patients with migraine headaches, percentages of headache reduction ranging from 45% to 47% were observed at 8-month,[101] 1-year,[102] and 3-year[103] followups. In addition to the improvements in headache activity, patients who had CBT for either tension-type or migraine headaches demonstrated a more positive appraisal of their headaches and reported more frequent problem-solving thoughts than patients who did not receive any headache treatment. This appears to be a central therapeutic mechanism of CBT.[91,107] Additionally, CBT has been shown to enhance the efficacy of unimodular psychophysiologic treatments such as biofeedback.[104-106]

APPLICATION TO HEADACHE AND INSOMNIA

CBT represents a wide variety of approaches including rational psychotherapies,[108] coping-skills therapies,[109] and problem-solving therapies.[110] Yet these diverse forms of CBT have several components of treatment in common that follow each other in a logical course of education and training.[8,111]

These phases of treatment are generally flexible enough that patients can move back and forth between them while progressing in the overall management of the symptoms or complaint.[112] The phases of treatment can be categorized into four overlapping stages:

1. Reconceptualization
2. Skills acquisition
3. Cognitive and behavioral rehearsal
4. Generalization and relapse management

Reconceptualization

The objective of this phase of treatment is to provide the patient with a rationale for CBT and to elicit and clarify the patient's expectation about treatment.[113] The patient and therapist engage in an exchange of ideas, information, and questioning. The patient is encouraged to be receptive to suggestions by the therapist while providing feedback to the therapist regarding what is being asked of the patient.[114] Successfully engaging the patient in the treatment process at this point enhances the likelihood that the patient will actively participate in subsequent stages of treatment.[113,114]

Education is important to headache sufferers.[115,116] A survey conducted by Packard[117] indicated that nearly 50% of the patients who consult for headaches do so mainly to obtain information about what is causing their pain. Therefore, as with all forms of therapy, headache treatment begins with education. This initial reconceptualization emphasizes three steps. The first step is to provide information about the etiology of headache, particularly the features that can be controlled by the patient. This information serves to combat the patient's feelings of helplessness and demoralization. Step two consists of informing the patient of the self-management approach he or she will be learning that will help manage the headaches. This approach encourages the patient to collaborate with the therapist. It assumes that the therapist may be an expert in the assessment and treatment of headaches but that the patient is an expert in the specific variables associated with his or her headache. The third step is explaining to the patient the procedures that will be used in the course of treatment. This includes the homework assignments the patient will be expected to complete between sessions.[118,119]

For insomnia, sleep education consists of introducing the patient to the basic tenets of sleep stages, sleep functions and effects, and developmentally related sleep changes.[120] Sleep hygiene is a sensible place to begin treatment and it also helps assess the patient's compliance and receptivity to a behavioral approach.[121] This approach is concerned with lifestyle factors, such as diet, exercise, and alcohol or caffeine use; and environmental factors, including mattress, temperature, and light that affect sleep. The approach is intended to inform patients who engage in activities that are detrimental to sleep or to encourage patients to refrain from practices that might interfere with sleep. Guidelines include the following:

1. Refraining from using caffeine and nicotine 4 to 6 hours before bedtime
2. Abstaining from alcohol around bedtime
3. Avoiding a heavy meal before bedtime and restricting liquid intake in the evening
4. Avoiding exercise too close to bedtime[82,122]

This phase of treatment is extremely important because it establishes the tone and pace for the remainder of the treatment.

Skill Acquisition

In this phase the objective is to promote the successful acquisition and use of adaptive coping strategies.[9] These strategies can be broadly grouped as behavioral or cognitive. Behavioral strategies are directed at reducing excessive autonomic arousal, eliminating maladaptive behavior patterns, and increasing the patient's self-efficacy for using constructive coping strategies. Cognitive strategies focus on maladaptive thoughts, beliefs, and appraisals that create heightened emotional and physical arousal or that interfere with the patient's employing adaptive coping strategies.

Relaxation strategies for headaches are then introduced to patients. Patients are also told how their headaches may be initiated, exacerbated, or maintained by a combination of excessive muscle tension in tension-type headaches, or general sympathetic arousal and vasoconstriction in migraine headaches.[116] Two useful models to discuss with patients are the stress-tension-pain cycle and the stress-headache-stress-cycle.[123] In the stress-tension-pain model, patients are asked to consider what happens to them when they are fearful or faced with an unpleasant task. Most patients can identify some area of their body that becomes tense, such as neck or jaw muscles. Most patients will accept the suggestion that this increased muscle tension can lead to an increase in their headache. The stress-headache-stress cycle emphasizes the role of the autonomic nervous system in precipitating a physiologic change, such as vasoconstriction, that may cause a migraine headache. In this model patients are educated about the fight or flight response in which stress elicits multiple changes in the body's physiology that influence headaches and perception of pain. Patients might be asked to consider what happens when they are faced with a very stressful experience such as awaiting an unpleasant medical procedure or being told that their workload at the office is being doubled. Most patients will understand this analogy and will acknowledge that they become emotionally distraught. They may say that they have noticed bodily changes such as feeling flushed, perspiring, having their heart race, or breathing rapidly and shallowly. Many patients will give their own examples of how emotional distress and stressful circumstances influence their headaches. Paying attention to the headache and noticing increased pain then acts as a stressor that evokes further emotional distress and autonomic arousal, thereby maintaining the cycle of stress, headache, and further stress.[123]

For patients with insomnia, a similar educational format is used to introduce the patient to the role of excessive autonomic arousal, whether emotional, physical, or cognitive, in creating a sleep disturbance. Patients will often admit that difficulty falling asleep on previous occasions creates a state of tension and anticipatory anxiety. This condition continues to inhibit relaxation, the necessary prologue to sleep.[120] Patients may also report difficulty in initiating sleep because their "mind won't slow down" or they feel "too wound up."

With this background established, patients with insomnia or headaches are informed that relaxation strategies can provide relief in several ways, including the following:

1. Reducing excessive muscle tension causing headache or sleep-onset difficulty
2. Reducing the patient's attention to pain or anxiety while attempting to focus on the relaxation procedure
3. Reducing the emotional arousal that can amplify pain perception or inhibit sleepiness
4. Promoting a feeling of control during episodes of pain or insomnia that further counteracts emotional arousal and muscle tension.[124]

It is extremely important to emphasize to patients that relaxation strategies are learned skills that require practice and use in the appropriate circumstances. It is also critical to encourage patients to notice any changes in their headache awareness, or other bodily changes such as reduced muscle tension. The patient should then attribute these changes to their efforts rather than to something that the professional did to them.

There are numerous relaxation strategies that can be taught to patients for either headache control or insomnia. Some methods, such as muscle relaxation, focus on the somatic level and others focus on the cognitive level to reduce the cognitive processes of worrying and ruminating. The most common techniques for treating headaches and insomnia are progressive muscle relaxation training,[125,126] autogenic training,[127] relaxation imagery, and variations on these techniques. Progressive muscle relaxation involves alternately tensing and then relaxing a series of muscles.[113] The purpose of initially tensing the muscle group is to train the patient to recognize what muscle tension feels like in his or her body and to discriminate between a state of tension and a state of relaxation. Tensing muscles and then abruptly relaxing those muscles also produces a more pronounced sensation of relaxed muscles. The therapist continually focuses the patients' attention on the sensations occurring in the muscle groups. When patients have developed confidence in identifying tension in muscles, the tensing portion of the exercise is eliminated.

Autogenic training[127] is a psychophysiological approach designed to simultaneously regulate cognitive and somatic functions through passive concentration on a phrase such as "my head is cool." The term *passive concentration* implies a casual attitude and functional passivity towards the intended outcome of the concentration. Conversely, active concentration is characterized by a person's concern, interest, attention, and goal-directed efforts towards the final functional outcome when performing a task.[127] The patient is instructed to follow a sequence of standard self-statements that describe sensations typically associated with the psychophysiological changes that occur during sleep and hypnosis, for example, warmth or heaviness. The patient is asked to visualize the relevant part of the body and then concentrate on the corresponding autogenic formula.[118] This approach can produce significant levels of relaxation, autonomic changes, and distraction away from painful sensations or distressful worries.

Imagery training is another behavioral strategy taught to patients with either headaches or insomnia. Imagery training can be categorized as incompatible imagery or transformative imagery.[118] Incompatible imagery is designed to compete with sensations of pain, awareness of distracting somatic sensations, or distressful thoughts and ruminations. Transformative imagery is designed to alter specific features of the headache or distressful physical sensations.

For a patient with insomnia, incompatible imagery training represents a form of mental relaxation that does not actively attempt to reduce muscle tension. Rather, the patient is taught to focus on images that are incompatible with those thoughts and ruminations that tend to increase autonomic arousal and, thereby, interfere with sleep onset. Meditation, which focuses a patient's attention on physical sensations such as respiration, often employs imagery training as well.[128] Woolfolk and McNulty[79] devised imagery training that used six images: a candle, an hourglass, a blackboard, a kite, a lightbulb, and a bowl of fruit. Patients were instructed to concentrate on the details of each item and to then practice visualizing the objects sequentially at home while lying in bed. They found this to be a particularly beneficial approach for patients who were distracted by intrusive thoughts of the past day or concerns about falling asleep.[79]

Transformative imagery is used more commonly with patients who experience headache pain. There are three versions of transformative imagery: contextual, stimulus, and response.[118,124] Contextual transformation requires patients to imagine their headache pain in a different environment or circumstance. A patient may accept that his or her headache pain does not represent a serious brain disease, but it may help more if the patient imagines that the headache is the result of intense concentration used to successfully solve a difficult problem. With stimulus transformation, the patient modifies the sensation of the headache. For example, a patient who describes his or her headache as a "tight band around my head" might imagine a tight cord around the head being gradually loosened, causing the headache pain to diminish. Response transformation refers to relabeling the sensation of pain to create a less distressful sensation. A patient complaining of a stabbing pain like a knife might use the imagery of the sensation of pressure on a muscle rather than a sharp object.

In another variation of incompatible imagery for headache pain, the patient is encouraged to visualize images that elicit emotional responses that are in-compatible with the distress associated with pain. The patient might imagine scenes that produce an affective response of humor, contentment, excitement, or sexual arousal.

Attention-diversion strategies are forms of behavioral intervention that are also used primarily with headache disorders and other chronic pain conditions.[118,124,129] Attention-diversion strategies, sometimes called distraction techniques, are directed at diverting the patient's attention away from the headache sensations.[124,130] Patients generally require a rationale for this approach given their conviction that they are unable to attend to anything but their headache pain. Patients are introduced to how attention can influence a person's perceptions either by selecting a focus of attention or by magnifying the awareness of a sensation. Patients might be asked to pay attention to the sensations of their bodies in the chair. They would then be told to notice that these sensations, such as the pressure and weight of their thighs on the seat of the chair, are obviously real and present even though they had not been noticed earlier. Patients can be offered the analogy of watching a television show and then changing the station to watch another show. The patients would be reminded that the previous show did not go off the air. Rather, the channel had simply been switched so they were no longer tuned in to the first show. Generally patients can remember at least one situation in which they were not as focused on their pain. Examples that have been offered by patients include being engrossed in watching a movie, absorbed in a book, engaged in watching a sporting event, or involved in an emotionally arousing interaction.[9,129]

Attention-diversion can be accomplished in several ways—by focusing on internal sensations and mental activity or by focusing attention on the external environment. Patients might focus on the internal sensations of breathing, as in meditation, or on parts of the body that are comfortable and relaxed. Some patients can successfully distance themselves from headache sensations by analyzing the sensation as if they were conducting a scientific experiment and being totally objective about the sensations. Focusing on mental activity might include having the patient plan a week's worth of activities, perform mental arithmetic such as serial subtractions, or recall the words to a favorite song or poem.[9,118] An external distracting focus would be instructing the patient to pay close attention to visual, auditory, tactile, and olfactory stimuli in the environment and to characterize each of the sensory experiences in great detail. Listening to music or studying artwork can also be effectively, if temporarily, distracting. All the attention-diversion strategies may not be effective for all patients all of the time. However, it is important to remind the patient that by developing a repertoire of techniques, there is a greater likelihood that at least one technique will provide some degree of relief.[9,118]

Stimulus control is a behavioral strategy developed for patients with insomnia that is directed at curtailing sleep-incompatible behaviors and regulating sleep/wake cycles. The main objective is to bring sleeping under the stimulus control of the patient's bedroom and bed.[130] Bootzin[72] established the following six rules for stimulus-control of insomnia:

1. Go to bed only when sleepy. The patient is instructed to use physical cues of sleepiness to signal when to go to bed. Bedtime should not be based on the evening hour.
2. Use the bed only for sleeping. This is to insure that the bed becomes strongly associated with falling asleep.
3. Get out of bed if unable to fall asleep.
4. Get out of bed if awakened and then unable to return to sleep. This rule is directed at helping patients cope with nocturnal wakefulness and not necessarily to promote sleep.
5. Get up at the same time each morning. This rule is to be followed regardless of how much sleep the patient has had. The patient is told not to remain in bed after awakening so the waking time is also the rising time. This rule is directed at establishing a strong biologic rhythm with a reliable anchor point.
6. Do not nap during the day. This is to further reinforce the association of sleep, nighttime, and the bed.[131,132]

Paradoxic intention is based on a theoretical rationale that sleep is basically an involuntary physiologic process, which cannot be placed under voluntary control.[77] Patients attempt to force themselves to fall asleep and become frustrated when they cannot. This leads to autonomic arousal that continues to interfere with efforts to fall asleep. Paradoxic intention is introduced to patients as an approach to permit them to learn how they fall asleep. Patients are instructed either to try to remain awake in bed and focus on their thoughts before they fall asleep or to apply relaxation in bed, increasing the number of steps in the relaxation exercise so that the time needed to fall asleep is increased. Another version requires the patient to lay in bed with his or her eyes open and to remain awake as long as possible, but without using any active methods to remain awake. This procedure eliminates the performance anxiety of patients who are exerting an effort to fall asleep since the instructions are to remain awake. Eventually, the arousal level is reduced and natural sleepiness takes over.[77]

Sleep restriction consists of curtailing the amount of time the patient spends in bed to the actual sleep time. This approach is based on the assumption that patients with insomnia spend an excessive amount of time in bed but not necessarily sleeping. With sleep restriction, individualized sleep/wake schedules are designed by adjusting the sleep period to the estimated total sleep time.[80,130] First, a consistent time for awakening each morning is established. Next, an average subjective total sleep time is established. Finally, the time for retiring is calculated so that the time between retiring and awakening will equal the established total sleep time. As the patient's sleep efficiency (time asleep divided by total time in bed times 100) increases to 85%, the allowed time in bed increases, usually by 15 minutes. If the sleep efficiency drops below 85%, then a 15-minute reduction of time in bed is required.[80]

Cognitive strategies for insomnia and headaches assume that a patient's cognitions, attributions, and beliefs can directly influence the patient's development, exacerbation, and/or maintenance of symptoms.

The use of cognitive strategies for insomnia is based on the established evidence that patients engage in dysfunctional cognitions that can exacerbate what would otherwise be transient sleep problems.[82] Faulty beliefs and attitudes play an important mediating role in insomnia, feeding on the vicious cycle of sleep difficulties, emotional distress, fear of sleeplessness, and more insomnia. Targets of treatment include unrealistic sleep expectations (e.g., "I must have 8 hours of sleep every night"); misconceptions about the causes of insomnia (e.g., "because I'm older, it is normal to have difficulty sleeping"); and misattributions or amplifications of its consequences (e.g., "having less than 8 hours of sleep will result in my getting ill and not being able to function at work").[130] Cognitive therapy for insomnia uses the following three-step process:

1. Identifying the patient's specific maladaptive sleep cognitions
2. Confronting and challenging those thoughts

3. Implementing methods for revising and altering those thoughts using more rational substitutes[130] Cognitive restructuring techniques teach patients to distinguish between normal sleep disturbances related to everyday stress or illness, and pathologic sleeplessness. The technique also attempts to help the patient alleviate anxiety about diminished sleep, thereby interrupting the cycle of anxiety about sleeplessness, emotional arousal, and further sleep disturbance.

Patients experience performance anxiety resulting from excessive attempts to control the process of sleep, and they develop learned helplessness associated with the perceived unpredictability of sleep.[130] Erroneous beliefs about sleep-promoting practices can also perpetuate sleep difficulties. For example, a patient might believe that the best way to get to sleep is to stay in bed and try harder to fall asleep or that the best coping strategy for minimizing the consequences of sleep loss is to take daytime naps.[82]

For the patient whose sleep disturbance is due primarily to intrusive thoughts, techniques such as thought stopping and articulation suppression[81] can be useful. In articulation suppression the patient is taught to control intrusive thoughts by repeating the syllable *the* to himself, pacing it in a nonregular manner. Worry control is another variant of these strategies. The patient is instructed to write down, early every evening, any problems that might turn up at bedtime. The patient is told to then write down a strategy for addressing each problem the next day. If the worry begins at bedtime the patient reminds himself or herself that things are under control.[133] These approaches work better for patients whose sleep is disturbed by trivial and incidental thoughts than by emotionally charged worries.[131]

The use of cognitive coping strategies for headaches is based on the understanding that the most common headache triggers are stress and dysphoric emotions such as anger, depression, or anxiety.[116] Headaches are aversive and stressful experiences. Therefore, cognitive interventions are directed at both the precipitating thoughts and appraisals that induce a headache and the maladaptive responses and dysfunctional thoughts about headaches that perpetuate them.

Cognitive restructuring is a specific application of a cognitive coping approach for headaches. Patients are asked to consider how their thoughts and appraisals influence their headache experience. A man may describe a scenario in which he wakes up with a headache and says to himself, "Oh no, not again, I thought this was going to be a decent day. I probably won't be able to go in to work today. I'll miss the important staff meeting. My work will pile up and I will get behind. My boss will probably be annoyed with me for being out again. What is the use of living like this?" The man then observes that he feels demoralized and anxious and finally notices that he begins to wonder if there may be something wrong in his head that the physicians have not diagnosed.[9]

This patient would be asked to consider how realistic these beliefs were about his headache and then to develop alternative views that could lead to less distress. In this example, the patient might consider that before he assumes he will not be able to go to work that he might wash up and then determine if he is feeling any better. Alternatively, the patient might decide to challenge the belief that there is anything seriously wrong with his head. He might remind himself that he has had the headaches for many years without any worsening of his symptoms and without developing any new symptoms.[9]

Cognitive restructuring enlists patients to challenge their beliefs or correct the distortions in their thinking. The therapist does not offer direct alternatives or tell patients what to do. Instead the therapist emphasizes a collaboration in which patients are helped in creating their own alternative views and competing thoughts or images.[133]

Cognitive and Behavioral Rehearsal

In this stage of CBT, patients are to integrate the skills they have acquired in the previous stage and practice these skills in their everyday lives. Several techniques are employed in this stage, including stress inoculation and role-playing. Stress inoculation is clearly applicable to both insomnia and headache treatment. Role-playing is an approach used for patients whose primary stress and headache precipitates tend to be conflictual interpersonal situations.

Stress inoculation follows logically from the strategy of cognitive restructuring in which patients become familiar with monitoring their thoughts, feelings, and behaviors when experiencing headaches or insomnia.[134,135] This approach introduces patients to a plan for problem solving concerning episodes of insomnia or exacerbations of headaches. Stress inoculation teaches patients how to break down episodes of insomnia or headache into several manageable steps. The first step is for patients to recognize that episodes of insomnia or the flare-up of a headache require a period of preparation, followed by an attempt to actually manage the headache or sleep difficulty. Next, patients make an effort to cope with thoughts and feelings at critical moments. Finally, patients review how they handled the episode and credit themselves for their efforts at coping. In the preparation phase, patients recognize that there are many periods during which they are not experiencing headaches or that there are nights when they sleep reasonably well. Patients are encouraged to recognize early signs of headaches or difficulty falling asleep and to maintain a positive attitude. Patients can say to themselves, "I am beginning to worry about the headache and I am becoming anxious, but I am reminding myself that I have ways to deal with the headache." Patients then notice an increase in the headache or sleep disturbance and confront these symptoms with the behavioral and cognitive coping techniques they have acquired. At this point patients could employ a combination of relaxation, imagery, and attention-diversion strategies. However, there will be times when the strategies do not work. When this happens, patients may become discouraged because the headache is increasing or fearful that the insomnia will return. At these critical moments the patient employs coping statements such as, "I may not eliminate the headache completely but if I persist I know I can make myself more comfortable," or, "If I let myself become too anxious I will have more difficulty falling asleep." Finally, after the episode resolves and symptoms diminish, patients are expected to review how the episode was handled and to consider what could be done differently the next time. Patients are also told that they must credit themselves with their efforts regardless of the relative effectiveness of the strategies.[9,134]

Role-playing is another approach directed at consolidating patients' coping skills. Patients identify situations in which interactions with another person consistently elicits increased distress or headache.[9,124] The situation is then reenacted, with the therapist assuming the role of the patient while the patient plays the role of the antagonist. The therapist attempts to model appropriate coping strategies including assertive communication, breathing exercises, and coping self-statements. A variation on role-playing is role-reversal in which the patient plays the therapist and the therapist assumes the role of a new patient consulting with the therapist. In this version of role-playing the patient has an opportunity to convince the therapist that he or she can learn to manage headaches. The patient might also teach the therapist, in the role-reversal, how to employ the various coping strategies the actual patient has learned.[9,124]

Relapse Management

In this final phase of C-B treatment patients are asked to focus on circumstances in which they might be prone to relapse.[107,124] This discussion is not intended to suggest to patients that they are expected to fail in managing their headaches or sleep disturbances. Rather, it is to recognize that they will likely experience exacerbations of their headache or recurrence of their insomnia and that these situations may challenge the patients' coping resources. Once these high-risk situations are identified, patients are encouraged to problem solve how they will handle particular situations. During this final stage of treatment patients are asked to review what they have learned and to compare how they were feeling and functioning at the beginning of treatment with how they are currently feeling and functioning. It is particularly useful for patients to review the headache logs or sleep diaries they have been maintaining since beginning treatment. Ultimately, the goal of this stage of treatment is to reinforce for patients the following:

1. They have developed a repertoire of coping strategies that have been effective in reducing their headaches or improving their sleep.
2. The success of these strategies has been a function of their efforts.
3. Their continued success depends on their continued adherence to these strategies.[107,135]

SUMMARY

CBT has been demonstrated empirically to be a therapeutic intervention for a wide variety of psychiatric[136] and medical disorders.[25-59] However, its clinical application to neurologic diseases has been limited, and research supporting CBT's efficacy has been demonstrated primarily in epilepsy, headache, and insomnia.[60-106] This chapter attempts to provide a conceptual model of CBT and to demonstrate its applicability to neurologic disorders. The intent is to inform concerning both the utility and practicality of CBT for neurologic disease. It is further hoped that the examples on applying CBT to headache and sleep disorders will inspire confidence in introducing and preparing patients with neurologic disease for referral for CBT when appropriate.

References

1. Blair DT, Ramones VA: Education as psychiatric intervention: the cognitive-behavioral context, *J Psychiatr Nurs* 35(12):29-36, 1997.
2. Bandura A: *Principles of behavior modification,* New York, 1969, Holt, Rinehart & Winston.
3. Beck AT: *Cognitive therapy and emotional disorders,* New York, 1976, International University Press.
4. Beck AT, Emery G: *Anxiety disorders and phobias: a cognitive perspective,* New York, 1985, Basic Books.
5. Michenbaum DH: *Cognitive-behavior modification,* New York, 1977, Plenum Press.
6. Michenbaum DH, Cameron R: Cognitive behavior therapy. In Wilson GT, Franks CM, editors: *Contemporary behavior therapy,* New York, 1982, Guilford Press.
7. Turk DC, Rudy TE: A cognitive-behavioral perspective on chronic pain: beyond the scalpel and syringe. In Tollison CD, editor: *Handbook of chronic pain management,* Baltimore, 1989, Williams & Wilkins.
8. Kendall PC, Braswell L: *Cognitive-behavioral therapy for impulsive children,* New York, 1985, Guilford Press.
9. Witkower A: Behavioral medicine assessment and treatment.
10. McKay M, Paleg K: *Focal group psychotherapy,* Oakland, Calif., New Harbinger.
11. Beck AT et al: *Cognitive therapy of depression,* New York, 1979, Guilford Press.
12. DeRubeis et al: A mega-analysis of cognitive therapy versus pharmacotherapy for severely depressed patients, Unpublished manuscript.
13. Hollon SD et al: Cognitive therapy and pharmacotherapy for depression: singly and in combination, *Arch Gen Psychiatry* 49:774, 1992.
14. Murphy GE et al: Cognitive therapy and pharmacotherapy, *Arch Gen Psychiatry* 41:33, 1984.
15. Rush AJ et al: Comparative efficacy of cognitive therapy and pharmacotherapy in the treatment of depressed patients, *Cogn Ther Res* 1:17, 1997.
16. Kovacs M et al: Depressed outpatients treated with cognitive therapy or pharmacotherapy: a one year follow-up, *Arch Gen Psychiatry* 38:33, 1981.
17. Simons AD et al: Cognitive therapy and pharmacotherapy for depression: sustained improvement over one year, *Arch Gen Psychiatry* 43:43, 1986.
18. Beck AT, Emery G: *Anxiety disorders and phobias: a cognitive perspective,* New York, 1985, Basic Books.
19. Chambless DL, Gillis MM: Cognitive therapy of anxiety disorders, *J Consult Clin Psychol* 61:248, 1993.
20. Arntz A, van den Hout MA: Psychological treatment of panic disorder without agoraphobia: cognitive therapy versus applied relaxation, *Behav Res ther* 34:113, 1996.
21. Barlow DH et al: Behavioral treatment of panic disorder, *Behav Ther* 20:261, 1989.
22. Klosko JS et al: A comparison of alprazolam and behavior therapy in treatment of panic disorder, *J Consult Clin Psychol* 58:77, 1990.
23. Williams SL, Falbo J: Cognitive and performance-based treatments for panic attacks in people with varying degrees of agoraphobic disability, *Behav Res ther* 34:253, 1996.
24. Clark DM et al: A comparison of cognitive therapy, applied relaxation and imipramine in the treatment of panic disorder, *Br J Psychiatry* 164:759, 1994.
25. Sharpe M: Cognitive behavior therapy for functional somatic complaints: the example of chronic fatigue syndrome, *Psychosomatics* 38:356-362, 1997.
26. Kroenke K, Arrington ME, Manglesdorf D: The prevalence of symptoms in medical outpatients and the adequacy of therapy, *Arch Intern Med* 150:1685, 1990.
27. Sharpe M, Peveler R, Mayou R: The psychological treatment of patients with functional somatic symptoms: a practical guide, *J Psychosom Res* 36:515-529, 1992.
28. Sharpe M: Cognitive behavior therapy. In Demitrack M, Abbey S, editors: *Psychiatric aspects of chronic fatigue syndrome,* New York, 1996, Guilford Press.
29. Sharpe M et al: Cognitive behavior therapy for chronic fatigue syndrome: a randomized controlled trial, *BMJ* 312:22-26, 1996.
30. Deale A et al: Cognitive behavior therapy for chronic fatigue syndrome: a randomized controlled trial, *Am J Psychiatry* 154:408-444, 1977.
31. Klimes I et al: Psychological treatment for atypical noncardiac chest pain: a controlled evaluation, *Psychol Med* 20:605-611, 1990.
32. Greene B, Blanchard EB: Cognitive therapy for irritable bowel syndrome, *J Consult Clin Psychol* 62:576-582, 1994.
33. Neff DF, Blanchard EB: A multicomponent treatment for irritable bowel syndrome, *Behav Ther* 18:70-73, 1987.
34. Blanchard EB et al: Two controlled evaluations of a multicomponent psychological treatment of irritable bowel syndrome, *Behav Res Ther* 2:175-179, 1992.
35. Warwick HM et al: A controlled trial of cognitive behavioral treatment of hypochondriasis, *Br J Psychiatry* 169:189-195, 1996.
36. Speckens AE et al: Cognitive behavior therapy for medically unexplained physical symptoms: a randomized controlled trial, *BMJ* 311:1328-1332, 1995.
37. Dobie TG, May JG: Generalization of tolerance to motion environments, *Aviat Space Environ Med* 61:707-711, 1990.

38. Dobie TG, Fischer WD, Bologna NB: An evaluation of cognitive-behavioral therapy for training resistance to visually-induced motion sickness, *Aviat Space Environ Med* 58:A31-41, 1987.

39. Reason JT, Brand JJ: *Motion sickness,* New York, 1975, Academic Press.

40. Burish TG, Snyder SL, Jenkins RA: Preparing patients for cancer chemotherapy: effect of coping preparation and relaxation interventions, *J Consult Clin Psychol* 59:518-525, 1991.

41. Greer S et al: Adjuvant psychological therapy for patients with cancer: a prospective randomized trial, *Br Med J* 304:675-680, 1992.

42. Blythe BJ, Erdahl JC: Using stress inoculation to prepare a patient for open-heart surgery, *Health Soc Work* 4:265-274, 1986.

43. Smith KE, Acherson JD, Blotcky AD: Reducing distress during invasive medical procedures: relating behavioural interventions to preferred coping style in paediatric cancer patients, *J Pediatr Psychol* 3:405-419, 1989.

44. Wells JV, Howard GS, Nowlin WF et al: Presurgical anxiety and post-surgical pain and adjustment: effects of a stress inoculation procedure, *J Consult Clin Psychol* 54(6):831-835, 1986.

45. Fawzy FI et al: A structured psychiatric intervention for cancer: Changes over time in methods of coping and affective disturbance, *Arch Gen Psychiatry* 47:720-725, 1990.

46. Fishman B, Loscalzo M: Cognitive-behavioural interventions in management of cancer pain: principles and applications, *Med Clin North Am* 4:71-82, 1987.

47. Telch CF, Telch MJ: Psychological approaches to enhancing coping among cancer patients: a review, *Clin Psychol Rev* 54:325-344,1985.

48. Pope AM , Tarlov, editors: *Disability in America: toward a national agenda for prevention,* Washington, DC, 1991, National Academy Press.

49. Bradley LA et al: Effects of psychological therapy on pain behavior of rheumatoid arthritis patients: treatment outcome and six-month follow-up, *Arthritis Rheum* 30:1105-1114,1987.

50. O'Leary A et al: A cognitive-behavioral treatment for rheumatoid arthritis, *Health Psychol* 7:527-544, 1988.

51. Bucklew SP, Parker JC: Coping with arthritis pain: a review of the literature, *Arth Care Res* 2:136-145, 1988.

52. Bennett P, Carroll D: Cognitive-behavioral interventions in cardiac rehabilitation, *J Psychosom Res* 38(3):169-182, 1994.

53. Freidman M et al: Alteration of type A behavior and its effect on cardiac recurrences in postmyocardial infarction patients: summary results of the recurrent coronary prevention project, *Am Heart J* 112:653-665, 1986.

54. Revel KF, Baer PE, Cleveland SE: Stress management in cardiovascular disease: postmyocardial infarction patients. In Russell ML, editor: *Stress management in chronic disease,* New York, 1988, Pergamon.

55. Langosch W et al: Behavior therapy with coronary heart disease patients: results of a comparative study, *J Psychosom Res* 26:475-484, 1982.

56. Oldenburg B, Perkins RJ, Andrews G: Controlled trial of psychological intervention in myocardial infarction, *J Consult Clin Psychol* 53:852-859, 1985.

57. Dunbar SB, Summerville JG: Cognitive therapy for ventricular dysrhythmia patients, *J Cardiovasc Nurs* 12(1):33-44, 1997.

58. Finkelmeir B, Kenwood N, Summers C: Psychological ramifications of surviving sudden cardiac death, *Crit Care Q* 7:71-79, 1984.

59. Vlay SC, Ficchione GL: Psychosocial aspects of surviving sudden cardiac death, *Clin Cardiol* 8:237-243, 1985.

60. Lesser RP: Psychogenic seizures. In Pedley TA, Meldrum BS, editors: *Recent advances in epilepsy: number 2,* Edinburgh, 1985, Churchill-Livingstone.

61. Goldstein LH: Behavioral and cognitive-behavioral treatments for epilepsy: a progress review, *Br J Clin Psychol* 29:257-269, 1990.

62. Montgomery JM, Espie CA: Behavioural management of hysterical pseudo seizures, *Behav Psychother* 14:334-340, 1986.

63. Fenwick P: Precipitation and inhibition of seizures. In Reynolds E, Trimble M, editors: *Epilepsy and psychiatry,* London, 1981, Churchill-Livingstone.

64. Fenwick PB, Brown SB: Evoked and psychogenic seizures: precipitation, *Acta Neurol Scand* 80:541-547, 1989.

65. Temkin N, Davis G: Stress as a risk factor for seizures among adults with epilepsy, *Epilepsia* 25:450-456, 1984.

66. Fenwick PB: Behavioral treatment of epilepsy, *Postgrad Med J* 66:336-338, 1990.

67. Aird RB: The importance of seizure-inducing factors in the control of refractory forms of epilepsy, *Epilepsia* 24:567-583, 1983.

68. Dahl J et al: Effects of a broad spectrum behavior modification treatment program on children with refractory epilepsy seizures, *Epilepsia* 26:303-309, 1985.

69. Dahl J, Melin L, Leissner P: Effects of a behavioural intervention on epileptic behavior and paroxysmal activity: a systematic replication of three cases of children with intractable epilepsy, *Epilepsia* 29:172-183, 1988.

70. Tan SY, Bruni J: Cognitive-behaviour therapy with adult patients with epilepsy: a controlled outcome study, *Epilepsia* 27:225-233, 1986.

71. Davis GR et al: Cognitive-behavioral treatments of depressed affect among epileptics: preliminary findings, *J Clin Psychol* 40:930-935, 1984.

72. Lundth L-G: Cognitive-behavioural analysis and treatment of insomnia, *Scand J Behav Ther* 27(1):10-29, 1998.

73. Liljenberg B et al: Age and prevalence of insomnia in adulthood, *Eur J Psychiatry* 3:5-12, 1989.

74. Mellinger GD, Balter MB, Uhlenhuth EH: Insomnia and its treatment, *Arch Gen Psychiatry* 42:225-232, 1985.

75. Borkovec TD, Fowles DC: Controlled investigation of the effects of progressive and hypnotic relaxation on insomnia, *J Abnorm Psychol* 82:153-158, 1973.

76. Bootzin RR: Stimulus control treatment for insomnia, *Proceedings of the American Psychological Association* 7:395-396, 1972.

77. Ascher LM, Turner RM: Paradoxical intention and insomnia: an experimental investigation, *Behav Res Ther* 17:408-411, 1979.

78. Hauri P: *The sleep disorders,* Kalamazoo, Mich., 1982, Upjohn.

79. Woolfolk RL, McNulty TF: Relaxation training for insomnia: a component analysis, *J Consult Clin Psychol* 51:495-503, 1983.

80. Spielman AJ, Saskin P, Thorpy MJ: Treatment of chronic insomnia by restriction of time in bed, *Sleep* 10:45-56, 1987.

81. Levey AB et al: Articulatory suppression and the treatment of insomnia, *Behav Res Ther* 29(1):85-89, 1991.

82. Morin CM: *Insomnia: psychological assessment and management,* New York, 1993, Guilford Press.

83. Morin CM, Culbert JP, Schwartz SM: Nonpharmacological interventions for insomnia: a meta-analysis of treatment efficacy, *Am J Psychiatry* 151:1172-1180, 1994.

84. Murtagh DR, Greenwood KM: Identifying effective treatments for insomnia: a meta-analysis, *J Consult Clin Psychol* 63:79-89, 1995.

85. Sanavio E et al: Behavior therapy for DIMS: comparison of three treatment procedures with follow-up, *Behav Ther* 18:151-167, 1990.

86. Lipton RB, Silverstein SD, Stewart WF: An update on the epidemiology of migraine, *Headache* 34:319-328, 1994.

87. Rasmussen BK et al: Epidemiology of headache in a general population: a prevalence study, *J Clin Epidemiol* 44:1147-1157, 1991.

88. Linet MS et al: An epidemiologic study of headache among adolescents and young adults, *JAMA* 261:2211-2216, 1989.

89. Holroyd KA, Andrasik F: A cognitive-behavioral approach to recurrent tension and migraine headache. In Kendall PC, editor: *Advances in cognitive-behavioral research and therapy,* vol 1, Orlando, 1982.

90. Mosley TH, Grothues CA, Meeks WM: Treatment of tension headache in the elderly: a controlled evaluation of relaxation training and relaxation training combined with cognitive-behavioral therapy, *J Clin Geropsychol* 1:175-188, 1995.

91. Gauthier JG, Ivers H, Carrier S: Nonpharmacological approaches in the management of recurrent headache disorders and their comparison and combination with pharmacotherapy, *Clin Psychol Rev* 6:543-571, 1996.

92. Holroyd KA, Andrasik F, Westbrook T: Cognitive control of tension headache, *Cogn Ther Res* 1:121-133, 1977.

93. Bakal DA, Demjen S, Kaganow JA: Cognitive-behavioral treatment of chronic headache, *Headache* 21:81-86, 1981.

94. Newton CR, Barbaree HE: Cognitive changes accompanying headache treatment: the use of a thought-sampling procedure, *Cogn Ther Res* 11:635-652, 1987.

95. Richardson GM, McGrath PJ: Cognitive-behavioral therapy for migraine headaches: a minimal-therapist-contact approach versus a clinic-based approach, *Headache* 29:352-357, 1989.

96. Holroyd KA, Andrasik F: Coping and the self-control of chronic tension headache, *J Consult Clin Psychol* 46:1036-45, 1978.

97. Holroyd KA, Andrasik F: Do the effects of cognitive therapy endure?: a two year follow-up of the tension headache sufferers treated with cognitive therapy or biofeedback, *Cogn Ther Res* 6:325-334, 1982.

98. McGrath PJ et al: The efficacy and efficiency of a self-administered treatment for adolescent migraine, *Pain* 49:321-324, 1992.

99. Richter IL et al: Cognitive and relaxation treatment of paediatric migraine, *Pain* 25:195-203, 1986.

100. Figueroa JL: Group treatment of chronic tension headache: a comparative treatment study, *Behav Modif* 6:229-239, 1982.

101. Sorbi M, Tellegen B: Differential effects of training in relaxation and stress-coping in patients with migraine, *Headache* 26:473-481, 1986.

102. Knapp TW: Treating migraine by training in temporal artery vasoconstriction and/or cognitive behavioral coping: a one year follow-up, *J Psychosom Res* 26:551-557, 1982b.

103. Sorbi M, Tellegen B, Du Long A: Long-term effects of training in relaxation and stress-coping in patients with migraine: a 3-year follow-up, *Headache* 29:111-121, 1989.

104. Blanchard EB et al: Placebo-controlled evaluation of abbreviated progressive muscle relaxation and of relaxation combined with cognitive therapy in the treatment of tension headache, *J Consult Clin Psychol* 58:210-215, 1990.

105. Murphy AI, Lehrer PM, Jurish S: Cognitive coping skills training and relaxation training as treatments for tension headaches, *Behav Ther* 21:89-98, 1990.

106. Tobin DL et al: Developmental and clinical trial of a minimal contact, cognitive-behavioral treatment for tension headache, *Cogn Ther Res* 12:325-339, 1988.

107. Holtzman AD, Turk DC, Kerns RD: The cognitive-behavioral approach to the management of chronic pain. In Holtzman, AD Turk, DC, editors: *Pain management: a handbook of psychological treatment approaches,* Elmsford, NY, 1986, Pergamon Press.

108. Ellis A: *Reason and emotion in psychotherapy,* New York, 1962, Lyle, Stuart, and Citadel Press.

109. Goldfried M: Systematic desensitization as training in self-control, *J Consult Clin Psychol,* 37:228-234, 1971.

110. Mahoney MJ: Personal science: a cognitive learning therapy. In Ellis A, Greiger R, editors: *Handbook of rational psychotherapy,* New York, 1977, Springer.

111. Bradley LA: Cognitive-behavioral therapy for chronic pain. In Gatchel RJ, Turk DC, editors: *Psychological approaches to pain management: a practitioner's handbook,* New York, 1996, Guilford Press.

112. Ott BD: Behavioral interventions in the management of chronic pain. In Aronoff GM, editor: *Evaluation and treatment of chronic pain,* Baltimore, 1992, Williams & Wilkins.

113. Bernstein DA, Borkovec TD: *Progressive relaxation training: a manual for the helping professions,* Champaign, Ill., 1973, Research Press.

114. Kroger WS, Fezler WD: Hypnosis and behavior modification: imagery conditioning, Philadelphia, 1976, Lippincott.

115. Blanchard EB, Andrasik F: *Management of chronic headaches: a psychological approach,* Elmsford, NY, 1985, Pergamon Press.

116. Martin PR: *Psychological management of chronic headaches,* New York, 1993, Guilford Press.

117. Packard RC: What does the headache patient want? *Headache* 19:370-374, 1979.

118. Martin PR: *Psychological management of chronic headaches,* New York, 1993, Guilford Press.

119. Holzman AD: Chronic headaches. In Holzman AD, Turk DC, editors: *Pain management: a handbook of psychological treatment approaches,* New York, 1986, Pergamon Press.

120. Espie CA: ABC of sleep disorders, *Br Med J* 306:509-511, 1993.

121. Lichstein KL, Reidel BW: Behavioral assessment and treatment of insomnia: a review with an emphasis on clinical application, *Behav Ther* 25:659-688, 1994.

122. Hauri PJ: Sleep hygiene, relaxation therapy, and cognitive interventions. In Hauri PJ, editor: *Case studies in insomnia,* New York, 1991, Plenum.

123. Belar CD, Kibrick SA: Biofeedback in the treatment of chronic back pain. In Holzman AD, Turk DC, editors: *Pain management: a handbook of psychological treatment approaches,* New York, 1986, Pergamon Press.

124. Turk DC, Michenbaum D, Genest M: *Pain and behavioral medicine,* New York, 1983, Guilford Press.

125. Jacobson E: *Progressive relaxation,* Chicago, 1938, University of Chicago Press.

126. Borkovec TD, Fowles DC: Controlled investigation of the effects of progressive and hypnotic relaxation on insomnia, *J Abnorm Psychol* 82:153-158, 1973.

127. Schultz JH, Luthe W: *Autogenic training: a psychological approach in psychotherapy,* New York, 1959, Grune & Stratton.

128. Woolfolk RL et al: Meditation training as a treatment for insomnia, *Behav Ther* 7:359-365, 1976.

129. Hanson RW, Gerber KE: *Coping with chronic pain,* New York, 1990, Guilford Press.

130. Morin CM, Mimeault V, Gagne A: Nonpharmacological treatment of late-life insomnia, *J Psychosom Res* 46(2):103-116, 1999.

131. Espie CA: *The psychological treatment of insomnia,* New York, 1991, Wiley.

132. Engle-Friedman M et al: An evaluation of behavioral treatments for insomnia in the older adult, *J Clin Psychol* 48:77-90, 1992.

133. Espie CA, Lindsay WR: Cognitive strategies for the management of severe sleep-maintenance insomnia: a preliminary investigation, *Behav Psychother* 15:388-395, 1987.

134. Meichenbaum DH, Turk DC: The cognitive behavioral management of anxiety, anger, and pain. In Davidson PO, editor: *The behavioral management of anxiety, depression, and pain,* New York, 1976, Brunner & Mazel.

135. Meichenbaum D, Turk DC: *Facilitating treatment adherence: a practitioner's guidebook,* New York, 1987, Plenum Press.

136. DeRubeis RJ, Crits-Christoph P: Empirically supported individual and group psychological treatments for adult mental disorders, *J Consult Clin Psychol* 66(1):37-52, 1998.

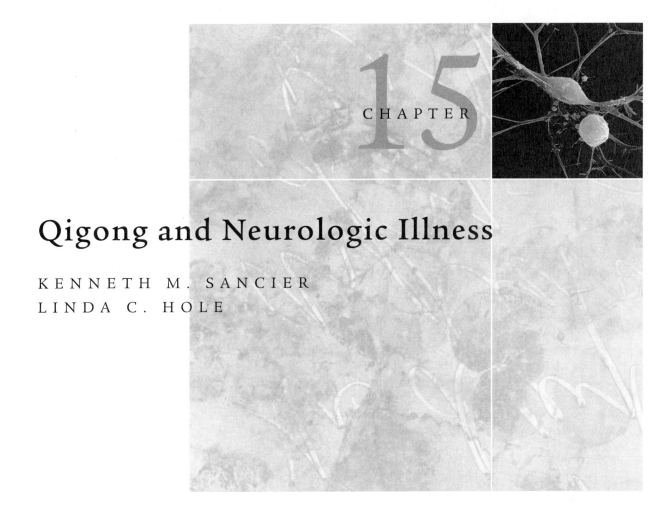

CHAPTER

15

Qigong and Neurologic Illness

KENNETH M. SANCIER

LINDA C. HOLE

SECTION 1: A SCIENTIFIC RESEARCH APPROACH

KENNETH M. SANCIER

Qigong is an ancient Chinese meditative moving exercise that is similar to, but more profound, than T'ai Chi Ch'uan. Qigong has been practiced in China for thousands of years to improve health and longevity.[1] There are many qigong clinics in China, and in some hospitals qigong is integrated with traditional Chinese medicine and conventional Western medicine. The practice of qigong is divided into three main applications: medical, spiritual, and martial. This chapter reviews clinical studies of qigong's effect on various neurologic illnesses and discusses mechanisms by which qigong promotes healing.

Recent scientific research has shown that qigong does indeed have profound health benefits and the author has published several experimental studies and reviews of clinical studies of qigong.[3-6]

The benefits of qigong can be achieved by self-practice, but for serious illness a qigong therapist may be required to diagnose the illness and recommend suitable exercises. In diagnosing, the qigong therapist senses the patient's body field for blocks to the flow of qi. The therapist may also diagnose according to traditional Chinese medicine by examining the tongue, eyes, and pulses at the radial artery of the wrist. Qigong therapy includes prescribed qigong exercises and treatment with emitted qi in serious cases. Qigong is well suited for treating chronic health problems such as hypertension, asthma, cardiovascular disease, stress, pain, and aging. It can also reduce the side effects of chemotherapy and radiation therapy. Qigong can increase the effectiveness of Western medications, even allowing the use of smaller doses, which reduces the risk of undesirable side effects.[5]

The basic principles of qigong—meditation, awareness, movement, and breathing—underlie several complementary energy exercises that are practiced in Western hospitals and are paid for by insurance. Among these exercises are yoga, therapeutic touch, T'ai Chi Ch'uan and mindful meditation. Yoga is prescribed as part of Dean Ornish's therapy for reversing heart disease,[8] and his cardiac health program is administered in hospitals and is covered by some major insurance companies.[9] Therapeutic touch has some of the elements of emitted qi wherein the therapist, often without touching, balances the patient's body energy. Therapeutic touch is taught to thousands of nurses and is practiced in about 100 health facilities[10] and 80 North American hospitals.[11] T'ai Chi Ch'uan, which derives from Chinese martial art, is considered an offshoot of qigong. T'ai Chi Ch'uan was included in a study of the effects of exercise in preventing falls by elderly patients.[12] John Kabat-Zinn's Mindfulness-Based Stress Reduction Therapy is a meditation exercise that promotes awareness of the mind and body, which is offered in many hospitals and clinics in the United States.[13] This therapy has been applied to physical pain.

SOURCES OF INFORMATION

This chapter endeavors to provide information from scientific research studies to help validate the healing benefits of qigong, but various obstacles to collecting high-quality research do exist. Until recently, almost all of the research on qigong was done by scientists in China, and these studies were reported mainly at scientific meetings. Few studies are published in China because suitable scientific journals are not available. The studies that are published are usually in Chinese. A rich source of information about research is the abstracts in English that are

printed in the proceedings of international conferences on qigong. These abstracts range in length from a paragraph to several pages. Some abstracts are minipapers with tables and statistical analysis, however many details are missing.

The abstracts in English since 1986 have been collected in the Computerized Qigong Database,™ which presently contains about 1660 citations taken from proceedings of meetings, scientific journals, and Medline.* Although there are many clinical studies of the benefits of qigong, too few meet current scientific standards. In addition, the English in the abstracts from proceedings often leaves much to be desired. However, these limitations should not be an obstacle to appreciating the significant body of research on medical applications of qigong. The reader is also asked to keep in mind the difficulties that the researchers in China encountered. For centuries qigong was a secret art passed on to only one person in a family. During the cultural revolution qigong was essentially outlawed and qigong masters were persecuted. In the late 1970s, after the cultural revolution ended, research was initiated to demonstrate that qigong was based in science rather than superstition, as the Communists feared. Many of the research studies were carried out in hospitals by staff members who were poorly trained in science, while many qigong masters worked full time in factories.

SCOPE OF REVIEW

Qigong has a wide scope of medical applications, and some studies that pertain to neurologic illnesses are discussed in the following sections. Searching the qigong database for selected neurologic-related words indicates the range of such studies. The number of references pertaining to selected neurologic terms that appear in the database are shown in Table 15-1.

Some terms relating to neurologic illness that do not appear in the database are brain damage, carpal, coma, chronic fatigue syndrome, multiple sclerosis, palsy, peripheral neuropathy, radicular, seizure, stress headache, and transient ischemic attack (TIA).

---

*For information about the Qigong Database, contact the Qigong Institute, 561 Berkeley Avenue, Menlo Park, CA 94025, or at http://www.qigonginstitute.org.

TABLE 15-1

The Number of References of Selected Neurologic Terms Appearing in the Qigong Database with References

Neurologic terms	Number	References
Anesthesia	7	14-20
Anxiety	14	21-34
Circulatory disturbance	5	35-39
Dementia	2	40, 41
Dizziness	4	42-45
Neuro (-pathy, -logic, -logical)	3	46-48
Neuromuscular	17	19, 37, 49, 50, 50-63
Pain	19	14, 16, 18, 37, 38, 49, 54, 57, 59-61, 63-70
Back	10	51, 57, 61, 63, 71-76
Headache	6	24, 53, 76-79
Migraine	2	80, 81
Neck and shoulder	2	54, 59
Paralysis	11	15, 82, 83, 83-90
Parkinson's Disease	2	91, 92
Psychosomatic	10	23, 24, 26, 30, 34, 93-97
Stroke	8	40, 79, 84, 98-102
Tinnitus	1	103
Vertigo	1	77

QIGONG'S EFFECT ON NEUROLOGIC ILLNESS

Some of the best clinical studies have been chosen to illustrate qigong's potential for treating neurologic illnesses. These studies are grouped under several main descriptors of neurologic disorders. For each clinical study, a brief description is provided of objectives, methods of treatment, and results. Where appropriate, present author has added comments about the study.

Paralysis

Hemiplegia and Paraplegia

Huang combined emitted qi with self-practice of qigong to treat paralysis in 19 cases of hemiplegia and 24 cases of paraplegia.[15] The Qigong masters emitted their qi to the acupuncture meridians of the patients two to three times a day. They also emitted qi while massaging energy (acupuncture) points of the patient once every other day. Under the instruction of a qigong master and according to the condition of the patient, the patients practiced qigong exercise one to two times a day. Improvements that were brought about by the qigong therapy are summarized in Table 15-2.

The authors report that the overall effect of treatment was excellent in 10 cases (23.3%), good in 20 cases (46.5%), fair in 10 cases (23.3%), and poor in 3 cases (7.0%). The total effective rate was 93.0% (excellent + good + fair). The authors also reported relief of symptoms in areas such as mental state, sleep, appetite, perspiration (limbs), and speaking ability.

Facial Paralysis

Xu reported that yoga is especially effective for treating facial paralysis.[83] Yoga, as it was used in this study, is similar to qigong because the therapists emitted energy from their fingers while massaging the patient. Therapists used contact or noncontact therapy to treat the disease. They tried to make the flow of energy (qi) rotate around the patient's face by using pushing, pressing, kneading, scrubbing, vibrating, and grasping manipulations. The massage points were mainly on the head at 13 acupuncture points associated with the

TABLE 15-2

Improvement in Conditions of Patients with Hemiplegia and Paraplegia after Therapy by Emitted Qi and Self-Practice of Qigong

Condition	Subjects	Improvements after therapy
Changes in myodynamics of paralyzed limbs	35	Increased range of motion from 0-2 to 3-5 degrees for 34 cases
Walking: Before treatment 37 of the 43 paralytic patients needed support	43	23 patients could walk without help, 20 patients still required crutches, but some only 1 crutch instead of 2
Managing daily life	43	Increased from 7 to 34 cases

meridians as described according to traditional Chinese medicine. The treatment focused primarily on the disordered side, and an accessory treatment, such as acupuncture, was applied to the healthy side of the face. While being treated, the patient could sit, lie, or stand. According to the author, the treatment relaxes muscles and tendons to open the meridians, activate blood circulation, and decrease stagnant energy conditions.

Of the 31 people who were treated, 22 were men and 19 women. The age range was 19 to 40 years in 22 cases, 41 to 55 years in 6 cases, and older than 60 years in 3 cases. Nine of the cases had been of a 10-day duration, six had continued for 6 months to 1 year, ten had lasted for 1 to 3 years, and six cases had endured for more than three years. Nine of the 31 cases had hemiplegia caused by cerebral hemorrhage complicated by facial paralysis that was marked by distortion of the mouth and eye and disturbance of speech. The total effective rate in the 31 cases was 96.8% and the failure rate was 3.2%.

Comments: This study indicates that some forms of paralysis can be treated successfully with a combination of emitted qi and self-practice of qigong exercises. Apparently, qigong was able to restore the damaged nervous system of paralyzed parts of the body. Perhaps limited by the nature of the abstract format, information was not included on the effectiveness of therapy according to duration and severity of the illnesses.

Pain

Spine-Related Diseases

Liu reported clinical studies of 292 cases of spine-related diseases that were treated with a combination of qigong and Chinese and Western medicines.[51] In these studies, the back was usually chosen as the treatment site when internal organs had problems. According to Chinese medicine many of the meridians associated with internal organs are located along the *Du* Channel, which runs down the back. To open up the meridians through which qi flows, treatments included traction by qigong, Chinese massage, and emitted qi. Results of the treatment of 18 diseases and conditions were reported. The total effective rate for all treatment of all 18 diseases was reported to be 97.7%. Data relevant to neurologic illness are summarized in Table 15-3.

Frozen Shoulder and Tennis Elbow

Gao reported on qigong's curative effect in treating 32 cases of frozen shoulder and tennis elbow.[59] The patients included 8 men and 24 women who were from 27 to 76 years old. Their histories of neuromuscular problems ranged from 1 week to 2 years. The author emitted qi for 5 to 10 minutes to the patient's shoulder or elbow without touching the patient. Acupressure and massage were applied after the external qi treatment. Shaking, vibrating, and other massage techniques were applied to the elbow or arm for approximately 10 to 30 minutes with treatments 2 to 3 times a week.

Most patients experienced relief from symptoms, such as insomnia caused by pain, difficulty in holding objects, or difficulty moving the shoulder or arm. Six patients (18.8%) received complete relief from the first visit; seven patients (21.9%) believed that most symptoms disappeared after 2 to 5 treatments; thirteen patients (40.6%) had noticeably effective or improved conditions after 6 to 15 treatments; four patients (12.5%)

TABLE 15-3

Clinical Effects of Treatments of Spine-Related Diseases by a Combination of Qigong and Chinese and Western Medicines

Disease	Total cases (No.)	Cured (No.)	Markedly effective (No.)	Improved (No.)	No effect (No.)
Prolapsed lumbar	108	95	10	2	1
Dislocated thoracic lumbar disks	26	12	5	7	2
Herniation cervical disk	70	59	7	3	1
Hyperostosis cervical spine	10	8	2		
Chronic lumbosacral pain	18	8	6	3	1

TABLE 15-4

Comparison of the Therapeutic Benefits of Qigong and Herbal Therapies for Cases of Ankle Joint Sprain

Group	Total patients (No.)	Marked effectiveness (No.)	Effective (No.)	Failure (No.)	Cure (%)
Qigong	50	39	8	3	94
Herbal	47	35	9	3	94

interrupted treatment after 2 to 4 treatments; and two cases failed (6.3%). The total effective rate was 81.2%.

Comments: Frozen shoulder and tennis elbow are difficult to treat by conventional medicine, but this study suggests that a combination of emitted qi and massage is beneficial.

Ankle Joint Sprains

Huang reported a clinical study comparing qigong and herbal therapies in cases of ankle joint sprain.[60] For the qigong group (n = 50) the average age was 30.2 years (range 16 to 43) and the average course of the injury was 4.5 days (range 1 to 15 days). For the herbal group (n = 47) the average age was 30.1 years (range 17 to 41) and the average course of the injury was 4.3 days (range 1 to 14). For both groups, the first step was bone setting. Qigong therapy consisted of emitting qi to the afflicted area while performing rotating and sweeping manipulations for 20 minutes a day for 7 days. Herbal therapy consisted of applying Chinese herbs to the affected areas once a day for 7 days. The results are summarized in Table 15-4.

Comments: A statistical difference was not found between the two groups (p > 0.05), so the results show

that qigong and Chinese herbs are both effective in treating injury of soft tissue.

Fibromyalgia

Singh et al. reported a pilot study of cognitive behavioral therapy for fibromyalgia, a syndrome characterized by widespread musculoskeletal pain, multiple tender points, high levels of self-reported disability, and poor quality of life.[104] In this pilot study, a mind-body approach (cognitive-behavioral therapy), which has been successful in treating chronic back pain, was tested to determine whether the therapy would improve function, decrease perceived pain, and improve mood state for fibromyalgia patients.

Twenty-eight patients participated in 8 weekly sessions of 2 1/2 hours each, with three components: an educational component focusing on the mind-body connection; a portion focusing on relaxation response mechanisms (primarily mindfulness meditation techniques); and a qigong movement therapy session. Data collection instruments were the Fibromyalgia Impact Questionnaire, the Health Assessment Questionnaire, the Beck Depression Inventory, the Coping Strategies Questionnaire, the helplessness subscale of the Arthritis Attitudes Index, the Medical Outcomes Study Short Form General Health Survey, and a double-anchored 100-mm visual scale to assess sleep.

Twenty patients completed the study. Standard outcome measures showed significant reduction in pain, fatigue, and sleeplessness; and improvement in functions, mood, and general health following the 8-week intervention. The authors concluded that an effective mind-body adjunctive therapy for patients with fibromyalgia should include patient education, meditation techniques, and movement therapy.

Slipped Disks

Noda describes a short, 1 to 3 minute, qigong treatment for slipped disks that usually result in painful pinched nerves.[57] While the patient lays supine with the arms of the upper body fixed with belts to a therapeutic bed, the qigong therapist focuses his or her qi to a point at the patient's upper chest (*Zhongfu,* lung l) and to a point above the knee (*Xuehai,* spleen l0). The patient's legs are first bent and then pulled straight and slightly upward. This procedure is repeated two or three times. Qigong is then emitted to the patient while he or she is lying on the floor to release concentrated qi to the low back. The released qi radiates within the entire body and moves all the muscles of the body. As the muscles move, the intervertebral disk tries to move back to its original place, pressure is reduced on the nerve fibers, and back pain is decreased. The patient can then freely bend the body forward and backward.

Among more than 2000 clinical cases, 70% were treated successfully by one to three treatments and 15% by four to five treatments. Of the remaining patients, improvement was seen in about 5%, no improvement was observed in about 5%, and the remaining 5% discontinued the treatment.

Comments: The treatment appears to be a combination of qigong and chiropractic therapies. Qigong relaxes the muscles so that a chiropractic maneuver proceeds more readily and effectively.

Arteriosclerotic Obstruction

Agishi reported the effects of emitted qi on 20 patients with arteriosclerotic obstruction.[38,39] Patients were seated with their lower extremities unclothed. The qi therapist held or moved his palms close to the patient's head, lower abdomen, and lower limbs, sometimes gently touching or rubbing. This was done for a period of 20 to 30 minutes, at weekly intervals for 1 to 8 weeks. The therapeutic effectiveness rates are summarized in Table 15-5.

The rise in leg temperature (2° C to 4° C) was measured by thermography, and peripheral blood flow by ultrasonic Doppler flow meter. Plethysmography indicated pulse amplitude and arterial notch.

Comments: This study provides evidence that qigong relieves leg pain due to arteriosclerotic obstruction. The authors propose that qigong improves blood circulation, which may help prevent the arteriosclerotic condition.

Intractable Pain

Omura discussed common factors contributing to intractable pain and approaches using qigong to alleviate pain.[79] He reported that it was possible to relieve pain and circulatory disturbances resulting from spastic muscles or arteries in vasoconstriction by applying qigongized paper, that is, paper to which he had emitted his qi, to an affected area of the body.[37] For a favorable effect, the qigongized paper should have (+) polarity. The polarity on the paper depended upon how the emitted qigong was applied to the paper and from which part of the body it emanated. The polarity on the paper was determined by the Bi-Digital O-Ring Test.

Comments: Omura suggests that the mechanism of qigong's action is to relax diseased or stressed tissues so that blood flow is enhanced to those areas of the body. Increased blood flow to those areas implies more efficient delivery of oxygen, nutrients, and pain-killing substances. This includes the delivery of drugs in the blood and the more efficient removal of metabolic waste products that could contribute to pain.

TABLE 15-5

Effect of Emitted Qi on Relieving Symptoms Associated with Arteriosclerotic Obstruction

Symptoms relieved	Therapeutic effectiveness (%)
Leg pain on walking, leg pain at rest, cold legs	83.3
Leg temperature rise (2° C to 4° C)	90.0
Peripheral blood flow	67.7
Improvement in plethysmography at the toes	72.4

Human Skin Pain Threshold

Zhang et al. reported on the analgesic effect of emitted qi on the human skin pain threshold using potassium mediated pain.[18] Subjects were divided into three groups. Group 1 received emitted qi from a qigong master, group 2 was treated by a non–qigong master, and group 3 was a control, not defined. The results of emitted qi on human skin pain threshold are summarized in Table 15-6.

The authors concluded that emitted qi had an obvious analgesic effect that raised the human skin pain threshold. Further studies of the influence of emitted qi on the cortical-evoked potentials elicited by c-fiber inputs (C-CEP as an index of response of somatosensory cortex to slow pain) in cats led them to suggest that endogenous opiate-like substances are associated with the analgesic effect of emitted qi.

Comments: The pain threshold increased with time after qi therapy, suggesting that the autonomic nervous system continues to respond to the stimulation of emitted qi.

Qigong and Psychotherapy

Mayer discusses an integrated approach to chronic pain relief that combines qigong and psychotherapy.[97] He also outlines an approach for working with anxiety disorders by integrating qigong with Western psychotherapy and hypnotherapy. One of his approaches to pain relief is using microcosmic and macrocosmic orbit breathing. In this form of qigong, subjects use their minds to focus on the breath and to imagine that the qi is circling continuously around the body. The circulating qi helps energy flow through blocks, which may be the cause of pain. Mayer also uses a balancing method that combines the Taoist concept of yin and yang with a hypnotherapeutic technique called "pain transferral." He discusses some case studies that illustrate these approaches.

TABLE 15-6

The Effects of Emitted Qi on Human Skin Pain Threshold

Time after qi emission (min)	Skin pain threshold (μA)	p-value
0	1525.4 ± 92.6	—
2½ to 5	1631.1 ± 89.1	< 0.05
7 to 10	1657.8 ± 93.3	< 0.01

Qigong Anesthesia

Lin reported clinical studies using qigong anesthesia (QA) during the resection of thyroid gland tumors and operations on tongue cysts.[14] The qigong doctor emitted qi from the center of the palm of his hand (*Laogong* point). Thirty-four cases of resection of thyroid gland tumors and cysts were successfully operated on under QA. Judging from the Anaesthetic Effect Standards stipulated at the National Conference of Acupuncture Anesthesia, 17 cases reached grade I, 14 cases grade II, and 3 cases grade III. Grades I and II combined accounted for an effectiveness of 91.1%, showing that QA was fairly effective as anesthesia during surgery.

Machi and Chu reported on physiologic changes that occur during qigong anesthesia.[105] Measurements were made of the physiologic changes that occurred in a qigong master and in the patient undergoing simulated qigong anesthesia, that is, without surgery. Simultaneous measurements included electroencephalogram (EEG), electrocardiogram (ECG), galvanic skin resistance (GSR), skin temperature (by thermography), respiration rate, and plethysmography of a finger. Some of the results observed during emitting and receiving of qi include the following:

1. The alpha waves increased and beta waves decreased in the frontal lobes of both the qigong master and the subject, indicating greater relaxation.
2. The GSR at first increased indicating some tension, but decreased strongly before the end of the anesthesia.
3. The thermography patterns of the face indicated that some areas increased in temperature.
4. Heart rate changes between therapist and subject were synchronized in the final stages of anesthesia.

These phenomena suggest that qigong can control the autonomic nervous system.

Parkinson's Disease

Chen studied the effects of emitted qi for treating Parkinson's disease.[91] He stated that over a period of more than 2 years, his qigong therapy cured hundreds of patients with Parkinson's disease. Chen's approach combined the theory of the Chinese traditional medicine and the basic principles for qigong treatment. The first principle was to establish a diagnosis and prescribe treatment based on an overall analysis of the illness and the patient's condition.

Among 15 patients who came for one course of 60 treatments, seven patients got an obvious effect (46.7%), five patients got a better effect (33.3%), and three patients got a general effect (20%). The definitions of these terms are as follows:

Obvious effect: The frequency and amplitude of tremble is diminished, the time interval between two attacks is obviously prolonged, and the duration of attack is obviously reduced.

Better effect: The tremble is obviously weakened; the patient walks more dexterously and more quickly, and speaks in a louder voice with clearer enunciation.

General effect: The tremble diminishes at the time of emitted qi therapy, but the patient relapses.

Zhang studied the effect of qigong on patients with Parkinson's disease by measuring brain waves according to the P33 auditory Event Related Potential (ERP).[92] A recording was made of the P_{300} of 24 normal controls and the P_{300} of 30 patients with Parkinson's disease before and after practicing qigong. The Webster scale was also recorded for 33 patients with Parkinson's disease who practiced qigong for 1 year.

The principal results were as follows:

1. In comparison with the normal controls, the P_{300} indexes of patients with Parkinson's disease exhibited a lengthening of the latency period and an increase in amplitude.
2. Comparing the records taken before and after patients with Parkinson's disease self-practiced qigong, the latency of target stimulating of P_{300} shortened significantly.
3. The Webster's score indicated that the clinical symptoms of Parkinson's disease improved for patients who practiced qigong.

Comments: This study shows that self-practice of qigong can alter the brainwaves of patients with Parkinson's disease. However, the question needs to be investigated of how changes in brain waves relate to improvements in clinical symptoms.

Drug Addiction

Finding effective and humane methods to help heroin addicts break the drug habit is a challenge to modern medicine. Li, Chen, and Mo compared the effectiveness of treating heroin addicts using qigong, regular medicine, and a control.[106]

Eighty-six heroin addicts who all met DSM-III-R substance dependence criteria in mandatory drug rehabilitation centers were randomly assigned to one of three groups.

1. Qigong treatment group (N = 34) practiced Pangu Gong for 2 to 2½ hours per day and had some adjustment by a qigong master (qi emission).
2. Medicine comparison group (N = 26) took detoxification pills (lofexidine-HCl, 0.2 mg) in a 10-day gradual reduction method.
3. Control group (n = 26) received basic care but no medicine.

Blood test, urine morphine test, ECG test, HAMA scale, and a withdrawal symptom evaluation scale were given before treatment and every day for 10 days during the study.

The results were as follows:

1. Withdrawal syndrome: From day one, the qigong group had significantly lower mean scores than the other two groups (p < 0.01). By day eight, 100% of the qigong group reported no withdrawal symptoms, but the other two groups still reported some at the end of the 10-day study.
2. Anxiety symptoms: Both the qigong and the medicine groups had much lower anxiety scores than did the control group (p < 0.01) on the fifth and tenth day of treatment. The qigong group had significantly lower anxiety scores than the medicine group (p < 0.01). The qigong group also reported more rapid improvement in sleep time and quality.
3. Urine morphine test: All subjects had a positive response to the urine morphine test before treatment. On the third day, urine tests were negative for 50% of the qigong group, 23% of the control group and 8% of the medicine group (p < 0.01). By the fifth day of treatment, the urine test was negative for all 34 patients in the qigong group, by the ninth day for the medicine group, and by the eleventh day for the control group.

The authors suggest that the mechanism of drug cessation depends on external qi breaking the combining power of the exogenous opium and human cells, and expelling the opiates from the body. They conclude that qigong treatment is an effective and safe treatment for detoxification and possibly for rehabilitation, with the additional benefits of low cost and no side effects.

Comments: The efficacy of a combination of qigong and drug therapy for detoxification of drug addicts should be investigated. This suggestion is based on reports that a combination therapy is better than drug therapy alone for treating hypertension and asthma.[5]

MECHANISM OF QIGONG HEALING

The research studies presented in this chapter provide evidence that qigong can alleviate symptoms of some neurologic diseases. Qigong can improve single symptoms, but it also has the potential to affect many functions of the body.[102] In this sense qigong is a holistic practice.

Qigong's role in affecting neurologic illness can be explained by a model that depends on qigong's ability to relax tissues, muscles, and tendons that are stressed, injured, or diseased. Once relaxed, the tissues permit greater blood circulation.[83,107] Enhanced blood circulation allows more efficient delivery of oxygen and nutrients to all cells of the body and increases the removal of metabolic waste products from the cells. As qigong increases blood circulation it also enhances the immune system and thereby improves health and healing. Several research studies have reported improvement in the immune system in humans and animals.[108-114]

Qigong helps relax the mind, muscles, tendons, joints, and inner organs of the body through exercises involving physical movements, focused meditation, breathing, and self-massage. One of the distinguishing features of qigong is that the mind can be trained to direct the flow of qi to any part of the body to relieve stress and pain. As the injured or diseased tissues become more relaxed, vasoconstriction is decreased and blood circulation is increased. Increased blood circulation may enable pain-inducing substances such as metabolic waste products to be removed from the tissues. It may also enhance the delivery, through the blood stream, of pain-killing substances such as endorphins or drugs to control pain.

During qigong meditation important changes can occur in the production of hormones. Higuchi studied the effects of qigong on hormone levels in the blood.[115] He measured the endocrine and immune responses of six qigong practitioners and seven nonpractitioners before and after 30 minutes of qigong meditation. Plasma cortisol, adrenaline, dopamine, and beta-endorphin levels decreased during meditation; although the beta-endorphin levels of a few qigong practitioners showed a slight increase. Apparently, qigong meditation decreases sympathetic nerve activity. These effects may be related to the effects of qigong meditation on brain waves[116,117] and on the synchronized brain waves of a qigong master and his subject during qigong anesthesia.[118]

Qigong's effect of enhancing blood circulation has been invoked by many researchers. For example, the effects have been shown in the removal of drugs from the bodies of drug addicts,[119] the delivery of drugs to diseased or stressed tissue,[37] and the increased blood circulation to the brain[120] and to the nailfolds of qigong practitioners.[121,122] A qigong master can increase the skin temperature of a subject without touching the subject,[123] evidence that the local blood circulation has been increased.

One of the main objectives of qigong is to balance the functions of the body so that organs are neither deficient nor overexcited. This balance can be assessed in a qualitative way using traditional Chinese medicine to read the pulses at the radial artery of the wrist. From the pulse reading, the therapist can deduce in a subjective way the condition of the 12 meridians and their corresponding organs of the body. Quantitative information on the condition of the meridians and their corresponding organs can be obtained by using Electroacupuncture According to Voll (EAV), which measures the electrical conductivity of acupuncture points on the meridians. A healthy, energetically balanced person will ideally have the same electrical conductivity for all 12 meridians and for the right and left side of the body. Sancier reported a pilot study in which EAV measurements were made on 11 subjects before and after the subjects practiced qigong of their own choosing for 10 to 15 minutes.[124] The results indicate that 7 of the 11 subjects balanced the functions of their meridians and organs. For example, the average reading of all 24 measurements was 69.0 ± 5.2 before and 51.4 ± 13.5 after the qigong practice. The EAV readings also provide other advantages, such as an insight into the condition of the individual organs and information about whether a given therapy is effective in balancing the organ.

A recent hypothesis attempts to explain distance and nontouch healing from a biophysic point of view. According to Gough, nonlocal inputs, that is, a healer's intentions, affect the shape of molecules such as DNA in the bodies.[125] Nonlocal input, such as emitted qi, provides guidance for maintaining the intercellular communication process essential for human growth and a healthy body. The intercellular communication between healer and healee, or the healing of oneself, is thought to involve increased coherence among cells. According to Gough, recent physics experiments strongly support the existence of the phenomena.

SUMMARY

Clinical evidence of the beneficial effects of qigong for treating some neurologic illnesses are presented in this chapter. There is a need for more rigorous methodologic controls in future studies to clarify putative qigong effects in neurologic disorders and to elucidate mechanisms.

The results of many studies offer promise that qigong can effectively complement orthodox medicine. For example, studies report that qigong decreases the drug dosage required to maintain patients with hypertension or asthma, helps drug delivery to stressed tissue, and assists detoxification of heroin addicts.

Qigong therapy has the additional benefits of being relatively inexpensive and often allowing patients to participate in their own healing process. For example, Reuther and Aldridge, who studied the effects of self-practice of qigong on asthma, reported improved breathing function and decreased drug dosages, hospitalization rate, sick leave, antibiotic use, and emergency consultation. These benefits resulted in significantly reduced treatment costs.[126]

Acknowledgments

The author gratefully acknowledges the insightful editorial comments of Ellen Friedlander and the suggestions and technical comments of James Lake, M.D.

References

1. Cohen K: *The way of qigong: the art and science of Chinese energy healing,* New York, 1997, Ballantine.
2. McGee CT, Chow E: *Miracle healing from China: qigong,* Coeur d'Alene, Idaho, 1994, MedPress.
3. Sancier KM, Hu B: Medical applications of qigong and emitted qi on humans, animals, cell cultures and plants: review of selected scientific research, *Am J Acupuncture* 19(4):367-377, 1991.
4. Sancier KM: Medical applications of qigong, *Altern Ther Health Med* 1(4),1996.
5. Sancier KM: Therapeutic benefits of qigong exercises in combination with drugs, *J Int Soc Life Inf Sci* 5(4):383-389, 1999.
6. Sancier KM: Anti-aging benefits of qigong, *J Int Soc Life Inf Sci* 14(1):12-21, 1996.
7. Genitoni V et al: Stomach vocal sound stimulation and E.A.V. measure of zusanli. Second Conference for Academic Exchange of Medical Qigong, Beijing, China, 1993.
8. Ornish D: *Reversing heart disease,* New York, 1990, Ballantine.
9. Ornish D: Healing of hearts, *Newsweek,* pp 50-56, March 16, 1998.
10. Krieger D: *Therapeutic touch inner workbook,* Santa Fe, 1997, Bear.
11. Field FD: Therapeutic touch in hospitals, *Columbus Dispatch,* pp 1-2, Aug 20, 1995.
12. Province M et al: The effects of exercise on falls in elderly patients, *JAMA* 273:1341-1347, 1995.
13. Kabat-Zinn J: *Wherever you go, there you are: mindfulness mediation in everyday life,* New York, 1994, Hyperion.
14. Lin H: Clinical and laboratory study of the effect of qigong anaesthesia on thyroidectomy. First Conference for Academic Exchange of Medical Qigong, Beijing, China, 1988.
15. Huang M: Effect of the emitted qi combined with self practice of qigong in treating paralysis. First Conference for Academic Exchange of Medical Qigong, Beijing, China, 1988.
16. Wang J, Li D, Zhao J: Experimental research on compound analgesia by qigong information treating instrument and acupuncture. Second International Conference on Qigong, Xian, China, 1989.
17. Lin M: The combination of qigong and acupuncture. Second International Conference on Qigong, Xian, China, 1989.
18. Zhang J et al: Analgesic effect of emitted qi and the preliminary study of its mechanism. Third National Academic Conference on Qigong, Guangzhou, China, 1990.
19. Zhang J, Hu D, Ye Z: Effect of waiqi (emitted qi) on experimental bone fracture in mice. Third National Academic Conference on Qigong, Guangzhou, China, 1990.
20. Inosuke Y: Fundamentals of qigong anesthesia and examples. Second Conference for Academic Exchange of Medical Qigong, Beijing, China, 1993.
21. Pavek RR: Effects of qigong on psychosomatic and other emotionally rooted disorders. First Conference for Academic Exchange of Medical Qigong, Beijing, China, 1988.
22. Tang C et al: The effects of qigong on reversal of aging process in some aspects of psychological functioning. Second International Conference on Qigong, Xian, China, 1989.
23. Li L et al: A comparative study of qigong and biofeedback therapy. Second International Conference on Qigong. Xian, China, 1989.

24. Shan H et al: A preliminary evaluation on Chinese qigong treatment of anxiety. Second International Conference on Qigong, Xian, China, 1989.

25. Yang S et al: Effect of treating neurasthenia with relaxation training and biofeedback therapy. Second International Conference on Qigong, Xian, China, 1989.

26. Du C et al: The correlation of individuality with types of disease and qigong-biofeedback curative effect. Second International Conference on Qigong, Xian, China, 1989.

27. Tsang R: Qigong, my experience and feeling. Second International Conference on Qigong, Xian, China, 1989.

28. Qin C et al: The research with the DQF-1 model multichannel qigong biofeedback apparatus. Second International Conference on Qigong, Xian, China, 1989.

29. Wu H et al: Study of the influence of Yuan Ji qigong on physical and mental health of students. Second Conference for Academic Exchange of Medical Qigong, Beijing, China, 1993.

30. Wang J: Role of qigong on mental health. Second Conference for Academic Exchange of Medical Qigong. Beijing, China, 1993.

31. Kato T, Numata T, Shirayama M: Physiological and psychological study of qigong, *Jpn Mind-Body Sci* 1(1):29-38, 1992.

32. Miyamoto T, Akasaka F, Oshima A: A measurement of physical and mental health at Hase Village in Nagano prefecture, *J Int Soc Life Inf Sci* 15(1):183-186, 1997.

33. Hutton D, Liebling D, Leire R: Alternative relaxation training for combat P.T.S.D. veterans. Third Conference for Academic Exchange of Medical Qigong, Beijing, China, 1996.

34. Geibler M: Qigong yangsheng application to psychotherapy. Third Conference for Academic Exchange of Medical Qigong, Beijing, China, 1996.

35. Chen C: Hypothesis about the mechanism of promotion of memory through qigong exercises. Second International Conference on Qigong, Xian, China, 1989.

36. Wang Y: Exploit of man's exploration of Mars and the contributions of Chinese taijiquan. Fourth International Conference on Qigong, Vancouver, BC, Canada, 1995.

37. Omura Y: Storing of qi gong energy in various materials and drugs (qigongization): its clinical application for treatment of pain, circulatory disturbance, bacterial or viral infections, heavy metal deposits, and related intractable medical problems by selectively enhancing circulation and drug uptake, *Acupunct Electrother Res, Int J* 15(2):137-157, 1990.

38. Agishi T: Evaluation of therapeutic external qigong from a viewpoint of the Western medicine, *J Int Soc Life Inf Sci* 14(1):102-103, 1996.

39. Omura Y, Beckman S: Application of intensified (+) Qi Gong energy, (−) electrical field, (S) magnetic field, electrical pulses (1-2 pulses/sec), strong Shiatsu massage or acupuncture on the accurate organ representation areas of the hands to improve circulation and enhance drug uptake in pathological organs: clinical applications with special emphasis on the "Chlamydia-(Lyme)-uric acid syndrome" and "Chlamydia-(cytomegalovirus)-uric acid syndrome," *Acupunct Electrother Res, Int J* 20(1):21-72, 1995.

40. Wang C: Effect of qigong on cardiovascular disease. Sixth International Symposium on Qigong, Shanghai, China, 1996.

41. Sun D: Senile dementia. Third Conference for Academic Exchange of Medical Qigong, Beijing, China, 1996.

42. Zhao G, Xie Q: A case of cerebral atrophy cured by qigong. First Conference for Academic Exchange of Medical Qigong, Beijing, China, 1988.

43. Jing G: Observations on the curative effects of qigong self adjustment therapy in hypertension. First Conference for Academic Exchange of Medical Qigong, Beijing, China, 1988.

44. Wong C: New qigong, an essential tool in healing and prevention of cancer. First Conference for Academic Exchange of Medical Qigong, Beijing, China, 1988.

45. Li S, Chen Z: 40 cases of coronary heart disease treated by qi operating method and its mechanism. Third Conference for Academic Exchange of Medical Qigong, Beijing, China, 1996.

46. Wu C, Xu P: Spontaneous dynamic qigong, involuntary motion qigong, and psychological medicine. First Conference for Academic Exchange of Medical Qigong, Beijing, China, 1988.

47. Zhang S: Observation of the curative effect of the eight diagrams qigong field on neuropathy. First International Congress of Qigong, UC Berkeley, Calif, 1990.

48. Hayashi S: Qigong and mental health: the positive effects of the state of rujing. Fourth International Conference on Qigong, Vancouver, BC, Canada, 1995.

49. Jia L, Jia J, Lu D: Effects of emitted qi on ultrastructural changes of the overstrained muscle of rabbits. First Conference for Academic Exchange of Medical Qigong, Beijing, China, 1988.

50. Cui Xi: Qigong's medical effect on the injured athletes during sports games. Fourth Conference for Academic Exchange of Medical Qigong, Beijing, China, 1998.

51. Liu L: Clinical research in treating spine-related diseases with qigong combined with Chinese and Western medicine. Fourth Conference for Academic Exchange of Medical Qigong, Beijing, China, 1998.

52. Ma D: Oral facial scar softened by qigong therapy. First Conference for Academic Exchange of Medical Qigong, Beijing, China, 1988.

53. Nakagawa S: Treatment method towards functional disease of the knee joint. First Conference for Academic Exchange of Medical Qigong, Beijing, China, 1988.

54. Wang F: Reports of treatments of shoulder inflammation by qigong tapping of insertion points and artificial

bleeding methods. Second International Conference on Qigong, Xian, China, 1989.

55. Yang S et al: Experimental research on the braking phenomenon of the upper limbs evoked by qigong waiqi (emitted qi). Third National Academic Conference on Qigong, Guangzhou, China, 1990.

56. Lee RH, Wang X: Use of surface electromyogram to examine the effects of the infratonic QGM on electrical activity of muscles, a double-blind, placebo-controlled study. Second Conference for Academic Exchange of Medical Qigong, Beijing, China, 1993.

57. Noda, Kozo: Study of the treatment of slipped disk. Second Conference for Academic Exchange of Medical Qigong, Beijing, China, 1993.

58. Omura Y et al: Unique changes found on the Qi Gong (Chi Gong) Master's and patient's body during Qi Gong treatment: their relationships to certain meridians and acupuncture points and the re-creation of therapeutic Qi Gong states by children and adults, *Acupunct Electrother Res, Int J* 14(1):61-89, 1989.

59. Gao Q: Qigong's curative effect on frozen shoulder and tennis elbow. Third Conference for Academic Exchange of Medical Qigong, Beijing, China, 1996.

60. Huang Y: Clinical observation of 50 cases of ankle joint sprain treated by qigong. Third Conference for Academic Exchange of Medical Qigong, Beijing, China, 1996.

61. Quan F: Observations of effect of qigong and acupuncture in treatment of lumbar sprain. Third Conference for Academic Exchange of Medical Qigong, Beijing, China, 1996.

62. Fukuzaki K: Some experiences about qigong therapy. Third Conference for Academic Exchange of Medical Qigong, Beijing, China, 1996.

63. Katayama T: From the balance of masseter to view the syndromes of sciatica. Third Conference for Academic Exchange of Medical Qigong, Beijing, China, 1996.

64. Yang K et al: Influence of electrical lesion of the periaqueductal gray (PAG) on the analgesic effect of emitted qi in rats. First Conference for Academic Exchange of Medical Qigong, Beijing, China, 1988.

65. Yang K et al: Analgesic effect of emitted qi on white rats. First Conference for Academic Exchange of Medical Qigong, Beijing, China, 1988.

66. Gao Z, Zhang S, Bi Y: Effect of emitted qi acting on zusanli point of rabbits on myoelectric signals of Oddi's sphincter. Third National Academic Conference on Qigong, Guangzhou, China, 1990.

67. Nishimoto S: Report on autonomic nervous system changes and pain reduction evinced by patients administered external ki therapy with alpha wave 1/f music, *J Int Soc Life Inf Sci* 14(2):259-262, 1996.

68. Yuen K: Qigong for the rehabilitation of acute and chronic pain. Third Conference for Academic Exchange of Medical Qigong, Beijing, China, 1996.

69. Nishimoto S: Report on the changing of the autonomic nervous system reducing pain of patients treated by external qi with alpha wave 1/F music. Third Conference for Academic Exchange of Medical Qigong, Beijing, China, 1996.

70. Ryu H et al: Comparisons of pain relief mechanisms between needling to the muscle, static magnetic field, external qigong and needling to the acupuncture point, *Acupunct Electrother Res, Int J* 24(2):119-131, 1996.

71. Liu X: Treatment of 19 cases of cerebral thrombosis by qigong therapy of insertion points and whole leading. Second International Conference on Qigong, Xian, China, 1989.

72. Wen R: Lumbar problems treated by qigong. Fourth Conference for Academic Exchange of Medical Qigong, Beijing, China, 1998.

73. He J: Qigong acupuncture therapy. Second International Conference on Qigong, Xian, China, 1989.

74. Yan B: Functions of qigong (breathing exercise) in clinical practice. Second International Conference on Qigong, Xian, China, 1989.

75. Wu H: Qigong exercise and health of elderly. Sixth International Symposium on Qigong, Shanghai, China, 1996.

76. Inosuke Y: Effectiveness of qigong therapy. Third Conference for Academic Exchange of Medical Qigong, Beijing, China, 1996.

77. Yan Q: Treating vertigo by qigong acupointing. Second International Conference on Qigong, Xian, China, 1989.

78. Jiang H: Therapeutic evaluation of 60 headache cases due to stagnancy of qi and blood treated by qigong. Second Conference for Academic Exchange of Medical Qigong, Beijing, China, 1993.

79. Omura Y et al: Common factors contributing to intractable pain and medical problems with insufficient drug uptake in areas to be treated, and their pathogenesis and treatment: Part I. Combined use of medication with acupuncture, (+) Qi gong energy-stored material, soft laser or electrical stimulation, *Acupunct Electrother Res Int J* 17(2):107-148, 1992.

80. Zhang S: Treatment of 126 cases of migraine with outgoing qi. Sixth International Symposium on Qigong, Shanghai, China, 1996.

81. Melchart D et al: Systematic clinical auditing in complementary medicine: rationale, concept, and a pilot study, *Altern Ther Health Med* 24(2):33-39, 1997.

82. Galashenburen: Concussion of brain treated by qigong. Fourth Conference for Academic Exchange of Medical Qigong, Beijing, China, 1998.

83. Xu X: Marked effect on facial paralysis treated by yoga. Fourth Conference for Academic Exchange of Medical Qigong, Beijing, China, 1998.

84. Zhang X, Weizhuang Z, Xinqu T: 147 cases of hemiplegia due to cerebrovascular accident treated by qigong. Fourth Conference for Academic Exchange of Medical Qigong, Beijing, China, 1998.

85. Wei S et al: A clinical observation on the recovery of extremity motion function in hemiplegic patients promoted by hypnosis and acupoint pressing. Fourth Conference for Academic Exchange of Medical Qigong, Beijing, China, 1998.

86. Lin H: Preliminary experimental results of the investigation on the basis of qigong therapy. Second International Conference on Qigong, Xian, China, 1989.

87. Lin Q: Facial paralysis treated by "external qi." Third International Symposium on Qigong, Shanghai, China, 1990.

88. Zhao Q: Treating bell's palsy through qigong. Third International Qigong Conference [in Chinese], Kyoto, Japan, 1992.

89. Liu J: Comprehensive treatment of spastic type cerebral palsy. Third International Qigong Conference [in Chinese], Kyoto, Japan, 1992.

90. Chow E: Chow qigong and rehabilitation: chronic degenerative diseases, paralysis and disabilities. Second World Congress Qigong, San Francisco, Calif, 1998.

91. Chen X: Exploration of using emitted qi of qigong for curing Parkinsonism. Second International Conference on Qigong, Xian, China, 1989.

92. Zhang J: Discussion of qigong effect on PD patients in clinic and P33 which is an auditory event related potential. Sixth International Symposium on Qigong, Shanghai, China, 1996.

93. Feng Y et al: Bidirectional influence on the electrogastric activity in man. First Conference for Academic Exchange of Medical Qigong, Beijing, China, 1988.

94. Cui R, Liu G, Zhang H: Neural mechanisms of qigong state: an experimental study by the method of visual evoked potential flash and pattern. Second International Conference on Qigong, Xian, China, 1989.

95. Qin C: Curative effect of qigong therapy for students with neurasthenia. Second International Conference on Qigong, Xian, China, 1989.

96. Kobayashi K, Itagaki Y: Double-blind test of qi transmission from qigong masters to untrained volunteers: (4) results of peripheral blood flow rate, skin electric potential, and meridian function measurements, during qi transmission, *Jpn Mind-Body Sci* 2(1):113-124, 1993.

97. Mayer M: Qigong and behavioral medicine: an integrated approach to pain, *J Tradit Eastern Health Fitness* 6(4):20-31, 1996.

98. Wang C et al: Research on anti aging effect of qigong. First Conference for Academic Exchange of Medical Qigong, Beijing, China, 1988.

99. Huang X: Clinical observation of 204 patients with hypertension treated with qigong. First International Congress of Qigong, UC Berkeley, Calif, 1990.

100. Wang C et al: Effects of qigong on preventing stroke and alleviating the multiple cerebro-cardiovascular risk factors—a followup report on 242 hypertensive cases over 30 years. Second Conference for Academic Exchange of Medical Qigong, Beijing, China, 1993.

101. Xing ZH, Li W, Pi DR: Effect of qigong on blood pressure and life quality of essential hypertension patients, *Chung Kuo Chung Hsi I Chieh Ho Tsa Chih* 13(7):413-414, 1993.

102. Kuang AK et al: Long-term observation on qigong in prevention of stroke—follow-up of 244 hypertensive patients for 18-22 years, *J Tradit Chin Med* 6(4):235-238, 1986.

103. Qing Liu Xiu D: Qing Liu electro-acupuncture therapy—treating tinnitus and failing hearing. Second International Conference on Qigong, Xian, China, 1989.

104. Singh B et al: A pilot study of cognitive behavioral therapy in fibromyalgia, *Altern Ther Health Med* 24(2):67-70, 1998.

105. Machi Y, Chu WZ: Physiological measurement for qigong anesthesia, *J Int Soc Life Inf Sci* 14(2):129-145, 1996.

106. Li M, Chen K, Mo Z: Qigong treatment for drug addiction. Third World Congress Qigong, San Francisco, Calif, 1999.

107. Agish T: Effects of external qigong on symptoms of arteriosclerotic obstruction in the lower extremities evaluated by modern medical technology, *Artif Organs* 22(8):707-710, 1998.

108. Feng L, Wang Y, Chen S, Chen H: *Effect of emitted qi on the immune functions of mice.* First World Conference, Qigong, Beijing, China, 1984.

109. Li, Caixi, Jinlong, Liu, Zhiyun, Zhao, Guang, Zhang, Yu, and Zhang, GuoxiXiyuan Hospital, China Academy of Traditional Chinese Medicine, Beijing, China [1] Effects of emitted qi on immune functions in animals, *1st World Conf Acad Exch Med Qigong Beijing, China 1988* 22.

110. Zhang, Li, Yan, Xuanzuo, Wang, Shuhua, Tao, Jundi, Gu, Ligan, Xu, Yin, Zhou, Young, and Liu, Dong: Institute of Qigong Science, Beijing College of Traditional Chinese Medicine, Beijing, China [1] Immune regulation effect of emitted qi on immunosuppressed animal model, *1st World Conf Acad Exch Med Qigong Beijing, China 1988* 27.

111. Feng, Lida, Wang, Yunsheng, Chen, Shuying, and Chen, Haixing: Beijing China Immunology Research Center, China [1] The effect on the immune functions in mice by qigong "waiqi," *2nd Int Conf on Qigong Xian, China 1989* 1.

112. Bi, Aihua, Fang, Jianming, Jiao, Qinan, Liu, Xiaoguang, and Feng, Wei: Dept Microbiology & Immunology, Tongji Medical University, China [1] The effect of the outgoing qi on the expression of surface antigens on human peripheral lymphocyte *2nd Int Conf on Qigong Xian, China 1989* 29.

113. Guan, Haoben and Yang, Jainhong: Guangzhou College of Traditional Chinese Medicine, Guangzhou,

China [1] Effect of qigong waiqi (emitted qi) on IL-2 activity and multiplication action of spleen cells in mice, *3rd Nat Acad Conf on Qigong Science*, Guangzhou, China 1990 84.

114. Higuchi Y et al: Endocrine and immune response during guolin new qigong, *J Int Soc Life Inf Sci* 15(1):138, 1997.

115. Ibid.

116. Kawano K, Kushita KN: The function of the brain using EEGs during induced meditation, *J Int Soc Life Inf Sci* 14(1):91-93, 1996.

117. Machi Y, Liu C, Wu RZ: Physiological measurements for the static qigong "Xiao Zhou Tian," *J Int Soc Life Inf Sci* 15(1):200-206, 1997.

118. Machi Y, Zhong CW: Physiological measurements under qigong anesthesia, *J Int Soc Life Inf Sci* 14(1):63-67, 1996.

119. Ou W, Li Ming: A preliminary exploration into the mechanism of drug cessation by pangu qigong. Fourth Conference for Academic Exchange of Medical Qigong, Beijing, China, 1996.

120. Liu Y, He S, Xie S: Clinical observation of the treatment of 158 cases of cerebral arteriosclerosis by qigong. Second Conference for Academic Exchange of Medical Qigong, Beijing, China, 1993.

121. Mo F et al: Study of prevention of microcirculating disorders of pilots in highlands by qigong. Second Conference for Academic Exchange of Medical Qigong, Beijing, China, 1993.

122. Wang C, Xu D, Qian Y: Effect of qigong on heart-qi deficiency and blood stasis type of hypertension and its mechanism, *Chung Kuo Chung Hsi I Chieh Ho Tsa Chih* 15(8):454-458, 1995.

123. Machi Y: Various measurements to qigong masters for analyzing qigong mechanism, *Jpn Mind-Body Sci* 3(1):65-87, 1994.

124. Sancier KM: The effect of qigong on therapeutic balancing measured by Electroacupuncture According to Voll (EAV): a preliminary study, *Acupunct Electrother Res, Int J* 9(2/3):119-127, 1994.

125. Gough WC: The cellular communication process and alternative modes of healing, *Subtle Energies and Energy Med* 8(2):67-101, 1999.

126. Reuther I, Aldridge D: Treatment of bronchial asthma with qigong Yangsheng: a pilot study, *J Altern Complement Med* 4:173-183, 1998.

SECTION 2: A CLINICIAN'S PERSPECTIVE

LINDA C. HOLE

The doctor who treats only physical illness is stupid.
Treating someone who is already ill is like waiting till you're thirsty to dig the well.
When you have a disease, do not try to cure it. Find your center, and you will be healed.

CHINESE PROVERBS

Each person carries his own doctor inside him. They come to us not knowing the Truth. We are our best when we give the doctor who resides within each patient a chance to go to work.

ALBERT SCHWEITZER, M.D.

What is qigong? Qigong is a powerful yet gentle paradigm shift tool in the New Millennium medicine. Qigong is the 5000-year-old Chinese energy healing system for body, mind, and spirit; and is practiced by more than 70 million people in China. In China qigong is an integral complement to the medical system, and in the West it is gaining widespread acceptance as well.

This section of the chapter is written by a clinician for clinicians. For a review of the scientific literature on qigong, see the beginning of this chapter written by Ken Sancier.

Qi (pronounced "chee") is breath or vital life force. Gong (pronounced "gung") is work. Qigong is the practice of cultivating qi, or vital life force through gentle breath and movement exercises and through healing meditation. There is also the discipline of living a life of qi.

Qi is also the Greek letter *chi,* or the cross. Qigong is thus also about staying centered in and open to universal Christ healing energy. Some say the greatest qigong master who ever lived is Christ. For many, qigong is the practice of breathing the breath of God, and it is taught in a number of mainstream Christian churches as a way of knowing God.

Qigong itself, however, is not a religion. Belief in God or religion is not at all necessary for qigong to work. Qigong is free and available to all. Within each and every one of us, there is a qigong master.

Qigong is documented to do the following:
- Strengthen the immune system
- Delay aging
- Prevent disease
- Relieve pain, stress, and paralysis
- Increase energy
- Promote peak performance

Qigong students and practitioners report profound healing and life-changing transformation, often where all else has failed.

As a free, simple, and effective tool to share with patients for their own self empowerment and healing, qigong is an HMO managed-care dream.

HARD VERSUS SOFT QIGONG

Hard qigong includes performance miracles such as qigong masters who light lightbulbs with their bare hands, affect instrument measurements and petri plate growth cultures from across a room, and move objects without touching them.

Soft qigong includes medical "miracles" that qigong masters routinely perform such as using medical X-ray intuitive vision, causing spontaneous cancer remissions, performing qigong anesthesia thyroidectomies, or directing external qi to lower a subject's blood pressure or increase a subject's EEG alpha waves.

One of the goals of this chapter is to take the mystique out of qigong and to present qigong as a healing modality that is available to anyone for the asking. The chapter focuses on soft medical qigong and

shares ways in which qigong can be integrated into one's life and practice.

I myself am a beginner, and no more a qigong master than you are. My youth, however, included vigorous scientific studies, such as honors physics taught by a Nobel Laureate.

Childbirth was my first direct life experience with qigong. When I allowed my mind to follow my thoughts and fears, the birth process was unspeakably painful. However, when I focused on my breath, surrendered my thoughts and fears to each breath, and used my breath to focus on each present moment of now, the natural birth process became pain free.

My more formal qigong experience includes studying with more than half a dozen world class qigong masters. Over the years, I have come to regard several of them as family. I have taught qigong since 1995. In addition to the school of life, my training has been primarily with Dr. Effie Chow in her integrated healing system of Chow qigong.

Along with information about the Chow qigong system, the material presented here includes pearls or wisdom gleaned from other teachers and from my own life experience as well. And, as is true in so much of medicine, my patients have been among my greatest teachers.

SOME CLINICAL VIGNETTES

In addition to qigong, I use a number of other healing modalities in my practice, including (KHT) Koryo Hand Therapy, homeopathy, nutrition, and prayer. Following are some clinical examples in which immediate results were obtained from qigong alone.

Headache in a 49-year-old white male veteran: I remember with fondness my first official qigong patient. He was a steak and potatoes veteran, and I remember wondering what on earth brought him to our holistic medical practice. He had suffered years of severe intermittent headaches, which had increased in severity and become constant over the last 5 weeks. The headaches were waking him from sleep and were no longer relieved by narcotic pain medications (T&C #4).

I had just attended my first introductory 1-day qigong workshop and was considering magnetic resonance imaging (MRI) to rule out a brain mass. I decided in the meantime to teach the patient the qi breath and the qigong "standing at the stake" posture. Within minutes, he broke out in a grin and said,

"What'd you do? My headache's gone!" That was nearly 5 years ago. The headaches he first presented with are still gone.

Migraines in 47-year-old white male blue-collar worker: The patient had a lifelong history of constant pressure with episodes of spiking pain, nausea, vomiting, lachrymation, and aura. The migraines had become progressively worse during the past year and he had been unable to work for the past 1 to 2 months. He had no relief with Demerol, Stadol, codeine, Norgesic forte, morphine, or a neurology consultation. With qigong breathing and meditation, the patient's pain level went from a 10 to a 2. With KHT, he left the office pain free and had remained headache free for 4 months when we last saw him in followup.

Transient ischemic attack (TIA) symptoms in 78-year-old widow: The patient had a 2-year history of fleeting episodes of ataxia, presyncopal lightheadedness, dizziness, and visual disturbance. Bilateral moderate carotid plaque and stenosis was discovered on carotid ultrasound. After just attending one of our introductory talks on qigong, she reported marked relief of her TIA-like symptoms for weeks afterwards.

Radiculopathy in 49-year-old professional artist with a long-standing history of right C5-6 herniated disk documented by MRI and neurology consultation: The patient had been experiencing a "pinched nerve in my neck" for several days and decreased mobility of the right upper extremity (RUE) with paresthesias and pain radiating to the RUE. With qigong, her mobility was restored and her pain was relieved within minutes.

QIGONG: ENERGY MEDICINE AND "MIRACLE HEALING"

Qigong is a truly powerful yet gentle tool for healing. I used to tell patients with severe "incurable" neurologic disorders that there was not much I could do for them. Using the traditional medical model, I could give them very little in the way of hope. I have since learned with qigong to let go of my own limiting medical beliefs, to just keep breathing, and to expect "miracles."

There are many "miracles" I could share with you, including the homemaker with diagnosed reflex sympathetic dystrophy (RSD) whose leg changed temperature, color, and diameter before my eyes; the retired minister with a long-standing benign essential

tremor, whose hands became still by the end of his first qigong exercise class; the child with cerebral palsy who, after his first introductory talk and treatment session, reached milestones within weeks at tasks he had struggled with for years; or the cerebrovascular accident (CVA) stroke survivor with aphasia and left hemiplegia, who with a multidisciplinary approach, made the news with his remarkable recovery.

With qigong, we have come to simply expect "miracles." We are amazed again and again at what can be done by simply teaching someone to fully breathe. Some "miracles" are dramatic, some subtle. A "miracle," however, may be as ordinary as a smile, a teardrop, or a ray of sunshine.

Qigong is a systematic way to learn how to practice energy medicine. Qigong "miracles," such as the ones I have shared with you from our classes and practice, are available to anyone, even ordinary beginners such as I. The profound healing possible with qigong is both humbling and uplifting.

CLINICAL APPLICATIONS AND EFFICACY OF QIGONG

We have used qigong to treat a full range of neurologic disorders with positive results. Those disorders include Bell's palsy, blepharospasm, carpal tunnel syndrome, cerebellar ataxia, cerebral palsy, CVA rehabilitation, deafness, diabetic and peripheral neuropathies, disk disease and injuries, headaches, migraines, multiple sclerosis, myopathies, neuralgias, neurasthesias, Parkinson's disease, post-polio syndrome, RSD, radiculopathies, sciatica, thoracic outlet syndrome, and tremors.

Dr. Effie Chow is an internationally recognized qigong master who is known for her experience and success in working with those suffering severe neurologic disorders, she also served on the original National Institutes of Health (NIH) Office of Alternative Medicine board. She has treated more than 200 patients with disabling neurologic disorders whose diagnoses included amytrophic lateral sclerosis, (Lou Gehrig's disease) brain injuries, cerebral palsy, multiple sclerosis, spinal cord injuries, Parkinson's disease, paralysis, reflex sympathetic dystrophy, and stroke.

Dr. Chow estimates that more than 95% of the 200+ patients she has seen with severe neurologic disorders have had positive results. The most remarkable successes have been in bringing a return of movement to patients with paralysis. Other results include increased sensation, decreased tremors, elimination of muscle spasms, decreased pain, and overall marked improvement in the sense of well being.

SEVERE NEUROLOGIC DISORDERS: SOME CLINICAL EXAMPLES

Dr. Chow's work with the severely neurologically disabled is remarkable. Rather than present formal cases, her patients and students best speak for themselves.

C-5 Quadriplegia in a 44-year-old Asian man:

I am a registered nurse and have been studying qigong with Dr. Chow for two and a half years. Two and a half months ago, a quadriplegic who had suffered a C-5 injury presented with severe uncontrollable muscle spasms. With even the slightest touch, his body would contort into uncontrollable spasms.

Within the 1st session, there was a marked decrease in muscle spasms, he was able to sit without outside physical support at the side of the bed for a minute at a time, and with qi, he was able to a degree, to actively move his legs. He continued qigong treatment, twice a week, two hours per session, and learned to control his spasms with his own breath.

With qi assistance, he is now able to roll on the floor, rock his hips, pull himself up to a sitting position, and sit balanced up to two and a half minutes at a time [Figure 15-1]. For the first time since the accident, he has independent active movement in his left index finger. Some of these changes have been documented by his occupational therapist. Most importantly, he now has hope, and has a happier more positive outlook on life.

Herniated disk with radiculopathy in 50-year-old white university professor:

In December 1995, . . . I was seriously injured in an auto accident. . . . My lumbar spine was badly damaged, leaving me with two ruptured disks and a fractured vertebrate. . . . The nerves in my lower spine had also been damaged, leaving me with constant back and leg pain, pronounced weakness on my left side, and areas of varying degrees of numbness and tingling. For the better part of the next eighteen months, I was bedridden and on high doses of medication.

Upon first meeting Dr. Chow, I did not tell her what my injury was, but as we were speaking she casually placed her hand on the small of my back. I immediately sensed a mild electric current, followed by warmth. . . .

Later, she used qi pressure on acupuncture points. . . . While she was working on my legs, I noticed several rather

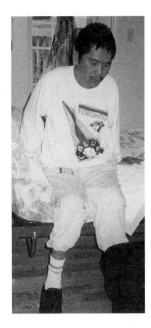

Figure 15-1 Quadriplegic patient is able to sit up after qigong treatment.

strange sensations of warmth, followed by a noticeable relaxation of the muscles, particularly in my left leg. On walking, I noticed that there was no longer a difference in the strength of either leg. I was absolutely flabbergasted, as my left leg had, since the time of the injury years ago, been markedly weaker. I walked around the room, to the amazement of myself, and the dozen other people in the room. I was so startled with the dramatic change in the strength in my left leg, that it took me a while to notice that the constant sciatic pain in both of my legs was gone as well!

My surgeons . . . were amazed at the objective documented changes in my mobility, flexibility, balance, and pain levels. . . . I have learned for myself that qigong breathing is the key to control of the emotions and pain. . . . Thank you for giving me new hope, empowerment, peace, and health.

Cerebral palsy in 3-year-old Tongan boy:

About three years ago, my wife and I became foster parents for a small huge-hearted island boy. . . . Setelo was born three months premature . . . barely larger than the size of a peanut. . . . In addition to roughly fifteen other diagnoses, he had meningitis . . . hydrocephalus . . . cerebral palsy . . . and two major cerebral hemorrhages motivating the Chaplain to read him his last rites. . . . I braced myself for the possible reality that Setelo would never sit up on his own or use his right hand . . . or ever walk.

When we found Dr. Chow and qigong three years later, we left her office with over 30 physical accomplishments Setelo had never before achieved. He began eating with his right hand for the first time. He began sitting up on his own. He learned to roll over multiple times on both sides. He started to walk without crossing his legs with remarkably less assistance than ever before. We had worked hard for almost three years to try to accomplish things that Dr. Chow was able to accomplish in just over three short days.

Physically, Setelo is growing, changing, and becoming proficient at things we previously dared not hope for . . . As participants of qigong, we neither have to change our religion nor abandon our Western medicine practices. . . . Setelo is a miracle. What Dr. Chow has helped us understand is . . . that with qi, there appears to be no limit to what Setelo can do.

QIGONG TOOLS FOR YOUR LIFE AND PRACTICE

There are literally hundreds of different traditions, schools, and teachers of qigong. The material in this section on qigong tools is from the classes I teach, from Chow qigong, and from other teachers as well.

These tools are for those who would like to use qigong to expand their lives and practice. Although we strongly recommend the discipline of daily practice, it is very possible to get remarkable results, even with very little formal practice. A single introductory workshop is often sufficient for students to successfully begin to diagnose and treat with qigong.

As scientists, we use basic kinesiology or muscle testing to demonstrate the efficacy of tools. Each of the following tools—qi, healing energy, and healing ability—when practiced correctly will increase strength. We invite you to see for yourself what qigong can do for you in your life, in your practice, and for your patients.

ACTIVATING YOUR QI

At the center of your palm is the *Lao Gong* point, or the "old worker." This point is also your hand chakra. On some of you, the *Lao Gong* may be a contrasting lighter area at the center of palm. This means that your healing channels are open and "turned on." In some paintings of saints, not only do the saints have halos, they also have golden beams of light, or qi, coming out of their hands from their *Lao Gong* points.

To activate your qi, rub your palms together back and forth at the *Lao Gong* points as if you are about to start a fire. Notice what you feel between your hands. Some people feel tingling. Some people feel a magnetic force. Some people feel a palpable live ball of energy. This is qi. The more you practice qigong and the more open you are, the bigger the ball of qi grows. As this ball of qi expands, your whole life changes and expands as well.

QI BREATH

The breath is key to qigong. In my own work I teach those who are ready that the qi breath is relaxing into the breath of God, and I use qigong as a tool for psychospiritual healing. Once again, for qigong to work a belief in God or any particular set of religious beliefs is not at all necessary. I, however, smile as I watch skeptics, agnostics, and atheists experience the healing of qigong.

Many people breath very shallowly, or barely breath at all. Many are totally unaware of their breath. Nonpermission and repressed emotions such as anger, grief, and fear are among the causes of shallow breathing.

The classic qigong breath cycle is the microcosmic orbit. For beginners, I first teach the qi breath as the Open Heart, Soft Belly Breath. That is, the open heart of compassion and the soft belly of letting go. Rather than using your chest and shoulder muscles to forcibly draw in the breath, keep an open heart, relax your abdominal muscles to allow your soft belly to expand, and draw the breath in via your diaphragm. We joke that correct qigong breathing is a belly-out contest.

The Open Heart, Soft Belly Qi Breath

1. Make sure your spine is aligned and stretched heaven to earth. Breathing is also done standing.
2. Open your heart and chest by rotating your shoulders back and dropping them down. Let your body, mind, and spirit relax.
3. Relax your abdominal muscles for a soft belly.
4. Draw your breath in via your diaphragm and allow your soft belly to expand.

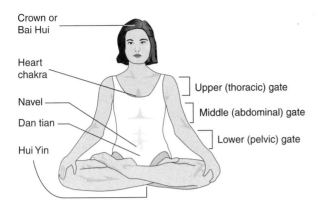

Crown or
Bai Hui

Heart
chakra

Navel

Dan tian

Hui Yin

Upper (thoracic) gate

Middle (abdominal) gate

Lower (pelvic) gate

Figure 15-2 Diagram of Qigong breathing.

5. With an open heart, imagine drawing the breath to your soft belly, down to your *Dan Tian,* which is the seat of energy two inches below your umbilicus.
6. Do not use your shoulder and chest muscles to draw in the breath. Hold your shoulders and chest wall still as you draw the breath into your soft belly.
7. As your belly expands, your chest cavity will naturally and gently expand as well. Allow your chest to passively expand as it fills with air.
8. Breath in through your nose, out through your mouth.
9. On the in breath, hold your tongue to the roof of your mouth. This connects all your qi energy meridian channels and potentiates healing.
10. On the out breath, release the breath through your mouth and drop your tongue. Let your body, mind, and spirit relax and let go.
11. As you grow accustomed to qi breathing, imagine breathing the qi into your heart as a funnel of light. Visualize this light in your heart, or qi, vibrating and expanding to fill your body and spirit, like a vase.
12. Relax and let this light in your heart continue to expand to cleanse, free, heal, and fill every cell and pore of your being with qi.

AWARENESS, CLEARING BAD QI, AND LETTING GO

Bad, stagnant, or blocked qi leads to physical pain and disease. To dispel bad qi, send a ball of light, or qi, to the affected body part or organ. Imagine the ball of light dissolving the bad qi away. Always be sure to replace bad qi with good qi and to completely fill any remaining empty space with good qi. This prevents bad qi from reentering,

The qi breath may bring to awareness unexpected tears. Tears are expressions of the deeper psychospiritual pain underlying the physical pain. This meltdown effect is a good sign. Allowing yourself to become aware of the tears of the spirit, and then releasing them, frees the body to heal. As one of my qi masters teaches, "99% of the battle is awareness. The rest is letting go."

QI CENTERING: HOW YOU STAND IN RELATION TO THE UNIVERSE

As with the Greek letter *chi,* or the cross, the qi stance is both centered and open. The Chinese character for king, I, or master, is a person standing centered between heaven and earth. Correct qi posture is standing centered and open, aligned between heaven and earth, open to the heavens above, and grounded to the earth below. Qi stance, posture, and centering are vital for opening to greater qi.

Ground, Let Go, Be Still, and Be Present

1. Imagine a silver thread stretching, opening, and aligning your spine from heaven to earth. Feel the silver thread supporting and connecting you.
2. At your *Bai Hui,* or crown, feel the silver thread lifting, connecting, and opening you and your spirit to the heavens (Figure 15-3).
3. At the base of your spine, visualize the silver thread grounding you and your body to the earth. Let this portion of the silver thread become a magnetic grounding cord. Let your grounding cord absorb and free you from whatever no longer serves you and from whatever you are ready to let go of. This grounding cord also acts as a lightning rod to ground out and protect you from whatever may harm you. Use your grounding cord to support you in standing your ground and staying centered in qi.
4. Remember Open Heart, Soft Belly: chest open, shoulders dropped back and down, abdomen soft, body relaxed.

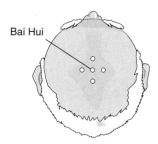

Figure 15-3 Bai Hui or Crown.

5. Remember to breath in light on the in breath and to let go on the out breath.
6. Be still, and with your breath, quiet your mind.
7. Be present in the "I am." With your breath, call back your spirit.

QIGONG MIND-BODY PRINCIPLES, POSITIVE MENTAL ATTITUDE, AND REFRAMING

Stressed is just desserts spelled backwards.

UNKNOWN

Love is the most important ingredient in healing.

EFFIE CHOW, Ph.D.

Qigong incorporates a whole set of mind/body principles as tools for healing. On this level, qigong is concerned with looking for the good and affirming the good, and about cultivating right thoughts and a Positive Mental Attitude (PMA). "Right" PMA thoughts do not imply any judgment or condemnation. Rather, "right" PMA thoughts are thoughts that make your heart sing, give you something to live for, raise your qi, make you stronger, and help move your immune system towards healing.

"Negative thoughts can negate all healing" is a corollary qigong teaching. One key to qigong healing is moving from the Western left-brained, problem-oriented approach of analyzing "What's wrong?" to a more heart-centered approach of remembering, acknowledging, and giving thanks for the good. Qigong reframes life. Rather than dwelling on and reinforcing the negative, qigong focuses attention and gives energy to the positive.

These concepts are obvious to parents. Focusing on a child's negative attention-seeking behavior accentuates the behavior. Giving the child unconditional love and PMA positive reinforcement within limits of heaven and earth, obviates the child's need for negative attention-seeking behavior. Disease is your body's negative attention-seeking behavior and its cry for help.

The Chinese word for *crisis* translates as either *danger* or *opportunity*. In qigong, we reframe the challenges of life's day-to-day stresses and crises as opportunities to grow, or as blessings in disguise, and simply give thanks.

Pure unconditional love is, of course, the most powerful qi tool for healing. Other qigong mind/body PMA tools include laughter, hugs, touch, reframing, clear intention, surrender, oneness, joy, and being thankful. The mind/body connection and how thoughts and emotions affect the immune system are well documented in psychoneuroimmunology. We can also demonstrate via kinesiology the power of these mind/body PMA tools of love, of thought forms, and of qi.

One benefit of sharing qigong with patients is the transformation of their attitudes. With qi, patients can reframe their lives in a new light. They often take on a refreshingly positive attitude towards their disease and towards life, and become more actively involved in their own healing process and in life itself.

QI EXERCISES

A day without dancing is a day lost.

UNKNOWN

There are literally thousands of different qigong exercises. My favorite is qi dancing. For medical qigong, the Chow qigong set of exercises is superb. Qi exercises open and free your energy channels to greater qi to greater energy, greater awareness, greater healing, and greater healing ability.

Infinity is a fun qi exercise. Align your spine on the silver thread. Imagine that your pelvis is loose on a ball and socket joint. Rest your palms on your sacrum parallel to your spine. Imagine a horizontal plane at the base of your pelvis, your *Hui Yin* or perineum. Rotate only your pelvis to draw an infinity sign on this horizontal plane. As you move your pelvis to the sign of infinity, remember to breathe into your heart, one breath for each infinity sign. Remember on the in breathe to hold your tongue at the roof of your mouth to connect all your qi energy channels. On the out breath, relax. This exercise frees the lower energy centers or chakras, helps open the energy channels between the lower and upper halves of your body, and most importantly helps open the energy channels to your heart.

QI MEDITATION

Be still, and know that I am.

PSALMS 46:10

One joy shatters a hundred griefs.

CHINESE PROVERB

Qi meditation is core to qi healing. Qi exercises open your energy channels in preparation for the healing of qi meditation. Qi meditation encompasses many of the same principles that are taught in Western schools of mindfulness, visualization, focusing, hypnosis, transcendental meditation, and centering prayer. As in centering prayer, qigong calls upon a greater energy, or universal qi, for healing. Qi, again, requires no particular belief system, religious or otherwise, and is available to all.

The qi "meltdown" effect: Qi frees, or melts down, walled off feelings, pictures, and memories and allows them to bubble up into your awareness. Give yourself permission to become aware of and to experience whatever surfaces, so that you can let it go. Especially give yourself permission to experience the uncomfortable feelings, for example buried anger, grief, pain, or loss. Then become a neutral, third party, detached witness and focus your attention on your breath. With your breath, simply observe the feelings and pictures, some of which may not even be yours. Do not allow yourself to get caught in thoughts, judgments, and emotions. Just surrender, release, breath it out, and let go.

Most importantly keep your heart, the heart of love and compassion, open. Visualize the qi as a funnel of light entering your heart. On the in breath, breathe in light and allow yourself to feel whatever you have to feel. On the out breath, breathe out whatever comes out . . . and let it all go.

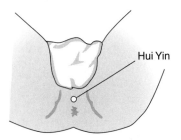

Figure 15-4 Hui Ying or perineum.

The MicroCosmic Cycle meditation and the Five Element meditation are specific and fundamental to qigong. For the meditations, remember the qi breath, qi centering, open heart, soft belly, and silver thread.

MicroCosmic Cycle Meditation

Visualize the qi circulating in a microcosmic cycle. On the in breath, visualize the qi as light flowing from your *Dan Tian,* the seat of energy two inches below your umbilicus, down to your *Hui Yin,* or perineum, then up the Governing vessel energy channel along your spine, through the Three Gates, and up to your crown or *Bai Hui* (Figure 15-4). On the out breath, visualize the qi flowing down the front of your body along the Conception vessel back to your *Dan Tian* (Figure 15-2).

The lower pelvic gate relates to fear, survival, sexuality, will power, and pelvic organs. The middle abdominal gate relates to power, control, resistance, judgment, empowerment, and abdominal organs. The upper thoracic gate relates to heart sadness and joy, speaking your truth, surrender, and thoracic organs. The *Bai Hui* or crown is your knowingness and connection to the heavens.

As the qi flows in this microcosmic cycle, visualize the qi clearing, cleansing, healing, and filling all your energy channels and centers with light.

Five Element Meditation

Each organ system is related to one of the five elements: fire, earth, metal, water, or wood. Each element governs a whole set of emotions. The body is about the five senses; the spirit is about the five elements. Beneath every pain, there is a psychospiritual wound.

Freeing the spirit frees the body. Meditating on the five elements helps free the spirit to free the body and is one of the most powerful, gentle, and effective tools in qigong healing. (See also KHT, Chapter Five, Element Therapy.)

Some Goals of Qi Meditation

A core goal of the qi meditation is self love, self acceptance, self forgiveness, and self worth. Self love is vital to healing. As Confucius taught, love first yourself, then your neighbor. True self love, self acceptance, self forgiveness, and self worth free you to love, accept, forgive, and give thanks for others, and thus give you internal peace, centeredness, balance, and power.

True freedom and staying centered are other goals of qi meditation. With practice, qi meditation brings a sense of peace and knowingness. This sense of peace frees you to stand centered in the universe and to move centered in the universe in a very clear and powerful way, amidst the chaos and stress of day-to-day life.

One last goal of qi meditation is to bring you to such a point of internal mind-body-spirit stillness, awareness, peace, and mastery that from a grounded space of complete centeredness and surrender, you can "command" the universe and heal.

DIAGNOSIS AND TREATMENT

Scanning Qi

As you become more sensitive and aware of qi, you can diagnose by sensing a person's qi, or energy field. This technique is called scanning. To scan, you simply run your hands about 6 to 12 inches over the patient's body. Over different areas of the body, you may feel different sensations. Some areas may feel hot and some cold. Some areas will seem to push your hands out and some will pull them in. Some areas may feel empty. These areas of different sensations invariably have to do with injuries or illnesses, or blocked, stagnant, or bad, qi. As you scan, you may intuitively "see" pictures, and "feel" feelings that are not necessarily your own, but have to do with the patient's imbalance, or "disharmonious" qi.

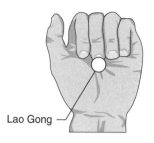

Figure 15-5 Lao Gong point.

Directing Qi

1. Simply brush away the excess or "bad" qi, or the areas that feel hot, and/or that push your hands out.
2. Pack in with "good" qi the areas that feel cold, empty, or pull your hands in.
3. You can also direct, send, and emit qi via your *Lao Gong* points or via your fingers (Figure 15-5).

Years ago, I brought my 12-year-old son to his first qigong workshop. He worked with an elderly gentleman with long-standing back pain. When I asked my son how the workshop was for him, to my astonishment he innocently replied, "Oh, you know that old man I worked with? Well, he was hot up top, nothing at the waist, then cold from the waist down. . . . So I brushed him off up top, packed him in at the waist. Then he was warm all over, and his back pain went away."

I have since both attended and given many introductory 1 to 2 hour qigong workshops, where participants have successfully sensed and directed qi. Just as we each have the five senses, we each have the ability to sense and direct qi as well. Once again, qigong as a healing modality is available to everyone.

QIGONG AND THE TRADITIONAL WESTERN MEDICAL MODEL

White man get headache, take aspirin, get stomach ache.

UNKNOWN

The whole Chinese medical system is based on the notion that the way you relate to other people, the way you think, and your emotions govern your health, . . . what kind of life you'll have, and what kind of health you'll have.

DAVID EISENBERG

The traditional Western medical model is problem oriented, problem solving, and deductive. The qigong model is remembering the good, affirming the good, raising the qi, and inductive. The Western model is organ centered with some outside intervention as the cure. The qigong model is qi centered and is about one's relationship with oneself and with the Universe. With qigong, clearing, balancing, and renewing qi is the cure.

In the Western model, the power to heal is outside the individual. In the qigong model, we honor the individual's inner knowing and inner power to heal. In the Western model, the cup is half empty. In the qigong model, the cup is half full. The Western model gives attention and energy to the problems. The qigong model gives attention and energy to the positive, and to the individuals universal innate ability to hear.

Qigong focuses attention on raising the qi, so that the problems simply melt away to make room for the miracles to unfold.

MORE TOOLS FOR GREATER QI AND HEALING: EMPTY VESSEL, BEING STILL, BEING PRESENT, AND CLEAR INTENTION

For greater qi and for greater qi healing, one must become a clear empty vessel for qi. One must surrender all ego, both the big ego of arrogance and conceit and the small ego of fear and inadequacy. Ego blocks qi. One must empty out all negative thoughts, feelings, limiting beliefs, and pictures. Surrendering all ego and releasing all negativity creates clear space for qi to go to work and heal.

One must be still and be present. Healing does not occur in the past or in the future. For qi healing, one must let go of both the past and future and be truly present in the still moment of now. Qi healing occurs in the stillness of the present moment.

One must have a clear intention, or *Yi Nian*, of what one would like to create, whether it be wholeness, wellness, and healing . . . or moving mountains. Hold your intention lightly and innocently, without ego or attachments. . . . And lightly, with qi, expect miracles.

A LIFE OF QI: RIGHT LIVING, THE WAY, AND DOING VERSUS BEING

The Way which can be spoken is not the Way.

LAO-TZE, TAO DE CHING

For committed qigong students and practitioners, qigong is far more than simply a set of breathing and movement exercises. Qigong, at its highest, is a way of life.

The way you think, the way you relate to your loved ones, the way you relate to your community, the way you relate to the world, the way you handle your emotions, the way you care for your body, the way you work, the way you stand in the universe, the way you commune with nature, the way you commune with God, and the way you love all determine your peace of mind, your state of health, and your state of qi. The choices you make about the way you live determine how you live; how you age; how you love; and how healthy, happy, and well you are.

For health, longevity, well being, and a life full of qi, one must practice right living, including right thoughts, relationships, love, livelihood, nutrition, exercise, practice, service, and communion.

The paradox, however, is that right living is about being rather than doing. The qi practice of right living, or doing qi, comes forth out of the qi practice of being in qi. Being in qi is being centered, being still, being present, being true to your inner knowing, and being true to who you really are.

First be. Then do.

In the context of medicine, qigong is a total wellness health program.

SUMMARY: APPLYING QIGONG TO YOUR LIFE AND PRACTICE

What more is there to say? Qigong changes lives and has made a tremendous difference in my life and practice, and in the lives of my patients. I share these simple yet profound tools with my patients, with the community, and with you.

What words are there to express how qigong can transform your life, your practice, and the lives of your patients as well?

I invite you to take a minute to be still, go within, and see for yourself.

Additional Readings

There are volumes of literature on qigong. For scientific reviews, Ken Sancier is the authority. For an introduction to qigong and energy medicine, the following are recommended:

Ballentine R: *Radical healing,* New York, 1999, Harmony Books.

Chow E, McGee C: *Qigong miracle healing from China,* Coeur D'Alene, Idaho, 1994, Medipress.

Cohen K: *The way of qigong,* New York, 1997, Random House.

Dossey L: *Reinventing medicine: beyond mind body to a new era of healing,* New York, 1999, HarperCollins.

Eisenberg D: *Encounters with qi,* New York, 1987, Penguin Books Ltd.

Gerber R: *Vibrational medicine, new choices for healing ourselves,* Santa Fe, 1996, Bear & Co.

Kaptchuk T: *The web that has no weaver,* Chicago, 1983, Congen & Weed.

Kushi M: *How to see your health: book of Oriental diagnosis,* New York, 1980, Japan Publications.

Lee PE, Richard H: *Bioelectric vitality: exploring the science of human energy,* San Clemente, Calif., 1997, China Healthways Institute.

Lee PE, Richard: *Scientific investigation into Chinese qi-gong,* San Clemente, Calif., 1999, China Healthways Institute.

Liu H: *Mastering miracles: the healing art of qigong,* New York, 1997, Warner Press.

Moyers B: *Healing the mind,* New York, 1993, Doubleday.

Sha ZG: *Zhi neng medicine 3396815,* Vancouver, BC, Canada, 1997, Zhi Neng Press.

The Role of Auricular Acupuncture in Neurologic Reflexes

TERRY OLESON

Of all the mysterious aspects of Chinese acupuncture, the use of acupuncture points on the external ear to control conditions in other parts of the body is one of the most enigmatic. Western-trained physicians find it very difficult to even conceive of the possible existence of anatomic pathways that could allow the ear to have an impact on distant regions of the body. The very foundation of neurophysiology is that specific somatic nerves from skin and muscle tissue project to specific neuroanatomic areas that are distinctly different from the parts of the brain that process sensory signals from the ear. However, practitioners of traditional Oriental medicine have extensive clinical experience in stimulating auricular acupuncture points to relieve a variety of somatic and neurologic illnesses. Skeptics might attribute such observations to the power of the placebo, but there is growing clinical evidence that acupuncture relief of pain is a verifiable phenomenon that cannot be so easily dismissed. The Oriental theory behind this type of treatment is that illness is due to a blockage of energy flow along lines of force known as meridians or channels. Stimulating acupuncture points on the body or the ear is said to alter this energy pattern, allowing for tissue healing and pain relief. This energetic theory may or may not ever be supported by sufficient scientific data. However, the many clinical benefits obtained with auricular acupuncture treatments must have some physiologic basis to explain its effectiveness in healing a variety of illnesses.

Ear acupuncture, also known as auriculotherapy, has origins in both Asia and Europe. Although ancient Oriental medical texts described the major acupuncture meridians as invisible lines of energy force extending throughout the body, only some of the primary meridians connected to the ear.[1] Classical use of ear acupuncture points was limited to a few medical conditions.

The auricular acupuncture practiced today is based principally on discoveries made by Dr. Paul Nogier of Lyon, France, in the 1950s. After observing a scar on a specific area of the upper, external ear in patients who had suffered from sciatica pain, Nogier[2] learned that the source of this scar was a cauterization treatment by a lay healer. More intrigued than appalled by such a barbaric treatment, Nogier performed a similar procedure on his own sciatica patients and found that the treatment did relieve their back pain. Nogier hypothesized that since the upper ear seemed to correspond to conditions in the lower back, the rest of the auricle could represent the rest of the body, but in an "inverted fetus" orientation. Because he had studied the works of the French acupuncturist Georges Soulie de Morant, Nogier was familiar with an energy meridian perspective of the human body. He knew that Chinese acupuncturists often used distal acupoints on the hands or feet to affect conditions in other parts of the body. The existence of this inverted fetus map on the ear was first reported at a 1957 acupuncture meeting in France. The map was then distributed internationally by an acupuncture journal published in Germany and was finally translated for acupuncture practitioners in Asia. In 1958, the Nanjing Army Ear Acupuncture Research Team conducted an evaluation of several thousand patients treated by "barefoot doctors" in China who successfully treated specific medical conditions according to the inverted fetus view of the ear.[3]

NEUROPHYSIOLOGIC PERSPECTIVES OF AURICULAR POINTS

In describing the basis for the benefits of auricular acupuncture, Nogier emphasized more neurophysiologic than energetic explanations for the manner in which pain conditions are alleviated. Nogier suggested that there are different regions on the external ear related to different types of nervous innervation. Both Dr. Nogier and Dr. Rene Bourdiol[4] of Paris have suggested that there are three different territories on the auricle representing three types of neurologic in-

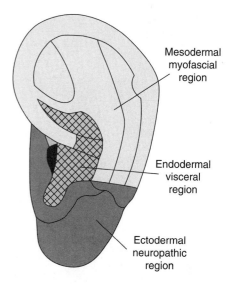

Figure 16-1 Embryologic regions on the external ear for endodermal visceral disorders, mesodermal myofascial tension, and ectodermal neuropathic problems.

put. Somatic nervous system control of myofascial pain is represented in one zone of the ear, autonomic nervous system control of visceral distress from internal organs is represented in a different auricular region, and central nervous system (CNS) regulation of neuropathic conditions is found in a third territory of the external ear. These three auricular regions are depicted in Figure 16-1. The central concha of the ear is the region concerned with autonomic nerves and internal organs. The surrounding antihelix and antitragus ridges of the ear represent somatic nerves and the musculoskeletal body. The outer helix tail represents the spinal cord and the spinal nerve roots emanating from it.[5] The ear lobe and adjacent antitragus represent the brain. All ear acupoints are said to activate autonomic or somatic spinal reflexes that affect the body by their connection to brain pathways. These pathways synapse in the reticular formation, hypothalamus, or thalamus.

Nogier's hypothesis that the somatotopic representation on the external ear could be perceived of as an inverted fetus is illustrated in Figure 16-2. The actual somatotopic representation on the auricle is not truly in the shape of a fetus, with its body curled in a concave, tuck position. Rather, the auricular body is curved in a backward, arching manner with the posterior spine extended in a position that could probably

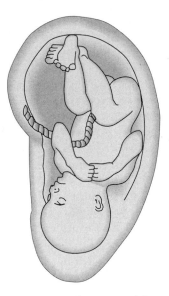

Figure 16-2 The concept of an inverted fetus pattern represented on the external ear.

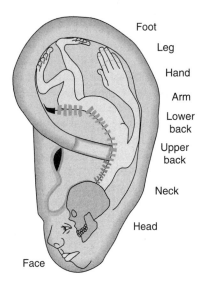

Foot
Leg
Hand
Arm
Lower back
Upper back
Neck
Head
Face

Figure 16-3 The curving somatotopic pattern on the ear that indicates areas of the auricle that correspond to specific areas of the body in an inverted orientation.

only be achieved by highly trained gymnasts or yoga masters (Figure 16-3). The head, skull, and brain are represented on the lower regions of the auricle; the lower back, legs, and feet are represented toward the upper regions of the ear; and the rest of the body is represented between the two. The somatotopic pattern that Pennfield and Rasmussen[6] first showed for the human cerebral cortex also depicts a convoluted perspective of the human body. The auricular somatotype could very well use this neurologic program in the brain. The combination of this somatotopic inversion pattern on the ear and the three different nerve projections to the auricle makes it possible to treat specific medical problems by stimulating ear points on specific areas of the auricle.[7]

The scientific credibility for this inverted, somatotopic perspective of the ear has been supported by objective measurements of the tenderness and the electrodermal activity of ear acupuncture points. Oleson et al.[8] conducted a double-blind, controlled trial of auricular diagnosis at the UCLA School of Medicine. Forty patients with musculoskeletal pain were interviewed by an independent evaluator to determine the physical locations of their pain. The patient and the practitioner of auricular diagnosis were not allowed to communicate with each other regarding the patient's medical history. Auricular points were identified as reactive by their tenderness to palpation and by electrical conductivity measuring more than 50 μA. There was a statistically significant 75.2% positive correspondence between reactive auricular points and the parts of the body where there was musculoskeletal pain. Nonreactive ear points corresponded to parts of the body from which there was no reported experience of musculoskeletal pain. Saku et al.[9] from Japan conducted a similar double-blind assessment of auricular points, but for visceral disorders rather than musculoskeletal problems. Reactive electropermeable points on the ear were defined as auricular skin areas that had conductance of electrical current greater than 50 μA. There was a significantly higher frequency of reactive ear points at the location of the Chinese heart point in the inferior concha for patients with myocardial infarctions and angina pain (84%) than for a control group of healthy subjects (11%). The frequency of electropermeable auricular points for the kidney (5%), stomach (6%), liver (10%), elbow (11%), or eye (3%) was the same for coronary patients as for individuals without coronary problems. Because there was no difference between the two groups in the electrical reactivity of auricular points that did not represent the heart, the study indicates the selectivity of auricular diagnosis procedures.

Experimentally induced changes in auricular reflex points in rats were examined by Kawakita et al.[10] The submucosal tissue of the stomach of anaesthetized rats was exposed, then acetic acid or saline was injected into the stomach tissue. A silver metal ball, which served as the search electrode, was moved over the surface of the rat's ear and a needle was inserted into subcutaneous tissue to serve as the reference electrode. Injection of acetic acid led to the gradual development of lowered skin resistance points on central regions of the rats' ears, the auricular areas that correspond to the gastrointestinal region of human ears. Low impedance points were rarely detected on the auricular skin in normal rats or in experimental rats before the surgical procedure. After experimentally induced peritonitis, there was a significant increase in low impedance points (0 to 100 kΩ) and moderate impedance points (100 to 500 kΩ), but a decrease in high impedance points (greater than 500 kΩ). These results demonstrated a reduction in the electrodermal resistance response to experimentally induced irritation of the internal organ corresponding to that auricular point. Histologic investigation could not prove the existence of sweat glands in the rats' auricular skin. The authors therefore suggested that the low impedance points are in fact related to sympathetic control of blood vessel activity.

MICRO-ACUPUNCTURE REFLEX SYSTEMS

The auricular acupuncture system has been described by Helms[11] as a "reflex somatotopic system," one of several micro-acupuncture reflex systems found on the hand, the foot, and other parts of the body. That there is a holographic homunculus pattern shown on the external ear and on other micro-acupuncture systems was first proposed by Ralph Alan Dale.[12] He hypothesized that ear acupoints have remote reflex connections to other parts of the body through neuronal pathways in the CNS. Dale has proposed that there are both organo-cutaneous reflexes, which allow the microsystem to reveal underlying body pathology; and cutaneo-organic reflexes, which enable micro-acupuncture stimulation to heal the pathologic condition. Foot reflexology, hand acupuncture, and scalp acupuncture are all said to serve as peripheral terminal microsystem inputs on the body that connect to a central brain computer that regulates pathologic conditions in all other parts of the body.

Tsun-nin Lee[13,14] has developed a thalamic neuron theory to account for reflex connections between acupuncture points and the brain. According to this theory, pathologic changes in peripheral tissue eventually leads to firing patterns in the correspondent neural microcircuits in the brain and spinal cord. The organization of the connections between peripheral nerves and the CNS are controlled by sites in the sensory thalamus that are arranged like a homunculus. The CNS institutes corrective measures intended to normalize the disordered neural circuits. However strong environmental stressors or intense emotions can cause the CNS circuitry to malfunction. If the neurophysiologic programs in the neural circuits are impaired, the peripheral disease may become chronic. Pain and disease is thus attributed to learned, maladaptive programming of these dysfunctional neural circuits. Stimulation of acupuncture points on the body or the ear can serve to induce a reorganization of these pathologic brain pathways. The spatial arrangement of these neuronal chains within the thalamic homunculus is said to account for the arrangement of acupuncture meridians in the periphery. The invisible meridians that purportedly run over the surface of the body may actually be due to nerve pathways projected onto neuronal chains in the thalamus. The auricular acupuncture system is more noticeably arranged in a somatotopic pattern on the skin surface of the external ear.

PAIN RELIEF BY AURICULAR ACUPUNCTURE REFLEX PATHWAY

The relief of pain by auricular acupuncture can best be understood using the theory of stimulation-produced analgesia. Liebeskind et al.[15] developed this theory to account for the pain-relieving effects of electrical stimulation of neurons in the brain. In addition to the classically known, ascending pain-sensation pathway, there is a descending pain-inhibitory pathway. The pain-inhibitory system travels from the brainstem down the spinal cord, then activates pain suppressive neurons in the dorsal horn of the spinal cord.[16] In their gate-control theory of pain, Melzack and Wall[17] had focused on the inhibition of input from nociceptive neurons by input from tactile neurons interacting through spinal cord interneurons. However, they further allowed that supra-spinal gates in the brain could produce descending messages to these same inhibitory interneurons, thus blocking the ascending pain signal. The most potent area for obtaining stimulation-produced analgesia in rats was the midbrain periaqueductal gray,[18] a region where there are neurons that are specifically responsive to noxious stimuli. Research in primates[19] has shown that deep brain stimulation in the subcortical thalamus is a more potent site for obtaining stimulation-produced analgesia in higher species. Examination of deep brain stimulation in human patients has shown similar findings.[20] Direct connections between auricular acupuncture points and antinociceptive brain pathways has not been investigated. However, neurophysiologic investigations of body acupuncture points suggest that the regions of the brain related to pain inhibition are also affected by the stimulation of acupoints.[21] Brain imaging research conducted by Cho et al. has provided the most conclusive evidence that needle stimulation of acupuncture points can selectively activate different areas of the brain.[22] Needles inserted into body acupuncture points used for visual disorders led to changes of functional magnetic resonance images (fMRI) only in the visual occipital cortex, whereas needles inserted into body acupoints used for hearing disorders selectively activated fMRI activity in the auditory temporal cortex.

Pain reduction by electrical stimulation of the brain has been associated with the CNS endorphinergic systems because of the reversibility of stimulation-produced analgesia by the opiate antagonist naloxone.[23] Pert et al.[24] showed that 7 Hz auricular electrical stimulation through needles inserted into the concha of the rat produced an elevation of hot plate threshold that was also reversed by naloxone. The behavioral analgesia to auricular electroacupuncture was accompanied by a 60% increase in radioreceptor activity in cerebrospinal fluid (CSF) levels of endorphins. This level was significantly greater than that found in a control group of rats. Concomitant with these CSF changes was auricular electroacupuncture-produced depletion in beta-endorphin radioreceptor activity in the ventromedial hypothalamus and the medial thalamus, but not in the periaqueductal gray. Supportive findings in human back pain patients was obtained by Clement-Jones et al.[25,26] Low-frequency electrical stimulation of the concha region of the ear led to relief of pain within 20 minutes of the onset of electroacupuncture. Accompanying the pain relief was an elevation of radioassays for CSF beta-endorphin activity in all 10 subjects. Abbate et al.[27] examined endorphin levels in six patients

undergoing thoracic surgery with 50% nitrous oxide and 50 Hz auricular electroacupuncture. He compared the patients with six control patients who underwent surgery with 70% nitrous oxide but no acupuncture stimulation. The auricular acupuncture patients showed a significantly greater increase in beta-endorphin immunoreactivity.

Kalyuzhnyi et al.[28] applied 15 Hz electrostimulation to the auricular lobe of rabbits, an area corresponding to the jaw and teeth in humans. They then measured behavioral reflexes and cortical somatosensory-evoked potentials in response to tooth pulp stimulation. Auricular electroacupuncture produced a significant decrease in both behavioral reflexes and cortical-evoked potentials to tooth stimulation. For most animals, the suppression of behavioral and neurophysiologic effects were reversed by injecting the opiate antagonist naloxone, suggesting endorphinergic mechanisms. In a few rabbits, however, auriculo-acupuncture stimulation did not induce this naloxone reversible effect. Instead, the naloxone injections themselves led to an analgesic effect. The authors suggested that this paradoxic effect could be explained by an inhibition of an antiopioid substance in select individuals.

Electrical stimulation of auricular acupuncture points on the ear lobes of rabbits, the auricular area that corresponds to the trigeminal nerve, was examined by Fedoseeva et al.[29] Auricular electroacupuncture led to a reduction in amplitude of the cortical somatosensory potentials that were evoked by tooth pulp stimulation. Intravenous injection of the opiate antagonist naloxone diminished the analgesic effect of auricular electroacupuncture at 15 Hz stimulation frequencies, but not at 100 Hz stimulation. Conversely, injection of saralasin, an antagonist for angiotensin II, blocked the analgesic effect of 100 Hz auricular acupuncture, but not 15 Hz stimulation. The amplitude of cortical potentials evoked by electrical stimulation of the hind limb was not attenuated by stimulation of the auricular area for the trigeminal nerve.

Simmons and Oleson[30] examined naloxone reversibility of auricular acupuncture analgesia to acute induced pain in human subjects. All 40 volunteers were assessed for tooth pain threshold by a dental pulp tester. Dental pain levels were determined before and after auriculotherapy and then again after double-blind injection of naloxone or placebo. Subjects were assigned to one of four groups: true auricular electrical stimulation (AES) followed by an injection of naloxone;

true AES followed by an injection of saline; placebo stimulation of the auricle followed by an injection of naloxone; or placebo stimulation of the auricle followed by an injection of saline. Dental pain thresholds were significantly increased by AES conducted at appropriate auricular points for dental pain. Pain thresholds were not altered by sham stimulation at inappropriate auricular points. Naloxone produced a slight reduction in dental pain threshold in the subjects given true AES, whereas the true AES subjects then given saline showed a further increase in pain threshold. The minimal changes in dental pain threshold exhibited by the sham auriculotherapy group were not significantly affected by saline or by naloxone.

Sjolund, Terenius, and Eriksson[31,32] noticed that pain threshold levels did not completely return to baseline after naloxone, suggesting that nonopioid as well as endorphinergic brain mechanisms underlie auriculotherapy. At the same time, auricular electroacupuncture and naloxone reversibility have been found to affect narcotic detoxification in animals[33,34,35] and in humans.[35]

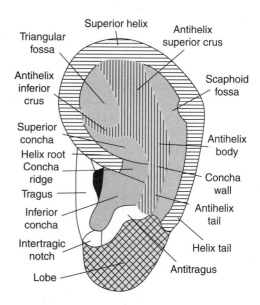

Figure 16-4 The specific anatomical regions of the external ear that distinguish different auricular structures and the terminology used to label them.

AURICULAR ANATOMIC REGIONS

The practice of auricular acupuncture begins with an in-depth appreciation of the complex curvatures that compose the anatomy of the external ear. In accordance with its purpose as the most distal component of the auditory system, the auricle of the ear is shaped to conform to the undulating waves of sound that arrive at the ear. International standardized nomenclature for these anatomic areas was agreed upon at a 1990 meeting of the World Health Organization.[36] The auricle consists of a series of circular ridges and valleys that focus sound input into the auditory canal at the center of the external ear. The most outer ridge of the auricle is referred to as the helix, which is a Latin term for a spiral pattern. An inner ridge within the outer rim is called the antihelix, indicating a spiral structure opposite to another spiral configuration. These two regions of the ear are illustrated in Figure 16-4. The helix is further subdivided into a central helix root, an arching superior helix, and the outermost helix tail. The subsections of the antihelix include an antihelix tail at the bottom; an antihelix body in the middle; and two branches from the antihelix body, the superior crus and the inferior crus. Between these two arms of the

upper antihelix lies the triangular fossa. The scaphoid fossa separates the antihelix from the helix tail. A fossa refers to a fissure or groove, and the scaphoid fossa is a long valley below the two circular ridges that constitute the external ear.

Covering the auditory canal is a flat section known as the tragus, which is a Latin term for a bendable flap. Opposite the tragus is another flap labeled the antitragus, which is a curving continuation of the antihelix. Below the antitragus is the soft, fleshy ear lobe, and between the antitragus and the tragus is an area known as the intertragic notch. The deepest region of the ear is called the concha, because it is shell shaped. The concha is further divided into an inferior concha below, a superior concha above, a concha ridge in between, and a concha wall that surrounds the whole concha floor. Two hidden areas of the ear are the subtragus beneath the tragus and the internal helix beneath the helix root and superior helix. The back side of the ear is referred to as the posterior auricle. This hind portion of the ear is subdivided into a posterior groove behind the antihelix, a posterior lobe behind the lobe, a posterior concha behind the concha, a posterior triangle behind the triangular fossa, and the posterior periphery behind the scaphoid fossa and helix tail. Taking the time to visually recognize and tactilely feel the different contours of the ear will assist greatly in applying the auricular somatotopic correspondences to specific anatomic structures.

AURICULAR MASTER POINTS

The first set of ear acupoints to be considered are the master points or tune-up points shown in Figure 16-5. These auricular points do not correspond to one specific body organ, but instead affect many different medical conditions. Thus they have a "mastery" over the general health of the body. Stimulating these master points serves to tune up or correct metabolic malfunctions. The first two master points, point zero and shen men, are used in almost all auriculotherapy treatment plans for the alleviation of most health disorders. Point zero, which was first described by Nogier, is found in a notch on the helix root as it rises from the concha ridge. It is located at the zero point connecting a vertical axis and a horizontal axis that meet at the center of the ear. Besides serving as an anatomic landmark that indicates the central most position from which other auricular points can be identified, point zero functions as a homeostatic point leading to a zero balance of dysfunctional conditions. The shen men point is similar in function to point zero, leading to a general balance of physiologic activity. It is used to alleviate stress, pain, tension, anxiety, depression, and substance-abuse disorders, which indicates that it is used to treat most medical problems. The English translation of shen men is *spirit gate,* suggesting that activation of this auricular point connects an individual to one's spiritual essence, enhancing the vital forces of life and one's general well being. The location of this auricular point is toward the tip of the triangular fossa, between the junction of the inferior crus and superior crus of the antihelix. Detecting auricular points by an electrodermal point finder typically finds both point zero and shen men to be electrically reactive in most patients.

The next master point is the autonomic point or the sympathetic point, referring to its use in regulating the autonomic nervous system. Although there are many physiologic disorders that involve hyperactive or hypoactive autonomic reflexes, the autonomic point is particularly useful for alleviating vasoconstrictive problems associated with hypertension and cardiovascular disorders. This point is also one of the principal auricular points used for drug detoxifica-

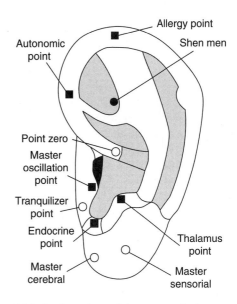

Figure 16-5 Surface view of the anatomical areas of the auricle indicating the location of master points on the ear. An open circle represents raised ridges on the ear, a closed circle represents deeper areas of the ear, and a black square represents hidden, vertical areas of the ear.

tion and substance-abuse treatment. Research by Young and McCarthy[37] has demonstrated evoked electrophysiologic responses following stimulation of the autonomic sympathetic point. As shown in Figures 16-5 and 16-6, the autonomic point is found on the underside of the internal helix where it meets the central-most portion of the antihelix inferior crus. These hidden points are represented by black squares, indicating that these auricular points are not normally visible because they are covered by another region of the ear, in this case the helix root. The next two master points, the thalamus point and the endocrine point, are represented by filled squares because they also are not visible without pulling the auricle outwards with retractors. The thalamus point is found on the base of the concha wall behind the antitragus, and the endocrine point is located nearby on the vertical surface of the intertragic notch. Another name for the thalamus point is the subcortex, indicating that this point connects to subcortical structures in the brain that are involved in neurologic dysfunctions and the reduction of pain sensations. The endocrine point represents the pituitary gland, the master control gland for all other endocrine glands and for the target hormones they release into the general blood supply of the body. An imbalance of circulating hormones accompanies most medical problems.

The next five master points are not used as frequently as the first five auricular points, but they are very important for certain medical problems. Superior to the endocrine point and beneath the lower knob on the peripheral edge of the tragus is the master oscillation point. This auricular point is used by European practitioners of auricular medicine to create a balance of left brain and right brain interactions. Oscillators are said to have a problem with laterality, that is, inappropriate control of cortical functions by the opposite cerebral hemisphere. On the underside of the apex of the external ear is the allergy point, named for its ability to alleviate allergies, arthritis, and inflammatory reactions. Toward the bottom of the tragus is the tranquilizer point, an ear acupuncture point used for sedating the mind and calming the body. The final two master points are located on the ear lobe. At the center of the lobe, vertically below point zero, is the master sensorial point used to alleviate any disturbing sensations. Central to this point on the lobe is the master

cerebral point, also referred to as the neurasthenia or worry point. It is stimulated to contain pathologic, obsessive, worry thoughts and generalized anxiety symptoms that accompany many chronic conditions.

SOMATOTOPIC MUSCULOSKELETAL AURICULAR POINTS

In his original text, *The Treatise of Auriculotherapy,* Paul Nogier[2] focused on auricular representation of the musculoskeletal body because a distinctive correspondence could be confirmed between anatomic areas of myofascial tension and specific regions of tenderness on the external ear. The somatotopic relationship of specific points on the auricle to specific areas of the musculoskeletal body is depicted in Figure 16-7. The cervical vertebrae are represented on the central side of the antihelix tail, the thoracic vertebrae are represented on the central side of the antihelix body, and the lumbo-sacral vertebrae are represented on the inferior crus of the antihelix. This pattern was first reported by

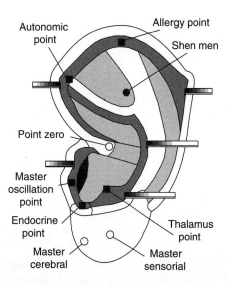

Figure 16-6 Hidden view of the anatomical areas of the auricle indicating the location of master points on the ear. An open circle represents raised ridges on the ear, a closed circle represents deeper areas of the ear, and a black square represents hidden, vertical areas of the ear. Retractors are used to suggest that the ear surface is pulled back to reveal underlying structures.

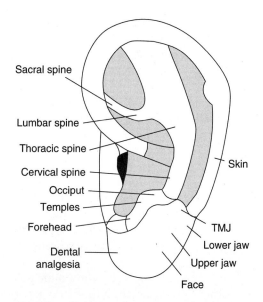

Figure 16-7 Musculoskeletal disorders related to the vertebral spine and the head shown on specific areas of the antihelix, antitragus, and ear lobe.

Nogier in 1957. The pattern is a slightly different configuration from the vertebral arrangement shown in many Chinese ear acupuncture charts. The French system of auriculotherapy of the musculoskeletal system seems to be more accurate for the alleviation of neck tension, back pain, and muscle tension. The posterior groove behind each level of the antihelix is also stimulated to effectively reduce pain from muscle spasms.

Auricular representation of the head and face is located toward the bottom of the ear, on the antitragus and the lobe (Figure 16-7). The occiput is appropriately represented on the antitragus region adjacent to the lowest portion of the antihelix tail that corresponds to the upper cervical spine. Toward the middle of the antitragus is the auricular microsystem point for the temples. Toward the base of the antitragus, near the intertragic notch, is the forehead point. The most reactive of these antitragus auricular points is used to treat both tension headaches and migraines. At the junction of the upper regions of the ear lobe and the lower sections of the scaphoid fossa is found the temporomandibular joint (TMJ) point, for relief

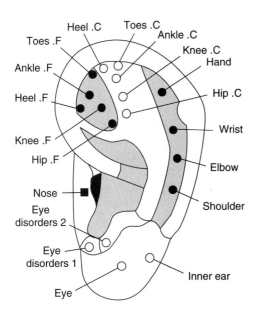

Figure 16-8 Musculoskeletal disorders related to problems with the lower and upper extremities are shown on specific areas of the superior crus of the antihelix, the triangular fossa, and the scaphoid fossa. ".C" indicates the Chinese designation for the area of the ear representing a specific area of the body. ".F" indicates the French localization of the auricular region corresponding to a given body area.

of tight and tense muscles of the lower jaw and upper jaw. Other aspects of the face are depicted on the central regions of the ear lobe. Sensory organs are also found on the ear lobe, including auricular points for facial tension and dental pain.

Figure 16-8 shows that there are both similarities and differences between the Chinese and the French systems of ear acupuncture for auricular representation of the lower extremities. In Chinese auricular charts, the hip, knee, ankle, and foot are represented in an upside down perspective on the superior crus of the antihelix. The somatotopic presentation of these same leg points in the French system are also found in an inverted orientation, but they are located in the triangular fossa. Some people find that the Chinese leg points most accurately correspond to auricular representation of their hip, knee, or foot problems. For other patients with lower extremity problems, greater tenderness and electrical activity is found on the corresponding French points in the triangular fossa. As with vertebral points, stimulation of the posterior side of the triangular fossa and the superior crus also serves to enhance the relief of myofascial pain in the legs or feet.

There are no discrepancies between French and Chinese ear charts depicting auricular representation of the upper extremities. (See Figure 16-8.) Treatment of shoulder problems is achieved by stimulating a point in the scaphoid fossa peripheral to point zero. The shoulder point is logically located next to the junction of auricular representation of the cervical spine and the thoracic spine. Since the somatotopic system on the ear is an inverted orientation, the elbow point is found in the region of the scaphoid fossa above the shoulder point. Ascending higher in the scaphoid fossa, one arrives at the wrist point and above that are several points for the fingers. Both the front and the back side of the ear are stimulated to relieve tennis elbow, carpal tunnel syndrome, and arthritic pain in the fingers. Figure 16-8 also shows areas on the external ear that are used to treat sensory dysfunctions related to the eyes, nose, and inner ears.

AURICULAR REPRESENTATION OF INTERNAL ORGANS

Visceral organs derived from endodermal embryologic tissue are found in the central valley of the auricle, the concha. The autonomic vagus nerve that regulates internal organs only reaches the superficial skin in the region of the concha floor. All of the digestive and thoracic internal organs are illustrated in Figure 16-9. In the inferior concha, below the helix root and near the opening to the actual auditory canal, is the opening to the digestive system, the mouth. These two points are used to alleviate sores affecting the lining of the mouth and throat. The esophagus point extends peripherally from the auditory canal and is used in the treatment of esophageal spasms. Of all the gastrointestinal points, the auricular point for the stomach is the most frequently used in auricular treatment plans. Located on the concha ridge, just peripheral to point zero, the stomach point is used to alleviate stomach aches, nausea, vomiting, ulcers, and weight-control problems. Shiraishi et al.[38] have demonstrated that stimulation of the auricular stomach point in animals reduces neuronal firing rates in the feeding center of the hypothalamus. Neuronal discharges in the satiety center of the hypothalamus are elevated by auricular stimulation. Auricular representation of the duodenum, the small intestines, and the large intestines is found in the superior concha. In Chinese auricular acupuncture, the ear points for the stomach, small intestines, and large intestines are said to connect to the energetic meridians of the same name. Stimulation of these points could thus relieve physiologic dysfunctions of each organ, such as

diarrhea or constipation, or they could alter the energetic function of the corresponding yang meridian. The auricular point for the rectum is found on the helix root and is used for problems of rectal pain.

The five-element Theory of traditional Oriental medicine suggests that five yin organs affect problems of energetic constitution unrelated to the known physiologic function of those organs. The kidney is related to bone problems and hearing disorders as well as urinary dysfunctions, the liver can affect tendon and ligament sprains as well as hepatitis, the spleen can reduce muscle spasms and lymphatic disorders, the lung not only relates to respiratory problems but also to skin disorders and drug detoxification, and finally, the heart is used for mental calming in addition to cardiovascular irregularities. The auricular point for the heart is found at the very center of the inferior concha, in the deepest region of the concha floor (Figure 16-9). This point is used to treat angina pain, hypertension, heart palpitations, and anxiety. Surrounding the heart point are auricular points for the lungs, which the Chinese further differentiated into lung 1, lung 2, and bronchi points. All of these lung points are used to alleviate respiratory problems, but lung 1 and lung 2 are also the principal ear points used to treat narcotic detoxification.

The ear acupoint representing the liver is shown in Figure 16-10. It is located on the concha ridge, pe-

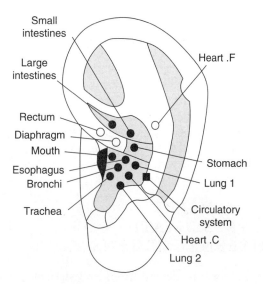

Figure 16-9 Auricular points for the digestive tract and thoracic organs.

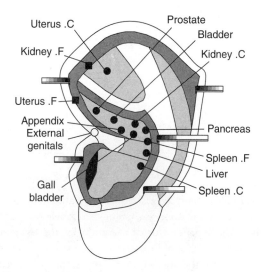

Figure 16-10 Auricular points for the abdominal and urogenital organs.

ripheral to the stomach point. Below the liver point in the inferior concha of the left ear is the Chinese location for the spleen point, whereas the French location for the spleen is on the left superior concha above the liver point. The auricular representation of the gall bladder is in the superior concha of the right ear. Nearby in the superior concha of both ears is the auricular representation of the pancreas, which is used in acupuncture treatments for diabetes.

Urogenital organs are represented on the external ear in either the superior concha below the inferior crus of the antihelix, or in the internal helix on the underside of the helix root. The Chinese auricular points representing the kidney are found in the upper regions of the peripheral superior concha. This ear point is frequently used to alleviate bone fractures, back pain, and hearing disorders as well as kidney dysfunctions. Nogier suggests that the kidney is represented in the internal helix region near the triangular fossa and, unlike the Chinese, believes it is used solely for kidney problems. Both the Chinese and the French localize the auricular bladder point to the region of the superior crus below the midpoint of the inferior crus of the antihelix. Both systems also include the bladder point in the treatment of urinary dysfunctions. One of the most frequently used points for female-related disorders is the Chinese location for the uterus. This rather amazing point has been successfully used for alleviating premenstrual syndrome, menopausal problems, and even infertility. In ancient China, this region of the ear was alluded to as the forbidden zone, since it purportedly lead to abortions in pregnant women. The French representation of the uterus is on the internal helix, below the region of the ear that represents the kidney. The external genitals are represented on the helix root, which is located on the external surface of the auricular region that corresponds to the internal genitals. The Chinese ear points for the external genitals is located higher on the helix root, where it crosses the inferior crus. However, the French representation of the external genitals is lower, where the helix root meets the tragus. Both of these points have been reported to alleviate impotency and genital pain.

NEURO-ENDOCRINE POINTS ON THE EAR

The master endocrine point in the wall of the intertragic notch has already been identified as the region of the external ear used to treat hormonal imbalances.

On auricular areas near the intertragic notch are points representing pituitary control of the adrenal gland and the gonads. The pineal gland is represented at the bottom of the tragus where it affects melatonin release and daily circadian rhythms. These auricular points are shown in Figure 16-11. The rest of the endocrine glands are represented on the concha wall adjacent to the antihelix areas corresponding to the vertebral regions of the body where those glands are found. The point for the thyroid gland is located in the neck near the cervical antihelix tail, the point for the thymus gland in the chest is near the thoracic antihelix body, and the adrenal gland's point is near the lumbar inferior crus. The ovaries and testes are represented on the internal helix beneath the helix root region that represents the external genitals. Stimulation of each endocrine point would lead to a balance of hyperactive or hypoactive hormone release by the corresponding endocrine gland.

Ear acupuncture points corresponding to the peripheral nervous system are found on loci all over the external ear, and the ectodermal CNS points are found on the outer rim of the auricle. The most commonly used auricular points for peripheral nerves are the

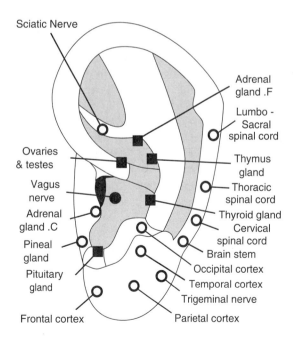

Figure 16-11 Auricular points for the endocrine glands, peripheral nerves, and central nervous system spinal cord and cerebral cortex.

sciatic nerve on the inferior crus, the vagus nerve on the inferior concha, and the trigeminal nerve on the peripheral ear lobe. These points are used for alleviating pain problems associated with sciatic neuralgia, autonomic dysfunctions, and trigeminal neuralgia, respectively. Peripheral neuropathies are treated by stimulating the corresponding auricular area where that body area is represented, and by stimulating the origin of the spinal nerves projecting to that body area and represented on the helix tail. The lumbo-sacral spinal cord is represented on the upper helix tail, the cervical spinal cord is represented on the lower helix tail, and the cervical spinal cord is in between. The ear lobe corresponds to the various lobes of the cerebral cortex, again in an inverted orientation. The motor frontal lobe is represented on the central lobe, near the jaw, but the somatosensory parietal cortex, auditory temporal cortex, and visual occipital cortex are represented on more peripheral regions of the lobe. These cortical points are used to treat neurologic disorders related to each respective cortex.

SUMMARY

There is not yet enough scientific research evidence to lead someone to easily accept the validity of the auricular acupuncture points that have been described. It may seem almost too good to be true that such a simple procedure as auriculotherapy could effectively alleviate pain and pathology in so many different parts of the body. Nonetheless, practitioners of this approach have repeatedly observed that specific areas of the auricle are more sensitive to pressure and more electrically active in a predictable pattern that conforms to the inverted fetus perspective that Nogier first discovered in the 1950s. Activation of these auricular points with needle insertion, transcutaneous electrical stimulation, or application of pressure pellets has been shown to alleviate physical symptoms in the corresponding part of the body. The use of auricular acupuncture to relieve chronic pain and to treat substance abuse has grown in China, Europe, and the United States because of the repeated clinical experience of the effectiveness of this technique. That neurologic reflexes could connect distant regions of the body to somatotopic microsystems on the ear suggests a whole new type of neuronal organization that needs to be fully understood by future studies.

References

1. Oleson T: *Auriculotherapy manual: Chinese and Western systems of ear acupuncture*, ed 2, Los Angeles, 1996, Health Care Alternatives.
2. Nogier P: *Treatise of auriculotherapy*, Moulins-les Metz, France, 1972, Maisonneuve.
3. Huang H: *Ear acupuncture*, New York, 1974, Rodale Press.
4. Bourdiol R: *Elements of auriculotherapy*, Moulins-les Metz, France, 1982, Maisonneuve.
5. Oleson T: Differential application of auricular acupuncture for myofascial, autonomic, and neuropathic pain, *Med Acupuncture* 9:23-28, 1998.
6. Pennfield W, Rasmussen T: *The cerebral cortex of man*, New York, 1950, Macmillan.
7. Chen H: Recent studies on auriculoacupuncture and its mechanism, *J Tradit Chin Med* 13:129-143, 1993.
8. Oleson T, Kroening R, Bresler D: An experimental evaluation of auricular diagnosis: the somatotopic mapping of musculoskeletal pain at ear acupuncture points, *Pain* 8:217-229, 1980.
9. Saku K et al: Characteristics of reactive electropermeable points on the auricles of coronary heart disease patients, *Clin Cardiol* 16:415-419, 1993.
10. Kawakaita K: Development of the low impedance points in the auricular skin of experimental peritonitis rats, *Am J Chin Med* 19:199-205, 1991.
11. Helms J: *Acupuncture energetics: a clinical approach for physicians*, Berkeley, Calif, 1995, Med Acupuncture Publishers.
12. Dale R: The micro-acupuncture system, *Am J Acupuncture* 4:7-24, 1976.
13. Lee T: Thalamic neuron theory: a hypothesis concerning pain and acupuncture, *Med Hypotheses* 3:113-121, 1977.
14. Lee T: Thalamic neuron theory: theoretical basis for the role played by the central nervous system (CNS) in the causes and cures of all disease, *Med Hypotheses* 3:285-302, 1994.
15. Liebeskind J, Mayer D, Akil H: Central mechanisms of pain inhibition: studies of analgesia from focal brain stimulation. In Bonica JJ, editor: *Advances in neurology*, vol 4, New York, 1974, Raven Press.
16. Basbaum A, Fields H: Endogenous pain control systems: brain stem spinal pathway and endorphin circuitry, *Ann Rev Neurosci* 7:513-532, 1979.
17. Melzack R, Wall P: Pain mechanisms: a new theory, *Science* 150:197, 1965.
18. Oleson T, Liebeskind J: Effect of pain-attenuating brain stimulation and morphine on electrical activity in the raphe nuclei of the awake rat, *Pain* 4:211-230, 1978.
19. Oleson T, Kirkpatrick D, Goodman S: Elevation of pain threshold to tooth shock by brain stimulation in primates, *Brain Res* 194:79-95, 1980.

20. Hosobuchi Y et al: Stimulation of human periaqueductal gray for pain relief increases immunoreactive beta endorphin in ventricular fluid, *Science* 203(46):279-281, 1979.

21. Kho H, Robertson E: The mechanisms of acupuncture analgesia: review and update, *Am J Acupuncture* 25:261-281, 1997.

22. Cho Z et al: New findings of the correlation between acupoints and corresponding brain cortices using functional MRI, *Proc Natl Acad Sci* 95:2670-2673, 1998.

23. Akil H et al: Enkephalin-like material elevated in ventricular cerebrospinal fluid of pain patients after analgesic focal stimulation, *Science* 209:463-465, 1978.

24. Pert A et al: Alterations in rat central nervous system endorphins following transauricular electroacupuncture, *Brain Res* 224:83-93, 1981.

25. Clement-Jones V et al: Acupuncture in heroin addicts: changes in met-enkephalin and beta-endorphin in blood and cerebrospinal fluid, *Lancet* 2:380-383, 1979.

26. Clement-Jones V et al: Increased beta-endorphin but not me-enkephalin levels in human cerebrospinal fluid after acupuncture for recurrent pain, *Lancet* 3:946-948, 1980.

27. Abbate D et al: A beta-endorphin and electroacupuncture *Lancet* 3:1309, 1980.

28. Kalyuzhnyi L: Analgesic naloxone's effect on acupuncture-resistant, acupuncture-tolerant, and acupuncture-sensitive rabbits, *Acupunct Electrother Res, Int J* 15:259, 1990.

29. Fedoseeva O, Kalyuzhnyi L, Sudakov K: New peptide mechanisms of auriculo-acupuncture electro-analgesia: role of angiotensin II, *Acupunct Electrother Res, Int J* 15:1-8, 1990.

30. Simmons M, Oleson T: Auricular electrical stimulation and dental pain threshold, *Anesthesia Prog* 40:14-19, 1993.

31. Sjolund B, Eriksson M: Electroacupuncture and endogenous morphines, *Lancet* 2:1985, 1976.

32. Sjolund B, Terenius L, Eriksson M: Increased cerebrospinal fluid levels of endorphins after electroacupuncture, *Acta Physiol Scand* 100:382-384, 1977.

33. Ho W: The influence of electroacupuncture on naloxone induced morphine withdrawal in mice: elevation of brain opiate-like activity, *Eur J Pharmacol* 49:197-199, 1978.

34. Ng L: Modification of morphine-withdrawal in rats following transauricular electrostimulation: an experimental paradigm for auricular electroacupuncture, *Biol Psychiatry* 10:575-580, 1975.

35. Ng L: Auricular acupuncture in animals: effects of opiate withdrawal and involvement of endorphins, *J Compl Altern Med* 2:61-64, 1996.

36. Kroening R, Oleson T: Rapid narcotic detoxification in chronic pain patients treated with auricular electroacupuncture and naloxone, *Int J Addictions* 20:1347-1360, 1985.

37. World Health Organization: *A standard international acupuncture nomenclature: memorandum from a WHO Meeting,* WHO Bulletin 68, Lyon, France, 1990, pp 165-169.

38. Young M, McCarthy P: Effect of acupuncture stimulation of the auricular sympathetic point on evoked sudomotor response, *J Altern Compl Med* 4:29-38, 1998.

39. Shiraishi T et al: Effects of auricular stimulation on feeding-related hypothalamic neuronal activity in normal and obese rats, *Brain Res Bull* 36:141-148, 1995.

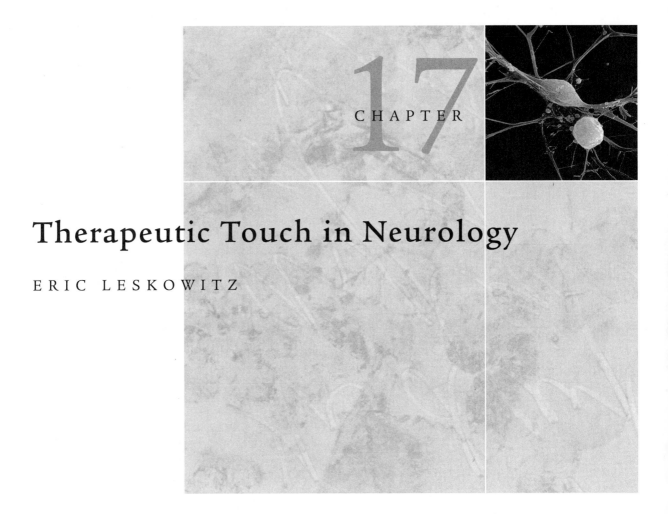

17

Therapeutic Touch in Neurology

ERIC LESKOWITZ

t is always a good idea to get a map before setting out for new territory. So before discussing this chapter's specific topic—the use of Therapeutic Touch (TT) in neurology—a brief overview of the field of complementary and alternative medicine (CAM) is in order. This overview is designed to emphasize the multidimensional nature of human beings and the importance of having a full spectrum of therapeutic approaches to deal with illness and health. This perspective is particularly important in considering therapies that seem to have no basis in scientific fact, according to the Western medical model.

THE MULTIDIMENSIONAL MODEL OF HUMAN FUNCTION

It is helpful to think of human beings as having four main levels of function and structure. The most concrete level is physiology, the major focus of medical school training and modern medical and surgical therapies. In the biomedical model, which focuses on this level, the human body is seen as a complex mechanism that is the source of illness and the target for treatments. The biomedical model focuses all its treatments, whether pharmaceuticals, surgery, radiation, or genetic manipulation, on this concrete level.

Emotions and thoughts constitute the next important levels. In some traditions, such as yoga and Theosophy, these are believed to be two distinct levels. However, for the purposes of this chapter, the realm of thoughts, beliefs, attitudes, and emotions are considered as one level. This dimension is addressed by psychotherapy and other mind-body techniques. A large body of knowledge in the field of psychoneuroimmunology has demonstrated that psychologic and emotional events can influence the onset and course of most important medical syndromes. A whole range of mind-body techniques that are discussed elsewhere in this book addresses this area. For example, hypnosis, biofeedback, meditation, imagery, and specific psychotherapies all fit into this second paradigm.

The last dimension is the spiritual. The most lasting value of holistic medicine may be that it finally bridges the long-standing gap between religion and science. We now have scientific data validating the clinical efficacy of interventions like prayer[1] and the laying on of hands,[2] two approaches that were formerly taboo for medical researchers to investigate, let alone prescribe. What these and other spiritually based therapies have in common is an insistence that human beings are animated by a special type of vital energy. This vital energy fills individuals up with health when they are inspired, and is drained when they are ill. Many cultures speak of the phenomenon in their own language. In China, the energy is called *qi;* in India, yogis call it *prana;* in Hebrew mysticism, it is called *ruach;* but in Western medicine there is no word or concept for this vital energy. The end result is called *homeostatic balance,* but there is no knowledge as to how it comes about.

A wide range of alternative medicine therapies deal with this dimension of subtle energy. These therapies tend to be the ones that are most controversial and the most difficult for mainstream science to make sense of. Some of the most prominent energy-based therapies are addressed elsewhere in this book, including acupuncture, qigong, homeopathy, shiatsu, and tai chi. The focus for this chapter is on one of the few Western-based techniques that acknowledges and harnesses this so-called subtle energy, Therapeutic Touch (TT).

HISTORIC PRECURSORS OF THERAPEUTIC TOUCH

To be fair, some of the medical renegades of the Western medical tradition did try to characterize this sub-tle life energy. Sigmund Freud talked of libido, Wilhelm Reich researched orgone, Henri Bergson wrote of élan vital, and most importantly for this chapter, Franz Mesmer tried to harness "animal magnetism." Although widespread opinion holds that Mesmer's work was that of a charlatan, his technique was actually a precursor of TT and was more valid than he was ever given credit for. In addition, the treatment he was given by the medical establishment of his time has interesting overtones considering the American Medical Association's (AMA) hostile reaction to CAM and the recent controversy over a widely publicized attempt to debunk TT.

Austrian physician Franz Anton Mesmer participated in the intellectual ferment that swept Europe in the late 1700s, in particular the interest in the newly discovered forces of electricity and magnetism.[3] He developed a wildly popular form of magnetic therapy that used magnetic stones and his own personal store of so-called animal magnetism to heal his wealthy aristocratic patients. The wide range of disorders that he healed would probably be labeled as conversion symptoms today. However, because the medical establishment was threatened by his runaway success, both medical and financial, King Louis XVI asked the Royal Society to investigate the claims of Mesmerism. These eminent scientists, including Lavoisier, Guillotine, and Ben Franklin, found that his patients did, in fact, get better, but only through the powers of imagination and suggestion. They discounted the magnetic fluidium that Mesmer claimed to transmit to his patient by making his famous Mesmeric passes. These passes consisted of stroking the air several inches from the patient's body in repeated downward movements. The fact that a commission completely vindicated Mesmer after his death was no solace, as he had effectively been run out of town, never again to recover his reputation or influence.

Two hundred years later, the twentieth century having drawn to a close, the tide has turned. Modern biomagnetism has documented that there is an energy field surrounding the human body.[4] The process has shown that purported energy healers emit measurable negative body potential surges of up to 90 volts under experimental conditions.[5] In the early 1970s, a team consisting of nurse Delores Krieger and medical intuitive Dora Kunz developed a standardized treatment known as Therapeutic Touch.[6] The purpose of TT was to allow medical professionals, particularly nurses, to harness some of the same subtle energies that saints and mystics and healers had been working with for centuries.

THE TECHNIQUE
OF THERAPEUTIC TOUCH

The standardized TT treatment protocol involves five steps.[7] The first and most important step is centering, in which the nurse healer takes a moment to quiet the mind and focus on a heart-centered wish to be of service to the patient. The second step is known as the assessment, in which the nurse scans the patient's external energy field by placing the palms of her hands several inches away from each part of the patient's body. The nurse tries to sense alterations in the subtle perceptions of tingling or temperature that are typically experienced in this process. These alterations are thought to reflect underlying physiologic problems and indicate the regions to be addressed in step three.

In the third treatment step, the nurse tries to unruffle and clear these apparent energy blocks with a series of slow, stroking movements down the patient's energy field. The nurse does not actually make any physical contact. These movements are identical in form to the Mesmeric passes. In the next step, the nurse focuses his or her hands on one particular region, and directs and modulates the flow of energy there. This balancing phase may also involve direct physical contact with the patient's body. In the final phase, the nurse evaluates the changes in the patient's energy field hoping to detect the symmetric and open flow that marks a successful treatment.

SCIENTIFIC STUDIES

In the past 20 years, a large amount of clinical literature has built up around TT. There are 129 references listed at the end of the Rosa article cited later, and Medlines gave 317 TT citations as of October 2000. The technique has been applied to a wide range of conditions, not only measuring subjective variables, such as pain, anxiety, and self-esteem, but also objectively measuring physiologic processes, including immune function, wound healing, and general medical conditions. Experimental rigor, as usually defined by clinical medicine, is hard to come by, in part due to the nature of TT itself. A sham TT technique has been developed in which patients can be blinded to TT. In this technique, nurses move their hands in the typical downward strokes of TT, but occupy their minds with mental arithmetic rather than the attitude of compassionate caring that marks true TT. Unfortunately, the nurse cannot be blinded to the treatment being given because, by definition, he or she is aware of which of these two states of mind is being used. Hence, TT research can at best be only single blind.

Two key physiologic studies follow as well as some case vignettes that illustrate how TT has been integrated into the Pain Management Program at Spaulding Rehabilitation Hospital (SRH) in Boston.

Stress is known to inhibit numerous physiologic processes. One such process that is susceptible to objective monitoring is wound healing, that is, the rate of repair of damaged skin. For example, the skin of people under high stress, in this case caregivers of Alzheimer's patients, heals much more slowly from punch biopsies than does the skin of matched controls.[8] In contrast, TT has been shown to accelerate the rate of wound healing in healthy volunteers. In an elegant study, Daniel Wirth[2] controlled for placebo and expectancy effects when he demonstrated that after 15 days, none of the 50 mm^2 biopsy wounds in the untreated control group had completely healed. However, 50% of the TT recipients had healed. The level of statistical significance was p < 0.0001. Unfortunately, this crucial study has never been replicated by independent researchers, but it provides a tantalizing clue as to how clinicians might someday be able to enhance the body's healing response after surgery or injury.

Another important study[9] showed that stress-induced immunosuppression could be reversed by TT, as measured by serum levels of immunoglobulins A and M in medical students during final exam time. Again, a clinically important physiologic variable was effected in a positive manner by a relatively brief course of TT. The potential clinical applications are intriguing, especially given the wide range of medical conditions that are characterized by immune dysfunction.

THERAPEUTIC TOUCH
IN NEUROLOGY

So it is possible to pick out important nuggets from the medical literature, some intriguing research data suggesting that TT can influence mind and body. But what about neurology? The next section focuses on several specific neurologic conditions and highlights some relevant research and clinical findings.

Peripheral Neuropathy

Two clinical vignettes from SRH highlight potential applications of TT to peripheral neuropathy; however, no formal research studies have yet been done with this specific syndrome.

Case 1: Dan was a 39-year-old man with AIDS-related peripheral neuropathy. His bilateral foot pain had not responded to opiates, tricyclics, or anticonvulsants. His primary nurse attempted to alleviate his attendant anxiety with a course of TT and found, much to her surprise, that not only did Dan's anxiety level decrease with TT, but his pain level went from a self-rating of "very bad" to "not much." Unfortunately, his pain returned the next day. He continued to respond favorably to each TT session, although his carryover only lasted several hours. He was lost to followup after discharge.

Case 2: Lillian was a 68-year-old woman who had developed neuropathic pain in the distribution of her femoral nerve, which had been accidentally injured during vascular surgery several years earlier. She was able to obtain only slight relief with standard medications for neuropathic pain. In addition, her allodynia was so severe that she could not participate in any form of rehab that involved direct physical contact, including physical therapy (PT) manipulation and tactile thermal desensitization. However, during the course of a TT treatment she felt the sensitivity decrease to such an extent that she allowed the TT practitioner to physically touch her leg. This was the first time she had allowed another person to touch her. This decreased sensitivity opened the door to a range of other standard pain management approaches, which were able to significantly decrease her discomfort. Interestingly, the other intervention that lessened her pain level was psychotherapy, during which she was able to express for the first time her rage and disappointment at the trusted surgeon who had damaged her nerve.

Phantom Pain

The SRH clinic has recently reported on the successful use of TT in treating cases of phantom limb pain.[10,11] A fascinating aspect of this work, which merits further

study, is the finding that the TT therapist can perceive the energetic outlines of the phantom limb in what appears to be empty space. The patient is also able to detect when the therapist's hands make contact with his phantom limb. These findings suggest validity to the notion that a subtle energetic anatomy exists independent of our physiology. The TT process, when successful, creates a feeling that has been described as draining the pain out of the affected limb. Benefits last from hours to days, and patients have been taught to administer this treatment to themselves for sustained long-term benefits.

Case 3: Mary was a 73-year-old woman who had a below-the-knee amputation of her left leg to prevent the worsening of peripheral-vascular-disease-induced gangrene. She had expected to lose only a toe, not a limb, and from the moment she awoke from surgery she experienced severe phantom pain in the toe that was gangrenous. No standard medications such as opiates, anticonvulsants, or antidepressants were helpful, but she responded almost immediately to TT. She felt the pain drain out of the bottom of her phantom foot and became pain free for the first time in more than a year. She could amplify the effects of this treatment by visualizing a soothing blue light coating her painful limb. She eventually learned to perform TT on herself and reported that she could start each day with a TT session and remain quite comfortable throughout the day, unless her stress level rose above a certain threshold.

Multiple Sclerosis

Several reports in the nursing literature describe the use of TT in the care of multiple sclerosis (MS) patients. One case study[12] highlights the adjunctive role of TT in MS care, noting in particular its benefits for such subjective symptoms as mood and comfort. Another paper[13] emphasizes the high rate of use of various alternative therapies by MS patients and indicates that TT is one of the most popular. Results are reported in terms of quality of life but are not quantitated by using, for example, the Schatsky functional rating scale or the Functional Improvement Measure (FIM). These simple steps could greatly strengthen the TT literature on MS. In addition, given the current conceptualization of MS as an autoimmune disorder, the previously mentioned demonstration of enhanced immune functioning following TT takes on added significance.

Dementia

No studies exist concerning the use of TT to reverse the dementing process, but several papers describe its use in bringing about behavioral changes in Alzheimer's patients. In one naturalistic study,[14] TT was introduced as a stress-management technique. It was found to induce a relaxation response in demented patients who had a history of agitated behavior, but it was not effective in decreasing the actual levels of these behaviors. Direct physical contact, as in hand massage, proved more effective than TT in reducing agitation in these patients suggesting that with a certain degree of brain damage, the effects of TT may be too subtle to translate into overt behavioral changes.

Headache

One of the best-designed TT studies ever performed looked at the effects of TT on tension headache pain.[15] By using the sham TT intervention mentioned earlier, expectancy and placebo factors could be taken into consideration. A matched group of 60 headache patients was studied, all of whom were naive to prior TT treatments. Ninety percent of the members of the active treatment group experienced improvements in symptoms following TT, averaging a 70% decrease in degree of symptom intensity. Of the control patients, 80% reported pain reduction that averaged only 37% in degree. It should be noted that both groups practiced deep breathing. Therefore the placebo group was actually receiving a treatment known to be somewhat helpful in itself for mild headache symptoms, and the treatment group actually received two treatments, TT plus breathing. Furthermore, this differential benefit was even more pronounced four hours after the initial treatment, again favoring TT over sham TT controls.

Postoperative Pain

In a single-blind clinical trial that measured postoperative pain in 108 patients, Meehan found[16] that a single TT treatment reduced the patients' need for analgesic medication, although reported pain levels were similar between patients who received genuine TT and those who received the sham TT control intervention. Presumably, the untreated patients used additional analgesics to make up for the differential im-

pact of TT. An extension of this work should look at the role of regular TT applications. Presumably there would be a sort of dosage effect, with greater impact coming from more regular application of the modality. The author cautiously notes that TT may be best conceptualized as an adjunctive pain therapy, rather than as a primary treatment modality.

Burn Pain

Pain, anxiety, and impaired immune function are all known to follow significant burns to the body surface. One study[17] measured the impact of regular TT treatments on these three variables on patients in a hospital burn unit. Again using sham TT control intervention, this single-blinded randomized clinical trial determined that 5 days of regular TT caused statistically significant reductions on self-reported pain (the McGill Pain Questionnaire Rating Index) and anxiety (the Visual Analogue Scale). Immune function was also altered, as reflected by a 13% decrease in CD8+ cell concentration, although the clinical significance of this cellular change was not clear. Again, the authors call for more studies to look at the long-term effects of ongoing TT and to control more tightly for behavioral variables that might influence outcome.

A RECENT CONTROVERSY

Despite this promising list of neurologic and other medical/physiologic processes that have been proven to be affected by TT, the general populace's view of this technique has recently become one of extreme skepticism. This stems in part from a lack of awareness of the body of research data cited previously. However, it stems more directly from the massive publicity given to a unique report—the *Journal of the American Medical Association's (JAMA)* recent publication of an 11-year-old schoolgirl's science fair project, titled "A Closer Look at Therapeutic Touch."[18] This study is important on so many levels that it is worth discussing in some detail.

At the level of basic science, this study is noteworthy for using an elegantly simple research protocol to test whether nurse practitioners of TT could in fact reliably detect the presence of the so-called energy field of their client. In this protocol, the nurses were effectively blindfolded and then asked to guess over which of their outstretched hands the researcher was placing her own hand. In other words, they were asked to sense the energy field emanating from the experimenter's hand. Interestingly enough, the nurses were only accurate 40% of the time in their guesses, indicating that they performed even more poorly in their energy assessments than would be expected with random guessing. The authors then concluded that because there was no experimental validation of the energy fields that purportedly underlie TT therapy, there could be no clinical effectiveness to TT as a treatment intervention. The *JAMA* editors joined in, urging patients to refuse to pay for such treatments until scientific evidence of its efficacy could be produced.

As a tide of rebuttal letters to *JAMA*[19] and editorial commentaries elsewhere[20,21] pointed out, there were numerous crucial methodologic flaws in the study. There were also logical fallacies in the conclusions reached by the authors and the editor. Of note, the degree of expertise of the TT volunteers was not reported, and they did not in fact enter into the true TT process outlined previously because they were never asked to elicit their inner intent to heal. This omission raises questions about what technique was actually being assessed. Many of the sessions were videotaped in a television studio, which could easily have generated performance anxiety. More importantly, there was no control for experimenter bias, a significant possibility given that the girl's parents, the article's co-authors, were members of Quackwatch Inc., an organization devoted to debunking alternative therapies.

Regardless, it is a basic tenet of energy-based therapies that the frame of mind of the healer influences the degree of energy effect he or she creates.[22] If the girl had been a master healer emitting huge bursts of energy, it would be striking that the success rates were so low. However, if she had at some unconscious or conscious level wanted negative results, she might have literally shut down her own energy field, making it even harder than normal to detect its presence. Perhaps this is the true significance of the low detection scores—the nurses may have been accurately responding to a negative alteration in the test energy field. Contrast these apparently negative data with results from an earlier study[23] that reported a successful detection rate of more than 65% using a similar protocol. Interestingly, this study was not referenced in the otherwise exhaustive TT bibliography cited in the *JAMA* paper. *JAMA* authors summarily dismissed this research literature as being without significant scientific merit.

Even more striking than these methodologic problems is the authors' unwarranted conclusion that TT is clinically useless. No clinical outcomes were assessed in this study, so no conclusions could logically be made in the domain of clinical efficacy. One wonders what led the usually judicious editorial staff of *JAMA* to make such an uncalled-for statement decrying the use of a therapeutic intervention. The resemblance to Mesmer's run-in with the Royal Society is striking: political influence attempting to destroy work that threatens the dominant medical paradigm.

SUMMARY

Certainly there has been a good measure of deserved resistance by the medical establishment to novel energy-based therapies like TT, but the tide is turning. The field of biomagnetics is documenting the existence of human subtle-energy fields. A rapidly growing body of evidence is proving that TT and its relatives can be effective in a wide range of clinical situations. In neurology, this includes most prominently a variety of pain conditions, as research on TT in other neurologic conditions is still in its infancy. Further research in neurology is needed to move beyond the reporting of subjective variables into the realm of functional measurements and biological parameters. The current situation is full of promise for future discoveries in the application of energy-based therapies to the problems of medicine, in general, and neurology, in particular.

References

1. Byrd R: The effects of intercessory prayer on patients in a coronary care unit, *South Med J* 81(7): 826-829, 1988.
2. Wirth D: The effect of noncontact therapeutic touch on the rate of healing of full thickness dermal wounds, *Subtle Energies* 1(1):1-21, 1990.
3. Ellenberger H: *The discovery of the unconscious*, New York, 1970, Basic Books.
4. Becker R: *Crosscurrents: the promise of electromedicine, the perils of electropollution*, Los Angeles, 1990, J Tarcher.
5. Green E et al: Anomalous electrostatic phenomena in exceptional subjects, *Subtle Energies* 2(3):69-81, 1991.
6. Wager S: *A doctor's guide to therapeutic touch*, New York, 1996, Perigee Books.
7. Mulloney S, Wells-Federman C: Therapeutic touch: a healing modality, *Cardiovasc Nurs* 28:117-125, 1998.

8. Kiecolt-Glaser J et al: Slowing of wound healing by psychological stress, *Lancet* 346:1194-1196, 1995.
9. Olson M et al: Stress-induced immunosuppression and therapeutic touch, *Altern Ther* 3:68-74, 1997.
10. Leskowitz E: Phantom limb pain: subtle energy perspectives, *Subtle Energy Energy Med* 8(2):125-152, 1999.
11. Leskowitz E: Phantom limb pain and complementary medicine: a case report, *Arch Phys Med Rehab* 81: 522-524, 2000.
12. Payne M: The use of therapeutic touch with rehabilitation clients, *Rehab Nurs* 14(2):69-72, 1989.
13. Fawcett J et al: Use of alternative health therapies by people with multiple sclerosis: an exploratory study, *Holist Nurs Pract* 8(2):36-42, 1994.
14. Snyder M, Egan E, Burns K: Interventions for decreasing agitation behaviors in persons with dementia, *J Gerontol Nurs* 21(7):34-40, 1995.
15. Keller E, Bzdek V: Effects of therapeutic touch on tension headache pain, *Nurs Res* 35(2):101-106, 1986.
16. Meehan T: Therapeutic touch and postoperative pain: a Rogerian research study, *Nurs Sci Q* 6(12):69-78, 1993.
17. Turner J et al: The effect of therapeutic touch on pain and anxiety in burn patients, *J Adv Nurs* 28(1):10-20, 1998.
18. Rosa L et al: A close look at therapeutic touch, *JAMA* 279:1005-1010, 1998.
19. Freinkel A et al: An even closer look at therapeutic touch, *JAMA* 280(22):1905-1908, 1999.
20. Achterberg J: Clearing the air in the therapeutic touch controversy, *Alt Ther* 4(4):100-101, 1999.
21. Leskowitz E: Un-debunking therapeutic touch, *Alt Ther* 4(4):101-102, 1999.
22. Brennan B: *Hands of Light,* New York, 1992, Bantam New Age.
23. Schwartz G, Russek L, Beltran J: Interpersonal hand-energy registration: evidence for implicit performance and perception, *Subtle Energies* 6:183-200, 1995.

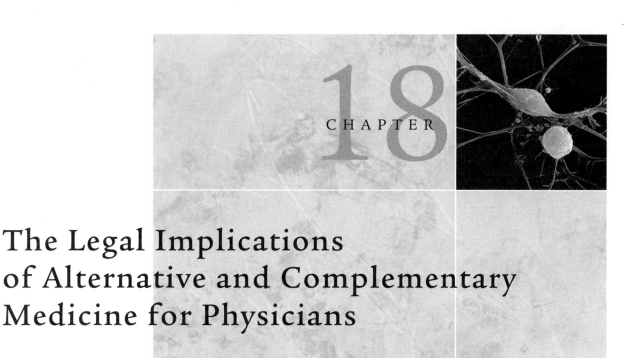

CHAPTER

18

The Legal Implications of Alternative and Complementary Medicine for Physicians

PAT LEPORE

lternative medicine is defined as "... medical interventions not widely taught in US
medical schools or generally available in
US hospitals."[1] Americans are turning to alternative,
or complementary medicine, including chiropractic,
acupuncture, biofeedback, massage, and nutrition
therapies, in record numbers.[1,2] Patient visits to alternative providers now outnumber visits to primary
care providers.[3] In a 1993 study published in the New
England Journal of Medicine, researchers concluded
that in one year alone, 427 million Americans or one
in every three, consulted alternative providers.[2] During the same time period, Americans paid $10.3 bil-
lion dollars out of pocket in professional fees for the
services of alternative medicine practitioners.[2] In contrast, only 388 million Americans made visits to their
primary care providers.[2] A follow-up study by the
same team of researchers showed that visits to alternative medicine practitioners increased to 629 million
by 1997, exceeding the number of total visits to all primary care practitioners in the United States.[4]

Some of this increase may be attributable to increased insurance coverage for nontraditional medical care. Until a few years ago, third-party reimbursement was available only for treatments and services
generally endorsed by the biomedical community. Responding to patient interest and recognizing the
lower cost frequently associated with alternative treatments, many insurance plans, particularly managed-
care plans, now reimburse for alternative therapies.[5]

Patients embrace alternative therapies for many reasons. Some people think that alternative methods are

more efficacious than traditional remedies. Others believe that alternative and complementary practitioners are more approachable than conventionally trained physicians, that the cost is less, or that the treatment is more accessible than conventional therapy.[6]

In response to this interest in alternative medicine, the federal government created the Office of Alternative Medicine (OAM) within the National Institutes of Health (NIH). Funds were appropriated to create OAM in 1992. Now called the National Center for Complementary and Alternative Medicine, the mandate of NCCAM is to "facilitate the evaluation of alternative medical treatment modalities" and to determine their effectiveness.[7] NCCAM also serves as a clearinghouse on alternative medicine and sponsors a research training program.[7]

Organized medicine, however, remains highly skeptical of the claims of alternative providers.[8] Through trade and professional associations as well as local legislatures, organized medicine has fought to restrict patient access to alternative health care providers.[6] Traditional medicine has used two approaches to limit access to nontraditional providers: licensing laws and insurance coverage. Medical licensing originated as a way to protect the public by driving unqualified personnel out of the profession. Anyone who did not train and graduate from an approved program of study was considered unqualified personnel. Where it was not possible to eliminate an alternative practice, such as with chiropractic, the licensing statutes acted to limit their scope of practice.

However, there are signs that conventional medicine is waking up to the trend towards alternative and complementary medicine. In 1998, 75 of 117 American medical schools that participated in a survey on medical school curriculum, indicated that some educational opportunities related to alternative and complementary medicine were available to students, although the courses were usually offered as electives.[5]

Patients are aware of traditional medicine's disregard for nontraditional practices. Consequently, patients do not typically share information about their use of alternative medicine with primary care practitioners. They also tend not to regard primary care practitioners as sources for advice or referrals when considering nontraditional medical approaches.[1] Researchers estimate that 90% of patients using alternative therapies are self-referred.[1]

The public has embraced alternative medicine. The government has established an office to study it, and insurers (particularly managed care plans) are beginning to reimburse for some nontraditional therapies.

Why then do physicians resist integrating nontraditional therapies into their practice? Certainly some resistance comes simply from a lack of knowledge about the efficacy of nontraditional methods of treating disease. A bigger concern for many physicians, though, is increased malpractice risk.[1] They believe that if they integrate nontraditional practices into their traditional approaches or if they refer patients to alternative and complementary medical providers, they will assume some liability for unsuccessful treatments or for nontraditional treatments that result in poor outcomes.

Is malpractice a significant risk? Are there other risks associated with integrating nontraditional approaches into traditional medical practice? And if there are risks, how can the risks associated with integrative medical practice be mitigated?

INCREASED MALPRACTICE LIABILITY

Malpractice is defined as any medical treatment that fails to conform to the standard of care within the profession and that results in injury to the patient.[9] All medical malpractice claims measure a physician's actions against this standard. The greater the deviation from the standard of care, the greater the physician's risk of malpractice.

Most alternative and complementary therapies are, by definition, outside the traditional treatments offered by physicians. Therefore, physicians believe that integrating alternative therapies into traditional medical practice brings with it an increase in malpractice liability. They may be correct. A court looks to the general medical community when evaluating a particular medical practice. Practices that are widespread, common, and accepted become part of the standard of care within that community.

Physicians may also face increased malpractice risk for referring patients to nontraditional providers. When patients suffer a negative outcome at the hands of an alternative practitioner, they may look to the referring physician for compensation under one of several theories of imputed or vicarious liability.

Integrating Nontraditional Therapies into Traditional Practice

When integrating nontraditional therapies into traditional practice, the malpractice risk arises from using or recommending alternative treatments, which frequently have little scientific data validating their usefulness, that then fail to cure or further injure a patient. For example, a physician recommends that a patient with coronary artery disease consider chelation therapy as an alternative to coronary artery bypass surgery.[10] Subsequently, the patient suffers a heart attack and sues the doctor for malpractice. Assume the patient was informed of the risks and consequences of undergoing the therapy and made a fully informed decision. What would be the result for the physician?

The plaintiff/patient in this case would argue that the physician was negligent by failing to provide medical treatment meeting the standard of care of medical practice within that locality. The plaintiff/patient would further argue that standard treatment for coronary artery disease includes bypass surgery. Chelation therapy is not standard therapy and, therefore, falls below the accepted standard of care. Many courts are tempted to equate unusual care with substandard care. Substandard care in any malpractice action constitutes negligence.

Therefore, under the traditional analysis applied to malpractice cases, the plaintiff/patient would prevail. The doctor failed to provide care according to the prevailing standards within the medical community, and the failure to provide appropriate care was a substantial factor in bringing about harm to the patient.

Referring Patients to Alternative Practitioners

What if the physician does not practice integrative medicine but refers patients to alternative medical practitioners? Does the referring physician assume any liability for making the referral? What are the possible actions physicians may face under this set of circumstances?

The general rule in malpractice cases asserting joint negligence is that the plaintiff must establish a relationship between the referring and treating physi-

cians.[9] There must be an ongoing relationship in which the referring physician continues to be involved in the treatment of the patient and exerts some control or influence over the course of treatment. Courts have generally been reluctant to impute liability to one physician for the actions of another.[10] It is more likely that a court would impute responsibility when a physician supervises other non–physician personnel, such as nurses or physician assistants. In these cases the physician has assumed responsibility for the overall care of the patient, and the other personnel involved in the care and treatment of the patient are assumed to be acting in accordance with the physician's orders. Therefore, referral to an alternative medicine practitioner is unlikely to provide a basis for a malpractice suit unless there is some ongoing, continual relationship between the practitioner and the referring physician involving the care of the patient.

Absent the relationship described previously, what liability does a physician assume for recommending an alternative practitioner? Physicians should be aware of a cause of action known as *negligent referral*. In this action, the plaintiff claims the referring physician assumes responsibility for the actions of the alternative practitioner because the referring physician should have known the following: (1) treatment by the alternative practitioner could be harmful to the patient and/or (2) the referring physician has a duty to refer only to skilled practitioners.[11]

Essentially, the court would evaluate the referring physician's ability to foresee harm to the patient based on the use of alternative treatment. If any harm, including harm resulting from a delay in conventional treatment, could be anticipated, the first part of the test is met.

The second element requires that referring physicians be knowledgeable about the care rendered by alternative practitioners. Referring physicians have a duty to the patient to recommend only highly skilled, competent practitioners. This is more difficult in the case of alternative and complementary practitioners because many are uncredentialled. Still, it would be prudent for physicians to make referrals only when they are comfortable with the level of expertise and skill of the provider.

No court has yet to entertain an action for negligent referral. Even though the risk may appear small, physicians interested in expanding their practice to include alternative practitioners would be wise to familiarize themselves with all possible areas of exposure. Referring only to licensed or credentialled practitioners and encouraging, even insisting, on conventional treatment when there is any possible risk to the patient's health is essential, both to protect the patient and to minimize any malpractice exposure.

Working with Alternative Providers

Physicians who choose to work in concert with alternative providers should be aware that they open themselves up to claims of "vicarious liability." Vicarious liability is the liability of one person for the actions of another.[12] Frequently, the other person is an employee or agent of the principal. In an action for negligence based on vicarious liability, the relationship between the parties is significant. Did one serve in a superior capacity to the other or control the actions of the other? Was the treating physician merely acting as an agent of the supervising physician? The likelihood of prevailing in a negligence suit based on vicarious liability is greater when the plaintiff can establish an unequal relationship between the parties and demonstrate that the actions were controlled by one party and merely carried out by the other.

Physicians working with alternative practitioners must be aware that relationships with alternative providers can give rise to a principal-agent relationship. Negligent acts of the agent, the alternative practitioner in this case, expose the physician to potential liability.

DEFENSES TO MALPRACTICE CLAIMS

Defenses that are available to claims of malpractice include assumption of the risk and the doctrines of the respectable minority, clinical innovation, and informed consent. All of these defenses are available to physicians involved in malpractice cases arising out of the use of nontraditional practitioners or referrals to these practitioners. Each is discussed in more detail in the following sections.

Assumption of the Risk

In the malpractice context, the doctrine of "assumption of the risk" recognizes the patient's responsibility for some treatment choices. Essentially, the doctrine acknowledges that an individual who knows and understands the risks associated with a particular therapy can consent to that course of treatment. By doing so, he or she implicitly recognizes the risk and agrees to assume responsibility for the decision to pursue that particular course of action. Assumption of the risk is doctrinally different from negligence because it shifts the focus of malpractice liability from the physician's treatment decisions to the choices the patient makes. The case of *Schneider v Revici* is illustrative.[13]

Mrs. Edith Schneider, the plaintiff in this case, rejected the advice of her physician and two surgeons, all of whom recommended the surgical excision of a breast mass. Instead, she consulted Dr. Revici who offered Mrs. Schneider a nontoxic, noninvasive therapeutic regime. After a 14-month course of treatment in which no improvement was noted, Dr. Revici also recommended surgery for Mrs. Schneider.

Mrs. Schneider had signed a consent form acknowledging the experimental nature of the treatments. The consent form also indicated that results could not be guaranteed. Nonetheless, Mrs. Schneider sued Dr. Revici for malpractice, fraud, and lack of informed consent.[13]

Assumption of the risk is an affirmative defense, meaning that if the defendant is successful in convincing the court that the plaintiff/patient assumed the risks of the treatment, no further action can be taken against the defendant. Mrs. Schneider won in the lower court but Dr. Revici appealed. The U.S. Court of Appeals for the 2nd Circuit concluded that Mrs. Schneider did indeed assume the risks posed by undergoing an experimental, unproven treatment and that she was fully informed when she consented.

Informed Consent

"Informed consent" refers to legal theories of recovery in medical malpractice cases that depend on the patient's right to make an informed decision regarding treatment options, rather than on the appropriateness of treatment.[14] Mrs. Schneider also asserted that she was not informed of the consequences of the experimental treatments in spite of the existence of a signed consent to treatment. The circuit court sided with the physician in this instance, believing that Mrs. Schneider was fully informed of the experimental nature of the treatment as well as the risks associated with a nontraditional approach to treating cancer.

Many physicians find little comfort in the doctrine of informed consent within the context of alternative and complementary medicine. The doctrine presumes competent individuals can decide on the best course of treatment for an illness by evaluating options most consistent with their beliefs and value system. However, most physicians recognize that there is much that is not known about risks and benefits of alternative and complementary therapies. In the absence of scientific evidence related to the efficacy of these treatments and their side effects, physicians are at a loss as to what to inform their patients about.

Respectable Minority

The "respectable minority" defense is available to physicians who choose to incorporate unusual but recognized treatment alternatives as options within an overall treatment program. Essentially, the physician would have to prove that a respectable minority within the profession who were faced with a similar set of circumstances would opt to treat the patient in the same manner as the physician in question. Establishing a respectable minority defense would not obviate a physician's liability but it would be one mitigating factor the court would take into account when assessing negligence.

The court in D'Angelis v Zakuto was presented with the issue of respectable minority.[15] The case involved a death resulting from undiagnosed pneumonia. One of the questions before the court was whether or not the physician's treatment was within the acceptable standard of care. Recognizing that experts might differ, the justices concluded that the respectable minority defense was allowable where the physician (1) followed a school of thought that had a reasonable number of supporters within the medical community, and (2) the school was reputable and respected by reasonable medical experts.[15,16] Essentially, the defense gives physicians latitude to choose among various treatment approaches as long as the approach selected is endorsed by a respectable minority of the medical community.

Clinical Innovation

"Clinical innovation" has not yet been tested but is a possible defense in malpractice actions involving al-

ternative and complementary medicine. The defense has been used in a very narrow set of circumstances, usually when the patient's situation is desperate and all traditional methods have been tried and have failed. As a final effort, a physician may prescribe a highly experimental course of treatment. Under these circumstances, the doctrine shields physicians from liability, however no court has extended the doctrine to cover the use of alternative and complementary treatments.[17]

OTHER RISKS

Revocation of License

Physicians who choose to integrate nontraditional therapies into traditional medical practice need to be aware of the licensing requirements in the jurisdictions in which they practice. Medical licensing laws have been used to restrict medical practice to traditional or allopathic treatments. Failure to conform to the licensing laws of the jurisdiction in which an individual practices could result in revocation of the license.

The case of Dr. George Guess illustrates some of the problems allopathic physicians encounter when they attempt to integrate homeopathic treatments into practice. Dr. Guess was licensed to practice family medicine in North Carolina. He regularly provided homeopathic remedies to his patients along with traditional allopathic treatments. In 1985 Dr. Guess was brought before the North Carolina Board of Medical Examiners for practicing homeopathy and thus failing to conform to the acceptable standards of medical care in the state. It should be noted that no patient ever complained about his or her treatment while in Dr. Guess's care. In fact, many of his patients testified on his behalf.

The issue before the Board was solely whether or not Dr. Guess, in his medical practice, conformed to the prevailing standard of care in North Carolina. At his hearing, Dr. Guess presented evidence on the efficacy of homeopathy and its acceptance in other countries. He failed to sway the Board of Medical Examiners with this evidence, though, and was ordered to cease all practice of homeopathy at once. He was also given a two-year probation. Alternatively, his license would be revoked.

Dr. Guess sued the Board of Medical Examiners. The case eventually made its way to North Carolina's Supreme Court, which sided with the Board. The Court refused to recognize any "fundamental right to receive unorthodox medical treatment."[18] Rather, the Court opined that the legislative intent behind the licensing statute was to protect the public by prohibiting unacceptable and unorthodox treatments and that this was true irrespective of any injury to patients.

Outraged, Dr. Guess' patients filed suit in Federal District Court against the Board. His patients were unsuccessful; the Court dismissed the case for lack of standing to sue. Undeterred, the patients lobbied the state legislature to amend the medical licensing law to prevent the Board from revoking a physician's license solely because he or she engages in ". . . experimental, nontraditional . . . medical practices."[19]

Licensing laws act as a limitation on a physician's ability to integrate nontraditional therapies into traditional practice. At a minimum, physicians should know and understand what is permissible within the jurisdiction in which they practice. More states are moving toward more expansive definitions of medical care. As of May 1997 at least eight states had adopted legislation permitting physicians to use alternative medicine without risking disciplinary action from medical boards.[20]

Fraud and Abuse Concerns

Fraud is defined as ". . . anything calculated to deceive."[21] In the context of health care, fraud includes the provision of treatments known to be useless and the submission of claims for medically unnecessary treatments. Most states have criminal and civil fraud laws, and state medical boards often sanction individuals who provide fraudulent treatments. The federal Medicare and Medicaid laws also contain provisions designed to protect patients from inappropriate, useless treatments. The Medicare program will only pay for services ordered by a physician that are both medically necessary and meet professionally recognized standards of practice.[22] Many alternative and complementary therapies are not generally accepted within the traditional biomedical community. Therefore, they do not by definition meet the recognized standard of care. Submitting a claim for payment of alternative services would be fraudulent, per se.

Private insurers also limit coverage to "medically necessary" treatments. Alternative treatments and experimental treatments that lack a strong scientific basis, frequently fail this test, and claims for these services are routinely denied. More important perhaps from the physician's perspective is that the continued use of unproven and experimental treatments can expose the physician to claims of fraud.[23]

Practitioners intent on offering alternative therapies to their patients should be very conscious of who they bill for what services. Failure to meet the medical necessity test could open physicians up to claims of fraud.

SUMMARY

Social and cultural indicators all point to continued growth in the use of alternative medical therapies by Americans. Third party reimbursement is becoming more commonplace, particularly for some of the more mainstream alternative practices. Organized medicine continues to examine the efficacy of alternative practices and most medical schools now include some instruction on complementary and alternative treatments. In short, the use and acceptance of alternative and complementary medical treatments is increasing.

Physicians are concerned and confused about the impact of this trend on traditional medicine. Some of the confusion is inevitable since legal principles in this area are not well defined. This situation is not likely to change until alternative and complementary therapies are integrated into the continuum of medical care. Nonetheless, physicians interested in integrating these methods into medical practice should be proactive in assessing the risk to their practice and their medical license. In general, the risks associated with expanding traditional practice to become more inclusive of other therapies appears to be minimal, particularly if physicians take the following precautions: refer to and rely on only experienced and credentialled providers, treat all emergent situations according to accepted medical practice, and know the billing rules and submit claims accordingly.

References

1. Studdert DM et al: Medical malpractice implications of alternative medicine, *JAMA* 280:1610, 1998.

2. Eisenberg D et al: Unconventional medicine in the United States: prevalence, costs, and patterns of use, *N Engl J Med* 328:246, 1993.

3. Ernst E et al: Complementary medicine, *Arch Intern Med* 155:2405, 1995.

4. Eisenberg D et al: Trends in alternative medicine use in the United States, 1990-1997, *JAMA* 280:1569, 1998.

5. Health Care Forum Journal, On the outside moving in: will the alternative medicine integration movement shape U.S. health care? 14–19, Nov/Dec 1998. Some of these plans include Kaiser Permanente, Aetna USHealthcare, UnitedHealth Group, and Blue Cross Blue Shield.

6. Boozang K: Western medicine opens the door to alternative medicine, *Am J Law Med* 24:185, 1998.

7. http://nccam.nih.gov/

8. *Wilk v American Medical Association,* 719 F2d 207, 1983; *Idaho Association of Naturopathic Physicians v FDA,* 582 F2d 850, 1978.

9. *Grady v New York Medical College,* 243 NYS 3d 940, 1963.

10. *Reed v Bascon,* 124 Ill. 2nd 386, 1988. Mrs. Reed sued Dr. Bascon, her general practitioner, claiming he was in part responsible for the negligent acts of the surgeon who treated her. Dr. Bascon referred Mrs. Reed to the surgeon but took no part in the actual surgery.

11. These two criteria are used by the court to evaluate "failure to refer cases" or cases where physicians should have referred a patient for more specialized treatment based on the severity or complexity of the patient's condition.

12. Vicarious liability is a form of strict liability in which the plaintiff need not prove fault. Participating in the activity or engaging in the conduct is enough in and of itself to establish liability.

13. *Schneider v Revici,* 817 F2d 987, 1987.

14. Informed consent is a common law doctrine that recognizes an individual's right to "bodily integrity." *See:*

15. *Schloendorff v Society of New York Hospital,* 105 N.E. 92, 1914.

15. *D'Angelis v Zakuto,* 556 A2d 431, 1989.

16. *Brook v St. John's Hickey Memorial Hospital,* 380 NE 2d 72, 1978. Mr. Brook sued a radiologist and hospital on behalf of his minor child, Tracey, who had been injected with a drug during a radiology procedure. The site of the injection was unusual. The court found for the defendant physician, noting that where there is an established mode of treatment, the physician is permitted to use his best judgment in the treatment of the patient.

17. Cohen M: *Complementary and alternative medicine: legal boundaries and regulatory perspectives,* Baltimore, 1998, Johns Hopkins University Press.

18. *In re Guess,* 393 SE2d 833, 1990.

19. GA Statutes 90-14(a)(6).

20. http://www.naturalhealthvillage.com/

21. Cohen M: *Complementary and alternative medicine: legal boundaries and regulatory perspectives,* Baltimore, 1998, Johns Hopkins University Press. Quoting Speiser S et al: *The American law of torts,* New York, 1992, Clark Boardman Gallagher.

22. 42 USC § 1320(c)(5).

23. See Cohen M: *Complementary and alternative medicine: legal boundaries and regulatory perspectives,* Baltimore, 1998, Johns Hopkins University Press, for a discussion on one of the leading cases in this area. Dr. Stanislaw Burzynski offered antineoplanton treatments to cancer patients. He sued Aetna USHealthcare when the insurer refused to pay claims in connection with these treatments. Aetna countersued, claiming not only that the treatments were medically unnecessary, but that they were fraudulent since there was no scientific evidence that the treatments had any medical value.

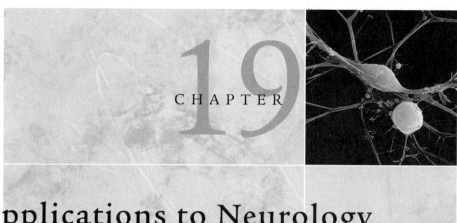

CHAPTER 19

Tai Chi: Applications to Neurology

T. C. HAIN
J. KOTSIAS
CLIVE PAI

ai Chi is an exercise discipline derived from the tradition of Chinese ethnomedicine and martial arts. Its historic roots go back more than 1000 years. Bodhidarma, founder of Zen Buddhism and abbot of the Shao Lin (or Shao-Lin) Monastery about AD 527, taught Changing Sinews, a stretching and strength exercise; Marrow Washing exercises to strengthen the bones and viscera; and an 18-movement technique of breathing and body control for relaxation and defense. Chang San-Feng, a somewhat legendary Taoist priest from about the thirteenth century, is honored by many as the systematizer of boxing and breathing exercises.[1] While the modern term for Tai Chi in the Orient is Tai Chi Chuan or Chinese Shadow Boxing, Tai Chi is presently used primarily as an exercise system.[2]

Tai Chi is generally practiced as a daily exercise routine, called a *form* or *style,* which consists of a sequence of movement modules. An average sequence of modules lasts about 30 minutes. The movements are typically slow and flowing. They are performed while standing and have an overall appearance that is similar to a slow dance. Tai Chi also commonly involves mental imagery including a visualization of life force, or Chi, as well as coordinated breathing. Figure 19-1 illustrates a typical Tai Chi movement. About 108 movements are available to the practitioner of traditional Yang style Tai Chi.

There are also several styles or schools of Tai Chi, each providing additional or variant movements. Yang style is the most popular (Table 19-1). This style was practiced among the royal families and by ordinary people who had not undergone rigorous martial arts training.[3] Some other styles were kept mainly within the circle of martial arts families. The Chinese government promoted the popularity of the Yang style by organizing the simplified and intermediate

forms for the Yang style. This organization made them more accessible to those who had limited time or were in poor health. For example, the 24 short form takes only 8 to 10 minutes to practice, the 48 intermediate form takes about twice that long, and the

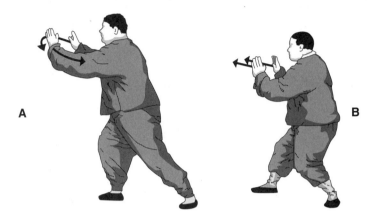

Figure 19-1 Turning the Wheel. This movement was adapted from the Yang school of Tai Chi. The student slowly shifts the body weight forward and backward while smoothly moving the arms in a circular fashion as if holding a handle on the rim of a wheel roughly 2 feet in diameter. In position A, the hands are extended at shoulder width and the trunk is forward. While moving the trunk backward to position B, the hands are brought slowly backward following a half-circular trajectory corresponding to the bottom half of the wheel. On returning to position A, the arms extend and hands are brought upward and forward, again following a half-circular trajectory corresponding to the top half of the wheel. The head moves on the trunk synchronously to keep the head horizontal in space. At least three repetitions are performed.

TABLE 19-1

Major Tai Chi styles (schools)

Originator	Characteristics	Different routines	Popularity
Yang Family	Open limb posture, slow practice speed	Simplified (24 forms), intermediate (48 forms), and long (e.g., 98 or 108 forms)	Popular and relatively standardized, especially the simplified and intermediate versions
Chen Family	Vigorous, deep squat basic posture, speeds range from slow and gentle to fast and vigorous	Long form (e.g., 71 or 83 forms) and many others	Less popular for health but popular for martial arts and competitions
Wu/Hao Family	Vigorous, small limb posture, emphasis on both attack and defense, and on posture; speed is usually slow	Long form (e.g., 96 to 108 forms)	Less popular

long form requires approximately 30 minutes or more. The purpose of this chapter is to review currently available evidence regarding Tai Chi's use as a treatment modality for neurologic problems.

DEFINITION AND ANALOGY WITH CONVENTIONAL MEDICINE

Despite the differences inherent in various styles and forms of Tai Chi, several principles are common to all. These common elements include the following:

1. A daily moderate exercise routine that may last about 30 minutes[4] and that incorporates both strengthening and flexibility.[5]
2. Slow and controlled movements performed in a circular fashion, as shown in Figure 19-1. This is called the principle of roundness. The shape of the major joints of the upper and lower limbs should present a visual sense of roundness rather than angularity. In other words, the joints are positioned at the middle of their corresponding range of motion, neither extremely extended nor extremely flexed. There is also a principle of change that requires the person to continuously move on to the next form, even though the speed is slow and the movement is not strenuous.
3. Mental imagery. A practitioner of Tai Chi is to empty the mind from daily stresses to experience the tranquility and to concentrate on the movement itself, the images of life force or Chi.
4. Positions involving alterations in stability through displacements of body mass. There is an emphasis on posture, with a straightened back and head combined with bent legs.
5. Relaxation through deep breathing, and slow and gentle movements.[6] The desired respiratory frequency is 11 breaths/min or less.[7]

In large part then, Tai Chi shows a close resemblance to Western physical therapy (PT), which might also include conditioning exercises and gait and balance training. The emphasis on slow and controlled movements is, however, unique to Tai Chi and could be a source of the differences in its effects from conventional PT. The use of relaxation, deep breathing, and mental imagery may contribute to its effects.

CARDIORESPIRATORY EFFECTS

As documented in the studies listed in Table 19-2, most Tai Chi styles involve a moderate exercise that, according to Zhuo,[4] is similar to walking at a speed of 6 km/hr. While most community Tai Chi classes do

TABLE 19-2

Cardiorespiratory effects of Tai Chi

Study	Population and design	Results	Comment
Brown[7]	6 Tai Chi practitioners	Respiration more efficient than cycle ergometry	Tai Chi exercise may have relaxation response
Lansheng et al[16]	100 volunteers	Heart rate increased 30 beats/min	Tai Chi is a light exercise
Lan[17,18]	22 Tai Chi practitioners (average 11.8 years) vs 66 sedentary seniors	Tai Chi subjects had more efficient oxygenation, greater flexibility, and lower % body fat; intensity is 52% to 63% of heart rate range	Tai Chi is a mild to moderate intensity exercise
Lai[19,20]	45 Tai Chi practitioners and 39 sedentary subjects	Tai Chi group showed much lower rate of decline of cardiorespiratory function	Tai Chi is a moderate aerobic exercise
Zhuo[4]	11 young men during long form of Yang style	Energy cost of 4.1 mets; mean heart rate was 134	Tai Chi (Long Yang Form) is a moderate exercise

not provide exercise as vigorous as that recommended for maintaining cardiovascular fitness, one must keep in mind that the alternative to Tai Chi might be no exercise at all. In addition, Tai Chi has other benefits, which will be documented.

BALANCE AND FALLING

As shown in Table 19-3, there are presently six reports suggesting that Tai Chi training improves or maintains balance and one study suggesting that Tai Chi reduces falling in the elderly. Improvement almost certainly derives in part from cardiovascular fitness and strengthening. However, there may be benefits related to other aspects of Tai Chi such as slowing of movement, stress management, practice with stabilizing sequences of movements, and better knowledge of personal limits of stability. Most studies to date have excluded individuals with neurologic disorders such as parkinsonism and cerebellar ataxia. Therefore, essentially no data exists

on any specific effects of Tai Chi on the unsteadiness that is common in these conditions.

There are several reasons why Tai Chi might improve balance. For example, in the lower limbs, the roundness principle requires a midjoint position for the hip, knee, and ankle. This requires adopting a squatting posture, which is difficult and can be demanding on one's strength. Generally, as a person practices, the squatting position becomes progressively deeper or closer to the ground demonstrating that the individual's ability to support his or her weight is improving. Therefore, the roundness principle promotes strengthening of the weight support muscles that enable an individual to resist limb collapse and falls.

The principle of change requires a person to move continuously. The essence of the control of balance is the location and speed of the body's center of mass (COM) with respect to the base of support (BOS), which is determined by foot placement. The need to take a step is dictated by the horizontal location and

TABLE 19-3

Studies of effects of Tai Chi on balance and falling

Study	Population and design	Results	Comment
Wolf[5,21,23,24]	Seniors, 72 Tai Chi vs balance training and discussion group	Fewer falls in Tai Chi group; no effect on sway; slowed gait velocity	Clear demonstration of benefit on reduction of falls
Hain[12]	22 unsteady subjects; before and after paired comparisons	Better balance (Romberg, posturography) after Tai Chi	Improvement may not be specific to Tai Chi
Tse and Bailey[25]	9 Tai Chi practitioners and 9 controls paired	Better balance in Tai Chi group	Tai Chi group may have differed from controls
Judge[26]	Seniors, 12 performed Tai Chi vs 9 sitting exercises	Increased gait velocity in Tai Chi group	Tai Chi component of exercise study was minimal; gait velocity finding differs from Wolf study
Schaller[27]	Seniors, 24 Tai Chi versus 22 controls	Improved single leg standing test	Selection of sample was not randomized
Wolfson et al[13]	Seniors, 110 divided into 4 groups with intensive training for 3 months followed by 6 months of Tai Chi	Tai Chi allowed maintenance of most gains obtained through intensive training	
Jacobson[28]	24 subjects, before and after Tai Chi	Better lateral stability	Improvement may not be specific to Tai Chi

velocity of the COM position.[8,9] Tai Chi promotes balance through continuous drill that enables a person to explore the interactions between the COM position and velocity.

To summarize, Tai Chi appears to be an established method of improving balance.[10] It may be particularly useful for individuals whose imbalance is mild,[12] or individuals for which long-term maintenance exercises are indicated.[13]

ARTHRITIS

Exercise has been shown to be beneficial in rheumatoid arthritis.[6] As a form of moderate exercise, Tai Chi appears to be safe and may serve as an alternative to exercise therapy and as part of a rehabilitation program for individuals with rheumatoid arthritis (Table 19-4). Tai Chi has also been advocated as a method of increasing range of motion in arthritis.[11] However, too little data is presently available to determine whether Tai Chi is actually beneficial.

PSYCHOLOGIC FUNCTIONING

The studies listed in Table 19-5 indicate that Tai Chi is approximately equivalent to brisk walking or meditation in usefulness for stress management. According to Weiser and associates[14] there are positive psychotherapeutic effects of martial arts physical training that occur immediately, as well as long-term benefits of increased self-esteem. There are also therapeutic effects that derive from the group experience

TABLE 19-4

Tai Chi studies in patients with arthritis

Study	Population and design	Results	Comment
Kirsteins[6]	45 subjects with rheumatoid arthritis and 20 controls	Safe for rheumatoid arthritis	Did not consider benefit
Koh[29]	Case report	Suggests greater benefit than conventional therapy for ankylosing spondylitis	

TABLE 19-5

Studies of Tai Chi for stress management

Study	Population and design	Results	Comment
Jin #81[30]	33 beginners and 33 practitioners	Mood became more positive and subjects reported less tension, depression, anger, fatigue, confusion, and state anxiety	Effect might also be found in other forms of moderate exercise
Jin[31]	96 Tai Chi practitioners randomized to Tai Chi, brisk walking, meditation, and neutral reading	Tai Chi stress reduction was similar to walking at a speed of 6 km/hr as well as other interventions	No differential effect of Tai Chi compared with exercise or meditation
Kutner[32]	160 seniors randomized into Tai Chi and computerized balance training	Tai Chi subjects reported enhanced balance in daily activities compared with controls	Documents that subjects enjoy Tai Chi

and from the positive role model of the instructor. To summarize, Tai Chi appears to be equivalent to regular exercise or meditation with respect to stress management.

DISCUSSION

The literature does suggest that Tai Chi exercise might be useful in certain medical settings, particularly as an adjunct or substitute for Western balance PT or as a method of stress management. Tai Chi has not yet been studied as a treatment in the West for many common neurologic problems such as headache, back pain, dementia, neuropathy, or vascular disease.

There are both advantages and disadvantages to Tai Chi as compared with conventional PT. One advantage of Tai Chi is that it may be less expensive than PT because it is normally practiced in a group setting. Second, because Tai Chi is suited to life-long practice and is commonly used that way, it may be more beneficial for maintaining health than brief periods of one-on-one PT. There is evidence that in some populations traditional PT to treat balance is helpful while being practiced, but that benefits are eliminated when PT is stopped.[15] Thus, for balance rehabilitation, it may be desirable to choose a modality such as Tai Chi that is suitable for long-term practice. Third, Tai Chi has been derived from a rich context of Chinese ethnomedicine and is intrinsically adaptable to a variety of clinical contexts. Therefore, it can draw from a large repertoire of exercise modules. A particular advantage is that some of the exercise modules of Tai Chi are quite challenging and may be suitable for individuals who are already functioning reasonably well but who wish to improve further. Fourth, Tai Chi offers a vehicle for meditation and relaxation training, which may be of additional benefit for certain populations of patients.

There are also several disadvantages of Tai Chi to one-on-one PT or counseling. First, safety may be a problem. Tai Chi is commonly performed either unsupervised or in a group setting where no medical personnel are available. While the risk may not be any greater than, for example, playing volleyball, the risk of falling is clearly greater than it is for sitting on the couch and reading a book. Second, one-on-one PT or stress counseling provides the opportunity for greater customization than do any sort of group sessions. Finally, one-on-one therapy allows closer monitoring of

patient progress and appropriate matching of the diagnosis to the form of therapy. Considering these problems, if Tai Chi is to be used as a vehicle for medical therapy, especially replacing PT, it would seem best to deliver it as a structured activity, supervised by health care professionals. There is a small but growing number of physical therapists who are incorporating Tai Chi into their practices.

Many questions remain open. How much of the benefit associated with Tai Chi training is related to physical conditioning, modification of movement patterns, or relaxation? What is the optimum duration of Tai Chi training? What is the optimum selection and sequence of movements? Should movements be individualized to patients or is use of a generic sequence reasonable? Is Tai Chi beneficial in patients with cerebellar disorders? Following stroke? With parkinsonism? It is hoped that answers to these questions will emerge in the form of controlled prospective studies.

ACKNOWLEDGMENT

Our research on Tai Chi was supported by grant 1R21RR0935-01 from the Public Health Service, Office of Alternative Medicine.

References

1. Ryan A: Tai Chi Chuan for mind and body, *Physician Sports Med,* pp 58-61, March 1974.
2. Koh T: Tai Chi Chuan, *Am J Chin Med* IX:15-22, 1981.
3. Jou TH: *The Tao of Tai-Chi Chuan: way to rejuvenation,* 1983. Rutland, VT: Charles E. Tuttle.
4. Zhuo D et al: Cardiorespiratory and metabolic responses during Tai Chi Chuan exercise, *Can J Appl Sport Sci* 9(1):7-10, 1984.
5. Wolf SL et al: Exploring the basis for Tai Chi Chuan as a therapeutic exercise approach [see comments], *Arch Phys Med Rehabil* 78(8):886-892, 1997.
6. Kirsteins AE et al: Evaluating the safety and potential use of a weight-bearing exercise, Tai-Chi Chuan, for rheumatoid arthritis patients, *Am J Phys Med Rehabil* 70(3):136-141, 1991.
7. Brown DD et al: Cardiovascular and ventilatory responses during formalized T'ai Chi Chuan exercise, *Res Q Exerc Sport* 60(3):246-250, 1989.
8. Maki BE, McIlroy WE: Postural control in the older adult, *Clin Geriatr Med* 12(4):635-658, 1996.
9. Pai YC, Patton J: Center of mass velocity-position predictions for balance control, *J Biomech* 30(4):347-354, 1997.

10. Pai YC, Patton J: Center of mass velocity-position predictions for balance control [published erratum], *J Biomech* 31(2):199, 1998.
11. Lumsden DB et al: T'ai Chi for osteoarthritis: an introduction for primary care physicians, *Geriatrics* 53(2):84, 1998.
12. Hain T et al: Effects of T'ai Chi on balance, *Arch Otolaryngol Head Neck Surg* 125(11):1191-1195, 1999.
13. Wolfson L et al: Balance and strength training in older adults: intervention gains and Tai Chi maintenance [see comments], *J Am Geriatr Soc* 44(5):498-506, 1996.
14. Weiser M et al: Psychotherapeutic aspects of the martial arts, *Am J Psychother* 49(1):118-127, 1995.
15. Comella CL et al: Physical therapy and Parkinson's disease: a controlled clinical trial, *Neurology* 44(3):376-378, 1994.
16. Lansheng JQ et al: Changes in heart rate and electrocardiogram during taijiquan exercise: analysis by telemetry in 100 subjects, *Chin Med J* 94(9):589-592, 1981.
17. Lan C et al: Cardiorespiratory function, flexibility, and body composition among geriatric Tai Chi Chuan practitioners, *Arch Phys Med Rehabil* 77(6):612-616, 1996.
18. Lan C et al: 12-month Tai Chi training in the elderly: its effect on health fitness, *Med Sci Sports Exerc* 30(3):345-351, 1998.
19. Lai JS et al: Cardiorespiratory responses of Tai Chi Chuan practitioners and sedentary subjects during cycle ergometry, *J Formos Med Assoc* 92(10):894-899, 1993.
20. Lai JS et al: Two-year trends in cardiorespiratory function among older Tai Chi Chuan practitioners and sedentary subjects, *J Am Geriatr Soc* 43(11):1222-1227, 1995.
21. Wolf SL et al: The Atlanta FICSIT study: two exercise interventions to reduce frailty in elders, *J Am Geriatr Soc* 41(3):329-332, 1993.
22. Province MA et al: The effects of exercise on falls in elderly patients: a preplanned meta-analysis of the FICSIT trials—frailty and injuries: cooperative studies of intervention techniques [see comments], *JAMA* 273(17):1341-1347, 1995.
23. Wolf SL et al: Reducing frailty and falls in older persons, an investigation of Tai Chi and computerized balance training: Atlanta FICSIT group—frailty and injuries: cooperative studies of intervention techniques [see comments], *J Am Geriatr Soc* 44(5):489-497, 1996.
24. Wolf SL et al: The effect of Tai Chi Quan and computerized balance training on postural stability in older subjects: Atlanta FICSIT group—frailty and injuries: cooperative studies on intervention techniques, *Phys Ther* 77(4):371-381, 382-384, 1997.
25. Tse SK, Bailey DM: T'ai Chi and postural control in the well elderly, *Am J Occup Ther* 46(4):295-300, 1992.
26. Judge JO et al: Balance improvements in older women: effects of exercise training, *Phys Ther* 73(4):254-262, 263-265, 1993.
27. Schaller K: Tai Chi Chih: an exercise option for older adults, *J Gerontol Nurs* 22(10):12-17, 1996.
28. Jacobson BH et al: The effect of T'ai Chi Chuan training on balance, kinesthetic sense, and strength, *Percept Mot Skills* 84(1):27-33, 1997.
29. Koh T: Tai Chi and ankylosing spondylitis: a personal experience, *Am J Chin Ed* 9:15-22, 1981.
30. Jin P: Changes in heart rate, noradrenaline, cortisol, and mood during Tai Chi, *J Psychosomatic Research* 33(2):197-206, 1989.
31. Jin P: Efficacy of Tai Chi, brisk walking, meditation, and reading in reducing mental and emotional stress, *J Psychosom Res* 36(4):361-370, 1992.
32. Kutner NG et al: Self-report benefits of Tai Chi practice by older adults, *J Gerontol B Psychol Sci Soc Sci* 52(5):242-246, 1997.

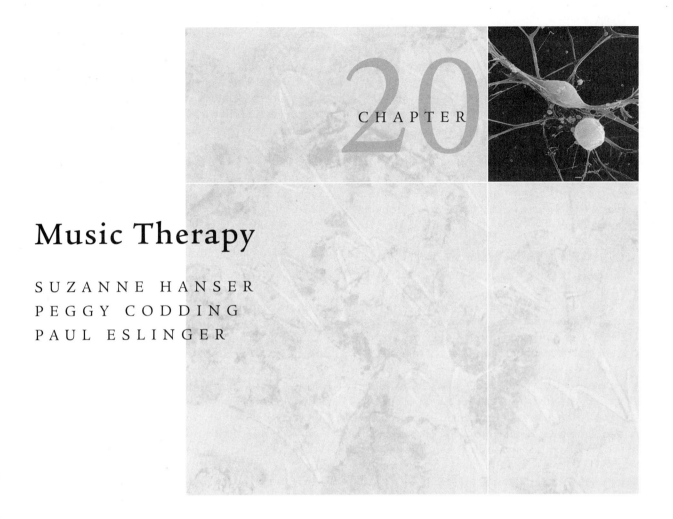

CHAPTER

20

Music Therapy

S U Z A N N E   H A N S E R
P E G G Y   C O D D I N G
P A U L   E S L I N G E R

Mary B. is a 59-year-old woman diagnosed with fibromyalgia. She has impaired mobility and experiences difficulty in performing many daily living skills, including dressing herself. She is extremely fragile and presents a rigid posture and gait, creating the appearance that she can hardly move. The severe, chronic pain throughout her body has contributed to her diagnosis of major depressive disorder. Her symptoms include hopelessness, insomnia, and dysphoria. Diabetes and sensitivities to a variety of medications prevent her from taking medications that are indicated for her condition.

Mary has little motivation to attend classes or support groups at the hospital, but she enjoys listening to music at home and reports that this is her only consolation. Her physician referred Mary to music therapy when he learned that music calmed her enough to lull

her to sleep at night. The music therapy assessment revealed that Mary had enjoyed piano lessons and had played frequently for friends until hand pain had incapacitated her. The music therapist taught Mary relaxation techniques that were cued by her favorite music. She resumed piano lessons on an electronic keyboard that enabled her to play with minimal pressure on the keys. Mary also began exercising to music in the morning and practicing deep muscle relaxation accompanied by a different kind of music at night.

Six months later, Mary still suffers from fibromyalgia, but she deals with her pain using music to relax her muscles and control her movements. She is motivated to dress and move more freely now that she attends weekly matinees and concerts. Other patients like Mary are also using music as therapy to facilitate their living with a neurologic illness. Many of

255

these patients experience relief from various symptoms and the ability to comply more easily with treatments that are paired with musical experiences.

AN INTRODUCTION TO MUSIC THERAPY

Anthropologists and enthnomusicologists say that music has been associated with the healing of the body and mind for centuries. Since the time of early nomadic civilizations, healers have incorporated music in their rituals "to solace the sick and weary, [and] to promote unspoken emotions." In some cultures, music was used in religious and healing rituals "for entreating the gods" to "exorcise malevolent . . . demon[s]" that many believed inhabited the body of any ill person.[1] Shamans used instruments, song, and dance to call up certain melodies and rhythms as healing medicine. The music corresponded to the spirits they thought were invading the bodies of the sick.

These practices were a natural healing response to a supernatural view of illness and health. Today, trained music therapists use music experiences to promote therapeutic change in a patient's symptomatology, coping skills, and quality of life. Generally, music therapists serve as members of the patient's treatment team within the hospital unit. Some music therapists work in private practice, accepting patients by physician referral. The growing body of knowledge derived from the empiric study of music and health supports the role of music therapy as a viable treatment alternative in the medical milieu.[2-6]

Music in some form has been used for nearly two centuries in hospitals throughout the United States. After the phonograph was invented in 1877, physicians sometimes made patient-preferred music recordings available to the sick. The music provided relief from the boredom of hospital routines and distracted patients from their physical discomfort or depression.[6] More recently, therapists have used live precomposed, improvised, or recorded music in individual or group music therapy sessions to reduce heightened feelings of fear or isolation, to promote mental focus, or to distract attention away from pain. Music therapists use music to facilitate physical activity during recuperation, to cue relaxation, and to mask unpleasant hospital sounds that cause patient stress. Some music therapists have also used music to promote essential coping strategies or to facilitate communication among family members regarding illness, treatment, or prognosis.[1]

Although acousticians frequently define music as organized sound and silence in time, twentieth-century pioneers of music therapy described the experience of music as much more. These early practitioners observed many people who were "under the influence" of music and found that listeners experienced music as a source of joy, a messenger of sadness with which they could identify, or a key to release the feelings of the moment. Music therapists have long understood that music is a powerful means of communication that is more subtle, more basic, and more personal than words. Music lyrics or melodies sometimes convey the unspeakable, or the clearly intimate that is almost inexpressible. Therapists have often seen familiar music allow an individual to elicit the memory of an important life event and to recall the very feelings that were felt at that moment. Music compels human beings to act by stimulating thought or mood, or by creating a need to move that can only be filled by the tapping of a foot or a quick step across the floor. Music, although not essential to human survival, exists and flourishes in all known cultures. It is the intimate personal expression of those who play it, and sometimes the spiritual salvation of those who hear it.

Music is a natural tool for therapy and alternative medicine because it is created by human beings to speak to human beings. Music draws attention to itself and is often useful for conveying ideas that are too difficult to express by speaking them aloud. Everyone can experience music in some form and participate successfully with whatever ability that is brought to the moment. People can listen passively to music while feeling calm or light, or they can use music actively to start moving. Music can be experienced alone, with someone who is well known to the patient, or in a new encounter.

In 1950, the National Association for Music Therapy established the field as an official discipline. The American Music Therapy Association, which was formed in 1998, along with its Standards of Practice and Code of Ethics, currently oversees 69 approved academic curricula in the United States and more than 150 approved full-time clinical internships. There are approximately 5000 professional and student music therapists who practice in schools, clinics, and community agencies; in hospitals; and privately.[6,7]

Music therapy is the application of specific music techniques to meet physical, social, emotional, and psychologic goals and objectives. Music therapists are qualified to practice in the United States when they have obtained a music therapy degree from an approved college, completed an approved clinical internship, and passed a National Board Certification Examination. The music therapist, after consulting with health professionals on the team, determines whether group therapy, individual work, or a bedside approach is most appropriate. In general, music therapy may be less effective for persons with hearing difficulties. However, many rhythmic and musical activities can still be enjoyed and appreciated by people with the most severe hearing loss. Because music is universal in its appeal, music therapy offers a viable methodology for individuals regardless of their functional abilities.

Music therapists assess each client's needs, establish goals and objectives consistent with the treatment team, and design strategies that incorporate nonverbal, creative ways to reach specified psychotherapeutic aims.[8] They may use any genre of music along with improvisation, singing, moving or dancing to music, playing instruments, composing music, talking about and analyzing music, learning music, or listening to music. Therapists use familiar, patient-preferred music as a nonthreatening means of establishing a clinical relationship with a new, anxious patient or as a stimulus to motivate the repetitive movement often essential to physical rehabilitation.[3] Music can encourage patients who are confused as a result of brain injury to focus their attention on something compelling and meaningful. The music therapist might also help patients with terminal illnesses to compose lyrics and music that express their feelings. Writing the piece structures emotional release and contributes to coping; sharing the music and lyrics with family helps to communicate love and loss.

MUSIC AND THE BRAIN

For much more than a century there has been a growing literature on music and the brain. Many observations have arisen from studying patients who had suffered a change in their musical abilities after cerebral damage from stroke. Such behavioral and cognitive alterations have been termed *amusias*. These acquired impairments include diverse performance deficits, such as in singing or instrumental skills; perceptual impairments, such as in pitch and rhythm discrimi-

nation, ability to read music, and recognition of melodies; and lost talent for composing music. Perhaps the best summary of such studies is in Critchley and Henson's[9] volume titled *Music and the Brain: Studies in the Neurology of Music.*

Many earlier brain-behavior studies supported a model of a select neural substrate for musical perception and processing residing primarily in the right cerebral hemisphere. For example, Milner[10] reported impairments in discrimination of timbre, duration, and tonal patterns following right temporal lobectomy in patients with intractable epilepsy. Others have reported impaired discrimination of melodies and pitch after right hemisphere damage.[11,12] In addition, case studies of musicians with acquired aphasias after left hemisphere damage from stroke have revealed that they may continue to perceive and evaluate critically, compose, and even read music although they are no longer able to comprehend and read language in comparable fashion.[13,14] Such observations have led to an intriguing but simplistic model of cerebral dominance, specifying that language and associated verbal processes are mediated through the left cerebral hemisphere. The model says that nonverbal musical processes are mediated through right hemisphere structures, particularly the temporal lobe where primary auditory cortex and auditory association cortices are localized. This verbal/nonverbal hemispheric dichotomy, as Zatorre,[15] and Hachinski and Hachinski[16] recently observed, is simply not supported by available data. These data suggest instead that complex and diverse interactions occur between the two cerebral hemispheres during musical behaviors and experiences.

The earlier right hemisphere model of music was important for providing an initial neural linkage between music and emotion, because this hemisphere has also been shown to play important roles in emotional perception and processing.[17-19] The medium of music may influence emotions in both direct and indirect ways, through overlapping or interactive neural activation and through powerful nonverbal symbolism that bypasses the pathways of language and verbal cognition. Recent studies in cognitive neuroscience have shown that a much broader array of neural structures participate in music behaviors and experiences than was previously thought. The most important of these structures include the frontal lobe, limbic system, and imagery-related cortical regions of the temporal, parietal, and occipital lobes.[15,20-24] These studies have been carried out in normal healthy volunteers who undergo functional brain scanning (Positron Emission Tomography, or PET) while undertaking music-related tasks. It is important to note that there is now scientific data supporting music stimulation effects in the frontal lobe and limbic system, which are key structures for emotional activation and experience of a diverse nature.[25,26] This provides a potential mechanism for musical influences on the regulation of emotions and on the autonomic centers that mediate respiration, heart rate, and so forth. Hence, there is a potential pathway for therapeutic change.

Thaut[27] has suggested that music may induce therapeutic change through its activation of affective systems. A structured approach to these systems and associated behaviors, such as through a music therapy program, may allow individuals with diverse neurologic conditions to experience, identify, express, and modulate emotions and physiologic responses in ways that are quite different from verbally mediated, insight-oriented, cognitive therapies. Moreover, music may provide a unique, complementary mode of stimulating emotions, emotional processing, and therapeutic emotional change.

MUSIC THERAPY IN MEDICAL SETTINGS

Research in music therapy as applied to medical settings has been reviewed by Standley.[2] A recent meta-analysis suggests the following generalizations about the response to music in medical treatment:[2]

- Based on a relatively small number of studies, women's response to music is somewhat greater than men's response.
- Children and adolescents are marginally more responsive to music than are adults. However, infants respond less to music than either of the other age groups, perhaps as a result of their having less experience with music.
- Live music performed by a music therapist results in a much greater effect on physical and psychologic states than does recorded music. However, patient-preferred music results in the greatest positive medical effect.
- Music has a greater effect when pain is present than when pain is not present. However, the positive effects of music seem to decrease as pain increases.

- The physiologic and psychologic effects of music vary according to the specific dependent measures used.

Greatest effects were reported for grasp strength in stroke patients, perceived effectiveness of music, EMG, self-report of pain, relaxation, and anxiety reduction. Least effects were measured by days of hospitalization, peripheral finger temperature, ease of childbirth, time of recovery from anesthesia, formula intake of neonates and neonate apnea.[2]

- "The least conservative measure of music's effect is patient self-report while systematic behavioral observation and physiological measures result in basically equivalent, conservative effect sizes. The most frequently utilized dependent variable is a physiological measure."[28]

MUSIC THERAPY TECHNIQUES FOR NEUROLOGIC ILLNESS

In 1994, a team of investigators at Hershey Medical Center undertook an initial research project on music therapy and brain injury that was funded through the Office of Alternative Medicine of the National Institutes of Health.[29] It had three aims:
1. Establish a scientific framework for investigating a music therapy intervention for psychologic impairments after brain injury.
2. Examine the effects of a specific improvisational music therapy program on empiric measures of self-perception, empathy, emotional processing, and social interaction.
3. Identify areas for future scientific study.

A stratified randomization procedure was used to assign adults with brain injuries to experimental and control groups. The 30 subjects were in the chronic phase of recovering from either traumatic brain injury (TBI) or stroke. No further medical therapies were available to address the residual social and emotional impairments that kept participants from returning to occupational activities. All subjects underwent preintervention neuropsychologic testing, with the experimental group receiving a 10-week therapy intervention and the control group meeting in similar fashion for casual support group sessions. The music therapy program was structured to address residual psychosocial impairments. Both groups were retested when the 10-week period ended. Results indicated that positive changes in emotional empathy, depression, and social behavior occurred in the music therapy group, particularly as noted by family members. Cognitive measures, as expected, did not change. The social support group also showed some positive changes in emotional empathy and a measure of daily competency, but no change was shown in depression. The findings suggest that positive changes in emotional processing, social behavior, and mood can be achieved through music therapy. Some of these effects could be achieved with socialization activities alone. However, the progress made by music therapy participants and the reports made by family members showed more evidence in social and emotional domains. It was clear from these pilot data that the length of the music therapy program—twice a week for 10 weeks—was too modest, particularly to address chronic psychosocial impairments after brain injury. In addition, it may be beneficial to combine music therapy with other modes of intervention such as social support groups, preoccupational training, and even individual psychotherapy to maximize social and emotional adjustment.

With patients who have neurologic illness, the research literature supports several music therapy strategies:

- Facilitating physical rehabilitation and communication
- Coping with pain by using music as a focus of attention and distraction
- Relieving anxiety and depression through music-facilitated stress management and coping techniques
- Improving orientation for people with dementia using structured, success-oriented musical experiences

Facilitating Physical Rehabilitation and Communication

As human knowledge about the relationship of brain function and psychophysiologic activity increases, so does the understanding of music perception and active response. Music therapists have used this developing knowledge to determine effective strategies for using music in the rehabilitation of persons with neurologic dysfunction attributed to traumatic brain or spinal cord.[29-33] In this setting, music applications are coordinated with other therapies to assist patients in reaching the sensory-motor, cognitive, communication, social, and emotional goals of rehabilitation.

Music strategies have also had many positive effects when applied to physical rehabilitation. A review of the experimental research that was available in English regarding music applications in rehabilitation generated 120 studies between 1950 and 1993.[3] According to this review, the settings in which music therapy has been implemented most frequently are general hospitals with rehabilitation units, state hospitals and schools, special education classes within public schools, and comprehensive rehabilitation centers or nursing/retirement centers. In these settings, music therapy has been implemented primarily for patients with cerebral palsy, developmental disabilities, orthopedic impairments, paralysis, and poliomyelitis. Other studies describe the effects of music in acute or chronic neurologic rehabilitation.[3]

Patients in rehabilitation commonly present a myriad of physical and communication disorders. Music therapy interventions in physical rehabilitation are most often used for two reasons: to distract the patient's attention away from the pain and to decrease the monotony of repetitive movements associated with rehabilitation while sustaining the patient's interest in the specific activities and their repetition.

Common uses of music therapy in rehabilitation include the following:

- Promoting neuromuscular coordination
- Structuring movement or muscle stimulation, such as in stretching, exercise, vestibular stimulation, and proprioceptive responses to stimulation
- Enhancing muscular and motor control, for example, with tremors
- Reestablishing neuromotor patterns to include basic motor skills or movement in rhythm
- Structuring muscular relaxation, including tension release of rigid or spastic muscles
- Improving joint mobility and agility, and preventing stiffness
- Improving muscle and joint strength
- Improving respiratory capacity and rate
- Improving balance and posture
- Increasing range of motion and the extension and flexion of limbs
- Enhancing muscle tone and counteracting atrophy
- Improving muscular endurance and reaction time[3]

Music has been described as a sensory medium capable of arousing the nervous system and cueing altered states of awareness in human beings.[34] A patient's state of awareness at any moment is influenced by the focus of his or her attention. The individual's attentional focus is altered by the characteristics of the presented stimulus as perceived, and finally he or she reacts to the sensory information.[35] When the most desirable sensory stimuli available to a patient at a particular moment is patient-preferred music, and when that music is presented at an amplitude that is pleasing to the ear, the music serves as a catalyst to do the following:

- Alter the patient's emotions by calling upon previous associations with the particular piece
- Channel the patient's cognitive focus away from hospital sounds and physical preoccupation and toward more pleasing and normalizing music stimuli
- Either command an immediate physical response to the music, with little to no preparatory thought, or facilitate more purposeful movement over extended periods of time.[3,28,36]

Speaking metaphorically, it has been said that, "one listens to music with one's muscles," that is, music commands human beings to react and to move.[35] Movement is a key to physical rehabilitation, as is the will to move.

Music motivates by arousing the human will to act. Human will is a key factor in physical rehabilitation and a possible predictor of patient success. It serves as the primary catalyst for actions that bring about desired physical change and psychologic health. Music has the power to focus attention, and to elicit, drive, and regulate movement.[34] Music therapists use music in rehabilitation to cue physical response, structure response completion, or reinforce occurrences of a particular nonmusic behavior.[37,38]

Music used as therapy can be directed toward the specific goals of physical rehabilitation. Preferred music accompanied by a verbal suggestion of progressive relaxation might be used to calm an anxious or distracted patient. Alternatively, music might be prescribed for the chronically fatigued or unresponsive patient to direct mental focus, motivate action, and structure repetitions of physical exercise. For example, when carefully selected rhythms are used to accompany gait irregularities in stroke patients, the structure provided by the repeated rhythm enables the patient to anticipate and thereby to prepare for movement structured in time, much like dancing. In other words, rhythms at movement-appropriate tempos are introduced to a patient to stimulate movement response or to reinforce patient gait. When

movement begins, the repeated rhythm helps structure repeated movements so the movements become synchronous with the rhythmic sound.[39] Although music therapists use the process of successive approximations to bring this about, the structure of the music, especially the rhythm, often forces physical precision in musical time for at least the duration of the musical stimulus. Gait-appropriate rhythms are encapsulated in patient-preferred live or recorded music and then played at a tempo that forces increasing precision in locomotor movement. This can result in more fluid and efficient movement. Rhythmic Auditory Stimulation (RAS), a music technique used to facilitate movement by providing an auditory structure to force precision, has been used to improve gait velocity, cadence, stride length, and symmetry in patients suffering TBI. Forcing the body to precision using auditory cues has been referred to as *entrainment*.[37] After repeated use and patient improvement, the music structure is withdrawn from walking activities using fading techniques. The patient has then relearned the essential skill of walking naturally to ability.[3,34,39]

Patient-preferred music is also used in physical rehabilitation to sustain physical posture. In this case, preferred-music listening is made to be contingent upon the patient's initiation and maintenance of a desired posture, such as holding the head up. For example, when the patient's head falls, the music stops; when the head position is returned voluntarily to the designated posture, the music begins again and continues to play until the head again drops.[40]

Music therapy applications may be adapted to individual patients working alone with a therapist, but some of these strategies are also useful in working with patients in small groups. Group participation by these patients can reduce feelings of personal isolation and hopelessness while urging them into a more normal social environment. These opportunities to provide the struggling patient with successful patient role models provides additional motivation and satisfaction.

Music therapy interventions can be applied to the rehabilitation of patients presenting with symptoms of TBI.[40-44] A review of the uses of music in the assessment and rehabilitation of speech disorders[34] revealed a small number of studies addressing specific rehabilitative needs of these patients. Twenty articles documented music therapy protocols in experimental or case studies. Of these, 12 studies described the use of music in the assessment of speech and language disorder. Another nine articles described music applications in the remediation of communication disorders. Subjects in the majority of these studies suffered from aphasia. The literature regarding music and TBI primarily describes the following:

- Music and speech/language rehabilitation
- Intervention models used
- Music-based clinical assessment of TBI[34]

A primary strategy among physicians, speech therapists, and music therapists for speech and language rehabilitation using music is Melodic Intonation Therapy (MIT). MIT is a structured music/language model designed for persons with aphasia. Short phrases and sentences are embedded in brief melodies with special attention to rhythm. Intoned syllables, then words, and finally phrases are used to gradually reintroduce simple speech, inflection, and rhythm to aphasic patients. As the patient experiences success in using expressive language by "singing" or intoning functional words and phrases, the music element is faded and speech often improves. MIT techniques generate improvement in speech rate, clarity, vocabulary, and inflection.[28,34,44]

The theory behind MIT is that speech functions that have been impaired by damage to one hemisphere of the brain might be relearned by other cells, possibly in the other hemisphere. If this is the case, return of speech capability might be a matter of retraining brain cells. Some patients maintain musical capacity, especially singing abilities, following TBI.[45-48] MIT techniques are used to retrain speech through simplified singing experiences in which singing is the obvious link to eventual speech. Other techniques that can be used with aphasia are presented in the literature.[30,42]

Coping with Pain

According to the popular gate-control theory of pain, a competing stimulus might be able to direct a person's concentration away from pain. Listening to music or, better yet, engaging in focused musical activity guides the attention to a positive stimulus. In this way, music is effective in distracting from pain. Pain mechanisms may be considered psychologic events that translate incoming pain signals in the spinal and thalamic areas of the brain.[49] Music and other stimuli that change the sensation, effect, and motivation associated with pain form a gate to the perception of pain. This perception may be modulated through the use of music.[50] Music also alters pain perception by changing the mood, diverting attention, focusing on taking control of pain, and using relaxation skills.[51] These cognitive and behavioral strategies have been successful.[52,53]

Music techniques have had many positive effects when applied to the pain and anxiety associated with a neurologic illness. A meta-analysis of music therapy research done before 1986 estimates effect sizes for 29 empiric research experiments that used music for medically diagnosed conditions or pain. A mean effect size of .98 was calculated for the reviewed studies.[54] Other reviews of the effect of music on pain and stress reduction reinforce the efficacy of music listening.[55-57] An updated meta-analysis through 1996 included 92 empiric studies. In these studies, patients who had been diagnosed with a variety of illnesses or who experienced real pain were exposed to music or music techniques.[2] These data yield effect sizes of 1.72 for headache patients, 1.26 for chronic pain patients, and 1.17 for physical rehabilitation patients. The results reflect greater responses from women than from men and stronger effects for live music presented by a qualified music therapist than for recorded music. Studies that apply music of the patient's personal preference show an effect size of 1.40. The effectiveness of music in diminishing pain decreases with the intensity of pain.

Controlled experimentation with hospitalized patients reveals many successful applications of music listening strategies, but there are mixed results in some studies. In general, music listening alone is effective in reducing pain and anxiety even when little emphasis is placed on the choice of music for a particular individual. Other applications of music are cited for such diverse conditions as chronic pain of rheumatoid arthritis,[58] pain related to cancer,[59] and anxiety of patients in a rehabilitation unit.[60]

Certain music therapy procedures designed to reduce pain have been particularly effective. Vibroacoustic therapy has been applied successfully in a large number of studies[61] as have other interventions by music therapists involving live music[62] and individualized approaches.[63,64]

Music therapy protocols for pain are diverse and incorporate techniques ranging from passive listening to active music making. Selected music therapy techniques include the following:

- **Movement to music.** Exercising muscles affected by pain while listening to music often creates a positive mood, distracts from physical discomfort, and structures exercise so that patients report a quick and pleasant passage of time. Performing physical therapy regimens while listening to preferred music or playing simple percussion instruments focuses attention on a stimulus that evokes pleasure and relaxation.

- **Breathing to music.** Pairing deep, relaxed breathing with rhythmic music provides cues for a regular breathing tempo. This, in turn, encourages the patient to maintain even respiration, which facilitates a relaxed body.
- **Imagery to music.** Guided imagery involves preparing patients by having them relax to programmatic music, close their eyes, and visualize various scenes and images. The music might take individuals to places where they would like to go, or it might conjure a familiar, soothing environment like home. With severe pain, music and imagery together may be contraindicated, but either used alone has been shown to be beneficial in many cases.
- **Listening to music.** Much of the research by professionals who are not music therapists involves having patients listen to music that is either self-selected or chosen by the researcher. Listening alone has been shown to be effective in reducing pain. Listening to music is a natural leisure activity used by people outside of the hospital to enhance their daily lives. When a hospitalized patient listens to preferred music, its familiarity often results in feelings of comfort and normalcy. When possible, music therapy procedures include listening to music and inducing relaxation training procedures before the onset of pain.
- **Improvising to music.** To break the cycle of recurring pain, music therapists use a projective technique of expressing feelings by playing music. Some patients find it cathartic to express themselves in this way.
- **Composing songs.** Writing about the experience of coping with pain is similar to communicating the feelings surrounding the experience of pain. Music therapists facilitate the process of songwriting or musical composition by probing for content and structuring the melodic, harmonic, and rhythmic aspects of the music.

Relieving Anxiety and Depression

Having a neurologic illness may mean living with pain, worry, and uncomfortable treatment, and the prospect of living with a severe or chronic condition. The following techniques may help to relieve anxiety and depression:

- **Taking control of feelings.** When patients find a piece of music that moves them deeply, relaxes them completely, or distracts them actively, they see how they can control their feelings quickly and relatively easily. Attending concerts, enrolling in a choir or community ensemble, or learning to play a musical instrument redirects attention to interests and skills.
- **Increasing pleasant events and mood.** Engaging in pleasant music-related activities has been shown to reduce depression when it is applied with other behavior therapy techniques.[65]
- **Focusing on abilities, talents, and strengths.** Retraining musical competencies or introducing new ones offers the patient with a degenerative condition the opportunity to witness growth and potential in contrast to the loss of abilities. Engaging in any form of preferred music activity in which the patient can demonstrate competence and mastery is indicated.[66]

Improving Orientation and Success

Loss of cognitive function occurs in age-related memory loss as well as in more devastating progressive illnesses such as Alzheimer's disease and Parkinson's disease. Music therapy is often considered the treatment of choice for cognitively impaired older adults who respond to music, but little else. Many individuals who are in advanced stages of dementia participate actively in music therapy using preserved skills such as singing familiar songs, performing well-known compositions, and providing rhythmic accompaniment to pieces of music. This ability to retain music competencies has been documented in several studies.[67-69]

Music therapy is used widely in long-term care settings with great success. There is a growing body of evidence supporting the efficacy of music therapy. Brotons, Koger, and Pickett-Cooper[71] reviewed 69 studies published between 1987 and 1997. A meta-analysis of this research[70] reveals an effect size of 0.79, thereby demonstrating a significant effect of music therapy on a variety of symptoms. Music therapy has been used to improve socialization,[72] cognition,[73] and quality of life,[74] and to manage disruptive and inappropriate behaviors such as agitation,[75-80] physical aggression,[81] wandering,[82,83] and sleeplessness.[84] It has been applied at all levels of care, from community senior centers to assisted and long-term care facilities. Techniques are diverse and depend on a comprehensive assessment of functional needs, musical abilities, and interests in music. The following are ways that music therapy is used both in groups and individually:

- **Music therapy in groups.**[85] When applied in groups, structured musical experiences offer a way for people with dementia to experience success and to orient to reality. Group participants may master and demonstrate musical skills such as singing, playing instruments, improvising, creating new songs or compositions, moving or dancing to music, and accompanying a song. Through this process, they are able to experience a sense of competence, which they may not feel in other areas of their lives. Music therapists create failure-free environments by demanding only what each participant is capable of performing. This may be accomplished by asking specific individuals to provide a steady beat on percussion instruments, to sing along, to solo, or to create new rhythms or simple patterns (ostinati) on tuned instruments. The success of a musical creation that can be recorded and played back for the group may lead to group cohesiveness, positive affect, and self-esteem while focusing attention on positive, creative actions.
- **Individual behavior management strategies.**[86] Music is effective in decreasing agitation[87] when its use is contingent upon appropriate behavior, when it is used as a comforting stimulus, or when it is used to attract attention. Music therapists may sing or play music for an individual to maintain a calm mood while the individual is engaged in activities of daily living. They may also redirect the attention of an agitated person who is in the throes of a catastrophic reaction by clapping and singing, thereby engaging the individual in a constructive and acceptable activity.

References

1. Davis WB, Gfeller KE, Thaut MH: *An introduction to music therapy,* ed 2, Boston, 1999, McGraw-Hill.
2. Standley JM: Music research in medical/dental treatment: an update of a prior meta-analysis. In Furman CE, editor: *Effectiveness of music therapy procedures: documentation of research and clinical practice,* Silver Spring, Md, 1996, National Association for Music Therapy.
3. Staum MJ: Music for physical rehabilitation: an analysis of the literature from 1950-1993. In Furman CE, editor: *Effectiveness of music therapy procedures: documentation of research and clinical practice,* Silver Spring, Md, 1996, National Association for Music Therapy.
4. Standley JM, Prickett CA, editors: *Research in music therapy: a tradition of excellence: outstanding reprints from the Journal of Music Therapy 1964-1993,* Silver Spring, Md, 1994, National Association for Music Therapy.
5. Radocy RE, Boyle JD: *Psychological foundations of musical behavior,* Springfield, Ill, 1997, Charles C Thomas.
6. Taylor DB: Music in general hospital treatment from 1900 to 1950, *J Music Ther* 18:62-73, 1981.
7. *AMTA member sourcebook,* Silver Spring, Md, 1998, American Music Therapy Association.
8. Hanser SB: Controversy in music listening/stress reduction research, *Art Psychother* 15:211-217, 1988.
9. Critchley M, Henson RA, editors: *Music and the brain: studies of the neurology of music,* London, 1977, Heinemann.
10. Milner B: Laterality effects in audition. In Mountcastle VB, editor: *Interhemispheric relations and cerebral dominance,* Baltimore, 1962, Johns Hopkins University Press.
11. Samson S, Zatorre RJ: Melodic and harmonic discrimination following unilateral cerebral excision, *Brain Cogn* 7:348-360, 1988.
12. Peretz M: Processing of local and global musical information by unilaterally brain damaged patients, *Brain* 113:1185-1205, 1990.
13. Luria AR, Tsvetkova LS, Futer DS: Aphasia in a composer, *J Neurol Sci* 2:288-292, 1965.
14. Gardner H: *Art, mind and brain: a cognitive approach to creativity,* New York, 1982, Basic Books.
15. Zatorre RJ: Functional specialization of human auditory cortex for musical processing, *Brain* 121:1817-1818, 1998.
16. Hachinski KV, Hachinski V: Music and the brain, *CMAJ* 151:293-296, 1994.
17. Blonder LS, Bowers D, Heilman KM: The role of the right hemisphere in emotional communication, *Brain* 114:1115-1127, 1991.
18. Borod JC: Interhemispheric and intrahemispheric control of emotion: a focus on unilateral brain damage, *J Consult Clin Psychol* 60:339-348, 1992.

19. Adolphs R et al: Cortical systems for the recognition of emotion in facial expressions, *J Neurosci* 16:7678-7687, 1996.

20. Sergent J et al: Distributed neural network underlying musical sight-reading and keyboard performance, *Science* 257:106-109, 1992.

21. Sergent J: De la musique au cerveau, par l'intermediaire de Maurice Ravel, *Med/Sci* 9:50-58, 1993.

22. Zatorre RJ, Evans AC, Meyer E: Neural mechanisms underlying melodic perception and memory for pitch, *J Neurosci* 14:1908-1919, 1994.

23. Platel H et al: The structural components of music perception: a functional anatomical study, *Brain* 120:229-243, 1997.

24. Liegeois-Chauvel C: Contribution of different cortical areas in the temporal lobes to music processing, *Brain* 121:1853-1867, 1998.

25. Blood AJ et al: Emotional responses to pleasant and unpleasant music correlate with activity in paralimbic brain areas, *Nat Neurosci* 2:382-387, 1999.

26. Eslinger, PJ, Leder L: Behavior and emotional changes after focal frontal lobe damage. In Bogorisslavsky J and Cummings JL, editors: *Behavior and Mood Disorders in Focal Brain Lesions,* Cambridge, 2000, Cambridge University Press.

27. Thaut MH et al: The connection between rhythmicity and brain function, *IEEE Eng Med Biol* 18:101-108, 1999.

28. Staugger, Rohrbacher, Eslinger, in preparation.

29. Adamek MS, Shiraishi IM: Music therapy with traumatic brain-injured patients: speech rehabilitation, intervention models, and assessment procedures (1970-1995). In Furman CE, editor: *Effectiveness of music therapy procedures: documentation of research and clinical practice,* Silver Spring, Md, 1996, National Association for Music Therapy.

30. Gilbertson S: Music therapy in neurosurgical rehabilitation. In Wigram T, Backer JD, editors: *Clinical applications of music therapy in developmental disability, paediatrics and neurology,* London, 1999, Jessica Kingsley.

31. Sandness MI: The role of music therapy in physical rehabilitation programs, *Music Ther Perspect* 13(2):76-81, 1995.

32. Staum MJ: Music for physical rehabilitation: an analysis of the literature from 1950-1993. In Furman CE, editor: *Effectiveness of music therapy procedures: documentation of research and clinical practice,* Silver Spring, Md, 1996, National Association for Music Therapy.

33. Tomaino CM: Music and memory. In Tomaino CM, editor: *Clinical applications of music in neurologic rehabilitation,* St Louis, 1998, MMB Music.

34. Sacks O: Music and the brain. In Tomaino CM, editor: *Clinical applications of music in neurologic rehabilitation,* St Louis, 1998, MMB Music.

35. Madsen, CK: Focus of attention and aesthetic response, *J Res Music Educ* 45(1):80-89, 1997.

36. Hurt CP: Rhythmic auditory stimulation in gait training for patients with traumatic brain injury, *J Music Ther* 35(4):228-241, 1998.

37. Madsen CK: *Teaching discipline: a positive approach for educational development,* Raleigh, NC, l998, Contemporary Publishing Company of Raleigh.

38. Madsen CK: *Music therapy: a behavioral guide for the mentally retarded,* Lawrence, Kan, 1981, National Association for Music Therapy.

39. Staum MJ: Music and rhythmic stimuli in the rehabilitation of gait disorders, *J Music Ther* 22(2):69-87, 1983.

40. Wolfe DE: The effect of automated interrupted music on head posturing of cerebral palsied individuals, *J Music Ther* 17(4):184-206, 1980.

41. Thaut MH: Music therapy in neurological rehabilitation. In Davis WB, Gfeller KE, Thaut MH, editors: *An introduction to music therapy theory and practice,* Boston, 1999, McGraw-Hill.

42. Barker VL, Brunk B: The role of creative arts group in the treatment of clients with traumatic brain injury, *Music Ther Perspect* 9:26-31, 1991.

43. Cohen NS: The effect of singing instruction on the speech production of neurologically impaired persons, *J Music Ther* 24(2):87-102, 1992.

44. Cohen NS: The use of superimposed rhythm to decrease the rate of speech in a brain-damaged adolescent, *J Music Ther* 25(2):85-93, 1988.

45. Galloway H: A comprehensive bibliography of musical studies referential to communication development, processing disorders and remediation, *J Music Ther* 12:164-197, 1975.

46. Kinsella G, Prior MR, Murray G: Singing ability after right and left sided brain damage: a research note, *Cortex* 24(1):165-169, 1988.

47. Jacome DE: Aphasia with elation, hypermusia, musicophilia and compulsive whistling, *J Neurol Neurosurg* 47(3):308-310, 1984.

48. Brust JC: Music and language: musical alexia and agraphia, *Brain* 103(2):367-392, 1980.

49. Filippini JF: Some useful basics of functional anatomy for a better understanding of the pain phenomenon, *Rev Laryngol Otol Rhinol* 117:75-78, 1996.

50. Wall PD: On the relation of injury to pain: the John J. Bonica lecture, *Pain* 6:253-264, 1979.

51. Magill-Levreault L: Music therapy in pain and symptom management, *J Palliat Care* 9:42-48, 1993.

52. Wolfe DE: The effect of automated interrupted music on head posturing of cerebral palsied individuals, *J Music Ther* 15:162-178, 1978.

53. Brown CJ, Chen ACN, Dworkin SF: Music in the control of pain, *Music Ther* 8:47-60, 1989.

54. Standley JM: Music research in medical /dental treatment: meta-analysis and clinical applications, *J Music Ther* 23(2): 56-122, 1986.

55. Maslar P: The effect of music on the reduction of pain: a review of the literature, *Art Psychother* 13:215-219, 1986.

56. Hanser SB: Music therapy and stress reduction research, *J Music Ther* 22:193-206, 1985.

57. Maranto CD: Applications of music in medicine. In Heal M, Wigram T, editors: *Music therapy in health and education,* London, 1978, Jessica Kingsley.

58. Schorr JA: Music and pattern change in chronic pain, *Adv Nurs Sci* 15:27-36, 1993.

59. Beck SL: The therapeutic use of music for cancer related pain, *Oncol Nurs Forum* 18:1327-1337, 1991.

60. Mandel SE: Music for wellness: Music therapy for stress management in a rehabilitation program, *Music Ther Perspect* 14:38-43, 1996.

61. Skille O, Wigram T: The effects of music, vocalization, and vibration on brain and muscle tissue: studies in vibroacoustic therapy. In Wigram T, Superstar B, West R, editors: *The art and science of music therapy: a handbook,* Chur, Switzerland, 1995, Harwood Academic.

62. Malone AB: The effects of live music on pediatric patients receiving intravenous starts, venipunctures, injections, and heel sticks, *J Music Ther* 33:19-33, 1996.

63. Standley JM, Hanser SB: Music therapy research and applications in pediatric oncology treatment, *J Pediatr Oncol Nurs* 12:3-8, 1995.

64. Michel DE, Chesky KS: A survey of music therapists using music for pain relief, *Art Psychother* 22:49-51, 1995.

65. Hanser SB, Thompson LW: Effects of a music therapy strategy on depressed older adults, *J Gerontol* 49:265-269, 1994.

66. Hanser SB: Music therapy with depressed older adults, *J Int Assoc Music Handicap* 4:16-27, 1989.

67. Crystal HA, Grober E, Masur D: Preservation of musical memory in Alzheimer's disease, *J Neurol Neurosurg* 52:1415-1416, 1989.

68. Beatty W, Zavadil K, Bailly R, Rixen L, Zavadil L, Farnham N, Fisher I: Preserved muscial skill in a severely demented patient, *Int J Clin Neuropsychol* 10:158-164, 1988.

69. Swartz, KP, Hartz EC, Crummer LC, Walton JP, Frisina RD: Does the melody linger on? Music Cognition in Alzheimer's disease, *Seminar on Neurology* 9:152-158, 1989.

70. Swartz KP, Walton J, Crummer, Hartz E, Frisina R: P3 event-related potentials and performance of healthy older adults and AD subjects for music perception tasks, *Psychomusicology* 11:96-118, 1992.

71. Brotons M, Koger SM, Pickett-Cooper P: Music and the dementias: a review of literature, *J Music Ther* 34:204-245, 1997.

72. Koger SM, Chapin K, Brotons M: Is music therapy an effective intervention for dementia? A meta-analytic review of literature, *J Music Ther* 36:2-15, 1999.

73. Pollack NJ, Namazi KH: The effect of music participation on the social behavior of Alzheimer's disease patients, *J Music Ther* 29:54-67, 1992.

74. Smith G: A comparison of the effects of three treatment interventions on cognitive functioning of Alzheimer patients, *Music Ther* 6A:41-56, 1986.

75. Lipe A: Using music therapy to enhance the quality of life in a client with Alzheimer's dementia: a case study, *Music Ther Perspect* 9:102-105, 1991.

76. Brotons M, Pickett-Cooper P: The effects of music therapy intervention on agitation behaviors of Alzheimer's disease patients, *J Music Ther* 33:2-18, 1996.

77. Clair AA, Bernstein B: The effect of no music, stimulative background music and sedative background music on agitation behaviors in persons with severe dementia, *Activities Adaptation Aging* 19:61-70, 1994.

78. Gerdner LA, Swanson EA: Effects of individualized music on confused and agitated elderly patients, *Arch Psychiatr Nurs* 7:284-291, 1993.

79. Goddaer J, Abraham I: Effects of relaxing music on agitation during meals among nursing home residents with severe cognitive impairments, *Arch Psychiatr Nurs* 8:150-158, 1994.

80. Tabloski P, McKinnon-Howe L, Remington R: Effects of calming music on the level of agitation in cognitively impaired nursing home residents, *Am J Alzheimer Care Relat Disord Res* 10:10-15, 1995.

81. Ward CR, Los Kamp L, Newman S: The effects of participation in an intergenerational program on the behavior of residents with dementia, *Activities Adaptation Aging* 20:61-76, 1996.

82. Thomas DW, Heitman RJ, Alexander T: The effects of music on bathing cooperation for residents with dementia, *J Music Ther* 34:246-259, 1997.

83. Fitzgerald-Cloutier ML: The use of music therapy to decrease wandering: an alternative to restraints, *Music Ther Perspect* 11:32-36, 1992.

84. Groene RW II: Effectiveness of music therapy: 1:1 interventions with individuals having senile dementia of the Alzheimer's type, *J Music Ther* 30:138-157, 1993.

85. Lindenmuth GF, Patel M, Chang PK: Effects of music on sleep in healthy elderly and subjects with senile dementia of the Alzheimer's type, *Am J Alzheimer Dis Relat Disord Res* 2:13-20, 1992.

86. Hanser SB, Clair AA: Retrieving the losses of Alzheimer's disease for patients and caregivers with the aid of music. In Wigram T, Saperston B, West R, editors: *The art and science of music therapy: a handbook,* Chur, Switzerland, 1995, Harwood Academic.

87. Hanser SB: Music therapy with individuals with advanced dementia. In Volicer L, Bloom-Charette L, editors: *Enhancing the quality of life in advanced dementia,* Philadelphia, 1999, Brunner/Mazel.

88. Hanser SB: Music therapy to reduce anxiety, agitation, and depression, *Nurs Home Med* 10:286-291, 1996.

Case Study in Music Therapy and Rehabilitation

SUZANNE HANSER

Ann C. is a 44-year-old woman who was admitted for evaluation after falling backwards from a 15- to 20-foot ledge in the mountains and landing on her back. The patient exhibited difficulty breathing and heart irregularities at the scene of the accident. Further diagnosis indicated a collapsed left lung, premature ventricular contractions, and rapid changes in blood pressure. Computerized tomography (CT) scan of the spine showed significant anterior column damage to thoracic vertebrae T7, T8, T9, T11, and T12 with compression. Also presented were a 3 to 4 mm retropulsion of the inferior portion of T7 at the spinal canal, and a 2 to 3 mm retropulsion of T9. A small linear fracture was observed at T1. Magnetic Imaging Resonance (MRI) scan of the thoracic spine indicated some compromise in the motion of her fractures, but no cord compression or gross intrinsic cord edema or hemorrhage. Ann reported that she had no feeling in her chest or in the area of her back surrounding the point of contact. Fractures were evident in posterior ribs 5, 6, and 7. There was no evidence of deep vein thrombosis of the lateral lower extremities. Hematoma was present in the right shoulder, and use of both arms was limited. There were contusions on the back of the skull and probable coronary contusions, but no evidence of internal hemorrhage.

Following examination in the emergency room, the patient was transferred by air to a multi-trauma hospital where she was reexamined and admitted to the critical care unit for a period of one week. Once stabilized, Ann was fitted for a Thoraco Lumbar Sacral Orthotic (TLSO) brace, admitted to a multi-trauma unit for an additional week, and finally released to a rehabilitation hospital for an additional 8 days of physical rehabilitation. Inpatient treatment occurred in three distinct phases:

Phase I: Critical care
Phase II: Multi-trauma
Phase III: Physical rehabilitation

Music therapies, physical therapies, and occupational therapies were incorporated into the treatment protocol. Sessions with a neuropsychologist were designed to support the development and use of the patient's coping skills.

Phase I: The patient was heavily medicated and disoriented for the first week following injury. Ann was unaware of the day, time, or place, and unresponsive when verbally prompted with questions or with commands to act. Staff reported one incidence of a panic attack in which Ann quickly attempted to remove medical apparatus from her body.

Phase II: When the patient's cognitive disorientation decreased and vital signs were stable, she was admitted to the multi-trauma unit of the hospital. Treatment objectives changed during this phase from stabilization to improvement of cognitive focus, increased physical exercise (first in bed) as a means of reducing muscle atrophy, and increased use of the upper body and limbs. Treatment objectives also included relearning daily living skills such as dressing; putting on her TLSO brace while lying down; eating using arms and hands; and moving, standing, and walking in her brace. Adaptive devices and strategies for accomplishing these skills were addressed in each therapy session. In all activities, purposeful and efficient use of movement and increased physical endurance were emphasized.

Pain management strategies first used by the patient during Phase II were intravenous administration of a combination of drug therapies followed by patient use of a morphine pump. However, allergy to selected drugs and their replacements resulted in severe and unrelenting nausea, vomiting, dehydration, and physical weakness shortly after introduction. The patient refused medication for pain management early in Phase II of treatment. She indicated that she would rather experience pain alone than pain with accompanying nausea. Ann was moved to a private room at this time to minimize environmental stressors resulting from the treatment activities and responses of patients in the same room.

Music therapy was used by Ann through all phases of hospitalization. Initially, she listened to music that was identified as preferred by a family member. Music listening was introduced during critical care as a means of assessing cognitive function and to cue any kind of response to stimuli. Familiar music was then used to stimulate long term memory and, thus, improve cognitive function. During Phase I, the patient, who is a musician herself, responded increasingly to music listening experiences and to topic-related questions with brief, but topic-specific verbalizations.

During Phase II, active music listening was used as a pain management strategy to focus attention away from pain and nausea for brief periods of time, and as a means of normalizing the hospital environment by masking stress-generating hospital sounds. Music used as a distractor from pain was an essential alternative to medication because it was implemented in the absence of medication for pain. Music listening was also used to calm the patient, reducing the possibility of an anxiety attack while intubated. No further anxiety attacks were observed. Additionally, music listening was employed to cue relaxation prior to sleep and whenever new IV lines were introduced, which occurred frequently.

As Phase II progressed, the strategies previously mentioned were continued, but additional music applications were also implemented. Music was used to focus Ann's attention on herself and her use of coping skills. This was important during the intensive daily 4-hour physical and occupational therapy sessions. Music was used prior to respiratory therapy to relax the patient for machine-accompanied deep breathing activities. These activities were designed to improve respiratory capacity that had been reduced as a result of the lung collapse and from being bedridden. Successful respiratory therapy was essential to this phase of treatment so that the patient could be removed from oxygen and become mobile. Tempo-appropriate music was also used intermittently during respiratory therapy to structure continued deep breathing and stamina during the procedure and to minimize anxiety.

Phase III: During physical rehabilitation, music was also added to the treatment protocol to motivate gross and fine motor and locomotor movement and to promote Ann's use of her upper body, especially her arms. Occupational therapists used tempo-appropriate music as a rhythmic structure for upper body movements during in-bed exercises. This music was also used to lengthen the time spent exercising and the fluidity of movement in space. Improvised piano music played by the music therapist was used to structure pacing in walking activities and to increase the amount of time spent walking.

An important use of music during physical rehabilitation was as an aid to psychological counseling. The neuropsychologist used music lyrics and recorded music to introduce topics for discussion that were designed to promote Ann's acceptance of her injury and its implications for the future. Through music experiences and counseling, Ann was encouraged to integrate her accident into her life experience and to make decisions aimed at improving her quality of life. For example, Ann reported that crying was not something she could do easily, but she believed that being able to cry would help her feel and to release her feelings about the accident. That, in turn, would enable her to grieve. She reported feeling emotionally "numbed" by the experience at that point. With Ann's help, music was selected that would cue intense feelings, thereby allowing her to cry and to feel the corresponding physical release that crying would bring. The patient also composed music lyrics as a means of self-disclosure once she was able to verbally communicate her feelings.

Near the end of her hospitalization, Ann was introduced to group music therapy to promote social interaction following the isolation of some therapy and prior to her release. Music therapy sessions were designed to expose Ann to appropriate peer role models who were, perhaps, further along in the process of rehabilitation. After 3 weeks in the hospital, Ann was released to continue her recuperation as an outpatient. She remained in her TLSO brace for several months and continued physical therapy under the care of her neurologist. One year later, Ann was walking, still struggling with pain management but with a modicum of prescription medications. She had returned to work full time in her continuing career as a music therapist.

In this case study, music therapy was used as a treatment alternative to do the following:
1. Assess cognitive function
2. Reduce patient stress
3. Distract attention from physical pain
4. Mask undesirable hospital sounds
5. Relax the patient prior to stressful procedures
6. Provide intermittent rhythmic structure for exhalation during respiratory therapy
7. Structure gross motor movement in marked time by forcing movement to (eventual) precision and prolonging time spent in repetitive exercise
8. Facilitate patient self-disclosure, initiate the grieving process, and/or provide an avenue for creative self-expression when used as a cue in psychotherapy
9. Provide a transitional structure for patient reintroduction into a social group; in this case, the transitional structure was in the form of peers serving as support and as models for proactive involvement in personal rehabilitation

This final step is one of the many small steps that physically injured persons must first choose to take, and then take, in the slow and arduous journey to improved health after trauma.

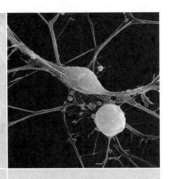

CHAPTER

21

Laser Biostimulation: A Novel Alternative Treatment in Neurologic Illness

MICHAEL I. WEINTRAUB

Knowledge, once gained, casts a faint light beyond its own immediate boundaries.
There is no discovery so limited as not to illuminate something beyond itself.

JOHN TYNDALL

The application of light for medicinal purposes (healing) has been used for thousands of years. The ancient Greeks believed that sunlight exposure induced strength and health. During the Middle Ages, the disinfectant properties of sunlight were used to combat plague and other illnesses, and in the nineteenth century, cutaneous tuberculosis (scrofula) was treated with ultraviolet exposure. Now light therapy is used to treat psoriasis, hyperbilirubinemia, and seasonal affective disorder (SAD).

WHAT IS LIGHT?

Light is electromagnetic waves consisting of photonic energy bundles that are divided by wave lengths. Visible light, called the visual spectrum, is 400 to 700 nm appreciated by the human eye. One nanometer (nm) equals one billionth of a meter. The smaller the wave length, the greater its ability to penetrate tissues. X-rays, gamma rays, ultraviolet rays, cosmic rays, and others all fall below visible light on the electromagnetic spectrum. Longer wave lengths such as infrared rays,

The author would like to thank David S. Casper for the use of the figures in this chapter.

microwaves, television transmissions, and FM/AM radio waves have different characteristics.

HISTORY

The atomic theories that lead to the discovery of lasers was established in 1917 by Albert Einstein. By 1960, the first practical ruby red laser was developed by T.H. Maiman[1] who used crystals and mirrors to produce a monochromatic, nondivergent light beam in which all waves were parallel and in phase. These characteristics were subsequently referred to as monochromaticity, collimation, and coherence, respectively. The original ruby red beam was a visible red light with a wave length of 694 nm. Since then, various crystals and gases have been used to expand the electromagnetic spectrum into the infrared and visible light lasers.

DEFINING LASER

Laser is an acronym for light amplification by stimulated emission of radiation. When light is directed onto an object, one of the following occurs:

1. The light is reflected.
2. The light is transmitted.
3. The light is scattered.
4. The light is absorbed.

Every object has optic properties that determine the effectiveness of light and the reaction of light on that object. For example, mid-infrared and far-infrared lasers, such as CO_2 and holmium, or yttrium-aluminum garnet (YAG), are primarily absorbed by water in the tissues. This absorption of the infrared light energy converts to heat, which leads to local vaporization that does not spread. Near infrared and visible-light lasers such as neodymium:YAG and argon are poorly absorbed by water but are rapidly absorbed by pigment such as hemoglobin and melanin. This optic property makes these lasers effective in the destruction of tissues that are rich in pigment such as retina, gastric mucosa, and pigmented cutaneous lesion. It is easy to see how these so-called high-powered surgical lasers, using heat and energy, lead to specific tissue changes. During the past 30 years, numerous animal and laboratory experiments were carried out using these high-energy lasers. These experiments produced results that have ultimately led to human testing and approval by the Food and Drug Administration (FDA) of the use of lasers on humans.

Despite more than 30 years of similar experiments using weak or low-level, nonthermal lasers, i.e., low level laser therapy (LLLT), there is still controversy concerning its effectiveness as a treatment modality, and the FDA has failed to approve its use. Some of the main reasons for this failure have been a literature filled with flawed methodology, various time and dosage schedules, and absence of strict placebo design.

Because the author believes that this novel approach is therapeutically valid, this chapter explores cold laser use in neurologic and generalized conditions.

THEORY OF COLD LASER

Cold laser, or LLLT, is based on the idea that monochromatic light energy, which is wave length-dependent for its penetration, can alter cellular functions. Because the original European studies on wound healing in animals was positive, it was described as a "bio-stimulation." Mester and coworkers,[2] and Lyons[3] found that light could be stimulatory at low powers and could elicit an opposite inhibitory effect at higher powers. In addition, the cumulative dosages of the radiation could sometimes be inhibitory. Today there are a variety of lasers, but the two most popular are helium-neon (He-Ne) and gallium aluminum arsenide (GaAlAs [830 nm]). In practice, these visible and infrared lasers have powers of 30 to 90 mW and deliver from 1 to 9 J/cm² to treatment sites. To date, they have been shown to be safe within this spectrum but they have also been used at higher dosages.

MECHANISMS OF ACTION

Musculoskeletal tissues appear to have optic properties that respond to light between 500 and 1000 nm. The sufficient specific laser dosage and the number of treatments needed are still the subject of controversy. It is hypothesized that light-sensitive organelles, or chromatophores,[4] absorb light and that ultimately the energy produces a biologic reaction. It has been suggested that chromatophores exist on the myelin sheath and mitochondria, and that monochromaticity wave length properties, rather than coherency and collimation, induce biologic changes. It is presumed that the collimation and coherency lead to rapid degradation by scatter.

TISSUE PENETRATION

Longer wave lengths penetrate more deeply than do shorter wave lengths. The shorter He-Ne laser beam (632 nm) penetrates several millimeters into tissue whereas the GaAlAs 830 nm/30 mW allows photons to penetrate more than an inch (3 cm). Several authors have stated that an infrared laser beam travels about 2 mm into tissue and that this represents one penetration depth with loss of 1/e (37%) of its intensity.[5] However, the shorter, visible, He-Ne red beam is attenuated the same amount in 0.5 to 1 mm.[6-8] How does one measure the decay in the amount of energy with distance? At the surface of the skin, the laser delivers from 1 to 9 J/cm^2. Karu[9] has demonstrated that 0.01 J/cm^2 can alter cellular processes. As a result, approximately six penetration depths (3 to 6 mm for He-Ne red light and about 24 mm for GaAlAs IR) are possible before the strength of the beam stream drops from 9 J/cm^2 to 0.01 J/cm^2. Thus, the threshold and specific therapeutic amount needed to stimulate the superficial nerve and tissues differs from the deeper structures. There is also a scattering of energy that influences nonneural adjacent tissues.

LASER RESEARCH

There have been many claims and studies regarding LLLT, but the varied quality of trials has led to controversy. Basford,[5,8,10] although a major critic of the deficiencies of many studies, does believe that LLLT research has developed along the following three separate lines:

1. Cellular function
2. Animal studies
3. Human trials

Perhaps the strongest and most well-established research has been on changes in cellular functions.

There is a strong body of direct evidence indicating that LLLT can significantly alter cellular processes (Table 21-1). Following are specific areas of treatment that have been cited:

- Stimulation of collagen formation leading to stronger scars[11]; increased granulation tissue and

TABLE 21-1

Cellular effects altered by low-energy irradiation

Phenomenon	Effect	
Collagen and Protein Synthesis	↑↑	↓↓
Cell Proliferation and Differentiation	↑↑	↓↓
Cell Motility	↑↑	
Membrane Potential and Binding Affinities	↑↑	
Neurotransmitter Release	↑↑	
Prostaglandin Synthesis	↑↑	
ATP Synthesis	↑↑	
Phagocytosis	↑↑	
Oxyhemoglobin Dissociation	↑↑	

fibroblasts[12]; increased neovascularization[13]; and faster wound healing[3,14,15]
- Pain relief analgesia and reduced firing frequency of nociceptors[16]
- Enhanced remodeling and repair of bone[4,15]
- Stimulation of endorphin release[17]
- Modulation of the immune system via prostaglandin synthesis[2,18]

Animal and Laboratory Studies

Basic animal and cellular research with red-beam, low-level laser has produced both positive and negative results. Passarella[19] believes that the optic properties of mitochondria are influenced by He-Ne laser irradiation, producing new mitochondrial conformations that ultimately lead to increased oxygen consumption. Walker[20] has suggested that He-Ne laser affects serotonin metabolism, and Yu[21] has demonstrated an increased phosphate potential and energy charge with light exposure. Further research continues at the cellular level. Fibroblast, lymphocyte, monocyte, and macrophage cells have been studied, and bacterial cell lines of E. coli have served as models of investigation.[22] The most popular laser in such cellular research has been the He-Ne laser with a wave length of 632.8 nm. However, some major discrepancies among the existing literature lie in the wide variation of laser parameters employed, particularly dose and treatment time. Because imprecise dosimetry has clouded the issues, the optimal dose for achieving a biologic benefit has yet to be determined.

Despite the problems posed by a lack of standardization, lack of controls, and imprecise dose and treatment schedules for in vivo experimental work, results from cellular research were extrapolated into research on animals. Subsequently, a wide variety of animal models were employed to assess the putative biostimulatory effects of laser irradiation on wound healing. Small, loose-skinned rodents, such as mice, rats, or guinea pigs have been used most often, but models using pigs have led to different results. It has been argued that pigskin represents a more suitable model for extrapolation to humans because it is similar in character to human skin.[10,23]

Baxter[24] provides an excellent review of the animal models used in the wound-healing literature. The details of experimental and irradiation procedures are so numerous and variable, however, that reproducibility and intertrial comparisons are usually not practical. Research groups reported either an acceleration in healing or no effect on the healing process. Two frequent criteria for assessing wound healing were collagen content and tensile strength. Rochkind[25] conducted one of the largest series of controlled animal trials on crushed sciatic nerves versus normal nerves in rats. Constant low-intensity laser irradiation (7.6 to 10 J/cm^2 daily for up to 20 days) with recording of compound action potentials demonstrated highly beneficial effects. Wound-healing rates in both irradiated and nonirradiated wounds were accelerated, but the amplitude of action potentials in crushed sciatic nerves were raised substantially only in the irradiated groups. The laser treatment also greatly reduced the degeneration of motor neurons and suggested that these results might be extrapolated for application in human research trials.

In conclusion, the information gained from in vivo animal trials exposed to laser photo biostimulation indicated that in certain animal models, wound healing could be achieved. Considerable skepticism still exists, though, due to variations among studies in such areas as methodology, techniques, dosimetry, exposure time, and frequency of treatments.

Clinical Studies

Despite the controversy, however, many groups of clinicians who were impressed and persuaded by the cellular and animal data, subsequently attempted human trials. A number of disorders, including neurologic, rheumatologic, and musculoskeletal have been treated with LLLT. Although some results are promising and extremely exciting, the FDA has not approved them and has maintained LLLT's "investigational" status. The FDA's skepticism has centered primarily on the absence of randomized, controlled trials; varied methodology; varied dosages and techniques; and the absence of objective parameters.

Neurologic Conditions

Compelling evidence exists that the distal median nerve at the wrist is very sensitive to LLLT both in patients who have carpal tunnel syndrome and in those who do not. Using only one joule of energy, Basford[26] found that he could statistically influence both sensory and motor distal latencies in normal volunteers. Basford's study was a double-blind control study using a GaAlAs percutaneous laser. Weintraub[27] used a similar laser, but at higher energy levels of nine joules, and Compound Motor Action Potential/Sensory Nerve Action Potential (CMAP/SNAP) electrophysiologic parameters to achieve a 78% success rate in resolving the symptoms of carpal tunnel syndrome. There were no controls in the study, but almost 1000 sensory and motor latencies of nerves were studied before and after each treatment. Particularly interesting was the fact that the distal latency was prolonged in 40% of subjects, yet they remained asymptomatic. This prolonged latency suggests that nonneural tissues were stimulated and could be responsible for symptoms of tendonitis. With this dosage, a significant number of individuals had immediate slowed prolongation of distal latency (nerve conduction). However, they remained asymptomatic and by the next visit, the distal latency was back to baseline or improved. This observation has also been noted by others.[28] For example, Padua[29] has validated Weintraub's study, and currently three placebo-controlled studies are being performed with preliminary results of 70% success.[30] Additionally, there are two reports using higher dosages of 10 to 12 joules of IR diode (40 to 50 mW) that reveal alterations of both the median and superficial radial nerve.[31-33]

Naeser[34] and Branco[35] used a combination of two non-invasive, painless treatment modalities, namely, red-beam laser and microamps transcutaneous electrical nerve stimulation (TENS), to stimulate acupuncture points on the affected hand. Sham controls were used. A significant reduction in median nerve sensory latencies in the treated hand and a 92% reduction in pain were observed. Postoperative failures also improved with this protocol.

Other superficial nerves also respond to laser bio-stimulation. Disorders such as meralgia paresthetica, cubital tunnel syndrome, tarsal tunnel syndrome, radial nerve palsy, and traumatic digital neuralgias have responded to this treatment.[36] Due to the small number of individuals treated, these observations are to be considered anecdotal. However, Weintraub believes that his observations of nonneural structures playing an important yet unappreciated role in symptomatic carpal tunnel syndrome, and probably other nerve entrapments, is indeed important. For example, the distal latency of the median nerve could be greater than 5 ms in patients who have become asymptomatic with laser treatment. Either a threshold exists for the median nerve, or the tendons and blood vessels surrounding the median nerve exert some influence. Franzblau and Werner[37] raised similar issues in a provocative editorial titled, "What Is Carpal Tunnel Syndrome?"

Neurogenic Pain

The efficacy of laser therapy in various pain syndromes has been investigated by several groups. Preliminary double-blind studies by Walker[20] demonstrated improvement in seven out of nine patients with trigeminal neuralgia. Two out of five patients improved with postherpetic neuralgia and five out of six patients improved with radiculopathy. Baxter[38] also believed that laser was effective for postherpetic neuralgia. Moore[39] investigated the efficacy of using GaAlAs laser in the treatment of postherpetic neuralgia in a double-blind, crossover trial on 20 patients. The result was an apparently significant reduction in pain. Hong[40] validated this study with 60% of the patients feeling improvement within 10 minutes. Friedman[41] used an intraoral He-Ne laser directed at a specific maxillary alveolar tender point to significantly abort atypical facial pain.

Trigeminal neuralgia was successfully treated with He-Ne laser by Walker.[42] In the 35 patients studied in this double-blind, placebo-controlled trial, he found a significant difference in visual analog scale (VAS) ratings between active and placebo-treated patients.

Using an intraoral He-Ne laser directed at the specific maxillary alveolar tender point (Figure 21-1), Weintraub was able to abort acute migraine headaches in 85% of cases with sham controls. These findings support the trigeminovascular theory of migraine with a maxillary (V2) provocative site.[48] These results rival pharmacotherapeutical results. Interestingly, Friedman[43] used the same maxillary alveolar tenderness

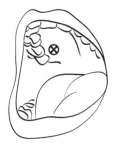

Figure 21-1 Laser site for migraine headache.

(MAT) point (Figure 21-1) to treat atypical facial pain and migraine headache cryotherapy (cold water). The treatment achieved a striking reduction in discomfort.

Radiculitis

Several groups have investigated the efficacy of laser therapy in the treatment of radicular and pseudoradicular pain syndromes. Bieglio[44] and Mizokami[45] reported positive effects. Low-power laser has also been used successfully to induce preoperative anesthesia in both veterinary practice and dental surgery.[46] In contrast to the numerous clinical human studies of laser-mediated analgesia, there have been relatively few laboratory studies. Most of the experiments have been completed in China using a variety of animals including rats, goats, rabbits, sheep, and horses. There are no English abstracts or translations of most of these works. Other studies published in English have reported variable findings using the tail-flick methodology.

Laser acupuncture using an He-Ne diode was reported to be successful in the treatment of experimental arthritis in rats. Vocalization and limb withdrawal were the parameters used in response to noxious stimulation.[47] Although it is clear that problems exist in extrapolating the findings of laboratory work to humans, Naeser[34] and Branco[35] were successful with this procedure in Carpal Tunnel Syndrome (CTS). Similarly, Weintraub[27] saw additional improvement when he incorporated Naeser's acupressure points (Figure 21-2) with his protocol (Figure 21-3).

Soft Tissue Healing

One of the major economic burdens in the United States has been caused by the high incidence of soft tissue injuries and low back pain and the subsequent

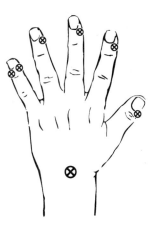

Figure 21-2 Dorsal hand.

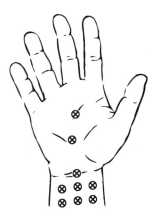

Figure 21-3 Volar wrist, palm.

loss of work. Numerous studies using He-Ne and infra-red (IR) laser diodes (830 nm range) have reported varying results,[8,10,49,50] but randomized control and blinded studies have been difficult to carry out.

Rheumatologists in this country have identified encouraging results in rheumatoid arthritis,[51] with similar results being reported in the Soviet Union, Eastern Europe, and Japan. Walker reported success after a 10-week course of treatment with He-Ne units. Using a GaAlAs 830 nm, Asada[52] found 90% improvement in an uncontrolled trial on 170 patients. Despite these generally positive results, Bliddal[53] did not see any significant change in symptoms of morning stiffness or joint function. However, there was slight improvement in pain scales. Similar positive results have been reported for osteoarthritis and other pseudoarthritic

conditions. Critics have argued, however, that because rheumatoid arthritis is a disease of exacerbation and remission, it is difficult to assess efficacy.

A number of reports document the apparent efficacy of laser therapy in reducing pain associated with sports injuries. These reports initially came from Russia and Eastern Europe and were subsequently confirmed by Morselli[54] and Emmanoulidis.[55] It is notable that in the latter study improvement was accompanied by a decrease in thermographic readings.

Tendinopathies, especially lateral humeral epicondylitis (tennis elbow) have been studied by numerous groups as well as the author. There has usually been a relatively rapid response to therapy, however Haker[56] failed to show any effect with laser acupuncture treatment for tennis elbow.

In summary, although a strong suggestion exists that laser therapy is beneficial for human pain, it is clear that the quality of the studies has been highly variable and that there have been few properly controlled clinical trials. Research designs show that a variety of wave lengths, power and energy densities, frequencies, and durations of treatment have been employed. Objectives such as optimum dosage treatment have not been achieved. In addition, several publications have reported a lack of benefit from the use of laser therapy. Laboratory investigations of laser-mediated analgesia are sometimes contradictory, and critics have found it difficult to correlate animal pain with the more complex aspects of human pain. Finally, the lack of an obvious pathophysiologic mechanism leads to confusion about such factors as the mechanism of action. It is hoped that future studies will be randomized and placebo controlled with a tight methodologic design as to wave length, frequency, and duration of treatment to determine efficacy for specific conditions.

Safety

No detrimental effects are produced by low-output, non-thermal lasers, although it is obvious that direct retinal exposure is to be avoided. Pregnancy does not appear to be a contraindication with LLLT, but investigators have been advised to avoid treating pregnant women and individuals with local tumors in the area of treatment. Individuals taking photosensitizing drugs such as tetracycline, or having photosensitive skin should probably avoid this treatment.

Neurologic Conditions with Possible Laser Benefit

Cerebral Palsy in Babies and Children

Asagai[57] performed LLLT on acupressure points in 1000 babies and children with cerebral palsy. The LLLT effectively suppressed tonic muscle spasms.

Stroke

Naeser[58] improved blood flow in stroke patients using laser acupuncture treatment and noted improvement in symptomatology.

Vertigo

Weintraub has achieved benefit by stimulating Naguien acupressure points with an 830-nm laser (Figure 21-4). Naeser,[59] in a review of the highlights of the Second Congress, World Association for Laser Therapy, reported that Wilden treated inner ear disorders, including vertigo, tinnitus, and hearing loss, with a combination of 630 to 700 nm and 830 nm laser. The total dosage was at least 4000 J. Daily 1-hour laser treatments to both ears were performed for at least 3 weeks. The lasers were applied to the auditory canal and the mastoid and petrosal bone. Wilden said that he used this approach for more than 9 years with 800 patients and, except in very severe cases, most patients reported improvement in hearing.

Acute Migraine Headache

Laser applied to the Hegu point (Figure 21-5) on the contralateral side may be effective for treating migraine headaches. Intraoral He-Ne along the zone of maxillary alveolar tenderness (see Figure 21-1) also achieves success in the range of 78%. Stimulation is repeated three times at 1 to 1 1/2-minute intervals.

Meralgia Paresthetica

Meralgia paresthetica is an often-disabling symptom that is due to compression of the lateral anterior femoral cutaneous nerve at the level of the inguinal ligament. The author has treated 10 patients with this condition by stimulating from the level of the inguinal ligament to the level of the knee anterolaterally (Figure 21-6). Significant pain reduction has been noted in 8 of the 10 patients by the fourth treatment, but there have been recurrences.

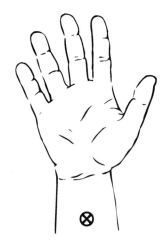

Figure 21-4 Naguien.

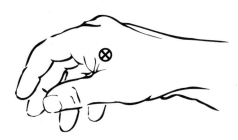

Figure 21-5 Hegu.

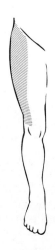

Figure 21-6 Laser site for Meralgia paresthetica.

Cubital Tunnel Syndrome

Compression of the ulnar nerve in the cubital tunnel may be associated with an epicondylitis. Anecdotal experience by the author has produced benefit in six patients.

Facial Palsy

Idiopathic Bell's Palsy or facial palsy both secondary to Lyme disease have been treated anecdotally with an 830-nm laser by the author. It is unclear whether this treatment has accelerated healing.

Tarsal Tunnel Syndrome

Compression of the medial and lateral plantar nerves at the level of the ankle has been attempted in two cases using 830 nm laser. There were no significant results.

Peripheral Neuropathy and Neuritis

The soles of the feet and various acupressure points were stimulated without relief in 10 cases of nondiabetic peripheral neuropathy.

Traumatic Neuritis

Traumatic neuritis secondary to dog bites in the limbs has been found to be sensitive to laser therapy in two cases by the author.

In conclusion, the neurologic community is faced with many conditions that respond poorly or marginally to pharmacologic therapy. Therapeutic laser treatment has been used successfully in a number of fields and is a popular modality worldwide. Critical analysis of the literature indicates that the majority of the studies suffer from methodologic flaws such as absence of controls, variable duration and intensity of laser treatment, and poor quality. Consequently, the majority of observations are to be considered anecdotal in nature until appropriate randomized control trials have been undertaken. In the interim, laser therapy appears to be safe and worthy of further neurologic investigation.

The creation of a thousand forests is in one acorn.

RALPH WALDO EMERSON

ACKNOWLEDGMENT

The author is indebted to Daniel S. Casper for his medical illustrations.

References

1. Maiman TH: Stimulated optical radiation in ruby, *Nature* 187:493-494, 1960 (letter).
2. Mester E, Toth N, Mester A: The biostimulative effect of laser beam, *Laser Basic Biomed Res* 22:4-7, 1982.
3. Lyons RF et al: Biostimulation of wound healing in vivo by a helium-neon laser, *Ann Plast Surg* 18:47-50, 1987.
4. Walsh J: The current status of low level laser therapy in dentistry: part I—soft tissue applications, *Aust Dent J* 42:247-254, 1997.
5. Basford J: Laser therapy. Paper presented at the fiftieth annual meeting of the American Academy of Neurology, Minneapolis, April 27, 1998.
6. Anderson RR, Parrish JA: The optics of human skin, *J Invest Dermatol* 77:13-19, 1981.
7. Kolari PJ: Penetration of unfocused laser light into the skin, *Arch Dermatol Res* 277:342-344, 1985.
8. Basford JR: Low intensity laser therapy: still not an established tool, *Lasers Surg Med* 16:331-342, 1995.
9. Karu TI: Photobiological fundamentals of low power laser therapy, *IEEE J Quantum Electron* QE-23:1703-1717, 1987.
10. Basford J: Low-energy laser treatment of pain and wounds: hype, hokum? *Mayo Clin Proc* 61:671-675, 1986.
11. Mester E, Mester AF, Mester A: The biomedical effects of laser applications, *Lasers Surg Med* 5:31-39, 1985.
12. Mester E, Jaszsagi-Nagy E: The effect of laser radiation on wound healing and collagen synthesis, *Stud Biophys* 35:227-230, 1973.
13. Mester E, Toth N, Mester A: The biostimulative effect of laser beam, *Laser Basic Biomed Res* 22:4-7, 1982.
14. Lam TS et al: Laser stimulation of collagen synthesis in human skin fibroblast cultures, *Lasers Life Sci* 1:61-77, 1986.
15. Rochkind S et al: Stimulating effect of HeNe low dose laser on injured sciatic nerves of rats, *Neurosurgery* 20:843, 1987.
16. Mezawa S et al: The possible analgesic effect of soft-laser irradiation on heat nociceptors in the cat tongue, *Arch Oral Biol* 33:693-694, 1988.
17. Yamada K: Biological effects of low-power laser irradiation on clonal osteoblastic cells (MC3T-E1), *Nippon Siekeigeka Gakkai Zasshi* 65:787-799, 1991.
18. Kubasova T, Kovacs L, Somosy Z: Biological effect of He-Ne laser investigations on functional and micromorphological alterations of cell membranes, in vitro, *Lasers Surg Med* 4:381-388, 1984.
19. Passarella S: HeNe laser irradiation of isolated mitochondria, *J Photochem Photobiol* 31:642-643, 1989.
20. Walker JB: Relief from chronic pain by low-power laser irradiation, *Neurosci Lett* 43:339-344, 1983.

21. Yu W et al: Photomodulation of oxidative metabolism and electron chain enzymes in rat liver mitochondria, *Photochem Photobiol* 66:866-871, 1997.

22. Karu TI. Molecular mechanisms of the therapeutic effect of low intensity laser irradiation, *Lasers Life Sci* 2:53-74, 1988.

23. Hunter J, Leonard L, Wilson R, et al: Effects of low energy laser on wound healing in a porcine model. *Lasers Surg Med* 3:285-290, 1984.

24. Baxter GD: *Therapeutic lasers: theory and practice,* New York, 1997, Churchill Livingstone.

25. Rochkind S et al: Systemic effects of low-power laser irradiation on the peripheral and central nervous system, cutaneous wounds and burns, *Lasers Surg Med* 9:174-182, 1989.

26. Basford J et al: Effects of 830 nm continuous wave laser diode irradiation on median nerve function in normal subjects, *Lasers Surg Med* 13:597-604, 1993.

27. Weintraub MI: Non-invasive laser neurolysis in carpal tunnel syndrome, *Muscle Nerve* 20:1029-1031, 1997.

28. Snyder-Mackler L, Bork CE: Effect of helium-neon laser irradiation on peripheral sensory nerve latency, *Phys Ther* 68:223-225, 1988.

29. Padua L et al: Laser bio-stimulation: a reply, *Muscle Nerve* 21:1232-1233, 1998.

30. Lasermedics: Personal communication, now Henley Healthcare 1999.

31. Walsh DM, Baxter GK, Allen JM: The effect of 820 nm laser upon nerve conduction in the superficial radial nerve. Abstract presented at fifth international Biotherapy Laser Association meeting, London, 1991.

32. Baxter GD et al: Effects of low intensity infrared laser irradiation upon conduction in the human median nerve in vivo, *Exp Physiol* 79:227-234, 1994.

33. Bork CE, Snyder-Mackler L: Effect of helium-neon laser irradiation on peripheral sensory nerve latency, *J Am Phys Ther Assoc* 68:223, 1988.

34. Naeser MA, Hahn KK, Lieberman B: Real vs. sham laser acupuncture and microamps TENS to treat carpal tunnel syndrome and worksite wrist pain: pilot study, *Lasers Surg Med Suppl* 8:7, 1996.

35. Branco K, Naeser MA: Carpal tunnel syndrome: clinical outcome after low-level laser acupuncture, microamps transcutaneous electrical nerve stimulation and other alternative therapies: an open protocol study, *J Alt Comp Med* 5:5-26, 1999.

36. Weintraub MI: Reply to Padua et al: *Muscle Nerve* 21:1233, 1998.

37. Franzblau A, Werner RA: What is carpal tunnel syndrome? *JAMA* 282:186-187, 1999.

38. Baxter GD et al: Low level laser therapy: current clinical practice in northern Ireland, *Physiotherapy* 77:171-178, 1991.

39. Moore KC et al: A double-blind crossover trial of low level laser therapy in the treatment of post-herpetic neuralgia, *Lasers Med Sci,* p 301, July, 1988 (abstract).

40. Hong JN, Kim TH, Lim SD: Clinical trial of low reactive level laser therapy in 20 patients with post-herpetic neuralgia, *Laser Ther* 2:167-170, 1990.

41. Friedman MH, Weintraub MI, Forman S: Atypical facial pain: a localized maxillary nerve disorder? *Am J Pain Manage* 4:149-152, 1994.

42. Walker JB, Akhanjee LK, Cooney MM: Laser therapy for pain of rheumatoid arthritis, *Lasers Surg Med* 6:171, 1986.

43. Friedman MH: Intra-oral maxillary chilling: a non-invasive treatment in acute migraine and tension-type headache treatment, *Headache Q Curr Treat Res* 9:274, 1998.

44. Bieglio C, Bisschop C: Physical treatment for radicular pain with low-power laser stimulation, *Lasers in Surg Med* 6:173, 1986.

45. Mizokami et al: Effect of diode laser for pain: a clinical study on different pain types, *Laser Ther* 2:171-174, 1990.

46. Christensen P: Clinical laser treatment of odontological conditions. In Kert J, Rose L, editors: *Clinical laser therapy: low level laser therapy,* Copenhagen, 1989, Scandinavian Medical Laser Technology.

47. Zhu L et al: The effect of laser irradiation on arthritis in rats, *Pain* 5(suppl):385, 1990.

48. Weintraub MI: Migraine: a maxillary nerve disorder? A novel therapy: preliminary results, *Am J Pain Manage* 6:77-82, 1996.

49. Klein RG, Eek BC: Low-energy laser treatment and exercise for chronic low back pain: double-blind control trial, *Arch Phys Med Rehabil* 71:34-37, 1990.

50. Gam AN, Thorsen H, Lonnberg F: The effect of low-level laser therapy on musculoskeletal pain: a meta-analysis, *Pain* 52:63-66, 1993.

51. Goldman JA et al: Laser therapy of rheumatoid arthritis, *Lasers Surg Med* 1:93-101, 1980.

52. Asada K, Yutani Y, Shimazu A: Diode laser therapy for rheumatoid arthritis: a clinical evaluation of 102 joints treated with low reactive laser therapy (LLLT), *Laser Ther* 1:147-151, 1989.

53. Bliddal H et al: Soft laser therapy of rheumatoid arthritis, *Scand J Rheumatol* 16:225-228, 1987.

54. Morselli et al: Very low energy-density treatment by CO_2 laser in sports medicine, *Lasers Surg Med* 5:150, 1985.

55. Emmanoulidis O, Diamantopoulos C: CW IR Low-power laser applications significantly accelerates chronic pain relief rehabilitation of professional athletes: a double-blind study, *Lasers Surg Med* 6:173, 1986.

56. Haker E, Lundberg T: Laser treatment applied to acupuncture point in lateral humeral epicondylalgia: a double-blind study, *Pain* 43:243-248, 1990.

57. Asagai Y et al: Application of low reactive-level laser therapy (LLLT) in the functional training of cerebral palsy patients, *Laser Ther* 6:195-202, 1994.

58. Naeser MA et al: Laser acupuncture in the treatment of paralysis in stroke patients: a CT scan lesion site study, *Am J Acupuncture* 23:13-28, 1995.

59. Naeser MA: Review of second congress: World Association for Laser Therapy (WALT) meeting, *J Alt Comp Ed* 5:177-180, 1999.

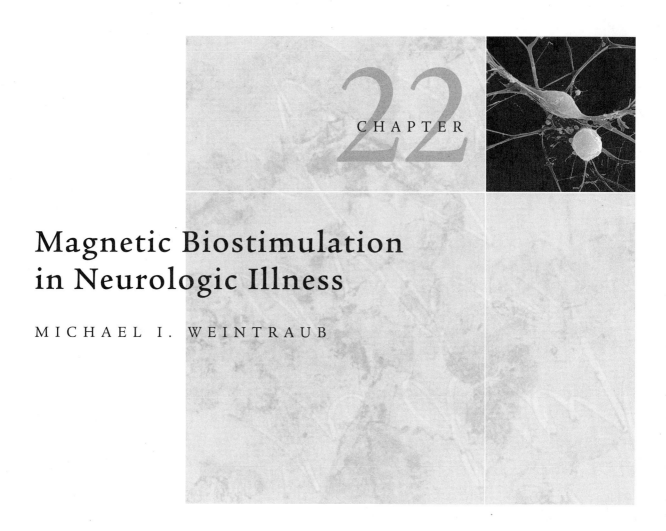

CHAPTER 22

Magnetic Biostimulation in Neurologic Illness

MICHAEL I. WEINTRAUB

To believe with certainty, we must begin by doubting.

KING STANISLAS I OF POLAND

Magnetic devices are a popular commercial method for achieving good health. Although their efficacy has previously been unproven, manufacturers and merchandisers advertise that applying static, permanent magnets produces "wellness" and "feeling good." Anecdotal endorsements by more than 70 sports figures from golf, baseball, football, and other sports, as well as word of mouth, has created a worldwide appeal prompting more than $2 billion in sales in 1998. Manufacturers have intentionally avoided making specific health claims because that would require Food and Drug Administration (FDA) testing and approval. Some people obviously believe in these products, so it is not surprising to find patients arriving at neurologists' offices wearing magnets to reduce their pain. Even though science has failed to validate the claims concerning magnetic devices and considers the claims to be speculative and unproven, there are many theoretic reasons why magnets may work. Because of their widespread use, high cost, and potential scientific merit, physicians should be challenged to determine whether indeed there is a scientific basis for magnetic therapy. Demystifying the role of magnets is not an easy task; the absence of scientific controlled studies and the public advocacy of magnetic devices only makes the task more difficult.

HISTORIC PERSPECTIVE

People's fascination with magnetism blends science, quackery, sensationalism, fashion, and controversy. Claims of magnetic healing have been traced back more than 2000 years. The term *magnet* was probably derived from Magnes, a shepherd who, according to legend, was walking on Mount Ida and was suddenly drawn to the earth by metallic tacks in his sandals. He began digging to find the cause of this phenomenon and discovered magnetite, the mineral lodestone containing a magnetic oxide of iron (FE_3O_4). Ancient humans also called these Herculean stones, lodestones, or live stones because they were meant to lead the way. The fact that lodestones could attract iron filings and that amber rods, when rubbed with fur, could attract paper and other objects, was considered a manifestation of the same phenomenon. Therefore, magnetism and electrostatic attraction were considered to be similar mechanisms. This connection has been maintained throughout history.[1-4]

The ideas expressed by the ancient Greek and Roman civilizations represent the historic origins of the "invisible movement of matter." Plato, Euripides, and others attributed various powers to magnets and sensed that lodestones could be put to practical use, such as building boats with iron nails and destroying the boats by putting them close to magnetic mountains of rocks. Healing properties of lodestones and amber were attributed to a "soul" and by A.D. 200, Greek physicians prescribed amber pills to stop hemorrhage and magnetic rings were sold in Samothrace to cure arthritis. Peter Peregrinus is credited with writing the first major treatise on magnetism in 1289. Lodestones were thought to have strong aphrodisiac powers, and curative powers for gout, baldness, and arthritis. The use of lodestones for drawing poison from wounds was even documented. Peregrinus's work also contains the first drawing and description of a compass in the Western world.

The Middle Ages witnessed a dark period for science during which an astounding number of beliefs and myths grew up about magnets. For example, it was believed that magnets could draw gold from wells and that garlic was an antidote for magnets. Paracelsus was a sixteenth century physician and alchemist who denounced Galenic medicine and made public displays of burning books. He investigated the medical properties of lodestones in the treatment of diseases such as epilepsy, hemorrhage, and diarrhea. Paracelsus combined mysticism with practical issues and, as a result, was a very controversial figure. One of his major beliefs was that every person is a magnet that can attract good and evil and that magnets are an important elixir of life.

By the middle of the sixteenth century, attempts were made to separate the magnetic phenomenon from the amber effect. William Gilbert (1533-1603), physician to Queen Elizabeth I of England, wrote his classic text *De Magnete* in 1600. The book described hundreds of detailed experiments concerning electricity using amber and electrons. He also described terrestrial magnetism, with the compass using the earth as a magnet. He debunked many quack medical uses of magnets and was responsible for laying the groundwork for future research and study. However, for almost 100 years after the publication of Gilbert's book, no major advancements were made in the study of magnetism.

Thomas Brown continued the attack on popular magnetic remedies and suggested that their putative healing power was due only to incorporated herbal and mineral compounds. He performed experiments that included demonstrating that lodestones retained their magnetism, that garlic could not destroy them, and that diamonds did not impede them.

In the early eighteenth century, significant interest in electricity and magnetism arose. An electrostatic engine was invented in 1705 by Francis Hauksbee. He mounted a glass globe on a spindle and rotated it at great speed while a woolen cloth was pressed against it by a strong brass spring. Hauksbee discovered that this apparatus produced a strong electric charge that could be transferred to other objects through a metal chain, or wire, connected to fine metal points suspended just above the glass globe's surface. This produced electric shocks. By 1743, showmen were traveling with electric machines throughout Europe and even went to the American colonies, giving people shocks for a small fee.

The same year, Benjamin Franklin's interest in electric and magnetic phenomena was aroused by an electrified boy exhibition in Boston by an itinerant electrician. In fact, much of the current terminology regarding electricity originated with Franklin, such as charge, discharge, condenser, electric shock, electrician, positive, negative, plus, and minus. Magnetism was not his major research area; instead, he distinguished himself in studies of electric fluid and charges. According to Franklin, all matter contains a magnetic field that is uniformly distributed throughout. When an object is magnetized, the fluid condenses in one of its extremities. That extremity becomes positively magnetized but the donor region of the object becomes negatively magnetized. The degree to which an object can be magnetized depends on the force necessary to start the fluid moving within it.

In Europe, Father Maximilian Hell was effecting medical cures with artificial lodestones, that is, pieces of iron that had been strongly magnetized through a process that had been developed between 1743 and 1751. His student, Anton Mesmer, obtained a supply of these magnets and began applying them to his patients, many of whom were experiencing hysterical or psychosomatic symptomatology. Consequently his cures appeared to be astounding but were, in fact, due principally to the power of suggestion. Mesmer then began to experiment with other objects, including nonmagnetic materials such as paper, wool, silk, and stone. He reasoned that he was not dealing with ordinary mineral magnetism but with a special kind that he called *animal magnetism*. He theorized that people who were ill could overcome diseases by mesmerizing their body's magnetic poles to induce a crisis, often in the form of convulsions. This crisis would then restore their health or harmony. In just a year, mesmerism and mesmeric cures became the rage of Vienna. In 1775, Mesmer published his first medical treatise on the "medicinal uses of the magnet." His exaggerated claims of success bordered on the theatric and forced the Royal French Academy of Science to convene a special study in 1784. The panel for the study included Anton Lavoisier, J. R. Guillotin, and Benjamin Franklin. In a controlled set of blinded experiments, patients were exposed to a series of either magnetic or sham-magnetic objects and were asked to describe the sensation. The committee concluded that the efficacy of the magnetic healing seemed to reside entirely within the mind of the patient; any healing was due to the power of suggestion in susceptible or naive individuals. Based on these findings in France, mesmerism soon came to symbolize medical quackery and was therefore scorned. Mesmer's theories were declared fraudulent and when the French Revolution began in 1789, Mesmer left France in disgrace.

Credit for discovering the true nature of electromagnetism goes to Hans Christian Oersted (1777-1851) who noted that a compass needle was deflected when a current flowed through a nearby wire. While experimenting, he discovered that not only did a current-carrying wire exert a force on a magnet but a magnet exerted a force on a coil of wire carrying electric current. The coil behaved like a magnet, as if it possessed magnetic North and South poles. Magnetism and electricity were somehow connected. Oersted was instrumental in creating a proper scientific environment that led to further progress. Subsequently the pace of scientific research on magnetism increased dramatically. Society embraced the use of magnets to treat illness, which in turn led to commercial enterprises.

The alleged benefits of magnetotherapy were summarized in a mail-order pamphlet printed in 1886 and distributed by Dr. C. J. Thatcher. He explained that magnetic healing provided a "plain road to health without the use of medicine and dependent upon the magnetic energy of the sun." He believed that the iron content of the blood made it the primary magnetic conductor of the body. The most efficient way to recharge the blood's magnetic field was by wearing magnetic garments, and Thatcher's Chicago Magnetic Company produced more than 700 individual magnetic devices and garments. The complete set was said to "furnish full and complete protection of all the vital organs of the body," but Thatcher was dubbed the "King of the Magnetic Quacks" by Collier's Magazine. However, by the late nineteenth century and early twentieth century, the medical establishment was beginning to accept electromagnetic approaches to the treatment of some diseases. In fact, a standard medical textbook from the period devotes an entire chapter to the use of galvanism and electromagnetic fields (EMF) in the treatment of neurologic disease. However, there were numerous skeptics who provided contradictory data, making it difficult for the medical establishment to either restrict or condone the practice of magnetic healing. Thus, magnetic devices were sold without regulation.

In 1896, D'Arsonval caused phosphenes, or stimulation of the retina, by placing his head inside a magnetic coil. However, many believe that the beginning of the era of modern magnetic stimulation was marked by critical reports by Bickford and Fremming,[5] who were able to twitch skeletal muscles by magnetic stimulation of peripheral nerves. Barker[6,7] and colleagues at the University of Sheffield developed the first commercial magnetic stimulator in 1986. As might be expected, stimulation of the central and peripheral nervous system using magnetic coils has been used worldwide for more than a decade and has created a new discipline for both diagnosis and therapy.

Similarly, the development of nuclear magnetic resonance (NMR) and magnetic resonance imaging (MRI) led to the application of imaging research to biologic systems. Hydrogen, sodium, and phosphorous were studied. Tissues would have a specific "signature" and these techniques have been further refined and are used by the neurologic community on a daily basis.

Pulsed electromagnetic field (PEMF) is another form of electromagnetic energy that influences biologic changes. This has been investigated at the cellular membrane level with ionic flux and with stimulating osteoblasts in nonunion fractures. In fact, the FDA has only approved PEMF for therapy. There is concern that exposure to various EMFs, such as high-voltage power lines and microwaves, may cause lymphoblastic leukemia and other malignancies. This was recently discussed in the New England Journal of Medicine.[8]

Since 1985, suprathreshold magnetic stimulation has been applied transcranially to the motor cortex and to the peripheral nerves to stimulate sensory and motor nerves. Unlike electric stimulation, magnetic stimulation does not rely on the direct passage of electric currents into the body from an external source.

The pulse of a magnetic field produces an electric current in tissue, which causes depolarization of a nerve membrane and the generation of an action potential. When used transcranially, it can cause a positive effect or disrupt a neural function, such as arresting speech.

When a time-varying, high-current electric pulse passes through a core of wires, it produces a magnetic field that passes unattenuated into the body. This magnetic pulse then produces a proportionate electric field in a direction opposite to the current in the core. The stimulated neurons may have either excitatory or inhibitory effects that may be either local or distant.

Repetitive electric stimulation of the cerebral cortex has long been known to interfere with speech processing. Other potential therapeutic applications are being explored in neuropsychologic disorders such as multiple sclerosis (MS), amyotrophic lateral sclerosis (ALS), ataxias, Parkinson's disease, epilepsy, dystonia, stroke, and obsessive-compulsive disorder.[9,10] From these data, an improved understanding of brain and peripheral nerve functions has produced a proper scientific foundation for future trials. As clinical trials are developed with diagnostic and/or therapeutic efficacy, speculation will be replaced by clinical relevance.

What about subthreshold magnetic devices influencing the same cellular mechanisms? Scientific advances are beginning to unlock the mysteries of pain, and research in cellular and molecular biology are defining the neuropathophysiologic basis of dysfunction. The linking of alleged benefits derived from static magnets to tissue and cellular pathophysiology is tenuous but needs to be explored.

The scientific community and most physicians are skeptical about the ability of permanent, subthreshold magnets to provide results similar to those discussed previously. However, there is enough theoretic information to suggest that these areas need to be studied. There have been numerous anecdotal observations of benefits, but critics have been quick to label them placebo effect. Although such a possibility surely exists and may be difficult to exclude, one cannot ignore significant literature showing reduction of pain, swelling, and ecchymosis in animals and infants. Therefore, the time is ripe to aggressively design studies that have valid and testable parameters for diseases with a known natural history. The scientific method cannot be abandoned. However, researchers cannot be held hostage to a rigid demand for evidence of objective cellular changes when they may not be obtainable. Methodologic shortcomings of earlier studies need to be resolved so that objective scientific data can be validated.

DEFINITIONS

Magnetic energy is part of the universe that surrounds the earth. The human body is also a magnet. Each cell has a positive and a negative field in the DNA that is paramagnetic. The term *biomagnetics* refers to the field of science dealing with the application of magnetic fields to living things. There are several different units of measurement for magnetic fields. The proper unit of measure is ampere per meter. More often, though, magnetic field strength is indicated by a related quantity called magnetic flux density, which is the number of field lines (flux) that cross a unit of surface area. This unit is usually described as Gauss (G) or Tesla (T). There are 10,000 G in each T. Because there is a logarithmic reduction of strength relative to the air space between skin and magnet, the objective is to keep the magnet close to the skin. Therefore, many magnets are taped on, but several are applied with a constricting velcro bandage or strap.

The magnitude of surface charge and internal cellular currents that are induced depend on numerous factors. The "Adey window"[11] has been proposed to explain the mechanisms of action that mediate the biologic effects of feeble electromagnetic forces that cannot be explained by Newtonian physics or by current laws of thermodynamics that govern ionic flux across cell membranes. This is basically at the atomic level. Adey emphasizes the role of free radicals, which form briefly in all chemical reactions and bonds that are essentially magnetic bonds. Thus, free-radical electrons are sensitive to both intrinsic and imposed magnetic fields. Adey believes that nitric oxide (NO) and the free radicals of oxygen and nitrogen play essential roles in health and disease. Thus, signal transduction can arise. Further study is needed to explain these mechanisms.

TERMINOLOGY

Magnetotherapy: Magnetotherapy has been defined as the use of time-varying magnetic fields of low-frequency values (3 Hz to 3 KHz) to induce a sufficiently strong current to stimulate living tissue.

Faraday's Law (1831): The induced (stimulating) current is proportional to the rate of change of the magnetic field. For a magnetic field to stimulate, it must be time varying. Initially it was thought that a static field did not stimulate; however, it is possible that a moving, excitable tissue such as blood or axoplasm in a static magnetic field could be stimulated.

Static Magnetic Devices: The strength of static magnetic devices varies from 300 to 700 G. The World Health Organization (WHO) has stated that there are no adverse affects on human health from exposure to static magnetic fields, even up to 2 T, which equals 20,000 G.

Hall Effect: When a magnetic field passes through ions in a direction that is perpendicular to the movement of the ions, a voltage (Hall) and heat are generated. It is presumed that this voltage might add to the nerve's resting potential of -70 mV and make it harder to depolarize. Once the resting potential rises from its normal undisturbed voltage of about -70 mV to a voltage of approximately -55 mV (threshold potential), an action-potential spike is initiated. Thus, a voltage is generated that is perpendicular to the flow of charged particles through a magnetic field. When ions move under the influence of a voltage, they become an electric current in which magnitude is determined by Ohm's Law, which states that electric current equals voltage divided by resistance. Mathematically, the Hall Effect can be represented as

E = BXVnq
E = electromotive force (voltage)
B = magnetic field intensity
XV = velocity of charged particles moving perpendicular to B
N = number of charged particles
Q = electric charge on each particle (ions)

The Lorentz force has been cited as the physical phenomena involved in the generation of a nerve action potential. Mathematically this force is represented as

F = qvXB
F = Lorentz force
q = electric charge (ion)
v = velocity of ion
XB = the perpendicular component of the magnetic field

Thus, the force acting on a charged particle is proportional to the strength of its electric charge, the velocity of its movement perpendicular to an applied magnetic field, and the strength of the magnetic field. The direction of the force is perpendicular to both the velocity and the magnetic force.

Magnetic design (static magnets): Permanent magnets are made up of different materials from those in the originally described lodestones. In addition to iron, they usually contain the rare earth metal neodymium and the mineral boron, which can be impregnated or combined as a ceramic or neoprene substance. Various commercial shapes and sizes exist. Manufacturers have claimed that combining several metals, such as gold, silver, copper, or copper zinc; and nickel or gold and aluminum, can create an augmented resonance characteristic known as *polarity agent effect*. Claims of increased benefit have not been proven.

It is important to recognize that all magnets are *not* equal. Three main geometric designs exist—unipolar, bipolar, and multipolar—with varying strength and deep field penetration. Each of these designs has proponents. For example, Philpott[12] claims that the unipolar magnets can improve health. Specifically, he claims that negative magnetic field energy fights infections, improves sleep, relieves pain, improves mood, and increases cellular oxygenation, whereas positive magnetic field energy overstimulates biologic systems to create an opposite effect. Philpott believes that the negative magnetic field is equivalent to the earth's north pole and the positive magnetic field equals the earth's south pole. He categorically states that most human illness, including seizures, psychopathology, infections, and toxic states, are driven by positive magnetic energy, or overstimulation. Philpott also advertises and sells magnetic products, but critics have argued about the lack of deep field penetration in his designs.

Kyoichi Nakagawa[13] believes that illness, including pain, headache, insomnia, dizziness, and constipation, is a "magnetic field deficiency syndrome." According to Nakagawa, one can achieve balance and ultimately help through the use of magnetic application.

In 1981, Arno Latske designed an alternating polarity magnet that relieved pain when placed over a specific area. Latske's design was improved upon by Horst Raermann, who used alternating concentric rings. This design generates parallel flux lines, which are most prevalent at the junction of opposing poles. Drs. Carlos Vallbona and Carleton Hazelwood[14] studied the use of these bipolar magnets for postpolio syndrome pain and noted significant relief. The patients who received sham magnets also improved but to a lesser degree. Recently Collacott and co-workers reported their negative experience in low back pain symptoms using bipolar magnets.[26]

The triangular board design consists of a patterned array of magnetic folds shaped like isosceles right triangles. Each pole is positioned adjacent and contiguous on each side to another identically shaped pole of opposite polarity. This design is commercially available. It has been said that this pattern optimally effects sensory nerves. Because sensory nerves tend to be randomly oriented in the human body, the angular arrangement of the alternating poles becomes an important factor. This is where parallel flux lines predominate. In addition, the steep field gradient has been reported to be greater with this design. A study by MacLean and coworkers demonstrated an enhanced blockade of sensory neuron action potentials using this design as compared with a unipolar design.[15] Using this specific geometric pattern, Weintraub reported benefits in diabetic peripheral neuropathy and carpal tunnel syndrome.[16]

In 1998, $200 million was spent in the United States and Canada and several billion worldwide on these magnetic devices, wraps, and bracelets. It is important to recognize that all of the previously discussed magnetic patterns are not equal in design, strength, and steep field penetration. Claims have been made by various manufacturers concerning the superiority of their product design or the benefit of applying a specific pole to the body. To date, however, there is no scientific evidence of significant biologic effects using these weak, permanent magnetic applications. Manufacturers tend to promote their products as ways to "feel good," and the FDA stands by to make sure that no irresponsible claims are made to dupe the public. The scientific community must remain skeptical regarding alleged benefits until a large, longitudinal cohort with a homogenous illness and strict methodologic controls of randomization and placebo can be performed. The results of such a study would determine whether there was a biologic effect and whether there is legitimacy to this novel approach to healing.

HYPOTHESIS

A time-varying magnetic field will produce an electric field in any volume through which it passes, irrespective of the conductivity of that volume. A variety of biologic effects have been attributed to the exposure of cells or organisms to extremely low-frequency EMFs. For example, it has been theorized that prolonged exposure to static magnetic fields causes nonspecific changes in membrane structure. Rosen believes that such exposure leads to the leakage of ions across cell membranes. This leakage causes a decrease in plasma sodium ($Na+$) levels, an increase in potassium ($K+$) levels, and an increase in metabolism to stabilize the new steady state. This essentially reduces the amplitude of action potentials and makes it harder to depolarize.[17] Additional changes include modification in the transport of ions and proteins across cell membranes; interference with DNA synthesis; alterations of mRNA transcription, disruption of normal cellular responses to hormones, neurotransmitters, and growth factors; and interaction with the kinetics of cancer cells.[18] It has been demonstrated that submaximal electric stimuli preferentially activate sensory rather than motor axons. Submaximal magnetic stimuli might do the same preferentially.

APPLICATIONS

Weintraub[19] used multipolar array permanent magnetic footpads (475 G) to treat peripheral neuropathy and burning feet syndrome in people with diabetes and with other etiologies. It was hypothesized that the potential neuroprotective effects of wearing magnetic footpads continually (24 hours/day) for 4 months would yield improvement. Pilot data demonstrated that six out of eight subjects (75%) with diabetes experienced reduction or reversal of symptoms, whereas only 50% in the group with other etiologies improved. Burning dysesthesia was reversed in all four subjects who had diabetes and in one subject who did not. The entire cohort (9 out of 14, or 64%) experienced an unexpected clinical benefit. Visual analog scale (VAS) pain scores were considered significant only in the diabetic peripheral neuropathy group. Electrophysiologic analysis using electromyography (EMG) and somatosensory-evoked potentials (SSEP) at the beginning and end of the study did not demonstrate any changes in the A-fiber conductions.

Based on this data, it was theorized that submaximal-constant magnetic stimulation appeared to selectively influence the C-fibers. However, there were no clinical or electrophysiologic changes in A-fiber function. A placebo effect could not be totally eliminated. Consequently, a randomized double-placebo controlled study was created in which 19 patients completed a 4-month trial. Ten patients had diabetic peripheral neuropathy (Stage II/III) and nine had nondiabetic peripheral neuropathy.[20] Significant statistical improvement was identified only in the diabetic cohort: 90% versus 33% at the end of 4 months ($P < 0.02$). During the first month, placebo effect was the same in both groups (22%) for the symptoms of burning, numbness, and tingling. In the second month, the placebo effect was greater in the diabetic cohort (38% versus 22%). This finding was thought to be an overshoot phenomenon and not representative of placebo effect. However, at the end of 4 months, the dysesthesias and diabetic neuropathic pain were significantly and dramatically reduced by the constant application of static magnetic footpads.

There were no significant electrodiagnostic changes noted on serial examination, although it is interesting to note that axonal damage was seen only in the diabetic group whereas demyelinative changes were noted in the non-diabetic group. This pathologic difference appears to be significant, with increased sprouting of neurons in diabetic peripheral neuropathy. The most plausible explanation of benefit was that the potassium internal rectifying channels were stimulated in the C-fibers producing repolarization and/or hyperpolarization.[21] No safety issues were considered, and this data needs to be validated by a larger longitudinal study. Unfortunately, blinding is almost impossible in these studies because patients are able to easily distinguish active magnetic properties from placebo.

Recently, Vallbona and colleagues[14] reported a reduction of pain over trigger points in postpolio patients with the application of concentric magnets. There was significant benefit within 45 minutes and no side effects were observed. This was a double-blind study and, even though it was an important study, it should be noted that the use of trigger points has been extremely controversial and has been rejected by many disciplines. It should be noted, too, that the sham group also improved within 45 minutes.

Weintraub[16] has also noted a 50% reduction in neuropathic pain in advanced cases of carpal tunnel syndrome. Despite this reduction in VAS scores, there was progressive prolongation of the distal latencies in 75% of the cases. This suggests that there is C-fiber modulation of pain, but that the underlying pathophysiology is unchanged.

Not all physicians agree that magnetotherapy produces a therapeutic effect. Hong and coworkers performed a randomized, double-blind study using a magnetic necklace to treat neck pain and concluded it was ineffective.[18]

Recently, a veterinarian critically assessed the literature and found the treatments to be harmless but was not persuaded that the treatments were effective.[22] However, since 1998 there have been $4 million in sales of magnets for veterinary medicine, much of it in the horse racing industry. Magnetic blankets to improve circulation and prevent soreness and stiffness are quite common in thoroughbred racing.

Anecdotal observations by Weintraub of individuals with a prior history of epidural fibrosis from failed back syndrome wearing magnetic back pads for 24-hour periods identified a 50% improvement. The prompt response observed by Vallbona in postpolio subjects has not been confirmed by most investigators. It is interesting, though, that the beneficial effects, especially in the feet and back, reappeared if the magnetic devices were not worn for several hours.

Some practitioners believe that magnets activate acupuncture points and meridians. Lawrence[23] has used permanent magnets over the Naguien point (P6) for stress reduction. Weintraub has also used these points anecdotally in cases of dizziness and vertigo with varying results. In Japan, tiny Tai Ki magnets have been designed to directly stimulate acupuncture sites. The former Yankee pitcher Hideki Irabu uses these magnets for enhanced performance.

Some authors have used small magnets around the temples for headache with variable results. Dr. John Warner[24] recently used bilateral magnet placement (> 1000 G) over the carotid bulbs in a case of supraventricular tachycardia. This presumably increased vagal tone leading to cardiac slowing.

Some practitioners have advocated the use of magnetic mattresses to treat fibromyalgia, a controversial condition that is not generally accepted by neurologists. Bohr[25] has been extremely critical of this diagnosis.

Currently, numerous studies have been undertaken to try to detect if there is any improvement in muscle contraction headaches or plantar fasciitis with the application of static magnets. These studies will also attempt to determine whether any neuroprotective prevention effect is experienced by wearing magnetic devices, compared with sham magnets, in chemotherapy-induced neuropathy. Recently Weintraub was contacted by an individual with spasmodic dysphonia who experienced significant improvement by wearing several magnets around the anterior portion of the neck while sleeping. She discussed this improvement with her support group and found that a total of five individuals used these magnets with benefit. Consequently, a multicenter study protocol was generated to determine whether these anecdotal results have any scientific merit or whether they represent a placebo or herd response. One of the major difficulties was obtaining objective parameters of improvement. Unfortunately, the grant protocol was not approved or funded.

PLACEBO EFFECT

Skeptics believe that any benefit from magnetic therapy is a result of placebo effect and pseudoscience. Claims of "increased circulation" and "reduced inflammation" or "speed recovery from injury" exist, but they are not supported by firm data. Ramey[22] acknowledges the widespread use of magnets in the vet-erinarian field, but is skeptical and encourages randomized, double-blind, placebo-controlled studies. Much of magnetic therapy has been alleged to be pseudoscience, similar to the claims of Mesmer. However, humans are at the threshold of improved scientific inquiry using new techniques such as threshold electrotonus, C-fiber analysis, transcranial magnetic stimulation, and neuromagnetic stimulation. It is hoped that these techniques will test Adey's hypothesis of cell membrane and free radicals. Some clinicians argue that even if the benefits are based on placebo effect, they can be positive, noting the important role the mind plays in experiencing pain. This point has been emphasized throughout this book.

SUMMARY

Although magnetic therapy is currently creating great enthusiasm in the area of alternative medicine, it is important to recognize that the scientific literature concerning magnetic therapy must be considered anecdotal at best. Until large cohort studies with randomized, placebo-controlled designs are performed in cases of homogenous disorders, there will continue to be speculation as to the efficacy of magnetic therapy. Currently, the major skeptic of magnetic therapy is the FDA. No indications have been accepted for the use of permanent magnets, and those who sell magnetic devices are only allowed to indicate that they may "relieve pain" or "feel good." Consumers must be cautious about these alleged claims. Additional questions that need to be addressed medically include whether the effects from permanent magnets can be improved by increasing the gaussian strength or by increasing field penetration. Progress in this area will only come about with appropriate funding for studies. Unfortunately, conservative health organizations and pharmaceutical companies have not supported such research, so the full potential of magnetic therapy has been inhibited. Magnetic therapy is still in the formative stages and all applications are to be considered anecdotal at this time.

CONCLUSION

Now, at the beginning of the twenty-first century, history has repeated itself but with more progress. Any serious student of neurology should remain skeptical but should keep an open mind. Science still does not have all the answers, but some people perceive magnetic devices to be safe and beneficial in promoting good health, and they are willing to spend their money.

He who influences the thought of his times, influences the times that follow.

ELBERT HUBBARD

References

1. Mourino MR: From Thales to Lauterbur, or from the lodestone to MR imaging: magnetism and medicine, *Radiology* 180:593-612, 1991.
2. Geddes L: History of magnetic stimulation of the nervous system, *J Clin Neurophysiol* 8:3-9, 1991.
3. Macklis RM: Magnetic healing, quackery and the debate about the health effects of electromagnetic fields, *Ann Intern Med* 118:376-383, 1993.
4. Armstrong D, Armstrong EM: *The great American medicine show*, New York, 1991, Prentice Hall.
5. Bickford RG, Fremming BD: Neuronal stimulation by pulsed magnetic fields in animals and man. In *Digest of sixth international conference on medical electronics and biological engineering* 112, 1965.
6. Barker AT et al: Magnetic stimulation of the human brain and peripheral nervous system: an introduction and the results of an initial clinical evaluation, *Neurosurgery* 20:100-109, 1987.
7. Barker AT: Introduction to the basic principles of magnetic nerve stimulation, *J Clin Neurophysiol*, 8:26-37, 1991.
8. Campion EW: Powerlines, cancer and fear, *N Engl J Med* 337:44-46, 1997.
9. Pascual-Leone A et al: Study and modulation of human cortical excitability with transcranial magnetic stimulation, *J Clin Neurophysiol* 15:333-343, 1998.
10. Cohen LG et al: Studies of neuroplasticity with transcranial magnetic stimulation, *J Clin Neurophysiol* 15: 305-324, 1998.
11. Adey WR: *Resonance and other interactions of electromagnetic fields, with living systems*, 1992, Oxford University Press (Edited by C Ramel, B Norden).
12. Philpott WA, Taplin SL: *Biomagnetic handbook,* 1992, Enviro-tech Production.
13. Nakagawa K: Magnetic field-deficient syndrome and magnetic treatment, *Jpn Med J* 274(5): 24-32, 1976.
14. Vallbona C, Hazelwood CF, Jurida G: Response of pain to static magnetic fields in post-polio patients: a double-blind pilot study, *Arch Phys Med Rehabil* 78:1200-1203, 1997.
15. McLean MJ et al: Blockade of sensory neuron action potentials by a static magnetic field in the 10 mt range, *Bioelectromagnetics* 18:20-32, 1995.
16. Weintraub MI: Constant median nerve exposure to a magnetic field in carpal tunnel syndrome: an electrophysiological and placebo analysis, in review.
17. Rosen AD: Magnetic field influences on acetylcholine release at the neuromuscular junction, *Am J Physiol* 262:C1418-C1422, 1992.
18. Hong CZ et al: Magnetic necklace: its therapeutic effectiveness on neck and shoulder pain, *Arch Phys Med Rehabil* 63:462-466, 1982.
19. Weintraub MI: Chronic submaximal stimulation in peripheral neuropathy: is there a beneficial therapeutic relationship? Pilot study, *Am J Pain Manage* 8:9-13, 1998.
20. Weintraub MI: Magnetic bio-stimulation in painful diabetic peripheral neuropathy: a novel intervention—a randomized double-placebo crossover study, *Am J Pain Manage* 1999; 9: 8-17.
21. Horn S et al: Abnormal axonal inward rectification in diabetic neuropathy, *Muscle Nerve* 19:1268-1275, 1996.
22. Ramey DW: Magnetic and electromagnetic therapy, *Sci Rev Alt Med* 2:13-19, 1998.
23. Lawrence R, Rosch PJ: *Magnetic therapy: the pain cure alternative*, Rocklin, Calif, 1998, Prima.
24. Warner J: Personal communication, April 1999.
25. Bohr TW: Fibromyalgia syndrome and myofascial pain syndrome: do they exist? In Weintraub MI, editor: Malingering and conversion reactions, *Neurol Clin* 13:365-384, 1995.
26. Collacott EA, Zimmerman T, White DW, Rindone JP: Bipolar permanent magnets for the treatment of chronic low back pain: a pilot study. *JAMA 2000;* 283: 1322-1325.

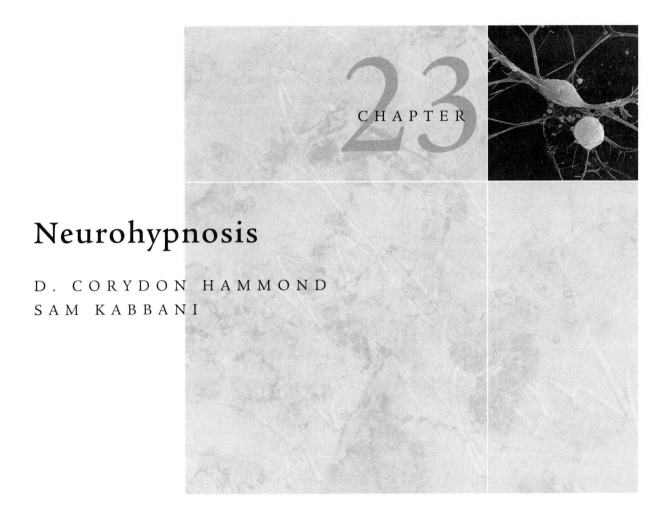

CHAPTER 23

Neurohypnosis

D. CORYDON HAMMOND
SAM KABBANI

ypnosis is best defined as a state of concentration and of very inwardly focused attention. Reviews[1,2] of electrophysiologic research show that highly hypnotizable individuals, whether in a nonhypnotic state or during hypnosis, experience more activity in the theta-2 range (5.5 to 7.5 Hz) and in the range of 40 Hz than do low hypnotizable persons. Extensive research[3,4,5] documents that both ranges of electrophysiologic activity are associated with intensely focused attention and arousal, which confirms clinical definitions of hypnosis.[6] In spite of the research, however, myths and misconceptions about hypnosis are often as widespread among professionals as they are among the public.

CHRONIC AND ACUTE PAIN

Hypnotized individuals are frequently able to reduce their perceived magnitude of pain and create an analgesia. It has been estimated that 70% to 80% of patients can obtain some degree of analgesia and a few patients can block all perception of pain and create an anesthesia. Hypnotic analgesia has proven to be extremely valuable in the management of problems such as chronic back pain, arthritis, migraine, obstetrical delivery, cancer pain, shingles, pain associated with burns, postsurgical pain, and acute pain associated with medical and dental procedures. Occasionally, chronic pain is known to have psychologic components. For example, pain may be an unconscious way for a patient to punish him- or herself or it may allow the patient to avoid doing certain things. When patients are responsive to hypnosis but the hypnosis does not successfully reduce their pain, rapid unconscious exploration of possible psychologic dynamics may also be done.

Hilgard's[7] carefully controlled studies suggest that mild to moderate experimentally induced pain may be reduced by 20% by using nonhypnotic cognitive strategies that do not require dissociative ability. Studies in clinical populations have found that such techniques as relaxation cognitive therapy, including attention diversion training, stress inoculation training, or positive self-talk and biofeedback may influence pain but do not seem to eliminate it.[8,9] In fact, these techniques appear to be substantially less effective than hypnosis and its German variant, autogenic training. In a review of published studies on nonsurgical and nonmedication treatments for pain, autogenic training (a structured form of self-hypnosis) and hypnosis were far and away the most effective nonmedication, noninjection methods of pain management.[10] The average effect size for hypnotic treatments was 2.7, but the effectiveness of other methods was much less. Biofeedback was only 0.95, cognitive therapy 0.76, relaxation 0.67, operant behavioral methods 0.55, transcutaneous electrical nerve stimulation (TENS) units 0.46, and a multicomponent treatment package 1.33. It is therefore unfortunate that hypnosis is dramatically underused in most pain clinic settings.

Cognitive-behavioral techniques are popular today and are often recommended in pain management. However, in support of meta-analysis findings,[10] Mauer[11] compared a cognitive-behavioral technique with a hypnotic technique (relaxation with guided imagery) and a control group for management of acute electromyographic procedure pain and anxiety. Pain and anxiety ratings were gathered from 45 EMG patients and observers for both nerve conduction and needle electrode components of the EMG exam. Only those in the hypnosis group significantly reduced pain and anxiety during the needle electrode portion of the procedure. One of the authors, Kabanni, routinely uses interactive hypnotic inductions during Peripheral Nerve Conduction Velocity (PNCV) and EMG studies with positive results. Patients often remark: "It didn't hurt like it did when the other doctor did it," or "Are you done?"

Another group[12] compared hypnosis to distraction in controlling pain and anxiety in children undergoing painful medical procedures. Hypnotizable chil-

dren had significantly lower pain, distress, and anxiety ratings than low hypnotizable children. Distraction produced significant positive effects only for observer ratings of distress in the low hypnotizable condition. Likewise, randomized controlled studies (RCTs)[13,14] have found hypnosis to be significantly more effective than cognitive behavioral therapy or a placebo-control condition in reducing pain and anxiety.

Clinical hypnosis clearly has more controlled research support than any other alternative medicine technique in the management of cancer pain. A recent survey[15] of health care professionals in two Ontario cancer centers determined that the five nonpharmacologic strategies of greatest interest for cancer pain management were acupuncture, massage therapy, hypnosis, therapeutic touch, and biofeedback. The authors conducted a systematic review and search for randomized controlled trials of each of the five strategies. The search yielded one RCT for acupuncture, one for massage therapy, and six for hypnosis. The studies of hypnosis suggested that there is much support for its use in the management of cancer pain, but evidence was either lacking, weak, or nonexistent for the other therapies examined. A variety of control group studies[16-22] have found substantive relief of pain (for example, in bone marrow aspirations), anxiety, and emesis in cancer patients who are taught to use self-hypnosis. In high-dose chemotherapy and radiation, oral mucositis almost always occurs. This condition requires narcotic infusions to control intense pain and makes most patients incapable of any oral intake until it dissipates. Hypnosis has proven valuable in controlling this type of pain also.[23]

A National Institutes of Health (NIH) review panel[24] concluded, "The evidence supporting the effectiveness of hypnosis in alleviating chronic pain associated with cancer seems strong. In addition, the panel was presented with other data suggesting the effectiveness of hypnosis in other chronic pain conditions, which include irritable bowel syndrome, oral mucositis, temporomandibular disorders, and tension headaches." Hypnosis is also very effective in controlling the side effects of chemotherapy.[25]

Available research suggests that the most substantial levels of pain relief seem to require the dissociative capacity possessed by highly hypnotizable subjects. One study[26] subjected very high and very low hypnotizable individuals to ischemic pain under three conditions:

1. A highly motivated waking baseline
2. Hypnotic analgesia

3. A placebo, administered double blind as a powerful analgesic medication

Researchers found that a placebo pill produced analgesia in both high and low hypnotizable subjects, demonstrating that the placebo response is not associated with level of hypnotizability. It is interesting to note, however, that the degree of relief obtained from placebo pill response among the low hypnotizable subjects was equal in magnitude and highly correlated with the degree of relief that low hypnotizable persons obtained with hypnosis. That is, equivalent nonspecific analgesic effects were obtained from a placebo pill and from hypnosis in subjects minimally responsive to hypnosis. However, some high hypnotizable subjects obtained much more substantial analgesic relief.

Other studies[7,27,28,29] have also documented that low hypnotizable patients receive equivalent nonspecific analgesic effects from placebo, cognitive-behavioral techniques such as stress inoculation training in positive self-talk, distraction, and relaxation,[30] acupuncture, or hypnosis. On the other hand, highly hypnotizable individuals receive much more profound analgesic relief from hypnosis—relief that has been found to be even more effective than morphine.[31] At a physiologic level, the amplitude of the evoked brain potentials has been found to increase during pain in which there is a suggestion of extra sensitivity and to decrease when experiencing pain with suggestions for analgesia.[32]

In followups of patients with refractory fibromyalgia,[33] hypnotherapy has proven more successful than physical therapy in treating sleep disturbance, reducing symptoms and medications, and helping patients cope with muscle pain and fatigue. Erythromelalgia is an unusual condition characterized by attacks of burning pain in the hands and feet, with local congestion and increased skin temperature. A case has been reported[34] involving transient hypertension and elevated urinary catecholamines that was successfully treated using hypnosis.

Illustrations of the potency of hypnosis in controlling pain are evident in the numerous reports of hypnosis being used as the sole anesthetic for both minor and major surgeries.[35] These surgeries have included mitral commissurotomy, coarctation of the aorta, hysterectomy, thyroidectomy, hemorrhoidectomy, transurethral resection, dilation and curettage, rhinoplasty, mammaplasty, amputations, cesarean sections, scar revisions, tonsillectomies, and cholecystectomy. Certainly the use of hypnoanesthesia as sole anesthetic is seldom necessary except under extenuating circumstances, but it is estimated that 10% of patients are so highly responsive that they could accomplish this. There is also evidence that when hypnosis is used to augment chemoanesthesia, less general anesthesia is needed. Hypnosis has also been shown to be very helpful when used in combination with local anesthesia.

There was speculation that endogenous opiates might create hypnotic analgesia because some studies suggested that placebo effects and acupuncture analgesia may be mediated through endorphins. Although one study produced partial support for this hypothesis, the weight of available data from six other studies suggests that this is probably not the mechanism of action in hypnotic analgesia. Logic also supports this conclusion since endorphins exert a general systemic effect, whereas hypnotic anesthesia may be localized according to suggestion and may be produced much more rapidly than would be anticipated from the release of opiates.

Reducing Inflammation and Facilitating Healing

Creating a hypnotic analgesia not only increases subjective comfort, but there is some evidence that it may also reduce inflammation and facilitate healing. In controlled research,[36] hypnotic analgesia has been found to block the production of the peptide bradykinin, thereby diminishing tissue damage and the histamine-mediated inflammatory response to burns.[37] Hypnosis has proved to be invaluable in assisting burn patients with pain and painful procedures like debridement, in enhancing appetite, and in helping to enhance self-esteem and motivation during rehabilitation.[38,39] For example, in one report[40] hypnosis helped with pain management in three out of four burn patients, with decreases in pain level of 50% to 64%. Hypnotic pain relief also seems to be most significant in patients reporting the highest levels of pain.[39] In another example[41] of hypnotic analgesia facilitating healing, the cutaneous pain threshold in 14 healthy and 13 atopic eczema patients was measured before, during, and after 10 sessions of hypnosis. A control group of 10 healthy subjects who were not hypnotized was also evaluated. Cutaneous pain threshold increase was correlated with improvement of eczema and with hypnotizability.

HEADACHE AND MIGRAINE

Hypnosis seems to be one of the most effective non-medication treatments for headaches. One study,[42] for example, compared the effectiveness of a hypnotic technique with a wait-list control condition in a single-blind controlled study. Subjects reported significant reductions in the number of headache days and hours, in the intensity of pain, and in anxiety. Another study[43] found that self-hypnosis training and autogenic training produced equivalent positive outcomes. Improvement at long-term followup was especially prevalent in patients who attributed the relief to their own efforts in using this self-management technique. Another group[44] also validated the efficacy of autogenic and self-hypnosis training at followup in a randomized, wait-list control group study of the treatment of chronic headaches. Olness[45] demonstrated the superiority of self-hypnosis over propranolol and placebo in the treatment of juvenile classic migraine. The mean number of headaches per child for 3 months during the placebo period was 13.3, compared with 14.9 during propranolol, and 5.8 during self-hypnosis.

Emmerson and Trexler[46] used group hypnosis with relaxation and had patients imagine that they were wearing cool helmets with freezer coils behind the protective covers. They then evaluated the effectiveness of hypnosis in reducing migraine duration, frequency, severity, and need for medication. Pretreatment trend and posttreatment effect were evaluated using a time-series design. During 12 weeks of pretreatment, the 32 patients recorded details about their migraines and medication use. Patients began the 12 weeks of treatment with a group hypnosis session and then patients were given prerecorded self-hypnosis tapes. Posttreatment duration of migraine was significantly shorter ($p < 0.0005$), frequency of migraines was significantly lower ($p < 0.0001$), severity of migraine was significantly reduced ($p < 0.0005$), and use of medication was reduced by almost 50% ($p < 0.0005$). The mean frequency of migraines decreased by 73%, the posttreatment duration of migraine showed a 40% reduction, the severity of migraines decreased by 68%, and medication use was reduced by about one-half.

The authors have their patients practice self-hypnosis daily for general stress reduction using an individualized audiotape. When a patient's headache is just beginning, he or she is asked to use a 10-minute self-hypnosis tape while wearing photic stimulation glasses with a gentle light pulsing at a frequency of 2 Hz. Encouraging patients to use this method when headaches are still mild eliminates about 80% to 90% of headaches. Adding gentle photic stimulation incorporates research by Solomon[47] who used 1 to 3 Hz stimulation for 5 minutes in the treatment of headaches. He found that 14 of 15 patients with acute muscle-contraction headaches and 5 of 6 patients with chronic muscle-contraction headaches obtained complete relief of headaches with the treatment. Three patients with acute sinusitis and four patients with migraines obtained no relief.

ANXIETY MANAGEMENT

Self-hypnosis training provides patients with anxiety management skills and is often used in treating various fears, such as test anxiety and fear of public speaking, as well as panic attacks. Several studies have suggested that patients with phobic disorders may have above-average hypnotic responsivity, making hypnosis a particularly helpful technique. Along with anxiety relief, suggestions are often routinely incorporated for enhancing self-esteem and increasing confidence.

Anxiety associated with medical procedures such as magnetic resonance imaging (MRI) and lumbar punctures may also be alleviated with hypnosis or self-hypnosis training, as was discussed in the section on hypnosis and pain. Lang[48] found in a randomized, control-group study that self-hypnosis reduced the need for intravenous sedation during radiologic procedures. All participants in the study had the capacity to administer patient-controlled analgesia. Patients were taught to use pleasant imagery and relaxation. If they experienced something unpleasant, they were told to allow an image to form in their mind representing the feeling, and then to transform the image to neutralize the emotion. If they experienced something painful, such as contrast medium injection, they were taught to imagine a competing feeling, for example, numbness. Compared with controls, hypnotized patients required fewer drugs (0.28 versus 2.01 drug units $p < 0.01$) and experienced less pain (median rating 2 versus 5 on a 0 to 10 scale $p < 0.01$). The control patients exhibited oxygen desaturation much more frequently and/or required interventions for hemodynamic instability. Anxiety ratings for the hypnotized patients were about half as great as those of the control patients. Benefits were unrelated to hypnotizability, indicating that patients did not need a significant degree of hypnotic talent to achieve this level of intervention, which focused on relaxation.

Sedation of medically compromised patients during medical procedures has increased the risk of adverse effects and the risk for liability. This includes geriatric patients and patients with cardiac, kidney, or liver diseases, or severe systemic conditions. Lu[49] treated 17 apprehensive dental patients with a combination of hypnosis and sedative drugs. Using hypnosis reduced the amount of sedative agent required and alleviated patient anxiety. Results indicate that hypnosis effectively allows a reduction in sedative dosage and provides successful and comfortable dental treatment.

INSOMNIA, BRUXISM, AND CLENCHING

The authors commonly use hypnosis to effectively treat sleep-onset insomnia. This condition usually arises from a combination of difficulty relaxing and an overactive mind. A 20 to 25 minute self-hypnosis tape is made containing procedures that focus on relaxation and pleasant imagery. In addition, techniques may be used that will clear the mind. For example, following a conditioned induction cue on the tape, the patient might be told the following:

I want you to focus on the sensations as you breathe, right at the entrance to your nose, right at the entrance to your nostrils, and that membrane between your nostrils. And breathe slowly, smoothly, and very deeply, not pausing or stopping at the top, or the bottom of the breaths, but just letting the inhalation flow into the exhalation [said as the patient is inhaling], and letting the exhalation flow into the inhalation, not pausing at the top or the bottom of the breaths. And each time you breathe in, I want you to think the syllable RE, RE, so that you're thinking, reeeeeeeeeeee, as you breathe in. And each time you breathe out, I want you to think LAX, as in 're-lax,' drawing that sound out over the entire exhalation. Breathing slowly, smoothly, and deeply, not pausing at the top or the bottom of the breath, and thinking RE as you breathe in, and LAX as you breathe out. And I'm just going to give you three quiet minutes to be absorbed in this way, while you drift deeper and deeper relaxed with every breath you take.

This method has been shown to not only produce physical relaxation from the deep breathing, but mental calm as well. It keeps the patient focused on so many things in the present moment, that it tends to clear the mind. This breathing exercise is followed by

suggestions for progressive relaxation[6] with a gradually softening voice. Further suggestions to facilitate relaxation and mental stillness are given with progressively longer pauses between softly verbalized, brief phrases. These pauses may last 15 seconds in the beginning and eventually increase to 60-second silences. The tape is left open-ended. This method, combined with practicing self-hypnosis during the day for general stress management, results in relief of insomnia in a majority of patients. Others[50-52] have also found hypnosis helpful in treating insomnia.

When headaches are often present upon awakening and then develop into migraines, it is usually the result of bruxism or clenching. In this case, suggestions such as the following are added to the tape that was described previously:

As you sleep, your jaw will remain loose, limp, and relaxed. If there is any inner need to clench anything, your unconscious mind will cause you to clench a hand into a fist, but your jaw will remain loose, relaxed, and at ease, free from tension and tightness.

Hypnosis has been used successfully to eliminate repetitive nightmares.[53] The successful treatment of a case of nocturnal "rocking"[54] has also been described, suggesting that hypnosis may be effective in disorders that occur at the interface between waking and sleep. The reader should also be aware that patients with somnambulism usually have high hypnotic ability.

TINNITUS

Forty-five patients with chronic tinnitus related to acoustic trauma were studied[55] and were assigned to one of three matched groups: self-hypnosis, masking, or a placebo-control condition consisting of attentiveness to patient complaints. The therapeutic stimuli in the masking sessions and the self-hynosis were recorded on audio cassettes and given to the patients to use when needed. The severity of tinnitus was significantly reduced by self-hypnosis, and partially relieved by receiving attention. Masking had no significant effect.

In a separate study[56] of 45 patients, a 68% improvement in tinnitus was reported after three sessions of hypnosis. Hypnosis was not as effective where there was hearing loss. Forty-six percent of the patients who did not benefit from hypnosis had a hearing loss of 30 dB or more in their better-hearing ear compared with 15% of the group that benefitted from hypnosis. Therefore, tinnitus patients without significant hearing loss may benefit from hypnosis.

RAYNAUD'S, HEMOPHILIA, AND SCLERODERMA

There are many case reports of the operative and postoperative control of bleeding through hypnotic suggestions, including reports of patients being saved from bleeding to death. In one controlled study[57] measuring surgical and postsurgical blood loss in patients undergoing bilateral molar extractions, the reduction of bleeding from using hypnotic suggestions was more than 65%. It is apparent that hypnosis can often exert considerable influence on vascular control.

In a patient with poor hand circulation due to Raynaud's disease, hypnotic suggestion produced a 400% increase in blood volume in the fingers within 45 seconds.[58] In using hypnosis to produce blood clotting in severe hemophilia patients, hypnosis has been found to be effective when compared with a control group,[59] with a significant correlation (0.56) between improved control of bleeding and the practice of self-hypnosis. Others[60] have also reported great success in their work with hemophilia.

The efficacy of hypnosis and autogenic training techniques focused on acral blood circulation and coping with scleroderma has been investigated.[61] In one experiment, significant increases in finger skin temperature were found after hypnosis was used for relaxation. The six patients in the experimental group then practiced autogenic training, with another six serving as a control. Finger skin temperature was significantly higher in the experimental group than in the control group. Long-term effects of the autogenic training were not found within the relatively short follow-up period of 4 months. However, two patients found that they could shorten the duration of Raynaud attacks through autogenic training. The use of hypnosis and autogenic training were recommended as complementary therapy in systemic sclerosis.

SPEECH AND SWALLOWING DYSFUNCTION

Gildston[62] used hypnosis to treat recurring juvenile laryngeal papillomatosis, which is generally resistant to cure. The condition usually requires multiple oper-

ations that can lead to extensive proliferation of vocal fold scar tissue. Severe hoarseness, sharply lower pitch, and weak loudness are common sequelae. Hypnotherapy was used to increase motivation for change, speed up the acquisition of vocal skills, and even facilitate or sustain remission of growths in selected patients. An 8-year-old girl with severe active eruptions went into remission after 16 sessions, and a 12-year-old boy, already in remission at the beginning of the intervention period, remained free of neoplasms throughout the regimen. Whether or not hypnosis contributed significantly to the sanguine results, it is probable that the hypnotic intervention at least facilitated the achievement of certain technical objectives in voice training.

There are also case reports of using hypnosis to treat psychogenic dysphagia.[63,64] One case history[63] demonstrated the successful use of hypnosis in treating psychogenic dysphagia in a 60-year-old cancer patient. He was first taught muscle relaxation, and then to imagine visual, olfactory, and gustatory sensations associated with eating. The patient practiced self-hypnotic relaxation at home with a tape, and subsequently was asked in the office to visualize eating a variety of favorite foods, imagining both their taste and smell. Finally, to desensitize, he was told to imagine the foods feeling stuck in his throat without feeling anxious or frustrated.

PSEUDOSEIZURE AND CONVERSION DISORDERS

Hypnosis has been used in treating pseudoseizures and conversion disorders for almost two centuries. Recently, Kabbani and others[65,66] have used hypnosis as a tool in the differential diagnosis of pseudoseizure.

Kabbani's Seizure Induction Technique

Before using seizure induction techniques, a good rapport must be established with the patient. The patient must be reassured again and again that he or she is in capable hands and that any emergency can and will be handled promptly and professionally. Reassure patients that they will always be in control and aware of what is going on and that their approval and consent will always guide your actions. If they wish to discontinue, they may do so. Again, reassure the patient that there is no danger and that the procedure is safe. A camera with picture-in-picture capability is directed at the patient so that individual body parts may be focused on. Technologists should be in a separate room. A nurse who has been instructed in the procedure then brings in a tray with two chemicals. One is labeled *seizure-inducing medicine* and contains bethadine, but the patient does not know this. The other bottle contains alcohol and is labeled *seizure-inducing medicine removal*. There are also two cotton balls and tape on the tray.

The patient is told that the red medicine has a seizure-inducing effect. Have the nurse pour it on a cotton ball in front of the patient. Explain that it is going to be placed next to the carotid arteries, where it will be absorbed transcutaneously directly into the bloodstream that goes to the brain. Tell the patient that within a few minutes, the medicine should contact his or her neurons and induce a seizure. Once again, reassure the patient that the procedure is safe. Instruct him or her to let the feelings be quite spontaneous. Encourage any feelings, telling him or her not to fight any sensation, whether it is numbness, tingling, a burning sensation, twitching, or jerking. Tell the patient that he or she is doing the right thing, is doing well, and is safe and secure. The physician may say, "If there is any problem, a whole medical team is available to handle it promptly. This procedure is safe and risk free."

After the seizure induction procedure is completed and enough EEG and video is recorded, tell the patient, "Just relax now. The seizure-inducing medicine is going to be removed," while placing the other cotton ball on the spot where the "seizure-inducing medicine" was put. Then say, "Within a few minutes this second medication will eliminate all the effects of the seizure-inducing medicine and all seizures will stop. Relax and be at ease. This second medication is taking away all the abnormal sensation and seizure activities." After completing this procedure, tell the patient, "You have done a wonderful job." Complement the patient and tell him or her that the procedure will be concluded after another half hour of EEG recording. Later, depending on the nature of the patient and whether the procedure was for diagnostic or therapeutic purposes, the patient may see the tape and/or discuss the findings. Naturally, this procedure should not be used unless the clinician is well trained and comfortable with it. In addition, written consent is always obtained before the procedure.

The literature on treating conversion disorders and on the use of hypnosis to treat conversion disorders, has been reviewed.[67] It has been found that the inclusion of hypnosis holds promise. It is widely believed that conversion phenomena result from dissociation and spontaneous use of self-hypnosis.

LEGITIMATE REFERRAL SOURCES AND TRAINING

Unfortunately, very few states have regulations governing hypnosis. Therefore, it is a buyer-beware marketplace in which numerous lay persons without legitimate credentials seek to practice medicine and psychology without a license. Therefore, it is vitally important to determine that referral sources for hypnosis possess advanced degrees and licenses in health care professions and not merely "certifications," which may be meaningless. Sources of high-quality training and referrals to legitimate professionals with advanced degrees may be obtained by contacting the following organization:

American Society of Clinical Hypnosis
33 West Grand Ave.
130 E. Elm Court, Suite 201
Roselle, IL 60172-2000
Phone: 630-980-4740

CONCLUSION

More research is available to support the validity and utility of clinical hypnosis than perhaps any other alternative medicine procedure. Hypnotic techniques, like any health care strategy, are not effective for every problem, and some patients are not responsive to hypnosis. However, a significant percentage of patients are likely to benefit from hypnosis. Treatment often requires only three to six sessions and, when hypnosis is unlikely to result in positive effects, it is generally apparent within one to two interviews. Clinical hypnosis is highly cost effective and focuses on teaching patients self-management skills. Neurologists who obtain training in clinical hypnosis often find that many informal hypnotic techniques can also be used conversationally during routine medical care.

References

1. Gruzelier J: A working model of the neurophysiology of hypnosis: a review of the evidence, *Contemp Hypn* 15:3-21, 1998.

2. De Pascalis V: Psychophysiological correlates of hypnosis and hypnotic susceptibility, *Int J Clin Experimental Hypnosis* 47(2):117-143, 1999.

3. Mizuki Y: Frontal lobe: mental function and EEG, *Am J EEG Technology* 27:91-101, 1987.

4. Schacter DL: EEG theta waves and psychological phenomena: a review and analysis, *Biol Psychol* 5:47-82, 1997.

5. Sheer DE: Focused arousal and 40-Hz EEG. In Knights RM, Bakker DJ, editors: *The neurophysiology of learning disorders: theoretical approaches,* Baltimore, 1976, University Park Press.

6. Hammond DC: *Hypnotic induction and suggestion,* Chicago, 1998, American Society of Clinical Hypnosis Press.

7. Hilgard ER, Hilgard JR: *Hypnosis in the relief of pain,* ed 2, Los Altos, Calif, 1983, William Kaufmann.

8. Turk DC, Genest M: Regulation of pain: the application of cognitive and behavioral techniques for prevention and remediation. In Kendall PC, Hollon SD, editors: *Cognitive-behavioral perspective,* New York, 1979, Guilford.

9. Turk DC, Meichenbaum D, Genest M: *Pain and behavioral medicine: a cognitive- behavioral perspective,* New York, 1983, Guilford.

10. Malone MD, Strube MJ: Meta-analysis of non-medical treatments for chronic pain, *Pain* 34:231-244, 1988.

11. Mauer DR: A comparison of cognitive-behavioral and hypnotic techniques in the management of electromyography pain, unpublished doctoral dissertation, Iowa City, 1991, University of Iowa.

12. Smith JT, Barabasz A, Barabasz M: Comparison of hypnosis and distraction in severely ill children undergoing painful medical procedures, *J Couns Psychol* 43(2): 187-195, 1996.

13. Syrjala KL, Cummings C, Donaldson GW: Hypnosis or cognitive behavioral training for the reduction of pain and nausea during cancer treatment: a controlled clinical trial, *Pain* 48:137-146, 1992.

14. Zeltzer L, LeBaron S: Hypnosis and nonhypnotic techniques for the reduction of pain and anxiety during painful procedures in children and adolescents with cancer, *J Pediatr* 101:1032-1035, 1982.

15. Sellick SM, Zaza C: Critical review of 5 nonpharmacologic strategies for managing cancer pain, *Cancer Prev Control* 2(1):7-14, 1998.

16. Hilgard J, LeBaron S: Relief of anxiety and pain in children and adolescents with cancer: quantitative measures and clinical observations, *Int J Clin Experimental Hypnosis* 30:417-442, 1982.

17. Katz E, Kellerman J, Ellenberg L: Hypnosis in the reduction of acute pain and distress in children with cancer, *J Pediatr Psychol* 12:379-394, 1987.

18. Liossi C, Hatira P: Clinical hypnosis versus cognitive behavioral training for pain management with pediatric cancer patients undergoing bone marrow aspirations, *Int J Clin Experimental Hypnosis* 47(2):104-116, 1999.

19. Zeltzer L: A randomized, controlled study of behavioral intervention for chemotherapy distress in children with cancer, *Pediatrics* 88:34-42, 1991.

20. Zeltzer L et al: Hypnosis for reduction of vomiting associated with chemotherapy and disease in adolescents with cancer, *J Adolesc Health* 4:77-84, 1983.

21. Zeltzer L et al: Self-hypnosis for reduction of pain and anxiety in adolescents with cancer, *Pediatr Res* 14:43, 1982.

22. Zeltzer L, LeBaron S: Hypnosis and non-hypnotic techniques for reduction of pain and anxiety during painful procedures in children and adolescents with cancer, *J Pediatr* 101:1032-1035, 1982.

23. Shum N: Hypnosis in the management of pain of oral mucositis associated with high dose therapy for cancer, *Aust J Clin Exp Hypn* 24(2):120-124, 1996.

24. NIH technology assessment panel on integration of behavioral and relaxation approaches into the treatment of chronic pain and insomnia, *JAMA* 276(4):313-318, 1996.

25. Walker LG et al: Hypnotherapy for chemotherapy side effects, *Br J Exp Clin Hypn* 5(2):79-82, 1988.

26. McGlashan TH, Evans FJ, Orne MT: The nature of hypnotic analgesia and placebo response to experimental pain, *Psychosom Med* 31:237-246, 1969.

27. Knox VJ et al: Analgesia for experimentally induced pain: multiple sessions of acupuncture compared to hypnosis in high- and low-susceptible subjects, *J Abnorm Psychol* 90:28-34, 1981.

28. Miller ME, Bowers KS: Hypnotic analgesia and stress inoculation training in the reduction of pain, *J Abnorm Psychol* 95:6-14, 1986.

29. Miller ME, Bowers KS: Hypnotic analgesia: dissociated experience or dissociated control? *J Abnorm Psychol* 102(1):29-38, 1993.

30. Meichenbaum, D: *Cognitive behavior modification,* New York, 1976, Plenum.

31. Stern JA et al: A comparison of hypnosis, acupuncture, morphine, valium, aspirin, and placebo in the management of experimentally-induced pain. In Edmonston, WE, editor: Conceptual and investigative approaches to hypnosis and hypnotic phenomena, *Ann N y Acad Sci* 296:175-193, 1977.

32. Arendt NL, Zachariae R, Bjering P: Quantitative evaluation of hypnotically suggested hyperaesthesia and analgesia by painful laser stimulation, *Pain* 42(2):243-251, 1990.

33. Haanen HCM et al: Controlled trial of hypnotherapy in the treatment of refractory fibromyalgia, *J Rheumatol* 18(1):72-75, 1991.

34. Chakravarty K et al: Erythromelalgia, *Postgrad Med J* 68:44-46, 1992.

35. Hammond DC: *Handbook of hypnotic suggestions and metaphors,* New York, 1990, WW Norton.
36. Chapman LG, Goodell H, Wolff HG: Increased inflammatory reaction induced by central nervous system activity, *Trans Assoc Am Phys* 72:84-109, 1959.
37. Ewin DM: Emergency room hypnosis for the burned patient, *Am J Clin Hypn* 29:115-118, 1986.
38. Crasilneck HB, Hall JA: *Clinical hypnosis:principles and applications,* Orlando, 1985, Grune Stratton.
39. Patterson DR, Ptacek JT: Baseline pain as a moderator of hypnotic analgesia for burn injury treatment, *J Consult Clin Psychol* 65(1):60-67, 1997.
40. Van der Does AJ, Van Dyck R, Spijker RE: Hypnosis and pain in patients with severe burns: a pilot study, *Burns Thermal Injuries* 14(5):399-404, 1988.
41. Hajek PR, Radil T, Jakoubek B: Hypnotic skin analgesia in healthy individuals and patients with atopic eczema, *Homeostasis Health Dis* 33(3):156-157, 1991.
42. Mellis PM et al: Treatment of chronic tension-type headache with hypnotherapy: a single-blind controlled study, *Headache* 31(10):686-689, 1991.
43. Spinhoven P, Linssen AC, Van Dyck R: Autogenic training and self-hypnosis in the control of tension headaches, *Gen Hosp Psychiatr* 14(6):408-415, 1992.
44. Ter Kuile MM et al: Autogenic training and cognitive self-hypnosis for the treatment of recurrent headaches in three different subject groups, *Pain* 58:331-340, 1994.
45. Olness K, MacDonald JT, Uden DL: Comparison of self-hypnosis and propranolol in the treatment of juvenile classic migraine, *Pediatrics* 79(4):593-597, 1987.
46. Emmerson GH, Trexler G: An hypnotic intervention for migraine control, *Aust J Clin Exp Hypn* 27(1):54-61, 1999.
47. Solomon GD: Slow wave photic stimulation in the treatment of headache—a preliminary report, *Headache* 25:444-446, 1985.
48. Lang EV et al: Self-hypnotic relaxation during interventional radiological procedures: effects on pain perception and intravenous drug use, *Int J Clin Experimental Hypnosis* 44(2):106-119, 1996.
49. Lu DP, Lu GP: Hypnosis and pharmacological sedation for medically compromised patients, *Compendium Continuing Educ Dent,* 17(1):32, 34-36, 38-40, 1996.
50. Anderson JA, Dalton ER, Basker MA: Insomnia and hypnotherapy, *J R Soc Hypn* 72:734-739, 1979.
51. Bauer KE, McCanne TR: An hypnotic technique for treating insomnia, *Int J Clin Experimental Hypnosis* 28:1-5, 1980.
52. Becker PM: Chronic insomnia: outcome of hypnotherapeutic intervention in six cases, *Am J Clin Hypn* 36(2):98-105, 1993.
53. Kingsbury SJ: Brief hypnotic treatment of repetitive nightmares, *Am J Clin Hypn* 35(3):161-169, 1993.
54. Rosenberg C: Elimination of a rhythmic movement disorder with hypnosis: a case report, *Sleep* 18(7):608-609, 1995.
55. Attias J et al: Comparison between self-hypnosis, masking and attentiveness for alleviation of chronic tinnitus, *Audiology* 32(3):205-212, 1993.
56. Mason J, Rogerson D: Client-centered hypnotherapy for tinnitus: who is likely to benefit? *Am J Clin Hypn* 37(4):294-299, 1995.
57. Chaves JF, Whilden D, Roller N: Hypnosis in the dental behavior sciences: control of surgical and post-surgical bleeding. In Ingersoll BD, McCutcheon WR, editors: *Clinical research in behavioral dentistry: proceedings second national conference on behavioral dentistry,* Morgantown, W Va, 1979, West Virginia University.
58. Conn L, Mott T: Plethysmographic demonstration of rapid vasodilation by direct suggestion: a case of Raynaud's disease treated by hypnosis, *Am J Clin Hypn* 26:166-170, 1984.
59. Swirsky-Sacchetti T, Margolis CG: The effects of a comprehensive self-hypnosis training program in the use of Factor VIII in severe hemophilia, *Int J Clin Experimental Hypnosis* 34:71-83, 1986.
60. LaBaw W: The use of hypnosis with hemophilia, *Psychiatr Med* 10(4), 89-98, 1992.
61. Selkowski K, Heber B, Haustein UF: Effect of hypnosis and autogenic training on acral circulation and coping with the illness in patients with progressive scleroderma, *Hautarzt* 46(2):94-101, 1995.
62. Gildston P, Gildston H: Hypnotherapeutic intervention for voice disorders related to recurring juvenile laryngeal papillomatosis, *Int J Clin Experimental Hypnosis* 40(2):74-87, 1992.
63. Kopel KF, Quinn M: Hypnotherapy treatment for dysphagia, *Int J Clin Experimental Hypnosis* 44(2):101-105, 1996.
64. Elinoff V: Remission of dysphagia in a 9-year-old treated in a family practice office setting, *Am J Clin Hypn* 35(3):205-208, 1993.
65. Bryant RA: Somerville E: Hypnotic induction of an epileptic seizure, *Int J Clin Experimental Hypnosis* 43(3):274-283, 1995.
66. Kuyk J et al: Pseudo-epileptic seizures: hypnosis as a diagnostic tool, *Seizure* 4:123-128, 1995.
67. Moene FC, Hoogduin DAL, Van Dyck R: The inpatient treatment of patients suffering from (motor) conversion symptoms: a description of eight cases, *Int J Clin Experimental Hypnosis* 46(2):171-190, 1998.

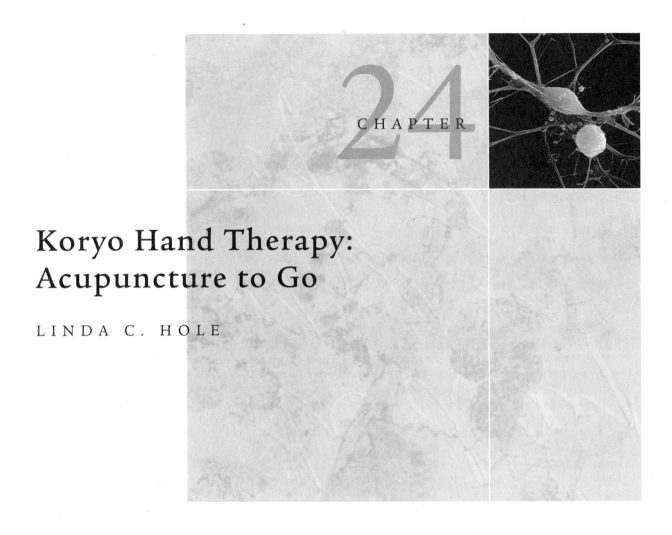

CHAPTER 24

Koryo Hand Therapy: Acupuncture to Go

LINDA C. HOLE

A wise man should consider that health is the greatest of human blessings, and learn how by his own thoughts to derive benefit from his illness.

HIPPOCRATES

Koryo hand therapy (KHT), discovered by Korean physician Tae Woo Yoo in 1971, is one of the most powerful and effective acupuncture microsystems known. KHT is based on a simple and systematic relationship between the body and the hand. It is noninvasive, effective without needles, and painless. Furthermore, KHT has no side effects, gives often-dramatic results within minutes, and is easy to both learn and apply. KHT is rapidly gaining worldwide recognition for its elegant methodic simplicity, immediate onset of action, and often near-miraculous results. Especially for those who have found little or no relief from other medical modalities, KHT is a real blessing.

Professor Yoo discovered KHT when he woke one night with a headache. According to Yoo, a thought occurred to him, inspired by God, to apply pressure to his third finger. He applied the pressure and received immediate relief from his headache. Thus, Koryo hand therapy was born.

CLINICAL APPLICATIONS OF KHT

We have used KHT in our practice for more than 10 years and have had positive results in applying KHT in a full range of neurologic disorders. These disorders include Bell's palsy, blepharospasm, carpal tunnel syndrome, cerebellar ataxia, cerebral palsy, cerebral vascular acciders (CVA) rehabilitation, deafness, diabetic and peripheral neuropathies, disk disease and injuries, hypothalamic syndrome, headaches, herpetic neuralgia and other neuralgias, migraines, myopathies, multiple sclerosis, Parkinson's disease, postpolio syndrome, Reflex Sympather Dystrophy (RSD), radiculopathies, sciatica, and thoracic outlet syndrome.

KHT is extraordinarily effective in the treatment of both acute and chronic pain, and pain that ordinarily requires medication, such as fractures, severe peripheral neuropathy, postoperative surgical pain, and terminal cancer bone pain. In general, we find that KHT frees patients, especially those with chronic pain, from dependence on long-term therapy and medication.

In his KHT Formulary for the treatment of neurologic disorders, Professor Yoo also has reported positive results using KHT to treat Bell's palsy, headaches, migraines, neurasthenia, numbness, paralysis, sciatica, seizures, stroke, and syncope.

Unlike Traditional Chinese Medicine (TCM) acupuncture, KHT requires no acupuncture or TCM training to learn or apply. However, for those with a TCM acupuncture background, KHT is based on the same principles as TCM acupuncture. The major exception is the KHT Kidney excess syndrome, which is a KHT addition to TCM's yin and yang syndromes.

Practitioners who have studied both KHT and TCM acupuncture find KHT superior for the following reasons:
1. More immediate onset of action, with results usually within minutes
2. Greater efficacy, depth, and breadth, and results even when other modalities including TCM have failed
3. Noninvasive and painless
4. Essentially has no side effects
5. Far less time required for treatment
6. Easier to learn and apply
7. Empowers patients to continue self-care KHT treatments at home

KHT is so elegantly systematic and easy to learn, that we routinely teach KHT to our students and patients for self-care empowerment. We have even taught children how to use KHT effectively. One 7-year-old boy successfully began treating his family and friends. The best way to learn KHT is to simply start practicing.

SOME KHT STUDIES

As an acupuncture microsystem, KHT works by the same biophysiologic mechanisms as acupuncture. Dr. Bruce Pomeranz, professor of physiology at the University of Toronto, carried out classic studies demonstrating that acupuncture stimulates the release of endorphins, dinorphins, serotonin, and norepinephrine. Research has since documented that acupuncture also induces vasodilation and vasoconstriction, and increases enkephalins, messenger RNA (mRNA), prostaglandins, and other antiinflammatory agents. Professor Yoo reports that stimulation of KHT hand points also augments electroencephalagram (EEG) Alpha 2 waves.

Dr. M.H. Cho in 1980 found that thermal stimulation of hand points produced an increase in temperature in corresponding KHT body parts. In Japan Dr. Yasu Mitsuo also demonstrated via thermography an increase in temperature of predicted corresponding KHT body parts using hand stimulation.

Effectiveness of KHT

KHT practitioners simply expect results. In speaking with licensed acupunctarist Dan Lobash, one of the leading pioneers in KHT, about designing studies to test the effectiveness of KHT, he joked, "A clinical study for KHT? Well, it'd be 100%. With KHT, our patients just all get better."

Pro Imura, Department of Health in Japan, reported the following results in 1987 for the treatment of injuries: 19.5% placebo response with random point stimulation versus 69.5% positive response with stimulation of indicated KHT correspondence points.[1]

Roberto Jordokovsky, pediatrician, reported in a 1999 pilot study, for the AAMA and *Journal of Physical Medicine,* of 106 children and adolescents who were treated with KHT[2]. In the 65% with painful acute conditions such as sprains, back pain, or headache he observed a nearly 100% positive response within one treatment session and no side effects. For the 35% with chronic conditions he noted significant improvement over time with repeated follow-up treatments.

Patrick Mok, anesthesiologist, pain management specialist, and one of the nation's most experienced teachers and practitioners of KHT, uses KHT to treat Attention Deficit Hyperactivity Disorder (ADHD), neuralgia, and myopathy. He reports, "Practically all patients will have positive results with KHT to different degrees, usually within 3 to 4 treatments." Dr. Mok's positive results for ADHD include "improvement in grades at school, and in interpersonal relationships." Positive results for neuralgia include "significant pain alleviation of varying degrees and duration, abolishment of acute exacerbations, and enhanced medication effect, with decreased doses of medication required." Myopathy results include "significant pain relief, and increased muscle strength, with a documented case of return to normal levels of CPK."

May Loo, professor of pediatrics at Stanford Medical School, likewise reports similar positive results in the treatment of pediatric neurologic disorders, such as ADHD, with KHT.

Like any competent KHT practitioner, we have similar results in our practice. In KHT, it is not uncommon for patients to require only one treatment to receive longstanding relief. KHT practitioners often see patients once and then hear about them years later. Usually a referred new patient says something like, "So and so saw you once for ___ years ago and it's been gone ever since. So here I am."

KHT CLINICAL VIGNETTES

Blepharospasm: A 67-year-old white man with a 3-year history of diagnosed blepharospasm, was unable to voluntarily open his eyes. Diagnosis and treatment were as follows: Diagnosis (Dx)—L and R Yang Syndrome, with Stomach excess; Treatment (Rx)—Sedate Stomach. Within minutes the man actively opened his eyes more than six times in a row for the first time in nearly 3 years.

Cerebellar ataxia: A 67-year-old festival president with a 1-year history of diagnosed cerebellar ataxia ("I walk like a drunk") with positive Romberg and positive finger to nose. Diagnosis and treatment were as follows: Dx—L and R Yin Syndrome, Bladder excess; Rx—Sedate Bladder. By the end of the session, the patient was able to walk steadily across the room. At followup, Romberg was normal, and the patient had walked a parade.

Diabetic peripheral neuropathy: A 53-year-old white CEO experienced constant pain, numbness, and sleeplessness even with medication. Diagnosis and treatment were as follows: Dx—L and R Yang Syndrome, with Large Intestine and Bladder excess; Rx—Sedate excesses. The pain was relieved and sensation returned.

Headache: A 23-year-old computer jock camp director presented with longstanding frontal headache radiating to the vertex. Diagnosis and treatment consisted of the following: Dx—Gall Bladder deficiency; Rx—Sedate Liver. The headaches were relieved. (See Chapter 15 on qigong for additional examples involving migraines and other headaches.)

Herpetic neuralgia: A 29-year-old health professional suffered from acute trigeminal herpetic neuralgia, which began after the death of a loved one. The patient was in tears with pain, and was unable to open mouth, chew, or smile. Diagnosis and treatment were as follows: Dx—L Yin Syndrome with Spleen and Lung excess, R Yin Syndrome with Gall Bladder and Bladder excess; Rx—Sedate excess organs. The patient left the office with full range of movement of the mouth and a happy smile as well.

Visual disturbance and eye pain: An artist, more than 50 years of age, attended her first qigong exercise class with visual disturbance and eye pain but no visible eye inflammation. Treatment consisted of the following: Rx—Applied Qi-KHT to sensitive eye correspondence point on hand. The pain was gone and her vision was clear.

Herniated disk: One of my favorite stories concerns a family friend who signed out against medical advice the night before his scheduled surgical repair. We found him prostrate at home on the floor with a porta-potty at his side. We treated him with Constitutional and Ring Therapy, and he was back at work within 2 weeks.

In contrast, one of our more difficult cases was a 30-year-old attorney with documented L-5 herniated disk, who complained of weakness, paresthesias, numbness, gait disturbance, and sciatica pain for 6 weeks. Treatment was as follows: Rx—Sedate Bladder, Liver, and Heart excesses. His case was unusual in that he required 7 KHT treatments over a 6-week period for his strength to return to normal and his symptoms to resolve.

Note: We use a number of modalities in our practice, but the immediate results of the previous cases and the cases we present throughout the chapter were primarily from the use of only KHT. The cases we present are typical for KHT practitioners. Similar KHT results are available to you for the asking.

KHT DIAGNOSTIC AND THERAPEUTIC (RX) APPROACHES

There are several levels of treatment in KHT, with Correspondence, Basic, and Formulary being the simplest. With a KHT atlas, the Meridian and Mo Yu levels are also straightforward. For more complex disorders, a more thoughtful, deeper approach is appropriate, such as Three Constitutions, Five Elements, or Birth Constitution Biorhythmic. With experience, combining different levels of the following treatments gives even more effective results.

Correspondence: This approach uses the corresponding or sensitive points on the hand to treat the affected target body area. This is the "aspirin" level of treatment; it is the simplest to learn and usually gives immediate and effective results.

Basic: The Basic approach energizes the upper, middle, and lower "heaters" or "burners." This set of points should be used in support of all other KHT treatments.

Meridian: This approach controls and balances the internal organs and meridians.

Three Constitutions: The Three Constitution balances the fundamental Constitution—the Yang, Yin, or Kidney—via the Extraordinary points and may be used in conjunction with Correspondence, Meridian, and Five-Element treatment.

Five Element: The Five-Element treatment balances the Five-Element energy channels and organs and is used for an even deeper-level treatment.

Mo and Yu points: Front Yin Mo and back Yang Yu points are used widely for both diagnosis and treatment, especially for pain.

Biorhythmic and Birth Constitution: This approach determines treatment according to the date and time of birth. In the hands of a competent practitioner, the Birth diagnosis matches the Three-Constitution, Five-Element diagnosis.

Formulary: Formularies are specific KHT point prescriptions formulated by Dr. Yoo for different conditions. This "cookbook" approach, based on Dr. Yoo's years of experience, is especially useful for those who are new to KHT.

Other KHT tools: Clear Intention Connecting Meridians, Four Gates, Hot versus Cold, Long versus Short Lever, Long Distance, Pendulum, Upside Down, and more. Although superbly effective and simple to learn, discussion is reserved for another time.

METHODS OF TREATMENT

Methods of treatment include the following:

Pressure pellets: Silver-colored pellets are negative and sedating, and gold-colored pellets are positive and tonifying. Current flows from negative silver to positive gold. The silver pressure pellets are applied directly to sensitive correspondence points daily for at least 30 minutes or as much as 2 to 3 hours at a time. On occasion, pellets are applied overnight.

Magnets: Magnets may be applied the same way pressure pellets are, using the north pole for sedation and the south pole for tonification. However, Professor Yoo advises caution in using magnets because of the possible side effect of shock.

E-Beam microcurrent: In this therapy, the black lead is negative, and the red lead is positive. Current is applied for 20 to 30 seconds to appropriate points and meridians. E-Beam, which is the deepest and most powerful method of treatment, is used for both acute and chronic disorders and is the treatment of choice for those with severe disorders.

Needles: Needles are inserted gently at a 90-degree angle, penetrating the skin no more than 1 to 3 mm. Best used for more acute conditions and injuries, needles are left in for 20 to 30 minutes.

Rings: Each finger controls a Five-Element organ pair, with the Fire element controlling an additional organ pair—the Pericardium as well as the Heart. The KHT control fingers do not correspond to the TCM body points. For example, the pinky is the location of TCM Heart (HT) points. However, it is the KHT control finger for the Water element organs, which include the hollow Yang Bladder (BL) and the solid Yin Kidney (KI). Silver rings are made especially for use in KHT to sedate the Yin organ.

Ring therapy continues and enhances treatment and is especially beneficial for those with deep or chronic illness. Rings are worn for 12 to 24 hours. See Table 24-1 for Five-Element finger controls.

Moxa: In moxa, KHT uses specifically placed, externally applied heat cones made of mugwort, to energize and balance the internal organs. The deeper the illness or more fragile the patient, the more sensitive the points are to heat. When moxa cones are used, they should always be applied to the Basic points as well. If the moxa cones become too hot, they are simply lifted off the skin surface and hand "stickers" specially made for use with moxa are used to buffer the heat for the next treatment. As the patient regains internal qi, the points become less sensitive. One to three courses of moxa are applied per treatment. Moxa is a must for those with deep or chronic illness such as cancer, HIV, AIDS, or autoimmune disorders.

Fingertip pressure and Qi-KHT: With fingertip pressure, preferably with qi, the sensitive correspondence point is gently stimulated with small circular fingertip motions until both the sensitive hand point and the corresponding body area are relieved. I personally find Fingertip Qi-KHT to be the most rewarding method. Patients often experience an "electric" tingling or warm sensation in the corresponding body part and sometimes even break out laughing.

Yi Nian or Clear Intention: Yi Nian means clear intention. When applying KHT, it is best to hold, without ego, a clear intention or picture of the patient being whole and well. Clear intention is not necessary for results, but it is so powerful that simply visualizing or drawing the treatment may be enough for a patient to experience significant relief.

Qi and/or IntraSound Applications: Applying some Qi-infused material, such as intrasound gel, directly to appropriate hand and body points may also potentiate the treatment for better results.

Five-Element "SEOM" food therapy: Specially formulated KHT Five-Element natural food packets enhance the KHT hand treatment. Sometimes just holding the correct Five-Element food packet relieves the symptom.

Cautions: Bad effects may occur secondary to overtreating, especially with magnets, or to misdiagnosing and applying an entirely wrong treatment prescription. There are also the obvious precautions concerning pregnancy and the possibility of burns using moxa. KHT is, however, by and large very forgiving and when practiced correctly has essentially no side effects.

CORRESPONDENCE THERAPY

A punch biopsy of any part of the body gives a hologram of the body. An embryologic cellular memory al-

TABLE 24-1

The Five-element finger controls

Digit number	Finger	Element	Yin organ	Yang organ
First digit	Thumb	Wood	Liver (LR)	Gall Bladder (GB)
Second digit	Index	Fire	Heart (HT)	Small Intestine (SI)
			Pericardium (PC)	Triple Heater (TH)
Third digit	Power	Earth	Spleen (SP)	Stomach (ST)
Fourth digit	Ring	Metal	Lung (LU)	Large Intestine (LI)
Fifth digit	Pinky	Water	Kidney (KI)	Bladder (BL)

lows cells to remember their origin, and how they relate to the whole. Well-documented microsystems include the scalp, eyes, ears, tongue, face, foot, and hand. The KHT hand microsystem, in which disorders produce sensitive or correspondence points on the hand, is one of the most therapeutically powerful.

The palm of the hand corresponds to the anterior or Yin surface of the body, such as the face, chest, abdomen, and knees. The dorsum of the hand corresponds to the posterior or Yang surface of the body, including occiput, spine, buttocks, and Achilles tendon (Figure 24-1).

The middle finger corresponds to the head and midline of the body, the second and fourth fingers (index and ring) to the upper extremities. The first and fifth fingers (thumb and pinky) correspond to the lower extremities (Figures 24-2 through 24-5 and Figures 24-6 through 24-12).

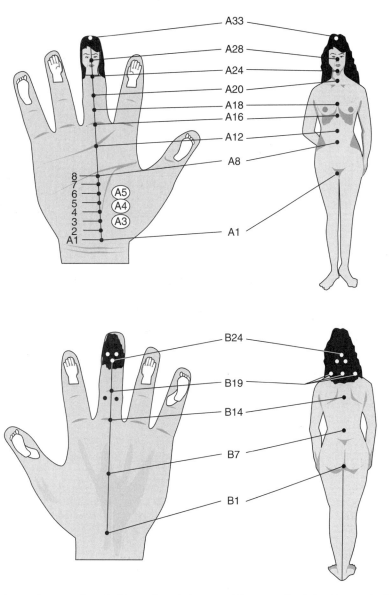

Figure 24-1 Correspondence points in Koryo hand therapy. (Courtesy Tae Woo Yo, used with permission.)

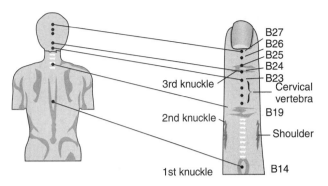

Figure 24-2 Correspondences of back with middle finger. (Courtesy Tae Woo Yo, used with permission.)

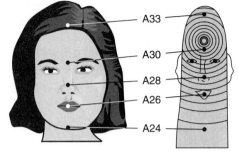

Figure 24-5 Face and the top of middle finger. (Courtesy Tae Woo Yo, used with permission.)

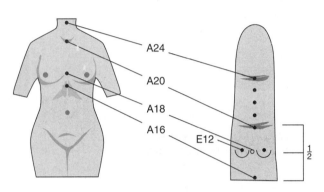

Figure 24-3 Correspondences of front with middle finger. (Courtesy Tae Woo Yo, used with permission.)

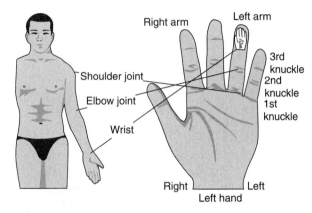

Figure 24-6 Correspondences of arm. (Courtesy Tae Woo Yo, used with permission.)

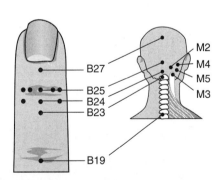

Figure 24-4 Back/side head and back/side of middle finger. (Courtesy Tae Woo Yo, used with permission.)

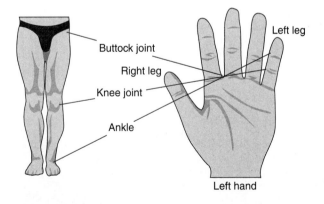

Figure 24-7 Correspondences of leg. (Courtesy Tae Woo Yo, used with permission.)

To determine left versus right, hold the hands palms out with the dorsal surface of both hands facing the body. The left side of each hand corresponds to the left side of the body, and the right side of each hand corresponds to the right side of the body. There-fore, for the left arm, go to either the left ring finger or the right index finger; for the right arm, go to either the right ring finger or the left index finger. Go to the left pinky or right thumb to treat the left leg, and to the right pinky or left thumb for the right leg.

The ipsilateral hand is usually used to treat disorders; that is, the left side of the left hand for left-sided disorders, and the right side of the right hand for right-sided disorders. For severe conditions, the contralateral hand, or long lever, is sometimes used. The contralateral long lever applies more healing force than the ipsilateral short lever. For example, if a severe right lower extremity neuralgia is not responding to ipsilateral treatment on the right pinky, the contralateral left thumb could be used for more effective results.

Each hand joint corresponds to a body joint. The distal interphalangeal, (DIP) joints correspond to wrist joints for the second (index) and fourth (ring) fingers, and to ankle joints for the first (thumb) and fifth (pinky) fingers. The proximal interphalangeal (PIP) joints correspond to elbow joints for the second and fourth fingers, and to knee joints for the first and fifth fingers. The metacarpal (MC) joints correspond to shoulder joints for the second and fourth fingers, and to hip joints for the first and fifth fingers.

For the third, or power finger, the head corresponds to the distal section, the neck to the middle interphalangeal (IP) section, and the thorax to the proximal section. The DIP joint corresponds to cervical vertebrate CV-2, the PIP joint to the cervical vertebrate CV-7, the MC joint to thoracic vertebrate T-4, and the midpoint of the MC bone to lumbar vertebrate L2.

The palm corresponds to all the internal abdominal and pelvic organs, with the corresponding umbilicus point being located at the center of the palm, at the level of lumbar spine L2.

Treatment on the correspondence level is straightforward. The sensitive points on the hand in the area corresponding to the affected body part is simply located and then stimulated. Fingertip pressure, Qi-KHT, pressure pellets, magnets, needles, or e-beams are all appropriate methods of treatment for correspondence therapy.

The more distal points on the fingers are used for more acute conditions, and the more proximal points for more chronic conditions. For example, the treatment of choice for a patient who has lost consciousness or is in shock, is to needle the very tips of the fingers.

The sensitive correspondence point on the finger can be extremely sensitive. The sensitivity is in direct relation to the severity of pathology of the target body area. As the corresponding target body area releases, the pain at the sensitive hand correspondence point also releases and becomes less sensitive.

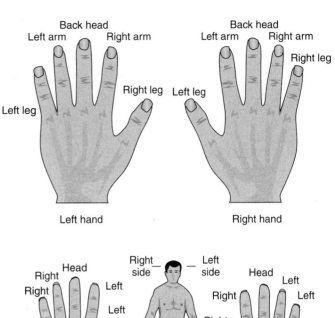
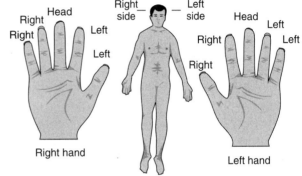
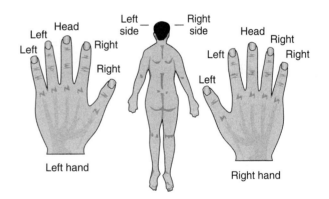

Figure 24-8 Allotment of right and left. (Courtesy Tae Woo Yo, used with permission.)

Correspondence Therapy Clinical Examples

For headache in a white, middle-aged man who was a blue collar worker, I applied needles to his sensitive correspondence points. He suddenly let out a very loud series of four-letter expletives for the whole office and waiting room to hear. Then with a sigh of relief, he said, "Whew! That sucker did it! My headache's gone."

For cervical disk disease with Raynaud's syndrome in a woman health professional, I applied fingertip Qi-KHT to correspondence points for her severe disabling neck pain, with points located on the dorsal surface of her middle finger. Within minutes her pain was relieved and for the first time in years, her hands were warm and pink. With only one treatment, her neck pain remained gone for months.

BASIC THERAPY

The Basic Therapy set of points should be used in conjunction with all treatments. The Basic points energize and balance the three heaters and the internal organs. The Lower Heater has to do with pelvic excretion and reproduction, with slightly different points for men versus women. The Middle Heater has to do with abdominal organs and digestion. The Upper Heater has to do with heart and lungs, circulation and respiration. For optimal results in any treatment, the three heaters should be balanced.

Professor Yoo recommends that practitioners use the Basic Treatment points as a foundation for all other treatments and for ongoing health maintenance as well. In Professor Yoo's clinical experience, the Basic Treatment points for health maintenance result in more restful sleep, increased overall energy, increased sexual energy, and a greater sense of well being. We find that the basic prescription not only increases energy and relieves fatigue, but usually results in increased alertness and clarity also.

MERIDIAN THERAPY

Meridian Therapy, which goes one level deeper than Correspondence therapy, is a safe and gentle method of controlling the six solid Yin and the six hollow Yang organs of TCM. Each meridian governs a set of coupled solid Yin and hollow Yang organs, and a body surface dermatome-like area specific for the meridian.

The first step in applying Meridian Therapy is to determine which body area or organ is affected and which meridian controls the body area and organ. Then the meridian is tonified or sedated. For body pain, this is relatively simple. There are many acupuncture atlases that illustrate the course of each meridian on the body, but for KHT purposes, Professor Yoo's text is the clearest. A practitioner can simply show the patient the KHT diagrams, ask the patient to point to the affected body area on the diagram, and then treat the indicated meridian according to the diagram. For pain, usually simple sedation of the indicated meridian gives relief.

To understand which direction the meridians flow, imagine a body with hands raised to the heavens with the palms Yin surface out and facing forward. Yang meridians run on the lateral and posterior Yang surface of the body. They correspond to the hollow Yang organs and flow from heaven to earth. Yin meridians run on the medial and anterior Yin surface of the body. They correspond to the Yin solid organs and flow from earth to heaven. Numbering of meridian points begins with number 1 at the origin and flows in the direction of lower to higher numbers. Yang flows from heaven to earth, and Yin from earth to heaven.

For example, Bladder is a solid organ and therefore Yang. As a Yang organ, the Bladder meridian runs from heaven to earth along the Yang dorsal surface of the body. The Bladder meridian starts at the top of the head, runs down the back, and ends at the fifth toe at TCM point B-67. The KHT Bladder "I" micromeridian on the hand begins at the top of the third finger at KHT point I-1 for the head. It runs down the dorsal aspect of the third finger to the third metacarpal for the back, and then up the fifth finger, or legs, ending at the toes at KHT point I-39.

The next question is whether to sedate or tonify the meridian. Sedating a meridian usually gives relief for someone with a normal energy level. If an individual, such as a cancer patient, has a depleted energy level, the better choice would be to tonify the coupled Yin or Yang meridian.

In my experience with KHT, pain is usually an excess. For example, if the patient complains of carpal tunnel pain along the body points of the Pericardium (PC) meridian, sedating the PC KHT micromeridian usually gives relief. For someone with low energy, tonifying the coupled Yang Triple Heater (TH) would be an even better choice. Once again the results of KHT are usually immediate and often dramatic, especially in the treatment of pain.

The choice of points for basic meridian sedation and tonification are the KHT points overlying the DIP and PIP finger joints. For the Bladder, the DIP and PIP KHT points are I-33 and I-37. Several methods may be

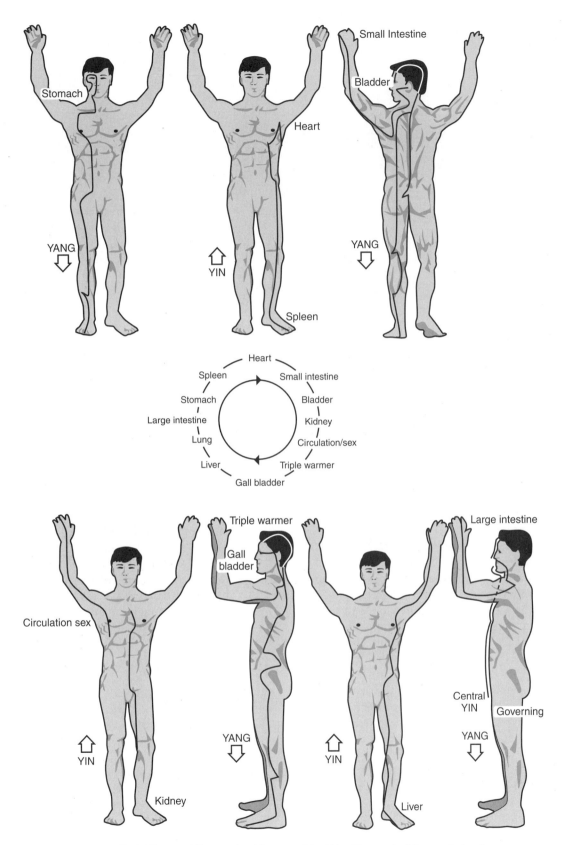

Figure 24-9 The meridian cycle. (Courtesy Tae Woo Yo, used with permission.)

305

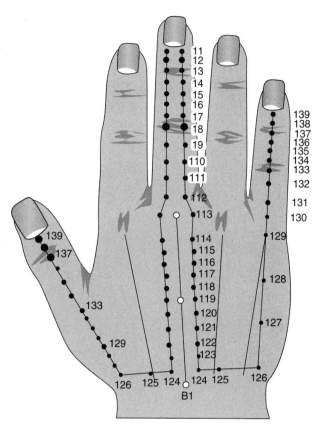

Figure 24-10 Meridian points. (Courtesy Tae Woo Yo, used with permission.)

applied to sedate or tonify the KHT micromeridians, including the following:

Pressure pellets, magnets, or e-beam: For toni-fication, pressure pellets, magnets, or e-beam are applied in the same direction as the meridian flow. The negative unit is at the lower num-bered KHT micromeridian point, and the pos-itive is at the higher numbered point. For sedation, application is against the direction of the meridian flow. The negative unit is ap-plied to the higher numbered micromeridian point, and the positive to the lower numbered point. Silver pellets are negative; gold are posi-tive. For magnets, north pole is negative; south pole is positive. The black lead for e-beam is negative and the red lead is positive.

Needles: Needles are angled in the direction of the meridian flow to tonify, and against the flow to sedate. Combinations of negative silver nee-dles and positive gold needles may be used in the same way as pellets, magnets, and e-beams.

Rings: For continued at-home treatment, apply a silver colored ring to the appropriate Yin or-gan control finger to sedate the Yin meridian and organ while tonifying the coupled Yang meridian. A gold-colored ring can be used to tonify the Yin organ while sedating the cou-pled Yang meridian, but it is not recom-mended for long-term use.

Fingertip pressure and Qi-KHT: Tonify by stroking the KHT micromeridian in the same direction as meridian flow. Sedate by stroking against the direction of the meridian flow. Se-dating or tonifying can also be accomplished by using a right-hand finger as a negative pole and a left-hand finger as a positive pole at the PIP and DIP points, remembering that current flows from negative to positive.

Yi Nian or Clear Intention: A skilled practitioner might also simply visualize the correct treat-ment, often with remarkable results. Dr. Yoo demonstrated this in a veteran who complained of more than 20 years of shoulder pain. Profes-sor Yoo drew the correct prescription on the blackboard: a simple arrow, pointing in the di-rection of the meridian flow. He then stroked the meridian on the blackboard in the correct direction, and the patient's pain was relieved. To prove the phenomenon, Professor Yoo erased the blackboard, drew the prescription again, stroked the blackboard in the opposite direc-tion, and the pain returned. Erasing the black-board one last time, Professor Yoo again drew the correct prescription and stroked the black-board in the correct direction. The patient's pain was again gone. A number of KHT practi-tioners have reported similar results.

Meridian Therapy Clinical Examples

A renowned author had experienced sciatica for months. I applied fingertip qi to sedate her Bladder meridian and stroked her pinky dorsal midline along her KHT Bladder micromeridian from distal tip to proximal MC joint. I then gave her a pinky copper ring to continue Bladder sedation tonification at home. For the first time in months, she was pain free, and she continued to be pain free for months afterwards.

Sciatic pain in KHT is often caused by a Bladder meridian excess. Yin and Yang organs are coupled, so tonifying the Yin organ also sedates the Yang organ. Bladder is the Yang hollow organ of the Water Element. Kidney is the Yin solid organ of the Water element. The pinky copper ring both tonified the Yin Kidney and sedated the Yang Bladder, thus giving the author continued pain relief.

A young woman with adult onset diabetes sought treatment for carpal tunnel syndrome, which is often caused by a Pericardium meridian imbalance. With a single KHT treatment, her physical therapist noted an increase in both muscle strength and mass.

THREE CONSTITUTIONS THERAPY

Three Constitutions Therapy is the next deeper level of KHT treatment. Three Constitution excess syndromes occur, namely Yang Excess, Yin Excess, and Kidney Excess. Within each syndrome are Yang types in which the excess organ is a hollow Yang organ and Yin types where the carotid pulse is greater than the radial. In Yin types the excess organ is a solid Yin organ, and the radial pulse is greater than the carotid.

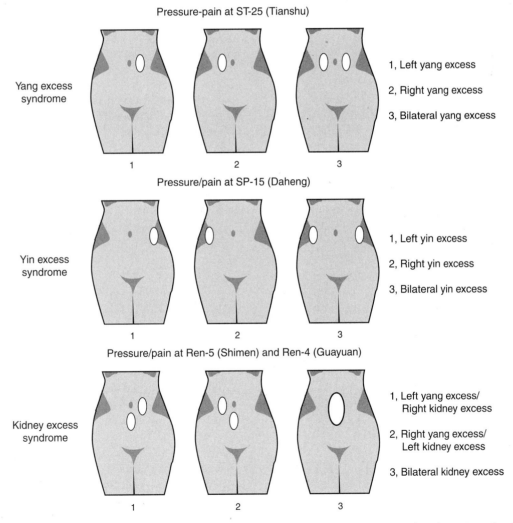

Figure 24-11 Patterns of pressure sensitivity used in abdominal diagnosis according to the Three Constitutions Theory of Korean Hand Acupuncture. (From Eckman P: Ayurveda and Korean hand acupuncture: a brief introduction to some similarities between constitutional typologies, *Am J Acupuncture* 23(2): 1995.)

The excess syndrome is diagnosed by palpating the abdomen. For each syndrome, there is a specific tender abdominal TCM point. These points are ST25 for Yang Excess Syndrome, SP15 for Yin Excess Syndrome, and CV4 for Kidney Excess Syndrome. Kidney Excess Syndromes may be tender at ST25 and SP15 as well.

For each of the three syndromes, there are specific sets of Extraordinary points for treatment. One set is for Yang types and another is for Yin types.

Individuals with Yang Excess Syndrome are characteristically thin, conciliatory, kind, left sided, and responsive to treatment. The major excess organs are the Large Intestine, Liver, and Heart. They are prone to dizziness, headaches, nervousness, fatigue, low back pain, sciatica, hemiplegia, and impotence. Their condition is aggravated by excessive drinking, sexual indulgence, emotional stress, unbalanced diet, and overeating.

Those with Yin Excess Syndrome are usually overweight and often greedy, tend to be big eaters and sleepers, and are responsive to treatment. The primary excess organ is the Spleen. They are especially prone to neuralgias, including trigeminal neuralgia, intercostal neuralgia, and lower extremity neuralgias that progress to loss of sensation. They are also prone to headaches, especially migraines; seizures; paralysis; and stroke.

By nature, individuals with Kidney Excess Syndrome like to save and spare; are preoccupied with their own troubles; tend to right-sided disorders; and are prone to disk disease and paralysis, and to allergic, rheumatic, and autoimmune disorders. The excess organ is Kidney, and these individuals are the most difficult to treat.

Diagnosing and treating the constitution is a must for those with deep or chronic disease. Using the Extraordinary points to balance the constitution frees Qi to catalyze the healing process. For significant disorders, I usually diagnose and treat on the Constitution level, then identify the unbalanced organs on the Meridian level, and finally treat Correspondence level points as necessary. The Extraordinary points alone may also give "extraordinary" results.

Three Constitutions Therapy Clinical Examples

Bell's Palsy: Professor Yoo once applied only the Three Constitutions Therapy treatment Extraordinary points to an elderly man with Bell's Palsy. The next morning, the class noted a significant improvement in his facial palsy.

Headache: Once when I was presenting at a medical symposium, a young woman with a 6-month history of constant severe throbbing headaches volunteered herself before the full audience for pain relief. I said to myself, "Uh, oh! Help!" but I applied only the four indicated Extraordinary points, and her headache was gone.

FIVE-ELEMENT THERAPY

Five-Element Therapy is a still deeper, more powerful, and effective level of treatment. When other levels of treatment are insufficient to fully alleviate the physical symptoms, the Five Elements should be used.

Each of the Five Elements governs a set of coupled Yin and Yang organs and a set of emotions, and has a whole set of characteristics. Each Meridian also has its own specific Five-Element points that are governed by both a Mother-Son Nourishing Cycle and a Control Cycle. In Five-Element Therapy, tonifying and sedating points are chosen according to the principles of these cycles.

Professor Yoo is extraordinary in his depth of medical knowledge and clinical details, and he also teaches that "The root of all disease is spiritual . . . in the mind and the emotions." For those who are ready, Five-Element principles can be used to address the deeper psychospiritual issues underlying the surface physical disorder.

Five-Element Clinical Examples

A 46-year-old woman, a professional artist, presented with MRI (magnetic resonance imaging documented disc disease, left upper extremity pain, and intercostal neuralgia. Heart sedation relieved her pain. The Five-Element Fire, or Heart, emotion is Sadness. Her underlying pain was caused by a deeply suppressed Sadness over the death of her father.

A 30-year-old woman, a health professional, complained of back pain, with radiating left sciatic pain. Left Bladder sedation relieved her pain and, on the right, she had a Large Intestine excess. Water, with the emotion Fear, is the Bladder element. Metal, with the emotion Grief, is the Large Intestine element. Her underlying issues were Grief over her father's illness, and the Fear that he might die.

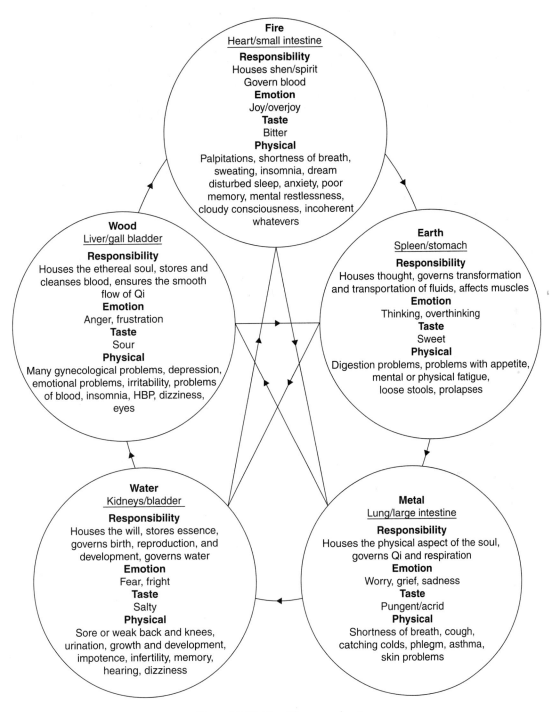

Figure 24-12 Five-Element chart.

Patients often present with a purely somatic complaint, in total denial of any underlying disturbance. In addition to using Five-Element theory in selecting points for treatment, I make it a practice to give patients feedback on their Five-Element issues. This feedback helps them become aware of the deeper psychospiritual pain underlying their presenting physical symptoms. With this awareness often come tears of release that are, in themselves, healing and that help facilitate a more rapid recovery.

ADDITIONAL SPECIAL POINTS, DIAGNOSTIC TOOLS, AND LEVELS OF TREATMENT

There are many other diagnostic and treatment approaches in KHT, such as the Four Life Saving points, Three Emergency Points, Four Gate points, Four Spiritual Points, Eight Extraordinary points, Twelve Source points, Five Su points, Mo and Yu points, and Special Points for Nervous Disease. Like much of KHT, these points are both highly effective and relatively simple to learn.

The Mo points can be especially helpful. Mo points are Yin gathering points on the palm of the hand for the Yin energy of the internal organs. The Mo point of the affected organ is tender. Stimulating the Mo point of the affected target organ augments treatment, especially in the treatment of pain. Yu points are the analogous Yang gathering points on the dorsal surface of the hand. With experience, the Mo and Yu points can greatly enhance KHT diagnostic and treatment skills.

CONCLUSION

KHT is a truly effective, easy to learn, rewarding, and empowering tool. I find tremendous gratification in practicing KHT. The look on a patient's face, when he or she realizes that the presenting symptom is suddenly gone, is priceless. Sometimes the reaction is amazement, sometimes disbelief, sometimes pure relief, sometimes laughter, and sometimes tears of release and gratitude. My hope in sharing these tools is that you yourself might have fun playing with some of these tools, and that you might see for yourself what a difference KHT can make in your own life, in your practice, and in the lives of your patients.

References

1. Eckman, P: The physiological basis of acupuncture microsystems, *AAMA Review* 3(2):7, 1991.

2. Jordokovsky, R: Hand acupunture experience in pediatric patients, *Medical Acupuncture* 11(1): 25.

The KHT literature available in English is scarce. Available texts include the following:

Yoo TWY: *Lectures on Koryo Hand Acupuncture*, vol 1, Seoul, Korea, 1977, Eum Yang Maek Jin (Edited by P Eckman).

Yoo TWY: *Lectures on Koryo Hand Therapy*, Seoul, Korea, 1976, Eum Yang Maek Jin (Translated into English 1993).

Articles available in English include the following:

Eckman P. "An Introduction to Koryo Sooji Chim: Korean Hand Acupuncture," *American Journal of Acupuncture,* 18(2): p. 135-139, 1990.

Eckman P: Ayurveda and Korean hand acupuncture: a brief introduction to some similarities between constitutional typologies, *Am J Acupuncture* 23(2): 153-158, 1995.

Eckman P: The Daoist concept of alarm points, *AAMA Rev* 6(1): 13-22, 1994.

Eckman P: The physiologic basis of acupuncture microsystems, *AAMA Rev* 3(2): 7-10, 1991.

Jordokovsky P: Hand acupuncture experience in pediatric patients, *Medical Acupuncture* 11(1): 22-28, 1999.

Omura Y: Effects of external Qigong on inanimate objects, *Acupuncture Electrotherapeutic Res Intl J* 15: 137–57, 1990.

Omura Y: Applications of Qigong-nized materials, *Acupuncture Electrotherapeutic Research Intl J* 17: 107–48, 1992.

For more resources and information, contact the author:
Dr. Linda Hole
2814 S. Grand Blvd.
Spokane, WA 99203
E-mail: AskDrLindaMD@aol.com
Phone: 509-747-2902 or 800-RxQIWAY (797-4929)
Fax: 509-838-3745

ACKNOWLEDGMENT

The author would like to thank Dan Lobash, LAC, May Loo, MD, Gene Liu, Patrick Mok, MD, and Tae Woo Yoo, OMD, PhD.

Index

Multiple sclerosis—cont'd
  Therapeutic Touch for, 237
  yoga for, 79, 82-83
Muscle energy techniques, 30
Muscle weakness, yoga for, 89
Muscular dystrophy, yoga for, 89
Music therapy, 255-63
  brain and, 257-59
  case studies in, 255-56, 266-67
  clinical applications of, 258-63
  definition of, 256-57
  with groups vs. individuals, 263
  history of, in U.S., 256
  in medical setting, 258
  as mind-body technique, 175
  practitioners of, 256, 257
  for rehabilitation, 259-61, 266-67
  research on, 257-63
Myasthenia gravis, chiropractic treatment
    of, 104
Myofacial pain syndrome, 31
Myofascial release, 29-30
Myopathy, yoga for, 89

N

Nadi Shodhanam, 82
Nadis, 80, 81
Nan Jing, 12
Nasal massage, 37
National Association for Music Therapy,
    256
National Center for Complementary and
    Alternative Medicine (NCCAM), 58,
    174, 242
National Certification Board for Thera-
    peutic Massage and Bodywork
    (NCBTMB), 29
National Institute of Neurological
    Disorders, 45
National Yoga Alliance, 90
Neck Disability Index, 102
Neck pain:
  acupuncture for, 23
  chiropractic for, 101-2
  yoga for, 87

Needles:
  in acupuncture, 15-16
    positioning of, 16-17
  in koryo hand therapy, 299, 306
Negligent referral, 243
Nei Jing, 12
Nerve root syndrome, osteopathic treatment
    for, 121
Nervous system, yoga and, 80
Neuralgia:
  koryo hand therapy for, 297
  massage therapy for, 33-34
Neurohypnosis; *see* Hypnosis
Nidana, 69
Nogier, Dr. Paul, 222, 228, 232
Non-adrenergic non-cholinergic nuclei
    (NANC), 168, 169
North American Society of Homeopaths
    (NASH), 55
Nyaya-Vaisesika, 69

O

Observational studies, 3, 4
Occipital neuralgia, acupuncture treatment
    for, 23
Ocean-sounding breath, 82
Odors; *see* Aromatherapy
Oersted, Hans Christian, 280
Office of Alternative Medicine (OAM), 58, 242
Organon of the Medical Art, 54
Osteopathic medicine, 109-23
  clinical applications of, 112-23
  history of, 109
  institutions for, 110
  licensure for, 110
  precepts of, 110
  principles of, 111-12
Outcomes studies, 20, 232
Over-the-counter (OTC) medications, 53

P

Pain:
  acupuncture for, 24
  aromatherapy for, 136-37